Healthcare Information Technology Exam Guide for CompTIA® Healthcare IT Technician and HIT Pro™ Certifications

Dr. Kathleen A. McCormick
Dr. Brian Gugerty

New York • Chicago • San Francisco • Lisbon
London • Madrid • Mexico City • Milan • New Delhi
San Juan • Seoul • Singapore • Sydney • Toronto

The McGraw·Hill Companies

Cataloging-in-Publication Data is on file with the Library of Congress

McGraw-Hill books are available at special quantity discounts to use as premiums and sales promotions, or for use in corporate training programs. To contact a representative, please e-mail us at bulksales@mcgraw-hill.com.

**Healthcare Information Technology Exam Guide for CompTIA®
Healthcare IT Technician and HIT Pro™ Certifications**

This book was written by Kathleen A. McCormick in her private capacity. No official support or endorsement by Science Applications International Corporation-Frederick (SAIC-F) is intended or should be inferred.

1234567890 DOC DOC 1098765432

ISBN: Book p/n 978-0-07-180277-2 and CD p/n 978-0-07-180278-9
of set 978-0-07-180280-2

MHID: Book p/n 0-07-180277-0 and CD p/n 0-07-180278-9
of set 0-07-180280-0

Sponsoring Editor	Acquisitions	Contributing Editors	Production Supervisor	Art Director, Cover
Meghan Riley Manfre	Coordinator	*Alisa Ryan, Sean Gugerty*	*James Kussow*	*Jeff Weeks*
	Stephanie Evans			
Editorial Supervisor		**Proofreader**	**Composition**	
Jody McKenzie	**Copy Editors**	*Paul Tyler*	*ContentWorks, Inc.*	
	Kim Wimpsett,			
Project Editor	*Barbara Gordon*	**Indexer**	**Illustration**	
Molly Sharp		*Jack Lewis*	*ContentWorks, Inc.*	

This book is dedicated to Francis McCormick, who is the Vis a Tergo, *the "force from behind." Kathleen is also supported by her sons, Francis and Christopher; her daughter-in-law, Ellen London McCormick; and her grandson Simon Francis McCormick.*

The book is also dedicated to Kathleen Bartley, whose constant support, encouragement, and occasional medical and health law advice enabled Brian Gugerty's participation in this book during an eventful year.

ABOUT THE LEAD AUTHORS

Kathleen A. McCormick, Ph.D., R.N., FACMI, FAAN, FHIMSS, is an author, senior practitioner, researcher, and policy executive in healthcare informatics and bioinformatics. She has authored or co-authored more than six books and hundreds of publications, including the McGraw-Hill title *Essentials of Nursing Informatics*, now in its fifth edition. She has a B.S. and M.S. in nursing and an M.S. and Ph.D. in physiology and has been involved in informatics since 1978. As a tenured scientist at the National Institutes of Health, she retired as a 06 Captain in the U.S. Public Health Service. Following her retirement, she has worked for the past 15 years in the healthcare IT industry as a scientist/executive contractor. Her fellowships in informatics include the College of Medical Informatics through AMIA, the American Academy of Nursing, and a fellow in Healthcare Information Management Systems Society (HIMSS). Dr. McCormick is an elected fellow in the prestigious National Academy of Sciences, Institute of Medicine (IOM). In addition, she is an author for and a member of the Medical Technology Policy Committee (MTPC) for the Institute of Electrical and Electronics Engineers (IEEE).

Brian Gugerty, DNS, R.N., is CEO of GIC Informatics, LLC, which assists physicians and clinicians to effectively and efficiently use EHRs during the critical EHR "go-live" period and then optimize EHR use on an ongoing basis. Dr. Gugerty has been in the clinical informatics field for 24 years. His experience includes teaching, clinical informatics research, clinical software development, and consulting to healthcare organizations. Dr. Gugerty has authored or coauthored more than 30 articles and book chapters on the theory, practice, and future of clinical informatics and is a frequent presenter of these topics both in the United States and abroad.

About the Part Editors

Part I: Healthcare Organizational Behavior

Janet Marchibroda, M.B.A., serves as chair of the Health IT Initiative for the Bipartisan Policy Center, a think tank formed by former Senate majority leaders that works to address key national challenges, including those related to democracy, economic policy, energy, national security, and healthcare. The initiative conducts research and engages stakeholders to make recommendations for the effective use of healthcare IT to support improvements in healthcare. Ms. Marchibroda serves as the executive director for Doctors Helping Doctors Transform Health Care. She supported the Office of the National Coordinator for Health IT and served as the Chief Healthcare Officer for IBM. She also served as chief operating officer of the National Committee for Quality Assurance and was the founding CEO of eHealth Initiative and the initial executive director for the Markle Foundation's Connecting for Health initiative. Ms. Marchibroda holds a B.S. in commerce from the University of Virginia and an M.B.A. from George Washington University.

Part II: Healthcare Regulatory Requirements

Donald T. Mon, Ph.D., is the senior director for the Center for Advancement of Health Information Technology (CAHIT). As the senior director, Dr. Mon leads the standards and interoperability practice in CAHIT. In this capacity, he represents RTI in key national and international standards development activities and directs RTI's business development and project implementations related to data and functional and interoperability standards. Additionally, Dr. Mon is chair of Health Level Seven International (HL7), co-chair of the HL7 EHR Work Group, president of the Public Health Data Standards Consortium, and subject-matter expert in the U.S. Technical Advisory Group (the U.S. representative to ISO Technical Committee 215-Health Informatics). Dr. Mon has more than 35 years of experience in the areas of health information management/technology and informatics practice, research, and advocacy. Prior to joining RTI, Dr. Mon was vice president of practice leadership at the American Health Information Management Association (AHIMA), where he led the implementation of AHIMA's top strategic national and international initiatives.

Part III: Healthcare Business Operations

Michael J. Beller, M.D., M.M.M., is vice president and chief medical officer for Cerner West. He is responsible for Cerner's larger clients located in the western United States and served as interim CMIO in 2011 for Genesis Healthcare, a Cerner client implementing CPOE. Dr. Beller joined Cerner Corporation in August 2001 as a sales physician executive. Prior to joining Cerner, he was a family practice residency director for Intermountain Health Care in Provo, Utah. He has published articles on CPOE, quality improvement, and management and has presented to audiences around the country on computerized provider order entry and quality of care. He received his medical degree from Creighton University and master's in medical management from Tulane University.

Part IV: Healthcare IT Security, Privacy, and Confidentiality

Lori Reed-Fourquet, M.C.S, is a principal at e-HealthSign, LLC, consulting in health informatics. She is the convener for ISO TC215, WG 4 on Health Informatics Security, Privacy, and Patient Safety. She is also a member of the IT Infrastructure Planning and Technical committees; IHE Quality, Research, and Public Health Planning and Technical committees; and the HL7 Security and HL7 Public Health and Emergency Response committees. Ms. Reed-Fourquet has been working in medical and health informatics for more than 20 years, serving in numerous leadership capacities creating successful collaborations involving diverse healthcare communities in competing markets. She was part of the contracting teams to the Office of the National Coordinator for Health Information Technology and the Security and Privacy and the Standards Harmonization initiatives as part of the U.S. efforts to advance nationwide interoperable health information technology. She serves as a technical assessor for the American National Standards Institute (ANSI), the U.S. Office of the National Coordinator (ONC) Approved Accreditor for the Permanent Certification Program for Health Information

Technology (HIT). She holds a master's of computer science degree from Rensselaer Polytechnic Institute.

Part V: Healthcare IT Operations

Andre Kushniruk, Ph.D., is a professor at the School of Health Information Science at the University of Victoria in Victoria, Canada. Dr. Kushniruk conducts research and consulting in a number of areas including evaluation of the effects of technology, human-computer interaction in healthcare, and other related areas. His work is known internationally, and he has published widely in the area of health informatics. Dr. Kushniruk has held academic positions at a number of Canadian universities and has worked with many major hospitals and health organizations in Canada, in the United States, and internationally on a range of health informatics projects. He holds under-graduate degrees in psychology and biology, as well as an M.Sc. in computer science from McMaster University and a Ph.D. in cognitive psychology from McGill University. Dr. Kushniruk was elected a fellow of the American College of Medical Informatics in 2009.

About the Contributors

Julia Adler-Milstein, Ph.D., is an assistant professor at the School of Information at the University of Michigan with a joint appointment in the School of Public Health (Health Management and Policy). Her research focuses on policy and management issues related to the use of IT in healthcare delivery. Her expertise is in health information exchange and the productivity and efficiency of electronic health records. Dr. Adler-Milstein graduated with a doctorate in health policy from Harvard University. Prior to graduate school, she worked at the Center for IT Leadership at Partners Healthcare in Boston and in the Health and Life Sciences Division of Accenture.

Chris Apgar, CISSP, CEO, and president of Apgar & Associates, LLC, is a nationally recognized information security, privacy, national identifier, HIPAA, and electronic health information exchange expert. He has more than 13 years of experience assisting healthcare organizations comply with HIPAA, HITECH, and other privacy and security regulations. Mr. Apgar also has assisted healthcare, utilities, and financial organizations implement privacy

and security safeguards to protect against organizational harm and harm to consumers. Mr. Apgar is also a nationally known speaker and author. Mr. Apgar has been a Certified Information Systems Security Professional since 2002. His education includes a bachelor's of science degree in psychology and an associates of science degree in accounting.

Leland A. Babitch, M.D., M.B.A., is a board-certified pediatrician and the chief medical information officer at the Detroit Medical Center, a part of Vanguard Health Systems. He did his undergraduate training at Northwestern University and received his medical degree from Wayne State University. After completing his residency at St. Louis Children's Hospital, he worked in private practice for three years before returning to Wayne State, where he remains an assistant professor of pediatrics. Concurrent with his return to Detroit, Dr. Babitch completed M.B.A. training from Michigan State.

Dixie B. Baker, Ph.D., M.S., M.S., FHIMSS, is a senior partner with Martin, Blanck &

Associates, where she provides consulting services to public and private clients in high-assurance architecture and technology, electronic health records, healthcare privacy and security, and health information technology standards. Since May 2009, she has served as a member of the Health Information Technology Standards Committee (HITSC), a Federal Advisory Committee (FACA). She chairs the HITSC's Privacy and Security Workgroup and the Nationwide Health Information Network (NwHIN) Power Team. She also serves on the HIT Policy Committee's Privacy and Security Tiger Team. Dr. Baker is a fellow of the Healthcare Information and Management Systems Society (HIMSS) and serves on the HIMSS Privacy and Security Committee. Dr. Baker holds a Ph.D. in special education and an M.S. in computer science from the University of Southern California, as well as M.S. and B.S. degrees from Florida State University and The Ohio State University, respectively.

Kimberly Baldwin-Stried Reich, M.B.A., M.J., PBCI, RHIA, CPHQ, FAHIMA, is a credentialed healthcare information management, quality management, case management, and healthcare compliance professional with more than 25 years of experience in a variety of healthcare settings. Ms. Baldwin-Stried Reich holds a master's of business from the Lake Forest Graduate School of Management, a master's of jurisprudence in health law and policy from the Loyola School of Law–Beazley Institute for Health Law and Policy in Chicago, and a post baccalaureate certificate in clinical informatics (PBCI) from the Johns Hopkins School of Medicine. Ms. Baldwin-Stried Reich is the first Registered Health Information Administrator (RHIA) to successfully complete the Johns Hopkins program and is a 2011 recipient of the AHIMA e-HIM Triumph Award. Ms. Baldwin-Stried Reich is currently employed as a compliance and case management professional for Lake County Physicians' Association in Waukegan, Illinois. She is the lead author of *E-Discovery and Electronic Records* (AHIMA Press).

Mike Beaver, Ph.D., CompTIA Healthcare IT Technician, is a professor within the School of Engineering Technology at the University of Rio Grande in Rio Grande, Ohio. Dr. Beaver currently teaches a course designed to prepare students for the CompTIA Healthcare IT Technician exam. Dr. Beaver's interests include virtualization technologies, Linux, computer network security, wireless computer networks, and cloud security. Dr. Beaver received his doctorate in higher education administration from Ohio University, with cognate areas of college teaching, industrial technology, and industrial and systems engineering. He also holds a master's of science degree in engineering management from Marshall University Graduate College and a bachelor of science degree in mathematics from University of Rio Grande. He holds the following certifications, among others: CompTIA Healthcare IT Technician, CompTIA A+, CompTIA Network+, CompTIA Security+, and CompTIA Strata IT Fundamentals.

Karen M. Bell, M.D., M.M.S., chair of the Certification Commission, has wide and varied expertise in health information technology, quality assurance, clinical practice, and public health in both the private and public sectors. Between 2005 and 2008, she was director of the Office of Health Information Technology Adoption in the Office of the National Coordinator (ONC), where she also served as acting deputy when the National Coordinator position was under recruitment. She was ONC's representative on CCHIT's Board of Commissioners from 2006 to 2008 and currently serves on the Massachusetts HIT Council. Dr. Bell has also been senior vice president of HIT Services at Masspro, division director in the Quality Improvement Group for the Centers for Medicare and Medicaid Services (CMS), and medical director of Blue Cross Blue Shield (BCBS) in Massachusetts, Maine, and Rhode Island. She also has served as an associate medical director, Partners Community Healthcare, Inc., and associate medical director, Harvard Community Health Plan/Pilgrim Health Care,

Boston, while maintaining a practice in internal medicine based at Massachusetts General Hospital.

David Blumenthal, M.D., M.P.P., is chief health information and innovation officer at Partners Health System in Boston and Samuel O. Thier professor of medicine and professor of health policy at Harvard Medical School. From 2009 to 2011, he served as U.S. National Coordinator for Health Information Technology under President Barack Obama. He is the author of more than 250 scholarly publications, including seminal studies of the adoption and use of health information technology in the United States.

Elizabeth Borycki, R.N., HBScN, M.N., Ph.D., is an associate professor at the School of Health Information Science at the University of Victoria in Victoria, British Columbia, Canada. Dr. Borycki is a nurse and health informatics professional. Her research interests include clinical informatics, health information systems safety, patient safety, human factors, and educating health professionals about electronic health records and health services research. Dr. Borycki has authored and co-authored numerous articles and book chapters examining the effects of health and clinical information systems upon health professional work processes and patient-care outcomes. Dr. Borycki currently represents Canada's Health Informatics Association (COACH) as the academic representative to the International Medical Informatics Association (IMIA). Dr. Borycki holds a Ph.D. in health policy, management, and evaluation from the University of Toronto and a master's of nursing from the University of Manitoba.

Jane M. Brokel, Ph.D., R.N., FNI, is currently an adjunct assistant professor for the University of Iowa College of Nursing and nurse for Heartland Home Care, Inc. She has taught nursing, research, and informatics courses the past six years. She serves on the executive committee and advisory council for the state of Iowa Health Information Network to represent nursing's perspective in developing health information exchange. Dr. Brokel is the current president of NANDA International, Inc., an international nursing organization defining nursing knowledge and has published on the experiences and findings with patient-centered workflows, clinical decision support knowledge development, and measuring patient-desired outcomes. She has more than 35 years of experience in various nursing roles, which includes 20 years using databases and health information technologies.

Braulio J. Cabral, M.S., M.S., is currently the SAIC-F, Inc., director for technical operations supporting the National Cancer Institute's Center Biomedical Informatics and Information Technology Program. Previously, he served as the director of the NCI-CBIIT Enterprise Security Program. In this role, Mr. Cabral coordinated activities related to security compliance with federal mandates such as FISMA, HIPAA, FIPS, and other governmental cybersecurity-related activities. Prior to joining SAIC-F, Inc., Mr. Cabral served in several IT positions at GXS, Inc. (formerly GE Information Services), a B2B consulting and service provider firm. Mr. Cabral holds a bachelor of science in computer and information systems from Strayer University, a master of science in management information technologies from Regis University, and a master of science in management information systems security and project management, and Mr. Cabral is currently a Ph.D. candidate in applied management and decision sciences at Walden University.

Dave deBronkart, better known as "e-Patient Dave," is the leading spokesperson for the e-patient movement: empowered, engaged, equipped, enabled. Mr. deBronkart unexpectedly gained national notoriety in 2009 when he tried to move his hospital records into Google Health and what came across was his insurance records, not clinical records; his blog post analyzing the failure was reported on page 1 of the *Boston Globe*. Before his 2007 cancer, he was a data user and marketing speaker, so his analysis of the data experience led him to become an international keynote speaker. In 2009 he was elected a founding co-chair of the Society for Participatory Medicine, and *Health Leaders* named him (and his primary, Dr. Danny Sands) to its annual list 20 People Who Make Health Care Better. Mr. deBronkart's TED Talk "Let Patients Help" is in the top half of the most watched TED talks of all time, and in 2012 the National Library of Medicine announced that it had begun capturing his blog into its History of Medicine division.

Charles Denham, M.D., is the founder of TMIT, a nonprofit medical research organization. He is editor-in-chief of the *Journal of Patient Safety* and has authored more than 100 publications. He is an adjunct professor at the Mayo Clinic College of Medicine in health systems engineering, has been a senior fellow of the Harvard University Advanced Leadership Initiative, and is a lecturer on the faculty of the Harvard Medical School. He advises the Institute of Medicine and National Academies of Science and Engineering on their President's Circle. He is ranked 38th in the list of 50 Most Powerful Physician Executives. He has chaired the Leapfrog Group Safe Practices program since 2003 and co-chaired the National Quality Forum (NQF) Safe Practices committee from 2004 to 2010. He leads the global TMIT Greenlight Program, which is validating high-impact innovations that drive quality up and cost down.

Floyd Eisenberg, M.D., MPH, FACP, is president of iParsimony, LLC, serving organizations or clinical system vendors interested in repurposing data for measurement, clinical decision support, reporting, and research. Dr. Eisenberg received his M.D. degree from Penn State University followed by a residency in internal medicine at Abington Memorial Hospital in Abington, Pennsylvania, and a fellowship in infectious diseases at Temple University. His experience includes ten years of clinical practice in Norristown, Pennsylvania;

network quality improvement activities at Independence Blue Cross; and EHR development at Siemens Medical Solutions Health Services. More recently at National Quality Forum, Dr. Eisenberg led the development of the quality data model to enable performance measurement directly from EHRs. He is currently a member of the Health Information Technology Standards Committee (HITSC) of the Office of the National Coordinator for Health Information Technology (ONC).

Cheryl A. Fisher, Ed.D., R.N.-BC, is currently the program director for Professional Development for Nursing and Patient Care Services at the National Institutes of Health Clinical Center in Bethesda, Maryland. She received her doctorate in instructional technology from Towson University and has a postgraduate certificate in nursing informatics from the University of Maryland and a post-graduate certificate in nursing education. Dr. Fisher is responsible for all the central nursing education at the NIH Clinical Center and is actively working to reconceptualize courses utilizing technology to increase accessibility of all educational offerings. She is an adjunct professor for the University of Maryland and teaches graduate courses in nursing informatics. Dr. Fisher is also board certified in nursing informatics.

Gregory Forzley, M.D., FAAFP, is chief medical information officer for Health Networks with Trinity Health, based in Livonia, Michigan. He is responsible for supporting the development, implementation, and use of clinical information systems to assist clinicians within the health networks in the delivery of the highest-quality and most appropriate patient care. Prior to this, he was CMIO at Saint Mary's Health Care in Grand Rapids, Michigan. Dr. Forzley chairs the State of Michigan Health Information Technology Commission. He is actively involved in health information exchange, serving on the board of Michigan Health Connect while chairing the MHC Provider Advisory Committee. A board-certified family physician with a graduate degree in informatics,

Dr. Forzley's past experience includes private medical practice, family medicine residency faculty, managed-care physician executive, and physician leader in community quality activities. He co-authored an article on meaningful use in January 2012's *Journal of Health Information Management.*

Michael Fossel, M.D., Ph.D., received his M.D. and Ph.D. from Stanford University and was a practicing emergency physician and a professor of medicine for 25 years. He worked for Cerner Corporation for six years and currently works for HPG Resources as a medical IT consultant. He is the author of dozens of articles and several other medical books, and his latest book, *EHR's: Strategies for Long-Term Success,* is due out early next year.

Lisa A. Gallagher, BSEE, CISM, CPHIMS, serves as HIMSS's senior director of Privacy and Security. In this role, she is responsible for all of the privacy and security programs and provides privacy and security content support for HIMSS's federal and state government relations/advocacy work. Ms. Gallagher currently serves on the ONC Standards Committee's Privacy and Security Work Group and the Patient Matching Power Team. Ms. Gallagher has a bachelor of science degree in electrical engineering, was a certified trust technology evaluator (NSA), and is a Certified Information Security Manager (CISM) (ISACA). She is also a Certified Professional in Healthcare Information and Management Systems (CPHIMS).

John Glaser, Ph.D., currently serves as chief executive officer (CEO) of the Health Services Business Unit of Siemens Healthcare, where he is responsible for heading Siemens' global healthcare IT business. Prior to joining Siemens, Dr. Glaser was vice president and chief information officer at Partners Health-Care, Inc. Previously, he was vice president of Information Systems at Brigham and Women's Hospital. Dr. Glaser was the founding chairman of the College of Healthcare Information Management Executives (CHIME) and

is the former chairman of the eHealth Initiative Board and the Board of the National Alliance for Health Information Technology. He is a former senior advisor to the Office of the National Coordinator for Health Information Technology (ONC). He is also past president of the Healthcare Information & Management Systems Society (HIMSS) and is a fellow of HIMSS, CHIME, and the American College of Medical Informatics. Dr. Glaser has published more than 150 articles and three books on the strategic application of information technology in healthcare. Dr. Glaser holds a Ph.D. in healthcare information systems from the University of Minnesota.

Kenneth W. Goodman, Ph.D., FACMI, is founder and director of the University of Miami Bioethics Program and its Pan American Bioethics Initiative and co-director of the university's Ethics Programs. Dr. Goodman is a professor of medicine at the University of Miami with appointments in the Department of Philosophy, Department of Health Informatics, Department of Epidemiology and Public Health, Department of Electrical and Computer Engineering, School of Nursing and Health Studies, and Department of Anesthesiology. He chairs the Ethics Committee of the American Medical Informatics Association, where he cofounded the Ethical, Legal, and Social Issues Working Group. He is a fellow of the American College of Medical Informatics. His research has emphasized ethical issues in health information technology.

Tasha Green, RHIA, is the program director for the Health Informatics Information Technology Program at the Community College of Baltimore County in Baltimore, Maryland. Prior to this, she was the program chair for health information technology at TESST College of Technology (Kaplan Higher Business Education) and also held the position of HIM director at Howard University Hospital. Ms. Green holds a master of science degree in management, information systems, from the University of Maryland University College and a bachelor of science degree in health information management from Northeastern University. She holds the Registered Health Information Administrator certification from the American Health Information Management Association (AHIMA).

Liz Johnson, M.S., B.S.N., FHIMSS, CPHIMS, R.N.-BC, is the vice president of applied clinical informatics at Tenet Healthcare Corporation. She is also a member of the ONC Standards Committee appointed by Secretary Sebelius. For both 2010 and 2011, she was ranked in the top 25 Clinical Informaticists in America by Modern Healthcare. In 2010, she won the HIMSS Nursing Informatics Leadership Award. Ms. Johnson is a healthcare executive with more than 35 years of experience who has responsibility for leading the strategy, visioning, and implementation of clinical informatics across 49 hospitals in 11 states. She speaks more than 25 times a year on all aspects of clinical informatics in national meetings.

J. Michael Kramer, M.D., M.B.A., is a senior vice president and the chief quality officer with Spectrum Health. As Spectrum's system chief quality officer, Dr. Kramer is the leader for Spectrum Health's Quality Outcomes and Electronic Medical Records teams. He is actively engaged in advancing the quality and informatics strategy of all Spectrum Health's businesses including the Hospital Group, Medical Group, Research Institute, and Health Care Insurer. In his CMIO roles, Dr. Kramer has been a national leader in designing methodologies for implementing and optimizing systems that assist clinicians in achieving high-quality care and evidence-based outcomes. Dr. Kramer brings to his role as CMIO more than 15 years of information systems. He previously taught applied clinical informatics at the University of Michigan. Dr. Kramer recently was the co-author of two articles regarding the HITECH Act and meaningful use in the *Journal of Health Information Management* in January 2012. In 2011, he published on process design

for clinical information systems and clinical decision support methodologies.

Daniel Lachance, MCITP, MCTS, CNI, IBM Certified Instructor, CompTIA A+, CompTIA Network+, CompTIA Security+, is a technical trainer for Global Knowledge and has delivered classroom training in a wide variety of products for the past 17 years. Throughout his career he has also developed custom applications and has planned, implemented, troubleshot, and documented various network configurations.

John R. LeMoine, M.D., FACP, graduated from Dalhousie University Medical School in 1974 and is board certified in internal medicine, pulmonary medicine, and critical-care medicine. He has been a faculty member at the University of California – San Diego and Dalhousie University. Dr. LeMoine is currently system medical director and chief medical information officer for Sharp Healthcare in San Diego and is responsible for providing medical direction and physician counsel for Clinical Effectiveness and Information Systems.

David Liebovitz, M.D., is the chief medical informatics officer for the Northwestern Medical Faculty Foundation, the full-time academic medical practice affiliated with the Feinberg School of Medicine at Northwestern University. In this role, he works to advance the development of the outpatient medical records system and optimize information exchange with Northwestern Memorial Hospital, where he serves as associate chief medical officer and medical director for Clinical Information Systems. Dr. Liebovitz is also the program director for the Northwestern School of Continuing Studies Master's Degree Program in Medical Informatics and an associate professor of medicine at the Feinberg School of Medicine. He also serves as an associate program director for the Internal Medicine Residency Program. Prior to his current ten years at Northwestern University, Dr. Liebovitz received his medical degree at the University of Illinois at

Chicago and his undergraduate degree in electrical/computer engineering at the University of Illinois in Urbana-Champaign. His current funded research relates to the areas of security and privacy.

Roman Mateyko has worked in the telecommunications industry in both management and engineering roles in the private and public sectors. After moving to Victoria, British Columbia, in 1988, he joined the Government of British Columbia where he worked in network engineering, service management, contract management, planning, strategy, and regulatory affairs. He is currently an executive director in the Strategic Partnerships Office, Office of the CIO, in the Ministry of Citizens' Services and Open Government responsible for architecture and planning coordination. Before joining government, Mr. Mateyko worked in the cellular industry and for a common carrier. Mr. Mateyko has a bachelor's of applied science degree in electrical engineering from the University of Toronto, is a professional engineer, is a member of the IEEE, and is currently an adjunct assistant professor at the University of Victoria in the school of Health Information Science.

John Moehrke is a principal engineer specializing in standards architecture in interoperability, security, and privacy for GE Healthcare. He is primarily involved in the international standards efforts related to GE's healthcare businesses. He is a member of the Privacy & Security Workgroup of the HIT Standards Committee and is co-chair of the HL7 Security Workgroup. Mr. Moehrke is an active member in the United States' national initiatives to create a Nationwide Healthcare Information Network for both the Exchange architecture and the Direct Project. He is a GE representative to DICOM, HL7, NEMA, ISO, and IHE. He has been active in the healthcare standardization since 1999, during which time he has authored various standards, profiles, and white papers. Mr. Moehrke has become a well-known security and privacy expert in the Standards Organizations and Government regulations. Mr. Moehrke graduated from the Milwaukee School of Engineering with a bachelor's of science degree in computer science and engineering. Mr. Moehrke has an internationally read blog, Healthcare Security/ Privacy.

Alex Mu-Hsing Kuo, Ph.D., is an assistant professor at the School of Health Information Science at the University of Victoria in Victoria, British Columbia, Canada. Dr. Kuo's research focuses on five areas: healthcare database/data warehouse management, health information exchange (data interoperability), data mining application in healthcare management, e-health, and clinical decision support systems. Dr. Kuo holds a Ph.D. from the Department of Computer Science at the University of Nottingham, United Kingdom.

Judy Murphy, R.N., FACMI, FHIMSS, FAAN, is the deputy national coordinator for Programs & Policy at the Office of the National Coordinator for Health IT, Department of Health and Human Services in Washington D.C. In this role, she coordinates federal efforts to assist healthcare providers and organizations in adopting health information technology to improve care and to promote consumers' greater understanding and use of health information technology for their own health. Ms. Murphy served on the American Medical Informatics Association (AMIA) Board of Directors and the Health Information and Management Systems Society (HIMSS) Board of Directors. She is a fellow in the American Academy of Nursing, the American College of Medical Informatics, and HIMSS. She received the 2006 HIMSS Nursing Informatics Leadership Award, was named one of the "20 People Who Make Healthcare Better" in 2007 by *HealthLeaders* magazine, and was selected as one of 33 Nursing Informatics' Pioneers to participate in the Nursing Informatics History Project sponsored by AMIA, NLM, AAN, and RWJF.

Sean Murphy, FACHE, CPHIMS, CISSP-ISSMP, is a vice president in the SAIC Health Solutions Business Unit and serves as the organization's HIPAA/health information security officer. A healthcare information security expert with 20 years of experience, he has had success at all levels of healthcare. Prior to joining SAIC, Mr. Murphy was a lieutenant colonel in the U.S. Air Force Medical Service Corps. His proudest professional accomplishment was his service as senior mentor to the Afghan National Police Surgeon General's Office in support of Operation Enduring Freedom. He has master's degrees in business administration (advanced IT concentration) from the University of South Florida and in health services administration from Central Michigan University. He's also an adjunct professor at Saint Leo University, a fellow at the American College of Healthcare Executives, and board-certified by the Healthcare Information & Management Systems Society. He's an active Certified Information Systems Security Professional and Information Systems Security Management Professional.

Donald Nichols, Ph.D., is a senior research associate and the Health Care Financing Practice Area lead at IMPAQ International, LLC, in Washington, DC. Throughout his nine years as an academic and social policy researcher, Dr. Nichols has gained experience with program evaluations, demonstration designs, performance measures, and pilot testing in the healthcare field, particularly healthcare financing. His research includes evaluations of the Maryland Multi-payer Patient Centered Medical Home (PCMH) demonstration and Medicare Acute Care Episode (ACE) demonstration (bundled payment). Prior to joining IMPAQ, Dr. Nichols was on the faculty of Washington University in the Department of Economics where he taught courses in health economics and econometrics. He completed his doctoral work in economics at Stanford University where he was the recipient of the National Science Foundation and the Ford Foundation fellowships. Dr. Nicholas received his Ph.D. in economics from Stanford.

Sheila Ochylski is the director of clinical transformation at Trinity Health, one of the largest Catholic health systems in the United States, working with the Clinical Informatics team since 2008. Ms. Ochylski is dedicated to leading transformation initiatives in clinical process. With a focus on incorporating evidence-based practice, Ms. Ochylski provides support for the coordination, integration, and analysis of clinical processes across Trinity Health system-wide. She earned her master's degree in nursing and business from the University of Michigan where she served an internship with the International Council of Nurses (ICN) and worked with the World Health Organization (WHO) in Geneva, Switzerland. Ms. Ochylski's experience includes working as a nurse entrepreneur for 16 years, clinical experience including emergency and intensive care, and various leadership roles for 27 years; she is also an adjunct professor teaching clinical informatics at the University of Detroit-Mercy.

J. Marc Overhage, M.D., Ph.D., is a general internist who also earned a doctorate in biophysics and completed a residency in internal medicine and fellowship in medical informatics. During his 25-year tenure at the Regenstrief Institute and Indiana University, Dr. Overhage, who served as the Sam Regenstrief Professor of Medical Informatics, practiced and studied a variety of informatics topics including clinical decision support, the impact of health information technology on providers, and health information exchange. During that time, he, with his colleagues, developed the Indiana Network for Patient Care and studied the role of health information exchange on public and population health. Subsequently, he founded and served as CEO of the Indiana Health Information Exchange before becoming the chief medical informatics officer for Siemens Healthcare.

Thomas Payne, M.D., FACP, has 23 years of experience with EMRs and clinical computing systems in private, federal, and academic medical centers. He attended Stanford University and the University of Washington School of Medicine, was a medical resident at the University of Colorado, and was an NLM fellow at Harvard. For 12 years he has served as medical director of Information Technology Services at the University of Washington in Seattle and is an attending physician in medicine at UW Medical Center and Harborview Medical Center. He is on the Board of AMIA and a fellow of the American College of Medical Informatics, the American College of Physicians, and the Royal College of Physicians (Edinburgh).

Gila Pyke, BCompSc software engineering, is the president of Cognaissance and senior consultant specializing in privacy, security, and risk management, as well as interoperability standards in the healthcare IT domain. She has been working in IT for close to 20 years, including 12 in healthcare IT. She has been instrumental in the creation of healthcare IT privacy, security, and risk management standards through organizations such as HL7, IHE, ISO, HITSP, and the Canada Health Infoway Standards Collaborative.

Bharat Rao, Ph.D., is head of the Center for Innovations for Siemens Health Services, which was established to foster HIT thought leadership for Siemens and to create a continuous innovation pipeline of new products. Before that, Dr. Rao was senior director and head of the Knowledge Solutions group, Siemens Healthcare, which developed data mining solutions that analyzed millions of patient records, including automated decision support from hospitals' EMRs, computer-aided diagnosis from medical images, and predictive models for personalized medicine. He has received several international awards, including the ACM SIGKDD 2011 Service Award for "service to society for pioneering data mining applications in healthcare." He was also named the Siemens Inventor of the Year in 2005. He has been granted 50 patents and

published 100 scholarly publications and one book. Dr. Rao received his B.Tech in electronics engineering from the Indian Institute of Technology, Madras, and his M.S. and Ph.D. in electrical and computer engineering from the University of Illinois, Urbana-Champaign.

Cary Sennett, M.D., Ph.D., is the president of IMPAQ International. Dr. Sennett has more than 20 years of experience working with both public-sector and private-sector organizations to use data and information technology to improve the quality and value of healthcare in the United States. As executive vice president, he played a leadership role in building out the National Committee for Quality Assurance's (NCQA's) national standard measurement set, HEDIS®, and establishing a value-based purchasing dynamic in managed care. Prior to joining IMPAQ, Dr. Sennett served as a fellow in the Economic Studies Program at the Brookings Institution and as managing director for Health Care Finance Reform at the Engelberg Center for Health Care Reform. He has also served as a senior leader at the American College of Cardiology and the American Board of Internal Medicine. Dr. Sennett earned his M.D. from Yale and his Ph.D. from the Sloan School at MIT.

Joyce Sensmeier, M.S., R.N.-BC, CPHIMS, FHIMSS, FAAN, is the vice president of informatics for HIMSS. In her current role, she is responsible for the areas of clinical informatics, standards, interoperability, privacy, and security. Ms. Sensmeier became board certified in Nursing Informatics in 1996, earned the Certified Professional in Healthcare Information and Management Systems in 2002, and achieved HIMSS fellowship status in 2005. Ms. Sensmeier is president of IHE USA and previously served as the standards implementation technical manager for the Healthcare Information Technology Standards Panel (HITSP). Ms. Sensmeier was recognized in 2010 as a fellow with the American Academy of Nursing, the highest honor in the field of nursing. She is also cofounder and ex-officio chair of the Alliance for Nursing Informatics.

Dennis Seymour, CISSP, ITIL, is the senior security architect at Ellumen, Inc., in Arlington, Virginia. He has more than 17 years of healthcare-specific security experience, including 12 years of experience at the enterprise level for the Department of Veterans Affairs, Veterans Health Administration, in the positions of technical security advisor and information security officer, with the responsibilities of policy development, system controls assessment and certification, and medical device security policy development and compliance with HIPAA, NIST, FISMA, and other requirements. Mr. Seymour is currently serving as the chairperson of the Health Information Management & Systems Society (HIMSS) Privacy and Security Steering Committee and has been a member of the HIMSS Medical Device Security Task Force, Mobile Security Work Group, and Risk Assessment Work Group. In 2010 Mr. Seymour was a finalist for the International Information Systems Security Certification Consortium, Inc. (ISC),[2] Government Information Security Leadership Award (GISLA) in the contractor division.

Michael Stearns, M.D., is a board-certified neurologist and informaticist with 15 years of direct patient-care experience in clinical and academic medicine and 15 years of involvement in several high-profile health information technology efforts. He has provided leadership to several high-profile clinical informatics projects at the National Library of Medicine, the National Cancer Institute, and the College of American Pathologists. He served as the international director of SNOMED, where he played a central role in the development of SNOMED CT. He has provided direction and leadership to two leading EHR vendors, has served as founding board president for the Texas e-Health Alliance, has served on numerous boards and committees, and frequently lectures on a variety of HIT topics. Dr. Stearns is a Certified Professional Coder with expertise in computer-assisted coding in EHRs and holds the HIT Pro Clinician/Practitioner Consultant certification. He played a central role in the formation of the University of Texas at Austin HIT certificate program, a nationally recognized model for HIT workforce development.

Robert Tennant, M.A., is the senior policy advisor with the Washington, D.C.-based Government Affairs Department of the Medical Group Management Association (MGMA), headquartered in Englewood, Colorado. MGMA, founded in 1926, is the nation's principal voice for medical group practice. MGMA's 22,500 members manage and lead more than 13,500 organizations in which more than 295,000 physicians practice. Mr. Tennant focuses on federal legislative and regulatory health information technology issues for MGMA, including HIPAA and the administrative simplification provisions of the Affordable Care Act of 2010, electronic health records, electronic prescribing, ICD-10, and other electronic health information technology issues. Mr. Tennant has participated with numerous industry efforts including the Workgroup for Electronic Data Interchange; the ICD-10 Coalition; the National Uniform Claim Committee; the e-Health Initiative; the Council for Affordable Quality Healthcare CORE initiative; the Certification Commission for Health Information Technology; and the Healthcare Administrative Simplification Coalition.

CompTIA.

CompTIA Healthcare IT Technician

The CompTIA Healthcare IT Technician specialty certification is a vendor- and technology-neutral exam designed to ensure IT professionals have the operational, regulatory, and security knowledge necessary to provide hardware and software support in medical environments where electronic health record (EHR) systems are being deployed or maintained.

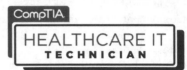

It Pays to Get Certified

In a digital world, digital literacy is an essential survival skill. Certification proves you have the knowledge and skills to solve business problems in virtually any business environment. Certifications are highly valued credentials that qualify you for jobs, increased compensation, and promotion.

Ten of the twenty fastest-growing occupations in the United States are healthcare-related, potentially yielding 3.2 million new jobs over the next decade.

- **U.S. HITECH Act**—funded imperative for U.S. healthcare industry
  - **Transition of paper records** to be completed in U.S. medical facilities by year-end 2015.

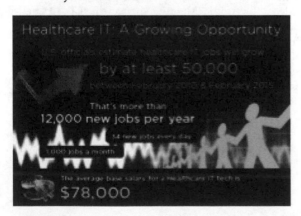

- **Individual physicians receive more than $40,000** for installing EHRs and demonstrating "meaningful use."
- **More than $88.6 billion** was spent by providers in 2010 on developing and implementing EHRs, health information exchanges (HIEs), and other HIT initiatives. HIT and consulting vendors expected to see a 10 percent to 20 percent hike in revenues in 2012.

How Certification Helps Your Career

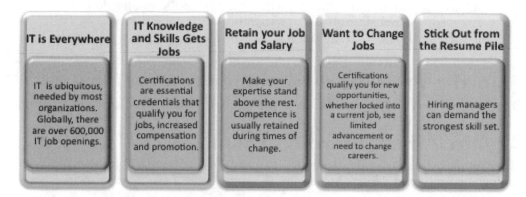

IT is Everywhere	IT Knowledge and Skills Gets Jobs	Retain your Job and Salary	Want to Change Jobs	Stick Out from the Resume Pile
IT is ubiquitous, needed by most organizations. Globally, there are over 600,000 IT job openings.	Certifications are essential credentials that qualify you for jobs, increased compensation and promotion.	Make your expertise stand above the rest. Competence is usually retained during times of change.	Certifications qualify you for new opportunities, whether locked into a current job, see limited advancement or need to change careers.	Hiring managers can demand the strongest skill set.

CompTIA Career Pathway

CompTIA offers a number of credentials that form a foundation for your career in technology and allow you to pursue specific areas of concentration. Depending on the path you choose to take, CompTIA certifications help you build upon your skills and knowledge, supporting learning throughout your entire career.

CompTIA HEALTHCARE IT TECHNICIAN™

HEALTHCARE IT SPECIALIST
CERTIFICATE

CompTIA A+

PC REPAIR AND SUPPORT
CERTIFICATION

POTENTIAL CAREER PATH

Steps to Getting Certified and Staying Certified

1. **Review exam objectives.** Review the certification objectives to make sure you know what is covered in the exam: http://certification.comptia.org/ Training/testingcenters/examobjectives.aspx.

2. **Practice for the exam.** After you have studied for the certification, take a free assessment and sample test to get an idea of what type of questions might be on the exam: http://certification.comptia.org/Training/testingcenters/samplequestions.aspx.

3. **Purchase an exam voucher.** Purchase your exam voucher on the CompTIA Marketplace, which is located at www.comptiastore.com.

4. **Take the test!** Select a certification exam provider and schedule a time to take your exam. You can find exam providers at http://certification.comptia.org/ Training/testingcenters.aspx.

5. **Stay certified!** Continuing education is required. Effective January 1, 2011, CompTIA Healthcare IT Technician certifications are valid for three years from the date of certification. There are a number of ways the certification can be renewed. For more information, go to http://certification.comptia.org/getCertified/steps_to_certification/stayCertified.aspx.

Join the Professional Community

The free online IT Pro Community provides valuable content to students and professionals. Join the IT Pro Community at http://itpro.comptia.org.

Career IT job resources include the following:

- Where to start in IT
- Career assessments
- Salary trends
- U.S. job board

Join the IT Pro Community and get access to the following:

- Forums on networking, security, computing, and cutting-edge technologies
- Access to blogs written by industry experts
- Current information on cutting-edge technologies
- Access to various industry resource links and articles related to IT and IT careers

Content Seal of Quality

This courseware bears the seal of **CompTIA Approved Quality Content**. This seal signifies this content covers 100 percent of the exam objectives and implements important instructional design principles. CompTIA recommends multiple learning tools to help increase coverage of the learning objectives.

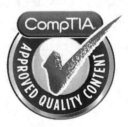

Why CompTIA?

- **Global recognition** CompTIA is recognized globally as the leading IT nonprofit trade association and has enormous credibility. Plus, CompTIA's certifications are vendor-neutral and offer proof of foundational knowledge that translates across technologies.

- **Valued by hiring managers** Hiring managers value CompTIA certification because it is vendor- and technology-independent validation of your technical skills.

- **Recommended or required by government and businesses** Many government organizations and corporations (for example, Dell, Sharp, Ricoh, the U.S. Department of Defense, and many more) either recommend or require technical staff to be CompTIA certified.

- **Three CompTIA certifications ranked in the top 10** In a study by DICE of 17,000 technology professionals, certifications helped command higher salaries at all experience levels.

How to Obtain More Information

- *Visit CompTIA Online* Go to www.comptia.org to learn more about getting CompTIA certified.

- *Contact CompTIA* Please call 866-835-8020, ext. 5, or e-mail questions@ comptia.org.

- *Join the IT Pro Community* Go to http://itpro.comptia.org to join the IT community to get relevant career information.

- *Connect with CompTIA* Find us on Facebook, LinkedIn, Twitter, and YouTube.

CAQC Disclaimer

The logo of the CompTIA Approved Quality Content (CAQC) program and the status of this or other training material as "Authorized" under the CompTIA Approved Quality Content program signifies that, in CompTIA's opinion, such training material covers the content of CompTIA's related certification exam.

The contents of this training material were created for the CompTIA Healthcare IT Technician exam covering CompTIA certification objectives that were current as of the date of publication.

CompTIA has not reviewed or approved the accuracy of the contents of this training material and specifically disclaims any warranties of merchantability or fitness for a particular purpose. CompTIA makes no guarantee concerning the success of persons using any such "Authorized" or other training material in order to prepare for any CompTIA certification exam.

CONTENTS AT A GLANCE

CONTENTS

FOREWORD

Healthcare in the United States is not what it should be. Our nation spends more on healthcare per capita than any other country, but we still lag far behind on many important measures of health. In 2010, the United States spent more than $2.6 trillion on healthcare, representing about 18 percent of our gross domestic product. But Americans receive only about half of the preventive, acute, and chronic care recommended by current research and evidence-based guidelines, and life expectancy in the United States is shorter than in many other countries. Cost is not the only issue. Access to both insurance and care itself has been an ongoing problem for millions of Americans.

The Patient Protection and Affordable Care Act of 2010, if implemented, will make coverage available to about 32 million people who were previously uninsured, bringing millions more Americans into regular contact with our healthcare system and making it more imperative than ever before to address cost and quality issues.

Addressing these problems will require innovation: innovation in the way we pay for, organize, and deliver care, as well as innovation in the information technologies we use to provide services every day.

Today, federal and private insurance programs typically pay for the *volume* of services provided, without regard to the quality or cost-effectiveness of those services. For example, doctors and hospitals are paid when they provide a service—a check-up, a procedure, a lab test—whether or not the patient benefited, the service was performed correctly, or the patient was harmed during the process. Finding ways to pay providers of care for quality rather than volume is now an area of active innovation within the federal government, within many states, and through commercial payers in the private sector.

Innovation in the organization and delivery of care is also needed to promote lower costs, higher quality, and better access to healthcare. New models of care that promote care coordination, accountability, and focus on the patient are now rapidly emerging. Governmental and private-sector entities are investing hundreds of millions of dollars to test new models of care, including accountable-care organizations, advanced primary care, the patient-centered medical home, and home-based care. These new models of care, it is hoped, will lower healthcare costs and improve quality by eliminating unnecessary procedures and emergency room visits and by increasing preventive care.

Effective use of information—enabled by technology—is foundational to innovations in all aspects of our healthcare system. Information is the lifeblood of healthcare. Those who deliver healthcare to patients cannot provide services effectively unless they know a patient's health history, health problems, laboratory and imaging results, medications, allergies, and other critical information. Bits of information about a patient usually reside in all the different settings where that patient has received care—and many times only on paper. Too often, vital information is unavailable to doctors and nurses when they need it most. Even patients themselves can have difficulty getting their own complete medical records, which impedes their ability to play a greater role in managing their care.

This is where information technology plays a critical role.

Information technology enables information about the patient to *follow* the patient across providers, settings, conditions, and time. Information technology helps clinicians and care teams provide integrated, patient-centered, and evidenced-based care— not only at the point of care but also between visits. Information technology also helps the patient by enabling more effective and efficient communication between the patient and the care team, by supporting new ways to access care when a visit is not needed, and by providing online and interactive educational tools designed to empower and educate patients about their health conditions and the strategies they can use to improve their health.

Information technology also enables the aggregation and analysis of data across patient populations, which is crucial to identifying trends, developing and implementing interventions to address areas that need improvement, and monitoring overall performance.

The Health Information Technology for Economic and Clinical Health (HITECH) Act of 2009 invested up to $30 billion in the adoption and use of health information technology to improve health and healthcare in the United States. A majority of this investment is in the form of financial incentives to healthcare professionals and hospitals that "meaningfully use" healthcare IT to improve care for their patients. Additional investments were made in programs designed to assure the adoption of standards for and interoperability of electronic health record (EHR) systems, support primary-care providers with the meaningful use of healthcare IT, improve privacy and security, facilitate the electronic exchange of information across care settings, and support the development of a workforce that will implement healthcare IT systems.

Moving healthcare from a paper-based system of "siloed" information to one robustly supported by health information technology will require a highly skilled workforce with new competencies and skills that have not been widely prevalent in healthcare. Healthcare professionals who are accustomed to working with paper systems—including doctors, nurses, and administrative staff—will need to learn new workflows and new systems for both clinical and administrative aspects of care. In addition, there is a growing and urgent demand for workers skilled in the implementation and maintenance of new EHR and health information technology systems. Already there is a significant deficit of healthcare IT workers in the United States; 67 percent of hospital executives reported a shortage of healthcare IT staff in a September 2012 survey conducted by the College of Healthcare Information Management Executives (CHIME). One study indicates that the healthcare IT workforce must increase by 38 percent, from the current number of 108,000 workers to nearly 150,000.

Through HITECH, the federal government has invested more than $180 million in various workforce development programs including curriculum and competency exam development, community college programs designed to educate healthcare IT professionals, and programs of assistance for university-based training.

Transforming our nation's healthcare system into one that reliably provides safe, effective, efficient, patient-centered, cost-effective care will require the focused commitment of professionals from many sectors. This book offers IT professionals an in-depth look at the needs and requirements of this critically important and growing field of healthcare IT. Becoming part of this new workforce will likely be challenging, exhilarating, and ultimately highly rewarding, as the positive impact of healthcare IT on our nation's healthcare system and on the health of the nation itself becomes unmistakably clear.

David Blumenthal, M.D., M.P.P.
Chief Health Information and Innovation Officer, Partners Health System
Samuel O. Thier Professor of Medicine, Professor of Health Policy, Harvard Medical
School. 2009–2011 U.S. National Coordinator for Health Information Technology
November 2, 2012

ACKNOWLEDGMENTS

The first acknowledgments go to the part editors of this book who worked on the chapters while they were supporting the healthcare informatics policy, industries, and academic institutions. Janet Marchibroda, Dr. Don Mon, Dr. Michael Beller, Lori Reed-Fourquet, and Dr. Andre Kuschniruk spent time shaping the outlines and the chapters that responded to the vision of providing one healthcare information technology book to prepare others in information technology to sit for the CompTIA and HIT Pro exams. The second round of thanks goes to the contributors who were equally stressed during this very intensive time in healthcare information technology to work over and above their work schedules to get this book delivered and out to the community. Working on project management from the beginning was Sean Gugerty, whom we wish success in his healthcare IT legal endeavors. Steadfastly facilitating editing and mapping was Alisa Ryan, who clearly became part of the team.

Behind all of us was a team from McGraw-Hill that is matched by no other in the dedication and commitment to pursuing what the healthcare information technology domain requires at this time. This team includes the leadership of Meghan Riley Manfre, acquisitions editor; Tim Green, executive acquisitions editor; and Stephanie Evans, acquisitions coordinator; and the legal department, which we challenged with more than 50 contracts. Meghan provided special leadership in creating a book that provides a vision in a creative way that is responsive to the CompTIA and HIT Pro exams.

When the production team started, we were joined by such specialists as Jody McKenzie, McGraw-Hill editorial supervisor; Molly Sharp, project manager for copyediting and page proofs; and her team, especially Kim Wimpsett and Barbara Gordon. What a dedicated team to maintaining quality, readability, and format.

Special thanks go to those who contributed to the content on the book's CD-ROM, especially Dr. Michael Stearns, Dennis Seymour, Dr. Mike Beaver, and Tasha Green.

Finally, the book's online learning center can be attributed to the dedicated team working with Megg Morin, acquisitions editor. Joining that team were Dr. Juliana Brixey, Jack Brixey, and Tasha Green.

INTRODUCTION

Kathleen A. McCormick

In the December 2011 issue of *Scientific American*, a lattice network diagram, created by scientist Hilary Mason, demonstrates how an analysis of the traffic on the World Wide Web has identified pathways that individuals are using to search the Web. The article refers to these pathways as "The Links We Love."[1] But this lattice could also have been titled "Where the Money Is!" Visible within the lattice is a thick line between health and technology, demonstrating a concentrated activity link. Conversely, distinct within the lattice network are outlier clusters of activity not in synchrony with health and technology: the computer science and engineering clusters. Looking at these clusters, it is apparent that if we continue in the pattern of these pathways, with computing and engineering existing autonomous of health and technology, the goal of quality, efficient, effective healthcare delivered at reasonable costs will be unachievable in the United States. The purpose of this book is to bridge this gap.

The Need for HIT Professionals

As substantiated by Mason's lattice network, the need for trained healthcare information technology (HIT) professionals is great. To put numbers to this need, the Bureau of Labor Statistics predicts that growth in HIT employment will increase 20 percent through 2018 (Occupational Outlook Handbook, 2010–2011 Edition),[2] with jobs for network and computer systems administrators growing by 28 percent.[3] The Bureau of Labor Statistics also suggests that 50,000 qualified HIT workers are needed to meet the demands of hospital and physician adoption of electronic health records (EHRs) and to connect to statewide health information exchanges (HIEs). These projections are corroborated by independent studies that also predict an HIT workforce shortage over the next five years.[4]

One organization active in the training of HIT professionals is the Healthcare Information and Management Systems Society (HIMSS). In 2012, HIMSS published its 23rd Annual HIMSS Leadership Survey reflecting the opinions of IT professionals in U.S. healthcare provider organizations regarding the use of IT in their organizations (HIMSS, 2012).[5] This study puts a finger on the pulse of HIT annually, with 302 HIT professionals surveyed for 2012 on a wide array of topics critical to HIT leaders including IT priorities, issues driving and challenging technology adoption, IT security, and IT staffing and budgeting plans. For the past several years respondents have identified the lack of adequate financial support as the top barrier to IT implementation. That is, until now. This year, 22 percent of respondents cited adequate staffing resources as their top challenge, followed by the lack of adequate financial support (14 percent) and vendors' inability to effectively deliver products or services to respondents' satisfaction (12 percent). The survey's healthcare CIO respondents believe that IT can have a positive impact on patient care, by either improving clinical/quality outcomes, reducing medical errors, or helping to standardize care by allowing the use of evidence-based medicine. Yet, as you can deduce, IT's ability to produce this positive impact depends upon the reality of the primary challenge: the lack of adequate staffing resources.

Preparing a Critical Mass

To meet this challenging and growing demand for HIT professionals, the Office of the National Coordinator for Health Information Technology (ONC), part of the U.S. Federal Government Department of Health and Human Services, has facilitated the entry of the Health Information Technology and Economic and Clinical Health (HITECH) Act. A portion of the nearly $30 billion grant provided by the act has gone to fund the Workforce Development Program.[6] The goal of this program is to train a new workforce of skilled HIT professionals who will be able to help providers implement EHRs and achieve meaningful use. It is hoped that ONC-funded programs will reduce the estimated workforce shortage by 85 percent.

The Workforce Development Program consists of four initiatives: University-Based Training, Curriculum Development Centers, the Community College Consortia, and the Competency Exam Program. It is the goal of the Community College Consortia to train more than 10,500 new HIT professionals annually in the roles of clinician/practitioner consultant, implementation manager, implementation support specialist, practice workflow and information management redesign specialist, technical/software support staff, and trainer. As a means of certifying individuals in each of these roles, six competency exams, one for each role, were developed by the Competency Exam Program. These exams are referred to en masse as the HIT Pro exams.

The Computing Technology Industry Association (CompTIA), a leading provider of technology-neutral and vendor-neutral IT certifications, has also undertaken the task of certifying HIT professionals with the CompTIA Healthcare IT Technician certification. Per CompTIA, "The CompTIA Healthcare IT Technician certification covers the knowledge and skills required to implement, deploy, and support healthcare IT systems in various clinical settings." The CompTIA exam is targeted at IT professionals because the certification is designed to ensure IT professionals have the "operational, regulatory, and security knowledge necessary to provide hardware and software support in medical environments where EHR systems are being deployed or maintained."[7]

Exam Guide and Reference Work

As is evident by the title, this book is designed to prepare you for the seven exams just mentioned: the CompTIA Healthcare IT Technical exam and the six HIT Pro exams. The scope of this book was defined by the objectives for these exams, and every objective from each exam is covered. Yet, rather than divide the book by exam, the objectives were organized into five categories: Healthcare Organizational Behavior; Healthcare Regulatory Requirements; Healthcare Business Operations; Healthcare IT Security, Privacy, and Confidentiality; and Healthcare IT Operations; with the result being an exam guide that doubles as a comprehensive introductory guide to HIT. Choosing to cover seven exams as opposed to one or two, we created an HIT reference work that will prepare you, the reader, for not only your certification exam but also a career in the burgeoning field of HIT.

Taken as a whole, this book serves as a reference work, but it is also an exam guide. For those who want to focus their studies on the objectives pertaining to a specific exam, two objective maps have been included as Appendixes A and B. Appendix A maps the coverage of each CompTIA exam domain to the chapters in which the domains are covered, and Appendix B does the same for each of the six HIT Pro exams.

The HIT Pro Exams

For those interested in taking a HIT Pro exam, free exam vouchers are available for students trained through the Community College Consortia and for other individuals with relevant experience, training, or education in healthcare or IT. Vouchers may be ordered by members of the Community College Consortia, other accredited academic institutions, state and local employment agencies, and healthcare providers. Shortly vouchers will be available through Pearson Vue's Voucher Store, www.pearsonvue.com/vouchers/. For those without an affiliation with one of these organizations, the cost of the first exam is $299. The cost for individuals re-taking an exam or taking an additional exam for another role is $199. Examinees can register to take any of the HIT Pro exams at one of Pearson Vue's 230 nationwide test centers. To make a reservation to take the exam, please contact Pearson Vue by telephone, 888-944-8776, or via its website, www.pearsonvue.com/hitpro/.

Each HIT Pro exam is a three-hour exam consisting of 125 multiple-choice questions. To pass an exam, you must achieve a scaled score of 500 out of 600. For more information on the passing score, as well as general exam information, please visit www.hitproexams.org/the-hit-pro-exams/.

The CompTIA Healthcare IT Technician Exam

The CompTIA Healthcare IT Technician exam is comprised of 75 multiple-choice questions that candidates have 60 minutes to answer. To pass the exam, you must achieve a passing score of 650 on a scale of 100 to 900. Like the HIT Pro exams, the CompTIA Healthcare IT Technician exam is given at Pearson VUE test centers within the United States. The cost of the exam is $100, and you may purchase exam vouchers through the CompTIA Marketplace, www.comptiastore.com. To register for the exam, visit www.pearsonvue.com/comptia/ to find the testing center nearest to you. For more information on taking the exam, visit http://certification.comptia.org/Training/testingcenters.aspx.

The purpose of this book is to prepare you for your future in healthcare information technology, for your certification exams, and beyond. On behalf of my fellow lead author, Brian Gugerty, the part editors, and the contributors, we wish you the best of luck.

References

1. Fischetti, M. (2011). Graphic science: The links we love. *Scientific American, 305*, 110.

2. Network and computer system administrators job outlook. Accessed on May 22, 2012, from www.bls.gov/ooh/Computer-and-Information-Technology/Network-and-computer-systems-administrators.htm.

3. Computer and information systems managers job outlook. Accessed on May 22, 2012, from www.bls.gov/ooh/Management/Computer-and-information-systems-managers.htm.

4. Skills for the 21st century: Health information technology. Accessed on September 18, 2012, from www.iowaehealth.org/documents/resource/38.pdf.

5. 23rd annual 2011 HIMSS leadership survey. (2012). Accessed on April 13, 2012, from www.himss.org/2012 Survey/.

6. Health and human services health IT initiatives. (2010). Accessed on June 1, 2010, from http://healthit.hhs.gov/portal/server.pt?open=512&objID=1487&parentname=CommunityPage&parentid=2&mode=2&in_hi_userid=10741&cached=true.

7. CompTIA healthcare IT technician certification information. Accessed on November 5, 2012, from http://certification.comptia.org/getCertified/certifications/hittech.aspx.

INSTRUCTOR AND STUDENT WEB SITE

Whether used as a self-study guide or a classroom text, this book is designed to prepare readers for the CompTIA Healthcare IT Technician and HIT Pro exams, as well as the field of healthcare information technology.

For those using this book in a classroom, please visit this book's Online Learning Center: http://mhprofessional.com/McCormickHITOLC.

McGraw-Hill's Online Learning Center is a web-based learning platform that connects instructors with support materials and students with assessments. On the student page, students will find quizzes for every chapter comprised of the end-of-chapter questions. The instructor-only page hosts a variety of resources available to instructors for download.

Additional Resources for Instructors

The Online Learning Center provides instructor support materials in a format that follows the organization of this book. On this site you will find the following:

- An instructors' manual that contains learning objectives, classroom preparation notes, instructor tips, and a lecture outline for each chapter
- Engaging PowerPoint slides on the lecture topics that include full-color artwork from this book
- Access to test bank files and software that allows you to generate a wide array of paper- or network-based tests and that feature automatic grading. The test bank includes the following:
  - Hundreds of review questions enabling you to customize tests to maximize student progress
  - Blackboard cartridges (other formats may also be available on request)

Please contact your McGraw-Hill sales representative for more information.

PART I

Healthcare Organizational Behavior

Janet Marchibroda, Editor

An Overview of Healthcare in the United States

Julia Adler-Milstein, David Blumenthal

Each of us comes into contact with the healthcare system at some point in life. Often it is for an emotionally charged event: a visit to the emergency room, the birth of a baby, a terminal illness diagnosis. These highly personal experiences powerfully shape our perceptions of where the healthcare system is functioning well and where it is broken. In this chapter, we offer a broader perspective on the healthcare system in order to go beyond personal experience and understand how the system is structured and how it is performing. At the outset, the system can seem daunting, and indeed it is highly complex. However, with a basic introduction to key concepts and frameworks, you will gain an understanding of the size, scope, organization, and performance of the healthcare system.

Macro View: What We Spend and What We Get

The performance of our healthcare system can be characterized along three dimensions: cost, quality, and access. In this section, we review each dimension and offer evidence on how the system is performing.

Cost

Compared to other sectors of the U.S. economy, health is distinguished by its rapid rate of growth in spending. Health spending is rising faster than income, which raises questions about how we will pay for future healthcare needs. The issue is particularly acute in the United States compared to other countries because we currently spend much more per capita *and* have one of the highest spending growth rates. In 2011, national health spending is estimated to have grown 3.9 percent and to have reached $2.7 trillion dollars, which comprises 17.9 percent of the gross domestic product (GDP). In the next decade, national health spending is projected to grow at an average annual rate of

5.7 percent, faster than the expected annual increase in the GDP. As a result, the health share of the GDP is projected to rise to 19.6 percent by 2021.[1]

Spending a lot on healthcare is not inherently problematic. We choose to spend money on the things we value, and our health is undoubtedly one of things we value most. However, as health spending grows faster than the GDP, consuming a greater relative proportion of it, the question we must ask is whether we value health *more* than other things, such as education, a strong military, and so on. This question has no right answer; it depends on the values of our society. To date we have allowed healthcare to grow at the expense of greater investment in other sectors, and it is not clear whether we will allow this to continue.

Quality

The issue of rising health spending is intertwined with a second and more clearly problematic issue: despite our higher spending, we as a country do not achieve better results than other nations on many important health measures; that is, we do not appear to be realizing great value for the money we spend on healthcare.

Evidence for this comes from a number of sources. For example, our country performs worse than many other developed countries on common measures of health status, such as life expectancy and infant mortality. However, many factors beyond the healthcare system itself contribute to these particular measures. Therefore, a better set of measures of healthcare system performance is one that assesses "the degree to which health services for individuals and populations increase the likelihood of desired health outcomes and are consistent with current professional knowledge." This definition of healthcare quality, from the Institute of Medicine (IOM), can be broken down into six characteristics of healthcare (Table 1-1) that better lend themselves to direct measurement.[2]

Quality Domain	Definition
Safe	Avoiding injuries to patients from the care that is intended to help them
Effective	Providing services based on scientific knowledge to all who could benefit; refraining from providing services to those not likely to benefit
Patient-centered	Providing care that is respectful of and responsive to individual patient preferences, needs, and values; ensuring that patient values guide all clinical decisions
Timely	Reducing waits and sometimes harmful delays for both those who receive and those who give care
Efficient	Avoiding waste, including waste of equipment, supplies, ideas, and energy
Equitable	Providing care that does not vary in quality because of personal characteristics such as gender, ethnicity, geographic location, and socioeconomic status

Table 1-1   Six Characteristics of Healthcare per the IOM[2]

Numerous studies have been done in each of these domains to assess how well the healthcare system is performing. For example, a landmark study assessing effective care examined the proportion of time that patients received recommended care (that is, for a given patient, care for which there is widespread agreement that it results in benefits for their specific condition). Overall, the study found that recommended care was delivered only 54.9 percent of the time. And this percent did not vary markedly by type of care (i.e., preventive, acute, chronic), function of care (i.e., screening, diagnosis, treatment, follow-up), or patient characteristics (e.g., education, income). The study therefore concluded that we are consistently failing to provide effective care to patients.

Across the six domains, we arguably have the most evidence on healthcare system performance in the safety domain. A series of groundbreaking studies over the past two decades documented the rate of adverse events—injuries or potential injuries due to medical care—and assessed how many were within the control of the healthcare system and therefore could have been avoided ("preventable"). For example, if a patient suffers from a reaction to a prescribed medication because of an *unknown* allergy (an unavoidable injury), this is different from the patient receiving the medication with a *known* allergy (an injury that could be avoided if the prescriber had checked the patient's record for allergies). In the hospital setting, a study in New York state estimated that adverse events occurred in 3.7 percent of hospitalizations, and 58 percent of the adverse events were preventable.[3] A second study found that after discharge from the hospital, 19 percent of patients suffered an adverse event,[4] and a third study found that 25 percent of physician visits led to an adverse event involving medications.[5] These studies also suggested that the healthcare system could avoid many of these adverse events and resulting injuries, leading to safer care.

While these studies suggest real problems with the quality of care in our country, the picture is not all bleak. First, these numbers are averages, and they therefore mask differences across organizations. Our country has some of the leading healthcare-delivery organizations in the world, and these organizations have learned how to consistently deliver high-quality care. The challenge is to help improve the many other organizations that are not performing at the same level as these leaders. Second, the evidence on quality of care that we presented is an assessment at a single point in time; that is, these studies ask, given what comprises high-quality care today, how are we performing? As a result, they do not capture substantial gains in quality of care over time. For example, because of better knowledge about and treatment of cardiovascular disease over the past 50 years (e.g., antihypertensive medications, coronary artery bypass grafts), today the average 45-year-old lives an additional 4.5 years.[6]

Access

While there are many opportunities to improve the quality of our healthcare system, these gains would be realized only by those able to access the system and receive care. The United States, unlike many other developed countries, does not guarantee access to healthcare for the entire population. Access can be thought of along two dimensions: access to health insurance and access to healthcare. These dimensions are clearly related; without health insurance, it is more difficult to afford healthcare, which limits access to care. There is an array of channels through which people obtain health insurance. Many people are covered by one of several government programs; the Medicare program covers the elderly, the Medicaid program covers poor and disabled populations, and the Children's Health Insurance Program (CHIP) focuses on poor children. Those who do not qualify for these programs may have insurance through their employers or choose to purchase coverage as an individual. This patchwork approach to insurance left nearly 50 million people without coverage in 2010. Lack of access to affordable insurance served as the primary motivation for the Patient Protection and Affordable Care Act of 2010, which aims to reduce the number of citizens without insurance to near zero.

Even if we are able to solve the issue of the uninsured by expanding access to insurance, there is a second dimension of access: access to care. Having health insurance does not guarantee that you will be able to see the doctor you want when you want. Studies suggest that access to care is influenced by factors such as where you live and the type of insurance you have. For example, in rural areas there are often shortages of both primary-care and specialist physicians, which can lead to delays in receiving needed care.[7, 8] People covered under the Medicaid program often report difficulty finding a doctor willing to see them.[9] This is because doctors are not required to accept Medicaid patients and because Medicaid often reimburses doctors at much lower rates than other payers. Even people covered by health insurance with more generous payments to doctors report problems accessing care. In 2010, 8 percent of Medicare beneficiaries reported access problems (unmet need or delay getting care), and 17 percent of those aged 55 to 64 with insurance reported access problems. The two types of access issues converge for the uninsured, of whom 41 percent report access problems.[10]

The Institutions and Individuals That Comprise Our Healthcare System

In the prior section, we discussed how our healthcare system is performing along three core dimensions: cost, quality, and access. In this section, we explore the types of organizations and professionals comprising the healthcare system. We begin by discussing the institutions that make up the infrastructure of our healthcare system. We then discuss the types of healthcare professionals working within and outside these institutions. We return later in the chapter to a discussion of the primary regulator of healthcare: the government (Figure 1-1).

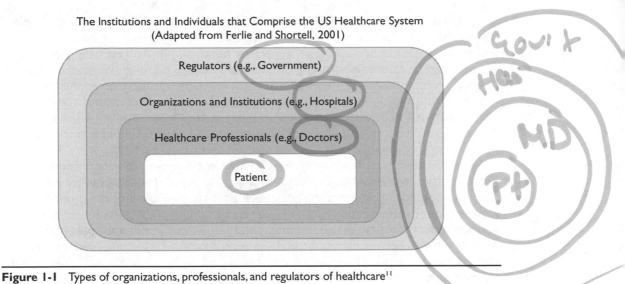

The Institutions and Individuals that Comprise the US Healthcare System
(Adapted from Ferlie and Shortell, 2001)

Regulators (e.g., Government)

Organizations and Institutions (e.g., Hospitals)

Healthcare Professionals (e.g., Doctors)

Patient

Figure 1-1 Types of organizations, professionals, and regulators of healthcare[11]

Organizations and Institutions

A comprehensive list of organizations and institutions that make up the healthcare system is long and diverse, ranging from large hospitals to your local pharmacy. We focus on those at the core of the system that directly provide care to patients: hospitals and physician practices. A critical distinction within the healthcare infrastructure is whether the setting is inpatient or outpatient (Table 1-2). Inpatient settings are those in which care is delivered in a clinical facility while the patient is residing there (i.e., admitted) as compared to outpatient (or ambulatory) settings in which care is delivered when the patient is not residing in the providing facility. Outpatient care may take place in a healthcare facility (e.g., a clinic or doctor's office) or the patient's home.

Setting	Definition
Inpatient	Inpatient care is care given to a patient admitted to a hospital, extended-care facility, nursing home, rehabilitation facility, or other facility. Long-term care is the range of services typically provided at skilled nursing, intermediate-care, personal-care, or eldercare facilities.
Outpatient	Outpatient care is any healthcare service provided to a patient who is not admitted to a facility. Outpatient care may be provided in a doctor's office, clinic, the patient's home, or hospital outpatient department.

Table 1-2 Definitions of Inpatient and Outpatient Settings

Hospitals are the emblematic type of inpatient setting, and numerous hospital types exist. General hospitals are set up to treat patients with many kinds of diseases and injuries. This is in contrast to a specialty hospital that delivers only certain types of care (e.g., a cardiac hospital) or treats only certain populations (e.g., a pediatric hospital). Hospitals also differ based on their ownership; there are public hospitals (government-owned) and private hospitals, which can be either nonprofit or for-profit. A third dimension of hospitals is whether they are a teaching hospital, which combines delivering care with teaching to medical students and nurses. These hospitals are often linked to professional schools, such as medical and nursing schools.

Similarly, there are different types of outpatient settings. The most common, the doctor's office, may be a single doctor or a large group of doctors practicing together. They may be generalists, treating patients for an array of conditions; specialists who focus on a particular clinical area (e.g., dermatology); or a combination of generalists and specialists. In some places, inpatient and outpatient settings are part of the same organization. When organizations that combine diverse types of care (such as inpatient and outpatient services) are well coordinated and reach a certain size, they may be referred to as an *integrated delivery system*.

Why do we have this range of settings? Inpatient hospitalization makes sense for major diagnostic, surgical, or therapeutic services, where the patient's condition or treatment requires complex care and close monitoring. Outpatient treatment is typically delivered in a doctor's office or multiphysician practice. This setting is the norm for most routine care. Home healthcare services are rendered to individuals who do not need institutional care but who need ongoing nursing services or therapy, medical supplies, and special outpatient services. They are typically delivered to patients who are confined to the home. Over time, advances in treatments and technology have enabled many tests and surgical procedures formerly conducted in the hospital to be done in an office setting. Since inpatient care, because of its intensity, is the most expensive care setting, one strategy for tackling rising healthcare costs is to reduce hospitalizations by identifying opportunities to manage more health problems in the outpatient setting or at home.

Healthcare Professionals[12]

Within the institutions that comprise our healthcare system, there is an array of professionals who deliver care. They are distinguished by their education, training, certification, and licensure, which shape the type of care they are qualified to provide. Doctors and nurses are the two most familiar categories, and within each of these there are many subtypes. For example, while there are only two degrees that a doctor may have—a medical doctor (MD) and a doctor of osteopathic medicine (DO)—doctors are distinguished by the clinical area in which they trained. They may be a more general, primary-care doctor or a more focused specialist. The term "generalist" often refers to doctors who train in internal medicine, family practice, or pediatrics. OB/GYNs are often included in this group, even though they specialize in obstetrics and gynecology, because many women use an OB/GYN as their primary-care provider. When a doctor chooses to become a specialist, which requires additional training, there are many areas in which they can specialize. Some examples include

- **Anesthesiology** The process of putting a patient into a painless sleep and keeping the patient's body working so surgeries or special tests can be performed
- **Cardiology** Heart disorders
- **Critical care** Intensive-care unit care
- **Dermatology** Skin disorders
- **Endocrinology** Hormonal and metabolic disorders, including diabetes
- **Gastroenterology** Digestive system disorders
- **General surgery** Common surgeries involving any part of the body
- **Hematology** Blood disorders
- **Immunology** Disorders of the immune system
- **Infectious disease** Infections affecting the tissues of any part of the body
- **Nephrology** Kidney disorders
- **Neurology** Nervous system disorders
- **Obstetrics/gynecology** Pregnancy and women's reproductive disorders
- **Oncology** Cancer treatment
- **Ophthalmology** Eye disorders and surgery
- **Orthopedics** Bone and connective tissue disorders
- **Otorhinolaryngology** Ear, nose, and throat (ENT) disorders
- **Physical therapy and rehabilitative medicine** For disorders such as lower-back injury, spinal cord injuries, and stroke
- **Psychiatry** Emotional or mental disorders
- **Pulmonary** Respiratory tract disorders
- **Radiology** X-rays and related procedures (such as ultrasound, CT, and MRI)
- **Rheumatology** Pain and other symptoms related to joints and other parts of the musculoskeletal system
- **Urology** Disorders of the male reproductive and urinary tracts and the female urinary tract

The field of nursing, like the field of medicine, encompasses many different types of specialties. However, unlike medicine, it includes many different types of degrees and licenses as well. Registered nurses (RNs) have graduated from a nursing program, have passed a state board examination, and are licensed by the state. Licensed practical nurses (LPNs) are state-licensed caregivers who have been trained to care for the sick but have a more limited scope of practice than RNs. Advanced-practice nurses have education and experience beyond the basic training and licensing required of all RNs. This includes nurse practitioners (NPs) who can serve as a primary-care provider in family medicine (FNP), pediatrics (PNP), adult care (ANP), or geriatrics (GNP). In some states, NPs can prescribe medications. Advanced-practice nurses also include the following:

- Clinical nurse specialists (CNSs) have training in a field such as cardiac, psychiatric, or community health.

- Certified nurse midwives (CNMs) have training in women's healthcare needs, including prenatal care, labor and delivery, and care of a woman who has given birth.

- Certified registered nurse anesthetists (CRNAs) have training in the field of anesthesia.

Beyond doctors and nurses, there are additional types of healthcare professionals found in care-delivery settings. A physician assistant (PA) can provide a wide range of services in collaboration with a doctor. Physician assistant education is based on the medical model, although unlike medical school, which lasts four years plus a specialty-specific residency, PA training is usually two to three years. And unlike physicians, who must complete a minimum of three years of residency after completing medical school, PAs are not required to complete such residencies. PAs may practice in any setting in which a physician provides care, and they are allowed to prescribe medications. Physician assistants are regulated at two different levels. They are licensed at the state level according to specific state laws. Certification is established through a national organi-zation.

Licensed pharmacists have graduate training from a college of pharmacy. They must graduate with a doctor of pharmacy (PharmD) degree from an accredited college of pharmacy, serve an internship under a licensed pharmacist, and pass a national exam. Pharmacists prepare and process drug prescriptions that were written by an authorized prescriber. They provide information to patients about medications, while also consulting with healthcare providers about dosages, interactions, and side effects of medicines. Pharmacists may also follow progress to check that patients are using their medications safely and effectively. There are other types of certified and licensed healthcare professionals who, like pharmacists, are specialized. Examples include clinical social workers, respiratory therapists, and occupational therapists.

Distinct from the types of professionals we just described, who have specific licensure and certification requirements, many types of healthcare workers do not hold a license or meet mandatory professional requirements but are trained to provide healthcare services. In some cases, they can choose to be certified, as is the case for medical assistants. In addition to medical assistants, *nursing assistant, nursing auxiliary, auxiliary nurse, patient-care assistant, patient-care technician, home health aide/assistant, geriatric aide/ assistant, psychiatric aide, nurse aide,* and *nurse tech* are all common titles of unlicensed assistive personnel, and they are collectively categorized as "personal care workers in health services." They typically work under the supervision of a licensed clinical professional, and their duties may include more clinically oriented tasks (e.g., assisting with motion exercises or collecting specimens for required medical tests) as well as more administratively oriented tasks (e.g., documenting clinical and treatment information).

There are also many nonclinical professionals who work in healthcare-delivery settings. Many of the leaders of healthcare organizations are laypeople who may or may not have advanced degrees in areas such as hospital administration, public health, or business. Both inpatient and outpatient settings have administrators who perform back-office work such as billing, facilities management, and procurement.

The scope of practice regulations governs what type of health professional can perform specific clinical tasks. However, there are no requirements about what types of professionals must be found in any given care setting or how different types of professionals work together. There are some norms, though; for example, a typical doctor's office will employ one or more nurses or medical assistants who will collect basic information and vital signs from the patient before the doctor sees them. Hospitals typically employ a wider range of professionals. Increasingly, there are doctors who treat only hospitalized patients (known as *hospitalists*), and they work alongside surgeons and other inpatient specialists. Similarly, there are many types of nurses in the hospital setting, ranging from highly specialized ICU nurses to RNs. Because of the complex nature of hospital care, coordination between the many types of professionals treating a given patient is critical. Often, this is accomplished through daily "rounds" in which the doctors and nurses (and in some cases others, such as pharmacists, therapists, and social workers) discuss each patient's care.

Types and Organization of Care

The prior sections discussed the varied settings and professionals who deliver healthcare. In this section, we discuss types of care as well as how care is organized. Perhaps the most important distinction is between chronic care and acute care. *Chronic care* addresses preexisting or long-term illness, and *acute care* is concerned with short-term or severe illness of brief duration. Examples of chronic medical conditions include asthma, coronary artery disease, congestive heart failure, chronic obstructive pulmonary disease, arthritis, hypertension, and diabetes. The prevalence of chronic illness has increased over time. It is estimated that almost half of all Americans are chronically ill,[13] and half of the chronically ill have more than one condition. As a result, chronic care currently accounts for the majority of healthcare spending. Examples of acute illness include appendicitis, pneumonia, an injury resulting from an accident, and stroke. Of course, acute illnesses can occur in combination with chronic conditions or can represent exacerbations of chronic conditions, so the distinction is not always clear.

Nonetheless, the conceptual distinction between chronic and acute care is important because people with acute conditions require different types of care than those suffering from chronic illnesses. Acute-care models are largely reactive—responding mainly when a person is sick—compared to chronic-care models that should be proactive and focused on keeping a person as healthy as possible. Acute-care models have not in the past been designed to give practitioners sufficient time to coordinate care across the multiple settings in which chronically ill patients receive care, follow up with patients to track the status of their condition over time, and train patients to manage their illness.

We have not adapted our healthcare system from a predominantly acute-care model to one that better serves the growing chronically ill population. How might we do this? One of the most widely cited models, known as the Chronic Care Model, is shown in Figure 1-2.[14] Table 1-3 defines the components of the model. The Chronic Care Model reflects the elements required in a system that better serves the needs of the chronically ill population: the community, health system, self-management support, delivery system design, decision support, and clinical information systems.

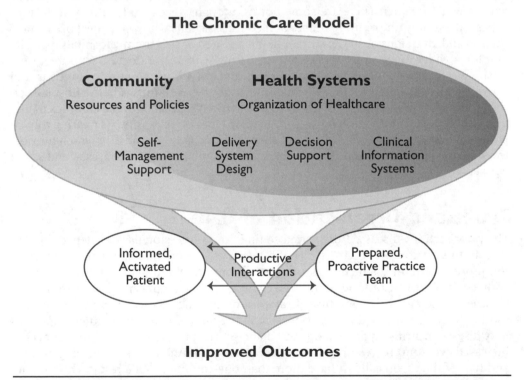

The Chronic Care Model

Figure 1-2 The Chronic Care Model. Reprinted with permission from Effective Clinical Practice, Chronic Disease Management: What Will It Take To Improve Care for Chronic Illness? Aug/Sept 1998, Vol 1, Figure 1.

Component	Definition
Health system	**Create a culture, organization, and mechanisms that promote safe, high-quality care** • Visibly support improvement at all levels of the organization, beginning with the senior leader • Promote effective improvement strategies aimed at comprehensive system change • Encourage open and systematic handling of errors and quality problems to improve care • Provide incentives based on quality of care • Develop agreements that facilitate care coordination within and across organizations
Delivery system design	**Assure the delivery of effective, efficient clinical care and self-management support** • Define roles and distribute tasks among team members • Use planned interactions to support evidence-based care • Provide clinical case management services for complex patients • Ensure regular follow-up by the care team • Give care that patients understand and that fits with their cultural background
Decision support	**Promote clinical care that is consistent with scientific evidence and patient preferences** • Embed evidence-based guidelines into daily clinical practice • Share evidence-based guidelines and information with patients to encourage their participation • Use proven provider education methods • Integrate specialist expertise and primary care
Clinical information systems	**Organize patient and population data to facilitate efficient and effective care** • Provide timely reminders for providers and patients • Identify relevant subpopulations for proactive care • Facilitate individual patient care planning • Share information with patients and providers to coordinate care • Monitor performance of practice team and care system
Self-management support	**Empower and prepare patients to manage their health and healthcare** • Emphasize the patient's central role in managing their health • Use effective self-management support strategies that include assessment, goal setting, action planning, problem solving, and follow-up • Organize internal and community resources to provide ongoing self-management support to patients
The community	**Mobilize community resources to meet needs of patients** • Encourage patients to participate in effective community programs • Form partnerships with community organizations to support and develop interventions that fill gaps in needed services • Advocate for policies to improve patient care

Table 1-3 The Definitions of Components in the Chronic Care Model

While the Chronic Care Model presents an integrated framework for delivering chronic care, it is virtually impossible to transform our healthcare system overnight from predominantly serving acute-care needs to predominantly treating those with chronic illnesses. The system is simply too large and complex. Therefore, in practice, we are moving toward a system better designed for chronic care in a slow, incremental way. For example, we are increasingly relying on a multidisciplinary approach to care in which a team of providers is responsible for patient care. Underlying this approach is the belief that no single healthcare professional can provide comprehensive care because each discipline brings unique knowledge bases and skill sets that together comprise optimal care. Under a multidisciplinary-care team approach, a physician-dominated model becomes a physician-directed model in which different members of the team are responsible for managing different aspects of the patient's care. For example, a registered dietician might work with a diabetic patient to modify their diet, and a pharmacist would monitor and suggest adjustments to the medication regimen. The team then works together to make care decisions under the guidance of the physician. This approach addresses many of the failures of the acute-care model to serve the needs of the chronically ill.

As our healthcare system evolves toward more multidisciplinary care, we are also seeing primary care evolve to play a more central role in coordinating patient care. This was in response to increasing specialization of care, which led to care that was fragmented. Patients often received conflicting recommendations and treatments from different specialists, which led to adverse events as well as waste and inefficiency. Those with chronic illnesses disproportionately suffer from fragmented care because many have more than one chronic illness and therefore see more than one specialist. The idea of primary-care-based care coordination has received significant attention in the past few years and has coalesced under the term "patient-centered medical home" (PCMH). The PCMH model is based on the following principles:[15]

- **Personal physician** Each patient has an ongoing relationship with a personal physician trained to provide first-contact, continuous, and comprehensive care.

- **Physician-directed medical practice** The personal physician leads a team of individuals at the practice level who collectively take responsibility for the ongoing care of patients.

- **Whole-person orientation** The personal physician is responsible for providing all the patient's healthcare needs or taking responsibility for appropriately arranging care with other qualified professionals. This includes care for all stages of life: acute care, chronic care, preventive services, and end-of-life care.

- **Care is coordinated and/or integrated** Across all elements of the complex healthcare system (e.g., subspecialty care, hospitals, home health agencies, nursing homes) and the patient's community (e.g., family, public, and private community-based services), care is facilitated by registries, information technology, health information exchange, and other means to assure that patients get the indicated care when and where they need and want it in a culturally and linguistically appropriate manner.

The patient-centered medical home model includes a multidisciplinary-care team (principle 2) and extends beyond it to focus on providing individualized, comprehensive, and coordinated care. The model does not, however, encompass all the elements of the Chronic Care Model. This reflects that we are still in an early phase of evolving our healthcare delivery system to meet the changing needs of the population, and we do not yet know the extent to which pieces of the model, such as the patient-centered medical home, will improve care.

While the predominant changes in our approach to healthcare delivery focus on better serving the needs of the chronically ill by shifting from acute to chronic care, there are also efforts to improve the delivery of two other types of care: preventive care and end-of-life care. *Preventive care* consists of measures taken to prevent diseases rather than curing or treating them. This contrasts with both acute and chronic care, which take place after someone is sick or hurt. Immunizations are a classic example of preventive care. Preventive care may also include examinations and screening tests tailored to an individual's age, health, and family history. Preventive care is typically delivered in primary-care settings. Despite the benefits of preventive care (avoiding or delaying illness), compliance with preventive care is inconsistent. There are efforts on both the provider side and the patient side to address this. For example, computerized reminders can alert the provider of recommended preventive care during the patient visit.

End-of-life care is distinguished from preventive care in that there is no longer the opportunity to prevent the clinical problem. It is distinguished from acute and chronic care in that the goal is not curative. Instead, end-of-life care seeks to relieve symptoms and suffering, making the patient as comfortable as possible (a feature of end-of-life care known as *palliative care*). End-of-life care is receiving attention because of the high costs incurred at the end of life that could potentially be avoided if palliative care was emphasized more and curative care less at this point in a patient's life. However, there are several challenges. Healthcare professionals are trained to provide curative care, and it is therefore hard to take actions that can be perceived as "giving up" on the patient getting better. In addition, it is difficult to accurately predict survival for a specific patient, and as a result, it can be difficult to judge when a patient has entered the end-of-life period. While there are few easy solutions, several efforts are underway to improve provider-family communication concerning end-of-life care, which can facilitate better decisions and higher-quality care.[16,17]

In this section, we discussed four types of care: acute, chronic, preventive, and end of life. While they are conceptually distinct, in practice they are often delivered by the same professionals and in the same delivery settings, and several types of care can be delivered at once. For example, a patient with emphysema (a form of chronic obstructive pulmonary disease) may receive chronic care in the form of regular medications, acute treatment with antibiotics for a pneumonia exacerbating his emphysema, preventive care in the form of influenza immunization to prevent acute episodes of influenza, and palliative care to manage chronic symptoms of breathlessness. Given the important differences and overlaps between these several types of care, an ongoing challenge is how to structure our delivery system in a way that performs each well.

The Role of Government

The governments at the national, state, and local levels play a substantial role in almost every dimension of our healthcare system. Together, they are the largest insurer in the country. They run public hospitals and clinics as well as entire delivery systems like the Veteran's Administration. They sponsor research that enables us to better understand diseases and treatments. In this section, we focus on one particular role of government: public health. Other important government roles will be discussed in more detail in later chapters.

Public Health

For the most part, our healthcare system focuses on treating individual patients. Government complements this by investing in public health in order to protect and improve the health of populations. This is done through a variety of activities, such as education, promotion of healthy lifestyles, research for disease and injury prevention, and disease tracking and surveillance. The public health system is built on the following components:[18]

- **Mission**   To ensure conditions in which people can be healthy.

- **Process**   The practice of public health can be thought of in terms of the key processes through which practitioners seek to identify, address, and prioritize community or population-wide health problems and resources and the outputs of these more fundamental processes, public health's interventions, policies, regulations, programs, and services. The processes of public health are those that identify and address health problems as well as the programs and services consistent with mandates and community priorities.

- **Outcome**   The immediate and long-term changes experienced by individuals, families, communities, providers, and populations are the system's outcomes, the cumulative result of the interaction of the public health system's structural capacity and processes. Outcomes can be used to provide information about the system's overall performance, including its efficiency, effectiveness, and ability to achieve equity between populations.

The public health system is comprised of agencies at the federal, state, and local levels that focus exclusively on public health. At the federal level, primary responsibility for public health lies with the United States Public Health Service in the Department of Health and Human Services (HHS), though other units also play important roles in public health. The Public Health Service consists of a subset of the entities that fall under the HHS. Examples include the Centers for Disease Control and Prevention (CDC), the National Institutes of Health (NIH), the Food and Drug Administration (FDA), and the Health Resources and Services Administration (HRSA).[19] Each entity focuses on a particular dimension of public health; for example, the CDC is the main assessment and epidemiologic unit that monitors and investigates health problems such as epidemics and outbreaks (among other things). Overall, federal activities can be characterized as either those that are conducted directly by the federal government (e.g., assessment, policymaking) or those that are contracted to state, community, and private organizations that are more focused on direct services.[20] Funding is authorized to each federal entity independently. The 2012 budget was $30.9 billion for the NIH, $8.4 billion for the HRSA, $6.9 billion for the CDC, and $2.5 billion for the FDA.[21]

States are the primary governmental entity responsible for protecting the public's health, and they therefore play an active role in the public health system. Each state has a health agency directed by a health commissioner or secretary of health. In some states, all public health activities are carried out by the state health agency, which operates any local health agencies within the state. In other states, local health agencies operate autonomously. The most common relationship between state and local health agencies is a hybrid model in which the state and the local agencies take on differing degrees of responsibility across an array of public health programs. Similar to the lack of uniform structure for public health within states, the range of issues that public health agencies target is varied. The most common areas for which state agencies report responsibility are bioterrorism, vaccines for children, injury control epidemiology, injury control and prevention, and breast and cervical cancer screening.[22] Public health agencies typically work closely with other public-sector agencies (such as schools, Medicaid, and environmental protection agencies) as well as private-sector organizations whose actions have significant consequences for the health of the public. Funding and other resources are determined by the state and vary with the size of the state and the scope of responsibilities carried out.

Local health departments directly deliver public health services to the population. While their scope of activities is dependent on the relationship with the state health agency, cities and towns may exercise powers autonomously as long as they do not conflict with the state. As a result, some locales may have a very active local health department, and others may be served only by the state health department. Common activities for local health departments include providing health education, offering screening and immunizations, and collecting health statistics.

Chapter Review

In this chapter, we covered key concepts about the structure and functioning of our healthcare system. We evaluated performance by examining three areas: cost, quality, and access. We then discussed the core types of institutions and healthcare professionals that are on the front lines of care delivery. We described four types of care (acute, chronic, preventive, and end of life) and the differences between them. We concluded with a discussion of the role of government, focusing on the multilevel effort to promote public health. Within each area we highlighted emerging trends. For example, we discussed the patient-centered medical home, a new approach to how care is organized and delivered. We touched on the recent Patient Protection and Affordable Care Act that seeks to improve access to care by expanding access to health insurance. There are, however, many other important emerging trends. Perhaps the most obvious is the rise in use of information technology to support care delivery, the topic that serves as the focus for the remainder of the book.

References

1. Keehan, S. P., Cuckler, G. A., Sisko, A. M., et al. (2012). National health expenditure projections: Modest annual growth until coverage expands and economic growth accelerates. *Health Affairs.*

2. Corrigan, J. M., Kohn, L. T., Donaldson, M. S., Maguire, S. K., and Pike, K. C. (2001). *Crossing the quality chasm: A new health system for the 21st century.* National Academy Press.

3. Brennan, T. A., Leape, L. L., Laird, N. M., et al. (1991). Incidence of adverse events and negligence in hospitalized patients. *New England Journal of Medicine, 324,* 370–376.

4. Forster, A. J., Murff, H. J., Peterson, J. F., Gandhi, T. K., and Bates, D. W. (2003). The incidence and severity of adverse events affecting patients after discharge from the hospital. *Annals of Internal Medicine, 138,* 161–167.

5. Gandhi, T. K., Weingart, S. N., Borus, J; et al. (2003). Adverse drug events in ambulatory care. *New England Journal of Medicine, 348,* 1556–1564.

6. Cutler, D. M. (2004). *Your money or your life: Strong medicine for America's health-care system.* Oxford University Press.

7. U.S. Department of Health and Human Services, Health Resources and Services Administration. Physician supply and demand: projections to 2020. Accessed September 5, 2012, from ftp://ftp.hrsa.gov/bhpr/workforce/ PhysicianForecastingPaperfinal.pdf.

8. U.S. Department of Health and Human Services, Health Resources and Services Administration. The physician workforce: Projections and research into current issues affecting supply and demand. Accessed September 5, 2012, from ftp://ftp .hrsa.gov/bhpr/workforce/physicianworkforce.pdf.

9. Berk, M. L., and Schur, C. L. (1998). Access to care: How much difference does Medicaid make? *Health Affairs, 17,* 169–180.

10. Cost and access challenges: A comparison of experienced between uninsured and privately insured adults aged 55–64 with seniors on Medicare. Issue Brief: Kaiser Family Foundation, Medicare Policy, 2010 Health Tracking Survey. Accessed on August 16, 2012, from www.kff.org/medicare/upload/8320.pdf.

11. Ferlie, E. B., and Shortell, S. M. (2001). Improving the quality of healthcare in the United Kingdom and the United States: A framework for change. *Milbank Quarterly, 79,* 281–315.

12. Types of healthcare providers. Accessed on August 16, 2012, from www.nlm.nih .gov/medlineplus/ency/article/001933.htm.

13. Anderson, G., Partnership for Solutions. (2004). *Chronic conditions: Making the case for ongoing care.* Johns Hopkins University.

14. Wagner, E. H. (1998). Adapted from Figure 1: Chronic disease management: What will it take to improve care for chronic illness? *Effective Clinical Practice, Aug/Sept 1998, Vol 1.* Accessed on August 16, 2012, from www.improvingchroniccare .org/index.php?p=The_Chronic_Care_Model&s=2.

15. Patient-Centered Primary Care Collaborative. Joint principles of the patient-centered medical home. Accessed on September 5, 2012, from www.pcpcc.net/node/14.

16. Curtis, J. R., Patrick, D. L., Shannon, S. E., Treece, P. D., Engelberg, R. A., and Rubenfeld, G. D. (2001). The family conference as a focus to improve communication about end-of-life care in the intensive care unit: Opportunities for improvement. *Critical Care Medicine, 29,* N26–N33.

17. Singer, P. A., Martin, D. K., and Kelner, M. (1999). Quality end-of-life care. *JAMA: The Journal of the American Medical Association, 281,* 163–168.

18. Public Health System concepts. Accessed on August 16, 2012, from www.hhs .gov/ash/initiatives/quality/system/index.html.

19. Organizational chart of HHS. Accessed on August 16, 2012, from http:/www .hhs.gov/about/orgchart/.

20. IOM. (1988). The future of public health. Accessed on August 16, 2012, from www.iom.edu/Reports/1988/The-Future-of-Public-Heath.aspx.

21. HHS budget. (2013). Accessed on September 5, 2012, from www.hhs.gov/budget/budget-brief=FY2013.pdf.

22. Beitsch, L. M., Brooks, R. G., Grigg, M., & Menachemi, N. (2006). Structure and functions of state public health agencies. *American Journal of Public Health, 96,* 167.

CHAPTER 2

An Overview of How Healthcare Is Paid for in the United States

Cary Sennett, Donald Nichols

In this chapter, you will learn how to

- Explain how Americans pay for the healthcare they receive
- Describe how health insurance plays a central role in healthcare payment
- Understand what Medicare, Medicaid, and commercial health insurance programs are and how they are similar and how they are distinct
- Describe the five major types of insurance products
- Explain how healthcare reform is likely to affect the organization of and payment for healthcare in the future

Healthcare is different from most other goods and services purchased in the United States in that the purchase of healthcare services involves, in almost all cases, the participation of a third party: the health insurance firm. While there are mechanisms to provide (and to pay for) care to those who lack health insurance—so-called funds for charity or uncompensated care—the care for the vast majority of Americans is paid for by the government (through the Medicare and Medicaid programs) or by private health insurance, which is almost always tied to employment. To understand how healthcare is paid for in the United States, it is necessary first to understand how insurance operates in the United States.

The Nature of Health Insurance

In theory, the objective of health insurance is to pool risk. Illness—particularly catastrophic illness that could bankrupt a family—is (fortunately) rare. Insurance is a vehicle that allows individuals to pay (for example, annually) a relatively small amount to an insurance pool, which covers the costs (of necessary services) for those individuals who are unfortunate enough to need care. It is important to note that insurance works only when there is broad participation and, in particular, only when individuals who are at low risk for illness participate (as well as those who are at high risk for illness). The cost of insurance—the insurance *premium*—is set based on predicted expenses (the so-called actuarially fair value, to which administrative costs are added) for all individuals in the covered population; if only high-risk/high-cost individuals participate in the insurance pool, the cost of insurance is likely to be perceived as prohibitive (and, in fact, the primary objective of insurance—to pool risk—is lost).

Initially, health insurance in the United States was designed to protect against potentially catastrophic expense, in particular, the cost of hospitalization or other care that was not routine. Over time, though, insurance has evolved from a risk-mitigation strategy to a prepayment strategy; that is, more and more, health insurance in the United States is designed to cover not only unexpected and potentially catastrophic healthcare needs but predictable healthcare needs (for example, preventive services).

For example, many economists—including us—argue that using insurance as a prepayment vehicle is not only inefficient (the economists' term) but wasteful. If an individual expects to have a service (for example, a woman expects to have a mammogram), bundling it into insurance means that the price of insurance rises by the expected cost of the mammogram *in addition to* the administrative fee that is loaded on by the insurance administrator. Using insurance to prepay for the mammogram simply adds that administrative cost. That said, the coverage by insurance of routine (preventive) services is now almost universal. Despite the theoretical argument that coverage for preventive care is not a goal of insurance, the marketplace appears to have spoken: the role of insurance has evolved from pure risk mitigation to include prepayment. The market for healthcare purchasing is complex; arguments about the proper role of insurance require consideration that is beyond the scope of this book.

The Structure of Health Insurance

Health insurance establishes rules for paying for healthcare, but at the end of the day, the dollars that are disbursed through health insurance systems come from other sources. It is important to take a brief look at who pays for what.

To begin with, Americans purchase (or, in some cases, receive as an entitlement) health insurance; when they do, they pay an annual premium, which typically depends on their family structure (whether they are purchasing insurance for themselves or for their family) and the nature of the insurance they are purchasing. When they use that insurance (to purchase or, more accurately, to obtain reimbursement for healthcare services that are covered by that insurance), they may also face costs (which depend on the nature of the insurance), in particular, a deductible and a copayment. The insurance *deductible* is a sum (that is tied to the structure of the insurance policy and hence to its price) that the insured must pay before insurance provides any coverage; in other words, it is a way of maintaining the original objective of insurance (to protect against very high costs). In addition to the deductible (which typically must be met on an annual basis so that insurance covers nothing until it is met, but once it is met, it need not be paid again in that year), there is typically a *copayment*: the consumer's share of the cost for every service that is reimbursable. Again, copayment levels vary across insurance contracts and clearly tie to price; the higher the copayment, the higher the consumer's share of the cost of the service and (importantly) the more likely it is that the consumer will forego a high-cost service (or substitute a lower-cost service for that high-cost one). So, the purpose of a copayment is less to transfer payment (cost) from the insurer to the insured than it is to increase the sensitivity of the insured to the cost of service and—through that—reduce demand for services (and especially reduce demand for high-cost services).

Insurance in the United States

With this brief overview of the nature and structure of insurance complete, we turn our attention to the insurance market in the United States.

There are three primary mechanisms through which Americans currently receive health insurance.

- **Commercial (private) health insurance**, which in the vast majority of cases is provided through an employer (employer-sponsored health insurance) but which can be purchased on an individual basis (typically at significantly higher cost). In 2010, the majority of Americans—approximately 196 million—were covered by private/commercial insurance programs,[1] with the vast majority of those (about 169 million, or 86 percent) through employer-sponsored health insurance.

- **The federally sponsored Medicare program**, which provides an insurance benefit to the elderly (Americans 65 and older), as well as to those who are disabled and those with end-stage renal disease (ESRD). In 2010, Medicare insured approximately 44.3 million Americans.

- **The Medicaid program**, which is administered by the states but funded by both the state and federal governments and which provides an insurance benefit to the economically disadvantaged as well as to certain categories of women (especially pregnant women) and children (through Medicaid or through a similar program called the State Children's Health Insurance Program [SCHIP], or now simply the Children's Health Insurance Program [CHIP]). In 2010, these programs insured approximately 48.6 million Americans.

In addition, nearly 13 million Americans receive health insurance/healthcare through the military healthcare system (including Tricare and programs offered by the U.S. Department of Veterans Affairs).

A significant number (approximately 50 million) Americans did not have health insurance in the most recent year for which data is available (2010). The Patient Protection and Affordable Care Act (PPACA or ACA)—President Obama's landmark health-reform legislation—is expected to reduce that, primarily through expansion of Medicaid but also through the application of an insurance "mandate" that will increase participation of low-risk individuals who currently opt out of the insurance market.

ACA includes a requirement that individuals who do not have health insurance provided through their employer or another source (e.g., Medicare or Medicaid) purchase health insurance (or pay a penalty that the Supreme Court of the United States has recently declared "a tax"): the so-called individual mandate. Subsidies are provided to those who are least able to afford that insurance. A policy goal of that "mandate" clearly is to reduce the number of individuals who are uninsured (and thereby to increase their access to care), but it is also to increase the size of the insurance risk pool (so that risk is spread across a larger group) and therefore to reduce the cost of insurance to the individual by bringing into the insurance pool low-risk individuals who historically have opted out of the insurance system. (By bringing that group in, average risk—and hence the actuarially fair value, or price—declines.)

Insurance Products

It is necessary, before going into more detail about how publicly and privately funded insurance programs pay for care, to point out that there are a range of insurance "products" that differ significantly in ways that affect payment. Although there is more variation (and arguably more innovation) across products in the commercial/private market, this product variation appears in both Medicare and Medicaid. To summarize, five major types of products are prevalent in the United States.

- **Traditional "open access"/fee-for-service (FFS) products**, which allow those individuals who are insured to obtain care anywhere they choose and reimburse providers on the basis of charges.

- **Preferred Provider Organizations (PPOs)/"tiered networks,"** which allow individuals to receive care from a network of "preferred providers"—typically hospitals and physicians with whom discounts have been negotiated. PPO agreements may (or may not) permit individuals to obtain care outside of the preferred provider network—at significantly higher cost to the individual seeking care (through a higher copayment).

- **Health Maintenance Organizations (HMOs)**, which significantly restrict access to care for insured individuals to a (typically relatively small) network of providers; which provide a range of value-added services including care-management services intended to improve quality and reduce cost by supporting patient self-management, preventive care, and coordinated care; and which often reimburse providers not on a fee-for-service basis but on a capitated (per-member per-month) basis to create incentives among providers for fiscally responsible care.

- **Point of Service (POS) plans**, which allow individuals to choose (at the point of service) whether to seek care under the PPO or under the HMO. POS plans typically offer more choice than HMOs but require that a patient have a primary-care physician (who serves as the "point of service contact"), so they typically offer less choice than a PPO.

- **Health Savings Accounts (HSAs)**, **High-Deductible Health Plans (HDHPs)**, **Consumer-Directed Health Plans (CDHPs)**, and other products that transfer much more of the financial risk to the consumer. This is a heterogeneous and rapidly evolving portfolio of offerings that currently constitutes a small share of the insurance market but that may become more important as insurers seek ways to make consumers more sensitive to the cost of the healthcare services they purchase.

Each of the main structures of insurance programs in the United States will be described in the following section.

Commercial (Private) Insurance in the United States

As noted, the majority of Americans receive health insurance through their (or a family member's) employer; health insurance as a benefit of employment has been the predominant form for several decades. Employer-sponsored health insurance has its roots in the wage and price controls that were in place during World War II and in favorable treatment under the tax code: employers offered richer health insurance benefits to attract and retain employees when wages were controlled and have added to the value of that benefit because the dollars that are set aside for health insurance benefits are effectively tax-free income to employees.

Employer-sponsored health insurance can follow either of two distinct (although, for employees and their families, often indistinguishable) paths: employers may purchase health insurance from an entity that pools risk and administers the health insurance program, or the employer may self-insure (that is, bear the risk itself) and hire (typically a health insurance firm to serve as) a third-party administrator (TPA) of its health insurance program. The TPA administers not only the basic mechanics of the insurance program (such as enrollment, payment of claims to providers, or reimbursement of payments made by consumers) but also a wide array of programs designed to improve health and/or manage cost (ranging from efforts to select and guide consumers to high-quality, cost-effective providers to programs intended to support consumer efforts to manage their own health and illness—so-called care, or disease, management programs). Many large firms elect to self-insure; smaller firms (which are not able to pool risk over a large population) will more often purchase insurance (although as the cost of healthcare and therefore the actuarially fair price of health insurance rises, many small firms are electing not to offer health insurance).

In either case, the health insurance benefit is typically structured as described earlier in the section "Insurance Products": employees have a choice as to whether to purchase insurance (which is heavily subsidized, as a benefit, by the employer, but the employee still pays, on average, between 15 percent and 25 percent of the premium), and employees often (but do not always) have a choice among insurance providers and/or insurance plans.

Commercial insurance plans/products will differ with respect to the extent to which they offer choice among providers, with respect to the nature and extent to which there are programs available to support employee or employer health-related goals, and (based on those) with respect to their premium, deductible, and copayment costs. Most employer-sponsored plans cover "major medical" (hospital and ambulatory service providers); coverage of prescription drugs is common but not universal.

Commercial products are as briefly described earlier in the section "Insurance Products." The majority (about 55 percent) of workers were, in 2011, enrolled in PPOs,[2]

17 percent were in HMOs, 10 percent were in POS plans, and 17 percent were in higher-risk plans (HSAs, HDHPs, CDHPs, and the like). Only about 1 percent of workers were enrolled in conventional open-access plans.

The distribution of workers across insurance products reflects what has been, over the past decade or more, a corporate priority of the first order: to control healthcare costs. That only 1 percent of workers purchase health insurance that provides open access undoubtedly reflects both employers' unwillingness to offer such open-access plans and the cost differentials that employees who choose them face. The preponderance of PPOs reflects the trade-off between choice and cost, which has been the conundrum; while PPOs offer significant choice among providers, there may be strong financial incentives to seek care in the PPO network so that choice is effectively constrained.

In the same way, the rapid growth of consumer-directed and high-deductible health plans—the penetration of which more than doubled between 2009 and 2011—reflects employers' interest in creating pressure for cost control, not by restricting access but by creating an incentive for employees and their families to purchase health services wisely. It seems very likely that this trend will continue—as will innovations in payment beyond discounted fee-for-service plans; current trends are discussed in the earlier section "Insurance Products."

Medicare

Medicare is the insurance program for Americans older than 64; it covers, as well, Americans who are disabled (receiving Social Security Disability Insurance for 24 months), including those disabled by Lou Gehrig's Disease and those with end-stage renal disease, which oftentimes requires dialysis.

Medicare pays for healthcare in two ways. The majority (about 75 percent) of beneficiaries choose to enroll in traditional Medicare, which reimburses for care on a fee-for-service basis. The remainder enroll in Medicare Advantage (managed healthcare; so-called Medicare Part C) plans, which collect premium from Medicare (on a risk-adjusted capitated basis; that is, they are paid a per-member per-month [PMPM] fee by Medicare and pay physicians, hospitals, and others providers on an FFS or PMPM basis for care of the beneficiaries that they manage with that premium).

Medicare FFS operates through three distinct benefit programs.

- **Medicare Part A**   Hospital insurance and covers inpatient and, in some cases, convalescent care in skilled nursing facilities. In the past, Medicare paid hospitals based on charges for every service provided. With rapid cost inflation, Medicare introduced a fixed-priced "episode-based" payment system using diagnosis-related groups (DRGs) in the 1980s. DRGs are severity and case-mix adjusted, and selected DRGs account for complications. DRG rates are updated regularly to assure that payment reflects changes in cost (as may, for example, follow the introduction of new technology related to the Health Information Technology for Economic and Clinical Health [HITECH] Act). DRGs are intended to capture the bundle of services typically provided to patients with specific conditions/receiving specific procedures/with specific predictable needs—for example, patients with pneumonia or who have a stroke or who have a joint replacement procedure. Paying the hospital a fixed fee for the bundle of services typically provided to such patients creates an incentive for hospitals to improve efficiency (and, in particular, to reduce the use of unnecessary, marginally valuable, or unnecessarily high-cost services). Because DRGs are set at the average cost for patients of a given type, hospitals will lose money on some patients (who have above-average service needs) but will make money on others (who have below-average service needs). For hospitals with reasonable volumes, the expectation is that (on average) DRG prices are fair.

- **Medicare Part B** Major medical; that is, it pays for covered services that are not under Part A (or medications, covered in the next bullet). In general, that includes ambulatory services (including physician services) and durable medical equipment (a major expense in the Medicare population).

  Medicare pays physicians and other qualified providers on an FFS basis, where fees are set (a Medicare fee schedule) based on a resource-based relative value scale (RBRVS). The RBRVS is an effort to estimate the resources required to deliver a given service (described by a code called a *current procedural terminology* [CPT] code; CPT codes in most cases define the billable service). These are defined in Chapter 12. Medicare's fee for a given service—the price it pays providers—is the product of the relative value units (RVUs) associated with that service (the CPT code for that service) and a "conversion factor", which effectively assigns a dollar value to an RVU. The RBRVS is updated annually by an RBRVS update committee (the RUC) that is comprised of 29 physicians— through a process that is often contentious because adjustments to the RBRVS are effectively a zero-sum game (an increase in the value of one service means that another service must be reduced in value).

- **Medicare Part D** Covers medications; it has since the Medicare Modernization Act of 2006. Medicare beneficiaries are eligible to obtain Part D benefits through stand-alone prescription drug plans (PDPs) or bundled with the Part C benefit (through a Medicare Advantage managed care plan). Unlike Part A and Part B (which provide standard benefits to all beneficiaries), PDPs (and MA PDPs) are able to offer a wide variety of pharmacy benefits—more or less inclusive, more or less generous, at different price points—to offer Medicare enrollees many options. Exceptions include medications administered in an ambulatory setting; for example, chemotherapy administered intravenously to a patient with cancer in a physician's office or day hospital is reimbursed under Part B, at 106 percent of the average sales price. In some cases, there has been concern that the number of options is overwhelming and that beneficiaries cannot understand what plan might be best suited for them.

Medicaid

Medicaid is a public insurance program available to low-income Americans including children, pregnant women, parents, seniors, and individuals with disabilities. It is jointly funded by federal and state governments but fully administered by states. The federal government provides a percentage (known as the federal medical assistance percentage [FMAP]) of the funding of each state's Medicaid budget. FMAPs vary across states and are determined by criteria such as a state's per-capita income. By law the minimum FMAP is 50 percent (a one-to-one match). In 2012, Mississippi has the highest FMAP at 74.18 percent. Thus, for every $1 contributed by Mississippi to Medicaid, the federal government contributes $2.87.[3]

As mentioned in the previous paragraph, Medicaid programs are administered by states. While there are minimum federal standards to which states must adhere in their eligibility rules and covered services, states have some liberty in the designs of their Medicaid programs through the use of waivers. Mandatory populations include children under age 6 below 133 percent of the federal poverty level (FPL), older children below 100 percent FPL, pregnant women below 133 percent FPL, and elderly and disabled Social Security Disability Insurance (SSDI) and the Supplemental Security Income (SSI) beneficiaries below 74 percent FPL. Mandatory benefits include inpatient and outpatient hospital services, physician services, nursing facility services, and home health services. Many states use waivers to expand their covered populations (e.g., have higher FPL thresholds) and covered services (e.g., prescription drugs, clinic services, and hospice services). In 2001, only about 40 percent of Medicaid expenditures were spent on mandatory services for mandatory populations.[4]

Like Medicare, Medicaid reimburses for care through two payment mechanisms: FFS and managed-care arrangements. Some states are also adopting integrated-care delivery models. Working within federal guidelines and approval, states design their reimbursement methodology. When determining their reimbursement rates for FFS, states may base them upon the costs of providing the services, the reimbursement rate of commercial payers in the private market, and/or a percentage of the reimbursement rate of Medicare. The reimbursement rate of Medicaid is typically significantly lower than that of commercial payers and Medicare.

States can make managed care enrollment voluntary or can seek a waiver from the Centers for Medicare and Medicaid Services (CMS) to require enrollment in a Managed Care Organization (MCO). Currently, most states have waivers to implement mandatory managed care in parts of their states or for certain categories of beneficiaries or to implement statewide mandatory managed-care enrollment as part of a demonstration.[5] Thus, the national Medicaid MCO enrollment rate is significantly higher (70 percent) than that of Medicare. Some states have managed-care enrollments rates that exceed 90 percent.

Medicaid's Role in Long-Term Care

Because of its inclusion of low-income elderly, its coverage of nursing home care and home healthcare, and the unpopularity of long-term care (LTC) insurance, Medicaid is a major player in the financing of long-term care. Forty-three percent of all long-term care is funded through Medicaid. Forty-eight percent of Medicaid expenditures purchase long-term care.[6] The quick growth in the percentage of Medicaid dollars spent on LTC has led to legislative attempts to contain the growth, such as the development of an LTC prospective payment system based on DRGs (vs. the previous fixed rates), certificate-of-need laws for the construction of nursing homes, and regulations on the "spending down" of wealth by the elderly to qualify for Medicaid.

Children's Health Insurance Program (CHIP)

Title XXI of the Balanced Budget Act of 1997 established the Children's Health Insurance Program (CHIP), formerly known as State Children's Health Insurance Program (SCHIP). This program is designed to provide health insurance for children from low-income households that earn too much to qualify for traditional Medicaid. Like Medicaid, CHIP is administered by states but funded jointly by federal and state governments. States receive an enhanced federal medical assistance percentage (eFMAP) to fund CHIP. The CHIP eFMAP is typically higher than the Medicaid FMAP (see Use Case 2-1). States that cover children with greater than 300 percent FPL receive their FMAP only for CHIP federal matching. However, unlike traditional Medicaid, federal dollars for CHIP are capped. Thus, each state is allocated part of this amount and must supply matching funds according to its FMAP.

Use Case 2-1: FMAP and eFMAP Rates

As mentioned in the text, Medicaid and CHIP are jointly funded by the federal and state governments. For both programs, the federal government provides a percentage of the funds. The percentages vary across states. FMAP is the federal government's contribution percentage toward a state's Medicaid program, and eFMAP is the contribution percentage toward a state's CHIP program. While the FMAP and eFMAP are not equal, there is a mathematical relationship between the two. A state's eFMAP is never less than its FMAP. The amount of additional percentage points of the eFMAP is equal to 30 percent of the difference between a state's FMAP and 100 percent. However, the maximum eFMAP is 85 percent. The following equation more clearly demonstrates the relationship between the two rates:

$$eFMAP = max[FMAP + 0.30 \times (100\% - FMAP), 85\%]$$

State's FMAP	FMAP + 0.30 × (100% − FMAP)	eFMAP
50%	50% + 0.30 × (100% − 50%) = 50% + 0.30 × 50% = 50% + 15% = 65%	65%
60%	60% + 0.30 × (100% − 60%) = 72%	72%
80%	80% + 0.30 × (100% − 80%) = 86%	85%*

*Recall that the maximum eFMAP is 85%.

The FMAP of a state is determined by a comparison between the state's per capita income and the nation's per capita income using the formula below. However, the FMAP must be at least 50%.

$$FMAP = 1 - 0.45 \times \frac{state\ per\ capita\ income^2}{national\ per\ capital\ income^2}$$

State Per Capita Income	$1 - 0.45 \times \dfrac{state\ per\ capita\ income^2}{national\ per\ capital\ income^2}$	FMAP
$38,263	$1 - 0.45 \times \dfrac{\$38,263^2}{\$40,584^2}$ $= 1 - 0.45 \times 0.8889$ $= 1 - 0.40$ $= 0.60$	60%
$27,056	$1 - 0.45 \times \dfrac{\$27,056^2}{\$40,584^2} = 0.80$	80%
$44,867	$1 - 0.45 \times \dfrac{\$44,867^2}{\$40,584^2} = 0.45$	50%

Uncompensated Care

Although healthcare providers are compensated for the majority of their services through commercial insurance, public insurance, or private payments, they do not receive payments for a significant portion of their services. This care is known as uncompensated care. In 2004, 2.7 percent of provided care was classified as uncompensated care. There are two sources of uncompensated care: charity care and bad debt. Charity care is care for which the provider never expected compensation because the patient is determined to be unable to pay. Bad debt is defined as services for which the provider expected reimbursement due to the insurance and/or financial status of the patient. Inability to collect the funds may result from an inability to collect co-payments and/or deductibles from insured patients, or to collect full payment from uninsured patients whose financial situation does not officially qualify them for charity care. Eligibility for charity care usually depends on factors such as individual and family income, assets, employment status, and the availability of alternative sources of funds.

Given the existence of the Emergency Medical Treatment and Labor Act, which mandates all emergency rooms to provide stabilizing care to patients with emergency conditions regardless of their ability to pay, and state laws such as New Jersey's N.J.S.A. 26:2H-18.64, which makes it illegal for any hospital to "deny any admission or appropriate service to a patient on the basis of that patient's ability to pay or source of payment," uncompensated care is an expected part of the healthcare system. Hadley and Holahan estimate that uncompensated care in the United States among the uninsured totaled $40.7 billion in 2004. Hospitals bear the bulk of these losses (60 percent), while physicians and clinics evenly split the remaining portion.[7] The AHA estimates that for the past 20 years, uncompensated care as a percentage of all hospital expenses has ranged between 5.1 and 6.2 percent.[8]

Hospitals typically do not write off the costs associated with uncompensated care. Rather, federal and state direct service programs reimburse hospitals via state and local tax appropriations, and/or cost-shifting to private payers. This means that uncompensated care is a problem that extends beyond providers and nonpaying patients.

One strategy that hospitals and physicians have tried to use to recover losses associated with uncompensated care (as well as to make up shortfalls when Medicaid payment rates fall below the providers' actual cost) is to raise prices to private payers. While providers do not have the ability to set prices unilaterally, they generally have more opportunity to negotiate with private payers than with Medicare and Medicaid. This "cost-shifting" raises insurance premiums, which ultimately is transmitted back to the employers who pay the largest portion of those premiums. This has an impact on their costs (therefore their profitability)—and is a force that can discourage employers from offering health insurance. It also drives them to shift costs directly to their employees— through higher premiums, higher deductibles, and higher co-payments. Cost-shifting is a serious concern, in a setting in which providers may be seeking to increase the revenue they derive from private payers, as public payers (Medicare and Medicaid) seek to reduce their costs. Shifting costs from Medicare to the private sector may preserve the Medicare Trust Fund—but it does not improve the efficiency of the healthcare system in the United States.

While cost-shifting is a significant concern, providers have other sources to cover the expenses related to the majority of their uncompensated care. In 2004, federal, state, and local governments did not fund 15 percent of the uncompensated care.[7] The largest sources of funding for uncompensated care are Disproportionate Share Hospital payments/adjustments through the Medicare and Medicaid programs. Hospitals that treat a large number of Medicaid, low-income, and uninsured individuals receive these payments, which help to preserve Medicare and Medicaid patients' access to care.

Trends in Payment/Payment Reform

Intense pressure on all payers—employers, the states, and the Medicare Trust Fund— has driven innovations in payment. These innovations have moved at a somewhat different pace across those three sectors. In general, the private sector has more aggressively sought change than have governments (both state and federal), but changes in the way the government pays for care (and, especially, changes in the way Medicare pays for care) have much more impact, given the scale of public programs.

While there have been a number of innovations in payment over the years, they can be grouped into three major categories.

- Pay-for-performance (P4P)/provider incentive programs
- Episode-based, or bundled, payment
- Payment reform coupled to delivery system innovation

Pay-for-Performance (P4P)/Provider Incentive Programs

Pay-for-performance programs are incremental innovations off of a fee-for-service payment platform. The idea of P4P is simple: the payer (private or public) offers providers additional payment for achieving performance targets, which are designed to improve quality but also achieve long-term reductions in cost. There are, for example, many short-term or physiologic health outcomes—hemoglobin A1c in patients with diabetes or cholesterol in patients with (or at high risk for) coronary artery (heart) disease—for which a strong logical case (and, in some cases, a data-driven empirical case) can be made that investing in care to achieve better outcomes will lead to improved health and lower total cost over time. By creating an incentive for providers to achieve health-related outcome targets, health can be improved (and costs controlled).

The introduction of P4P programs had to wait for the development and diffusion of quality metrics that could support the setting of performance targets. That was led by the Joint Commission and the National Committee for Quality Assurance (NCQA) through the development and deployment of a set of standard metrics for hospitals (ORYX) and health plans (the Healthcare Effectiveness Data and Information Set [HEDIS]). HEDIS metrics—which include statistics that address clinical quality, member satisfaction, and utilization (and will likely include measures of efficiency in the future)—permitted employers (and their employees) to select health plans (initially HMOs, but over time PPOs as well) based on both price and quality ("value") rather than on price alone. But they also permitted the setting of performance targets, which strategy has diffused, over time, both to the interface with providers and to the public sector. So, for example, P4P has diffused rapidly into FFS arrangements with physicians and hospitals in the private sector.[9] The Centers for Medicare and Medicaid Services has introduced quality payment differentials to hospitals based on hospital scorecards and has begun to introduce quality incentives to physicians through the Physician Quality Reporting System (PQRS; initially, the Physician Quality Reporting Initiative [PQRI]). That said, the performance of P4P programs (for achieving real improvements in value) has been described as "lackluster."[10] So, policymakers—in both the public and private sectors—have sought more powerful payment reforms.

Episode-Based, or Bundled, Payment

Many would argue that any payment innovation that begins with FFS—that is, a system that intrinsically motivates the delivery of more, and more intensive, care—will not achieve the results necessary to create a sustainable, high-performing healthcare system in the United States.[10] As a result, there have been innovations that begin with a radically different approach to payment—one that creates incentives that are in the opposite direction of FFS (and hence drives intrinsically toward lower cost).

Such approaches "fix price." That is, they are designed to provide a fixed fee that will cover all services (defined in some way) rather than reward the provider for each service independently. The first—and arguably strongest—such payment innovation is capitation, which is payment of a fixed amount on a per-member per-month basis for all services a member may require.

Capitation was prevalent in the early 1990s, with the introduction of HMO-style managed care. And capitation continues to be prevalent, at the point at which employers (and/or governments) pay health plans.

But capitation did not work well at the physician level—for many, many reasons. Physicians, especially in the early 1990s, were inexperienced with (and lacked the tools they needed to manage) the clinical risk that accompanied the financial risk inherent in capitation, and physicians have limited control over costs (for example, once a patient is hospitalized). So—although we may see and are, in fact, seeing capitation of providers reemerge (see the section "The Accountable-Care Organization")—there have been efforts to create payment strategies that are more discrete (and clinically manageable) than capitation.

Important among those are episode-based, or bundled, payments. The notion of a bundled payment is to offer a fixed fee—not for all services that a patient may require in a month (or over a year) but for the set of services a patient typically requires when they have a particular condition or procedure. To the extent that care is predictable for (for example) patients who are having elective surgery, or even for patients with conditions like diabetes, it should be possible to predict the needs (and therefore the costs) for patients during the course of a specific episode of care.

This is not a new idea; in fact, as discussed previously, it is the foundation of Medicare's DRG system for paying for hospital care, and it is the basis for which Medicare pays for outpatient dialysis for patients with ESRD. But what has emerged is broadening the scope of payment bundles and extending the "bundle" from the inpatient (or facility) stay (alone) to an interval that includes both pre- and posthospital care. By setting a fixed fee for a bundle that includes, in particular, postdischarge events, the provider bears risk for the costs that would follow an adverse outcome (such as a complication requiring significant ambulatory care or even a rehospitalization). So, the bundled payment creates a potentially strong incentive to optimize prehospital care (so that the patient is well prepared and the hospital stay can be minimized), to optimize care over the inpatient stay itself (so that the patient is not discharged prematurely and does not develop a complication or return to the hospital), and to optimize the postdischarge interval (so that gains achieved in the hospital are maintained and the discharge plan carefully executed).

There is considerable interest in, and innovation regarding, bundled payment. In the private sector, some provider organizations (notably, Geisinger Health System in Danville, Pennsylvania) have moved proactively to offer fixed-price bundles to payers through their ProvenCare program.[11] There are private-sector pilots underway in many parts of the country to evaluate bundled payment strategies that may be more realistic in markets in which provider organizations have not achieved the level of integration that Geisinger has; notable pilots include those led by PROMETHEUS Payment in five sites across the country and those led by the Integrated Healthcare Association (IHA) in California. That said, bundled payment remains, as of 2012, the exception and not the rule in the private sector.

Medicare has tested bundled payment strategies in two large demonstrations: one in the 1990s (the Medicare Participating Heart Bypass Center Demonstration)[12] and one that began in 2009 (the Acute Care Episode Demonstration).[13] In addition, the Center for Medicare and Medicaid Innovation (CMMI) has recently launched a Bundled Payment for Care Improvement initiative,[14] which offers organizations the opportunity to test a broad range of approaches to bundled payment. Finally, Section 2704 of the ACA establishes a demonstration project for Medicaid programs in up to eight states to evaluate bundled payments. So, the expectation is that there will be, in the public sector, testing and evaluation of bundled payment approaches, but it may be some time before they have moved into the mainstream.

Payment Reform Coupled to Delivery System Innovation

A primary objective of payment reform (including P4P and bundled payment) is to drive changes in the processes through which care is delivered—to increase coordination, eliminate redundancy, and thereby enhance quality and eliminate waste. That transformation of the care-delivery system will almost certainly require some restructuring of it. So, we expect—and in fact have seen—changes in the structure of the healthcare marketplace, where payment reform is underway.

On the other hand, there has been innovation in the delivery system, driven by the primary interest providers have in improving the quality and efficiency of care. The risk in such innovation is that it will in fact improve efficiency—so that providers that operate in an FFS environment will (as a consequence) see their revenue and profits fall.[15]

As a result, there is a clear need to link delivery system innovation to payment reform. There are two important delivery system innovations that are now linked to payment reform; it is important to briefly discuss these.

- The patient-centered medical home (PCMH)
- The accountable-care organization (ACO)

The Patient-Centered Medical Home (PCMH)   The PCMH is a "health care setting that facilitates partnerships between individual patients, and their personal physicians, and when appropriate, the patient's family, with the goal of providing comprehensive primary care for children, youth and adults."[16] Originally conceived and advanced by the medical societies representing the primary-care disciplines (the American Academy of Pediatrics, the American Academy of Family Physicians, the American College of Physicians, and the American Osteopathic Association),[17] the concept has been embraced widely—at least among those who pay for healthcare.

The detailed requirements that describe a PCMH can be found elsewhere;[18] what is important for the purposes of this discussion is that the providers must invest (significantly) in the infrastructure (including the HIT infrastructure) required to achieve the functionality, which is the PCMH. The rate at which the PCMH concept diffused was limited by the lack of a return on that investment. In response, many private payers have begun to offer a per-member per-month fee to practices that are certified PCMHs, which recognizes the additional capabilities (to improve care and reduce cost) that are expected in practices that achieve that recognition. That (patient management) fee is in addition to the FFS payment the practice earns when it sees a patient; the expectation is that a patient (or "case") management fee will be more than recovered through reductions in expenditures for other healthcare services (such as inpatient hospital stays).

Medicare is testing the PCMH through two demonstrations: the Advanced Primary Care Practice Demonstration and the Federally Qualified Health Centers Advanced Primary Care Practice Demonstration. In addition, CMMI is testing the PCMH model through a Comprehensive Primary Care Initiative that provides for multipayer support of primary-care practices to support their efforts to offer more effective and coordinated primary care. Finally, PCMHs are being evaluated at the state level (for example, a multipayer initiative in Maryland).[19] One can expect that, at least in the short run, payment of a PMPM management fee to qualified PCMHs will be more prevalent and a more important part of the revenue stream for primary-care practices.

The Accountable-Care Organization   The system for delivering healthcare in the United States is poorly organized, with weak relationships among the many providers and sites at which patients receive care. As a result, care is poorly coordinated and often redundant, patient outcomes suffer, and precious resources are wasted.

Many believe that solving this problem requires the creation of strong incentives and the infrastructure needed to drive care coordination and integration across providers. This has led to the articulation of the concept of an accountable-care organization (ACO). While ACOs are defined in different ways, what is common to all definitions—and is at the core of the concept—is that it is a delivery system entity that is prepared to accept accountability for the clinical and financial outcomes of the patients to whom it delivers care.

ACOs are emerging in both the public and private sectors.[20] There are two especially important innovations—that link ACOs to changes in Medicare payment—that we would like to call out.

- **Medicare Shared Savings Program (MSSP)**   A payment innovation linked to the operations of ACOs.[21] The program was mandated by the ACA, regulations describing the program were released in late 2011, and delivery systems are organizing to participate in 2012. Participation is voluntary, it requires the creation of an entity that includes primary-care physicians (and typically includes hospitals), and it creates a payment environment in which the ACO is paid on a discounted FFS basis (and providers that are part of the ACO are paid by the ACO according to agreements that operate within the ACO) but in which Medicare shares "savings" that derive from the ACO's efforts to deliver high-quality, coordinated, cost-effective care. "Savings" are calculated as the difference between what spending would have been (for those Medicare enrollees for whom the ACO is responsible) and what spending actually was, adjusted for factors that are beyond the control of the ACO. The ACO's share of savings depends on a number of factors, including (very importantly) how the ACO performs on a set of quality metrics designed to assure that savings are not generated by withholding (or "stinting") on care.

  The MSSP ACO is, then, a delivery system innovation tightly linked to a change in the way care is paid for. In its current form, it builds off of an FFS payment model; it is, in some ways, "simply" a P4P program with strong incentives to achieve financial (as opposed to only quality) performance targets, and it operates to create incentives across provider types (in particular, to align incentives for hospitals and physicians). It is important to note that, in the best case, ACO revenue will be less than pure FFS revenue. (The ACO incentive is to reduce Medicare's cost relative to projected FFS cost in a given year; to the extent that it does, it receives some share—up to 50 percent—of that difference. But that will always be less than it would have received had there been no ACO.) So, the ACO is able to succeed economically only if it can reduce production cost more than it reduces billings. This is likely to be a challenge for many organizations—and it is yet unclear how many organizations will participate in the MSSP.

- **Pioneer ACO Program (Pioneer)**[22]   An alternative to the MSSP. Unlike the MSSP (which is not a pilot or demonstration; any organization that qualifies can participate), Pioneer is a pilot run out of CMMI; 32 organizations were selected on a competitive basis to operate as ACOs in a payment environment that creates much greater opportunities for shared savings (but also much greater downside risk in the event that savings are not realized) but also intentionally moves toward a "population-based payment model" (that is, a per-member per-month payment; previously called *capitation*) that creates even more powerful incentives for cost control. Like the MSSP, there are strong protections to assure quality; in addition, there are incentives to encourage Medicare Pioneer ACOs to develop performance-based payment arrangements with other payers.

  The Pioneer program represents an important opportunity to allow healthcare organizations that have developed advanced care management/care coordination infrastructure to capture the financial gains associated with the effective use of that infrastructure. Whether organizations will succeed—and, importantly, whether (or how quickly) the model can scale (beyond the relatively small set of organizations that is the first set of Pioneers)—is a question that will be answered over the next several years. But, in any event, the Pioneer program sends a signal that CMS understands that there is a need to consider a move away from FFS Medicare, if Medicare is to achieve its triple aim of better care, better health, and lower cost.

Chapter Review

This chapter described the complex systems through which healthcare is paid in the United States. In particular, it described how insurance works and how costs are shared by the ultimate payers of care (the federal and state governments, employers, and individual Americans themselves), and it expanded on the main structures of programs. The chapter defined the major payers and the types of insurance products offered. Finally, the chapter discussed changes in the way care is paid for and delivered as part of healthcare reform or that may be accelerated by healthcare reform.

Questions

To test your comprehension of the chapter, answer the following questions and then check your answers against the list of correct answers at the end of the chapter.

1. Who pays for healthcare in the United States?

    A. The federal government, through the Medicare and Medicaid programs

    B. The states, through the Medicaid program

    C. Private corporations, by providing health insurance to their employees and their families

    D. Individual Americans

    E. All of the above

2. Which of the following is true about the source of insurance?

    A. Most Americans receive health insurance through Medicare.

    B. Most Americans receive health insurance through Medicaid.

    C. Most Americans receive health insurance through employer-sponsored health insurance.

    D. Most Americans buy health insurance policies as individuals.

    E. Most Americans do not have health insurance.

3. Which of the following is true?

    A. Individuals pay a relatively small percentage of the annual cost of their insurance.

    B. Individuals pay a copayment that is a relatively small percentage of the cost of most services they use.

    C. Individuals with private health insurance—particularly those with employer-sponsored health insurance—pay (and are likely to pay in the future) a larger share of the cost associated with their healthcare than individuals with Medicare or Medicaid.

    D. All of the above.

4. Which of the following are not insurance products commonly offered in the United States?

    A. Traditional/open-access health insurance plans

    B. Preferred Provider Organizations (PPOs) and Health Maintenance Organizations (HMOs)

    C. Independent Practice Associations (IPAs) and Patient-Centered Medical Homes (PCMHs)

    D. Consumer-Directed Health Plans (CDHPs) and Health Savings Accounts (HSAs)

5. Which of the following is true of the Medicare program?

A. All Americans older than 64 must participate.

B. The distribution of its beneficiaries across insurance products is very different from private insurance.

C. It has, since its inception, covered hospital care, ambulatory care, and prescription drugs.

D. It is administered by the federal government but jointly financed by the states and the federal government.

E. All of the above.

6. In general, Medicare pays physicians

A. Based on what physicians charge.

B. Based on fees that are negotiated with physicians.

C. Based on a fee schedule that is based on the resources required to deliver different services.

D. On a capitated (per-member per-month [PMPM]) basis.

E. Physician services are not covered by Medicare.

7. In general, Medicare pays hospitals

A. Based on what hospitals charge for each service they provide.

B. Based on fees that are negotiated with hospitals for each service they provide.

C. Through a shared savings program that rewards hospitals for saving money.

D. Through a "bundled payment" system that offers a fixed price for all hospital services delivered during a hospital stay.

E. Hospital services are not covered by Medicare.

8. Which of the following is true?

A. Accountable-care organizations (ACOs) are delivery system entities that are emerging in response to financial incentives to reduce the cost and improve the quality of healthcare.

B. Patient-centered medical homes (PCMHs) are nursing homes that are designed to assist patients to make the transition from hospital care to home care.

C. The Medicare Shared Savings Program (MSSP) is a way that Medicare beneficiaries can share in savings that derive from their efforts to take better care of themselves.

D. Bundled payment programs are an exciting innovation, but to date there is very little experience with them.

E. All of the above.

9. Which of the following is true of the insurance mandate in the Affordable Care Act?

   A. It will mean that the federal government and the states will no longer need to provide Medicaid.

   B. It should increase the efficiency of insurance by bringing more (and lower-risk) Americans into the insurance risk pool.

   C. It is unconstitutional, because the federal government cannot require Americans to buy anything (even health insurance).

   D. It does not support delivery system innovations such as ACOs.

   E. None of the above.

10. What is the minimum FMAP that will qualify a state for the maximum eFMAP?

   A. 85%

   B. 78.57%

   C. 98%

   D. 100%

Answers

1. **E.** Healthcare in the United States is paid for largely through insurance, which is provided to most employees by the company for which they work, to older Americans through the federal Medicare program, and to disadvantaged and vulnerable populations through the Medicaid program (and other programs like it) that are jointly financed by the federal and state governments.

2. **C.** Although many Americans receive insurance through the public programs of Medicare and Medicaid—and (because those who do may have relatively greater needs), expenditures for these programs outweigh expenditures for those with private health insurance)—the majority of Americans obtain insurance through a policy provided as a benefit of employment.

3. **D.** Individuals with private insurance typically pay less than 25 percent of their annual premium, and Medicare and Medicaid enrollees pay less than that. Similarly, copayments—though rising and often perceived as high—are typically far less than the cost of the service provided. As costs (and therefore insurance premiums) rise, insurance products are evolving to shift costs to individuals, both to reduce the employer (or public) contribution to care and to create an incentive for individuals to use care wisely.

4. **C.** IPAs are groups of individual physicians and medical practices that provide services to managed-care organizations. PCMHs are medical practices that have put in place the infrastructure needed to coordinate care. IPAs and PCMHs will often contract with managed-care organizations (in particular, PPOs and HMOs), but they do so to provide care (not to provide insurance).

5. **B.** Traditional (open-access, FFS) care dominates Medicare. That is very rare in the private sector. The distribution of its beneficiaries across insurance products is very different from private insurance.

6. **C.** Physicians are paid based on the Medicare fee schedule, which in turn is based on a resource-based relative value scale (RBRVS).

7. **D.** Medicare has paid hospitals for more than two decades using diagnosis-related groups (DRGs) that cover hospital—but not physician—services provided during a hospital stay. Increasingly, hospital reimbursement can be enhanced (or threatened) by quality performance. The Medicare Shared Savings Program (MSSP) is a voluntary program that gives hospitals (through establishing accountable-care organizations) the opportunity to improve profitability by generating savings (but only if they reduce their own production costs as well).

8. **A.** PCMHs are primary-care practices, with infrastructure designed to coordinate care (primarily ambulatory care, although transitions from hospital to home are important as well); they are not nursing homes. The MSSP is a program that permits providers (and, in particular, ACOs)—not patients/beneficiaries—to share savings with the Medicare program. There is considerable experience with bundled payments already—through hospital DRGs and through Medicare and private-sector pilots and demonstrations from the 1990s and early twenty-first century.

9. **B.** The Affordable Care Act should increase the efficiency of insurance by bringing more (and lower risk) Americans into the insurance risk pool.

10. **B.** The maximum allowed eFMAP is 85 percent; thus, to find the answer, the following algebra equation must be solved for x:

$$x + 0.30 \times (100\% - x) = 85\%$$

References

1. Census data number of insured (Table C-1). Accessed on September 8, 2012, from www.census.gov/prod/2011pubs/p60-239.pdf.

2. Commercial product statistics. Accessed on September 8, 2012, from http://ehbs.kff.org/pdf/2011/8225.pdf.

3. ASPE Medicaid. Accessed on September 8, 2012, from http://aspe.hhs.gov/health/fmap12.shtml.

4. Henry Kaiser Foundation Medicaid overview. Accessed on September 8, 2012, from www.kff.org/medicaid/upload/Medicaid-An-Overview-of-Spending-on.pdf.

5. Medicaid and managed care fact sheet. Accessed on September 8, 2012, from www.kff.org/medicaid/upload/Medicaid-and-Managed-Care-Fact-Sheet.pdf.

6. Medicaid's long-term care users: Spending patterns across institutional and community-based settings. Accessed on September 8, 2012, from www.kff.org/medicaid/upload/7576-02.pdf.

7. Hadley, J; Holahan J. The cost of care for the uninsured: What do we spend, who pays, and what would full coverage add to medical spending? Accessed on September 8, 2012, from www.kff.org/uninsured/upload/the-cost-of-care-for-the-uninsured-what-do-we-spend-who-pays-and-what-would-full-coverage-add-to-medical-spending.pdf.

8. American Hospital Association. Uncompensated hospital care cost fact sheet, December 2010. Accessed on September 8, 2012, from www.aha.org/content/00-10/10uncompensatedcare.pdf

9. Schneider, E., Hussey, P. S., and Schnyer, C. (2011). Payment reform: Analysis of models and performance measurement implications. Technical Report. RAND Corporation.

10. Rosenthal, M. B., Landon, B. E., Norman, S. L. T., Frank, R. G., Epstein, A. M. (2006). Pay for performance in commercial HMOs. *New England Journal of Medicine, 355*, 1895–1902.

11. Geisinger proven care program. Accessed on September 8, 2012, from www.geisinger.org/provencare/.

12. Cromwell, J.; Dayhoff, D. A.; McCall, N. T.; Subramanian, S.; Freitas, R. C.; Hart, R. J.; Caswell, C.; and Stason, W. (1998). Medicare participating heart bypass demonstration, executive summary. Final Report. Waltham, MA: Health Economics Research, Inc.

13. Medicare demonstration project on acute care episode. Accessed on September 8, 2012, from www.cms.gov/Medicare/Demonstration-Projects/DemoProjectsEvalRpts/downloads/ACE_web_page.pdf.

14. CMS bundled payment of care initiative. Accessed on September 8, 2012, from http://innovations.cms.gov/PPha.initiatives/bundled-payments/index.html.

15. Redesigning care delivery in response to a high-performance network: The Virginia Mason Medical Center. Accessed on September 8, 2012, from http://content.healthaffairs.org/content/26/4/w532.full.pdf+html.

16. Patient centered medical home. Accessed on September 8, 2012, from www.pcpcc.net/content/joint-principles-patient-centered-medical-home.

17. Sia, C., Tonniges, T. F., Osterhus, E., & Taba, S. (2004). History of the medical home concept. *Pediatrics 2004, 113*, 1473–1478.

18. (1)Defining the patient-centered medical home. (2012). Accessed on October 18, 2012, from http://pcmh.ahrq.gov/portal/server.pt/community/pcmh__home/1483/pcmh_defining_the_pcmh_v2. (2)Patient-centered medical home (PCMH) standards and guidelines. (2012). Accessed on October 18, 2012 from https://inetshop01.pub.ncqa.org/Publications/deptCate.asp?dept_id=2&cateID=300&sortOrder=796&mscssid=#300796.

19. Maryland multipayer initiative. Accessed on September 8, 2012, from http://mhcc.maryland.gov/pcmh.

20. Accountable care organization. Accessed on September 8, 2012, from www .brookings.edu/about/centers/health/accountable-care-organization-learning-network-releases-aco-map.

21. Medicare shared saving program. Accessed on September 8, 2012, from https://www.cms.gov/Medicare/Medicare-Fee-for-Service-Payment/ sharedsavingsprogram/index.html?redirect-/sharedsavingsprogram.

22. Pioneer accountable care organization program. Accessed on September 8, 2012, from http://innovations.cms.gov/initiatives/ACO/Pioneer/index.html.

Ethics and Healthcare: Focus on Information Technology

Kenneth W. Goodman

In this chapter, you will learn how to
- Recognize the difference between law and ethics
- Identify core components of professionalism in health information technology
- Identify leading ethical issues that arise in the use of health information technology
- Make and defend ethical arguments using some standard methods
- Explain to colleagues how an "appropriate uses and users" approach provides ethical guidance in a variety of circumstances and situations

Law, Ethics, and Professionalism

The question how one ought to behave is as old as civilization and as new as today's headlines. Humans have for millennia been concerned about ethics both for its own sake—how should I make my way in the world?—and because life is better, safer, and happier when people follow certain rules. Generally speaking, *morality* can be thought of as a community's set of rules for proper conduct. *Ethics* is the study or analysis of those rules, including reasons for following them, their interrelationships, and what to do if they are in conflict or when different communities (or cultures) have different rules.

Some people argue that good behavior is self-rewarding. That is, it is just a better way to live. But it also has good consequences for both the actors and their community. Some actions are universally regarded as so seriously bad and destructive that the actors must be punished. Legal systems have evolved to identify, select, or make clear which actions will be required and which prohibited and to carry out the punishments for those who do what they should not or for those who do not do what they should.

Put this way, it is clear that ethics precedes the law. Legislatures would not know what to require or prohibit if they could not figure out what was right or wrong in the first place. Some do a better job of this than others; some are no good at it at all. Indeed, many political and policy debates turn on disputes over what should be made illegal.

It is easy to see how there might be some actions that are wrong but not illegal (generally, lying is a good example of this). But the history of legal systems also gives us many examples of wrongs that were permitted or required but should not have been (think of slavery or segregation).

For our purposes, the health professions are a rich source of ethical issues. These range from traditional standards to contemporary moral issues, elicit examples of frank wrongdoing and virtuous action, and touch on a large ensemble of policy stances and challenges. Many of these can be rendered as questions: Why does informed consent matter? Why should privacy and confidentiality be protected? When is it permissible to treat a patient based on the output of a decision-support system? We return to these issues shortly.

Professional Standards and Values

In addition to broad social custom and legal mandate, some subgroups adopt additional obligations and prohibitions based on various skills, education, values, and traditions. From antiquity, people with special training or knowledge have by virtue of that training or knowledge been expected to hew to additional rules and standards. These people are *professionals*, and their rules have come to be called *professional standards*.

Some of these standards and values are based on common sense, some are just stipulated, and some are both. In the Hippocratic tradition, for instance, physicians are enjoined from having sex with patients, are required to protect patients' "secrets," and are told not to practice beyond their capacity. But they are also told not to perform abortions and to teach medicine without compensation to the male offspring of other physicians. Clearly, professional values evolve and are subject to constant analysis and scrutiny. Further, there are many values that are trans- or interprofessional: veracity, transparency, and accountability are the best known among these. These values apply to health professionals—including those who build or use health information systems—as much as they apply to others.

While some historians believe that there was no such person as Hippocrates, to whom the famous oath is attributed, it is clear that there is a powerful and longstanding desire to expect more from specially trained people than from others. If that training is in the health professions, the expectations are greater still. Attempts to codify those expectations in oaths or codes are therefore attempts to make explicit what it means to be a professional. Put differently, it has been suggested that the presence of an oath or code is itself among the hallmarks of a profession.

The reasons for demanding higher-than-usual standards for nurses, physicians, health informaticians, and others are generally based on the same foundations as laid by the ancients: patients are vulnerable, the well-educated are often more powerful, and the ability to help others often entails an obligation to do so. These are very powerful reasons. It follows that if one respects reasons, then professionals are duty-bound to demonstrate and live by the values of their profession. My unwillingness to embrace my profession's values suggests that I might have settled on the wrong profession.

In addition to questions of daily practice, some organizations commit their members to ideals of social justice and the reduction of health disparities, to the growth of knowledge, and to an emphasis on patient-centeredness.[1,2]

In health and biomedical informatics, a number of organizations have developed codes of ethics in an attempt to make explicit the values undergirding this comparatively new profession. It could be argued that professionals should be familiar with and, when asked, to contribute to the development of these statements.[3, 4]

 HIT PRO EXAM TIP Ethical elements of healthcare professionalism are usually straightforward and longstanding.

Tools for Ethical Analysis

Many people have opinions about ethics, and some of these opinions are quite reasonable if you think about them a little. Some do not make any sense at all. What is important to realize about ethics, however, is that opinions as such do not carry much weight unless they can be supported by reasons. Ethics is overwhelmingly about reasons, including figuring out which reasons are better than others. If you have no reasons to support your position, that position cannot be taken seriously.

So, what counts as a good reason in ethics? This can be a difficult question, and it has been the focus of work by philosophers for thousands of years. Nevertheless, there are areas of general agreement, and some of the ways nonphilosophers can do ethical reasoning are often unremarkable. Many ethics teachers like to make sure students are familiar with at least two main historical approaches to ethical reasoning; these methods can be quite useful in making at least some decisions. What follows are brief, potted, and oversimplified versions of these approaches. They cannot substitute for serious study and structured learning.

A duty-based approach to ethics requires that we always treat people as ends in themselves and never as means to an end; that is, don't use people. Relatedly, a good reason for an action is that it is an action you would—if you had the power—require everyone to do. Robbing people uses them for their money, and one would certainly not want to live in a world full of robbers. So, robbery is wrong. A reason why you should protect a patient's privacy is that violating privacy for some other purpose (selling patient names to a pharmaceutical corporation, say) uses them in a different way; moreover, imagine a world full of privacy violators. So, protecting privacy is good, and violating it is wrong. (We get into interesting territory with those cases in which one might want to promote other values—public health, say—over privacy. These require more nuanced argumentation; I address these cases later in this section.)

A consequence-based approach makes rightness or wrongness a calculation of whether the consequences of an action are, on balance, more beneficial than not or less harmful than otherwise. Some traditional utilitarians contend that actions should be weighed by their effect on the collective happiness. So, robbers harm people and make the rest of us fearful; therefore, robbery is wrong. Protecting privacy engenders trust and, in clinical contexts, entails that patients are more likely to tell nurses and physicians the truth, supporting more accurate diagnoses; therefore, protecting privacy is a good.

Note that in our oversimplified accounts here, both approaches give the same answer. This could be evidence we are on the right track. Increasingly, many people like a resource that combines elements of both approaches. In the estimation of one philosopher, if one is weighing the correct course of action, she should imagine advocating it in public to someone she cares about.[5] (That is, imagine, with the news cameras running, asking Mom to drive the getaway car for the bank robbery you are planning—or, in front of the same cameras, urging your son the nurse to find out your hospitalized boss's HIV status.)

The main point here is that we are entitled to hold any ethics opinions we like, but we are not to be taken seriously unless we can produce good reasons for those beliefs.

Appropriate Uses and Users

Health information technology raises as many interesting and important ethical issues as any other domain in the health professions. In this section, we are guided by an early and important analysis[6] that inaugurated an era of thinking about ethics and computers in clinical care, in part by drawing attention to questions of *appropriate uses* and *appropriate users* of decision support systems.

This has a number of advantages, not least that the history of bioethics has generally been shaped and driven by advances in technology: hemodialysis, end-of-life care, organ transplantation, genome science, and so on.

What is significant about smart machines is that unlike other technologies, which provide tools for our hands, ears, and eyes, computers are also tools for our brains.

Decision-Support Systems

It is well established that computerized decision-support systems, diagnostic expert systems, and prognostic scoring systems are often more accurate than human experts. This can be exciting, unsettling, or both. The very idea that a machine might do as good a job as a human at rendering a diagnosis (and at ranking differential diagnoses) raises what are arguably some of the most important questions in the history of the health professions:

> What does the practice of medicine or nursing consist in if a machine
> can do it as well as a human? And if these tools are so good, when are
> we doing wrong by not using them?

Let's begin to answer these questions by looking at other clinical and surgical tools and by considering their appropriate uses and users (arguing by analogy to settled cases can be very effective in ethics). Start with stethoscopes and scalpels. Appropriate employment of the former is uncontroversial: auscultation is an important clinical function, and stethoscopes are the tool we use. Their uses—listening to lungs, bowels, and hearts, for instance—are well established and of no concern. (Try to think of an inappropriate use of a stethoscope....) Now, who is an appropriate user of a stethoscope? Nurses? Physicians? Ethics committee members? Lawyers? Computer scientists? The correct answer must be this: one who uses the device with the intention of actual physiologic monitoring, checking a vital sign, or rendering a diagnosis (these being straightforward and appropriate uses) must be trained in the use of the device. So, an appropriate user is one who is trained to use the device as it was designed and for which it was intended. An appropriate use of a scalpel is, generally, to cut bodies open or parts off or out. An appropriate user is a surgeon whom we presume is adequately trained.

Note that any inappropriate use or user of a stethoscope or scalpel is likely to violate the rule-based and harms-avoiding ethics tools introduced earlier. For our purposes, "appropriateness" is an ethical concept.

A diagnostic expert system might be designed to educate students about differential diagnoses, in which case a student (construed broadly) is an appropriate user. A third-year medical student who uses the device to elicit a diagnosis to present at morning report is likely using it inappropriately. A prognostic scoring system designed exclusively to predict mortality in critical-care units is likely being used inappropriately if its scores are the only information used to decide to withdraw treatment at the end of life.

It gets a little more complicated when smart machines are used as intended by adequately trained personnel. Apropos our earlier questions, what do we need humans for if computers can do as good a job? The best response to this is wise and simple: we need humans because humans practice medicine, and nursing and machines—no matter how smart—do not.[7] Look at it another way. There is a lot more to the practice of nursing and medicine than making calculations or performing complex inferences. The health professions are occupied by people, who bring other skills and traits to bear. These skills and traits include the capacity for empathy, the capacity to understand why a side effect of antihypertensives in men engenders noncompliance, and the ability to recognize that when a patient says "yes" he might mean "I'm not so sure." There is good reason to believe that these skills are essential to successful clinical practice.

If, however, a smart machine can improve outcomes, then it probably becomes an obligation to use it—with appropriate training, of course. As computerized decision-support systems, diagnostic expert systems, and prognostic scoring systems become more common, it will be a great and interesting challenge to ensure they are used when appropriate and by appropriate people. Sorting out these limits and obligations will be one of the greatest challenges of twenty-first-century healthcare.

 HIT PRO EXAM TIP   Focus on the important role of education in assessing appropriate use.

Use Case 3-1: Using a Prognostic Scoring System

Your institution has purchased a well-known prognostic scoring system, which among other things calculates the likelihood of patients dying in your critical-care unit (CCU). The system was purchased to enable administrators to track CCU quality over time; the percentage of patients with similar physiologic profiles who died last year can be compared to the percentage who died this year, giving some evidence that care improved, declined, or remained the same. One day an intensivist in the unit asks for the score of a current patient. She wants the information because it appears the patient is dying, and if the computer gives a low score, it can be used to support termination of treatment.

Electronic Health Record Data

If you work in a hospital, then your institution either has installed an electronic health record system, is in the process of trying to make it work properly, or is planning to install one. There is no getting around this. The time has long passed when we could effectively store patient information on paper. Indeed, use of an electronic health record has become one of those duties that new technology thrusts upon us. That is, if a hospital is not using an electronic record, then it has fallen or is falling behind in the standard of care.

An electric health record is a very powerful tool, but it increases the challenges faced by clinicians and administrators. Failing to use the tool is blameworthy, and using it correctly is difficult. I now address some of the "appropriate uses and users" issues raised by electronic health records.

Appropriate users of these systems seem obvious: those who are involved in patient care and, perhaps, those who evaluate or oversee those who take care of patients. As with paper records, any other users must have a very good reason, and there should be a process to review requests to access patient records. Criminal investigators backed up by subpoenas or court orders would be an example. Marketing companies, pharmaceutical reps, and curious clinicians in other buildings would not be credible users. Note that audit trails to monitor access to electronic records are intended in part to ensure that only those with a credible reason to access a chart can actually access the chart. Others, sightseers, can be out of bounds even if they are clinicians. Giving in to the temptation to view the chart of a VIP, for instance, is a surrender to unprofessional desires; it is also wrong, according to duty-based ethics, because it fails to respect another person; it uses her as a means to (cheap and tawdry) ends. That makes it wrong, even if the patient is not harmed and even never finds out about it.

Consider appropriate uses. Generally, appropriate uses require more or less direct contributions to patient care, such as the following:

- Storing clinical notes, lab reports, and so on
- Monitoring, analyzing, and referring to these entries
- Making clinical inferences, developing treatment plans, and so on

In other words, use the electronic record in the same way that patient records have been used for centuries.

Here are some examples of inappropriate uses:

- Selling information to the medical device industry
- Learning why your brother-in-law had an appointment at the STD clinic
- Blackmailing someone

These are simple examples. Yet each one can help make clear that those who are entrusted with access to patient records acquire special responsibilities. Moreover, such responsibilities require that one must be trained or in training before accessing an electronic health record for clinical care (as opposed to some kinds of approved research). Indeed, that training should include a nontrivial commitment to ethical issues. This is in part why the accreditation of nursing and medical schools and residency programs includes requirements for education in ethics and professionalism.

Quality Assessment, Error Reduction, Outcomes, and Research

The obligations to improve quality, make fewer errors, assess outcomes, and even conduct formal research emerge from the uncontroversial recognition that yesterday's (or yesteryear's) standards can and therefore should be improved on. The history of the health professions is in many respects a history of self-improvement. How could it be otherwise? Willful ignorance is difficult to defend in ordinary contexts—it is impossible to defend when lives are at stake.

Many health information technology tools are available to foster this improvement. I consider three in the following sections: electronic health records, personal health records, and public health databases.

Institutional Records and Research

You've seen how consideration of appropriate uses and users can contribute to the employment of the electronic health record in the care of patients. This approach can also guide us when it comes to research or the collection and analysis (or selection and analysis) of health information. A randomized clinical trial, for instance, elicits, collects, and analyzes information; a review of preexisting information selects or identifies it for analysis. The information in electronic health records was for the most part collected for patient care and so existed before anyone decided to study it.

As a source of knowledge about treatment effectiveness, patient outcomes, and the internal workings of healthcare institutions, patient records are invaluable. It follows that we ought to use them to study how best to improve care and reduce error. These are appropriate uses because they will improve healthcare. Inappropriate uses of data from electronic health records might include assays to identify patients with poor outcomes so we can refuse future services, track patterns of pharmaceutical use to inform market speculators, or monitor frequency of medical device use to tip off device company sales representatives. It would also be inappropriate to suppress or hide information that would contribute to improved care.

In this context, appropriate users are those who are authorized to use the system and who do so with the intent of improving healthcare. Such authorization might include permission to view records with identifiable information about patients. Note here the importance of intentions in arriving at an ethically appropriate decision. In some or many cases, rightness or wrongness can be inferred from a user's intentions.

Personal Health Records

The increasingly widespread use of personal health records presents exciting new opportunities for patients to interact with clinicians.[8] These tools raise a number of interesting ethical issues, including those related to privacy, changes in the patient-clinician relationship, and some decision-support functions.[9] They also give us an opportunity to apply our rubric to a new and rapidly evolving technology.

Personal health records, which can reside on the Web as well as USB drives, smartphones, and other devices, enable patients to participate in health recordkeeping and broaden modes of communicating. Individual patients use these records to track medication, daily experiences, self-test results, symptoms, and other health information and to transmit it to clinicians; and clinicians can respond with advice, education, and instructions. Only a patient or designated surrogate should use that patient's personal health record—it makes no sense to suppose anyone else should. The class of appropriate users will include caregivers and indeed anyone who was an appropriate user of the patient's information in the electronic health record.

Moreover, and with adequate consent measures in place, researchers should be able to study personal health record data, both to assess their efficacy and to learn what they can about patient care and perhaps public health.

Public Health Databases

While hospital and other institutional electronic health records are valuable sources of information for epidemiologists and public health authorities and researchers, these agents themselves create and monitor stores of health data. This is necessary to protect public health by identifying, tracking, and warning of disease risks; predicting and responding to emergencies; and shaping education and policy.[10] It should be emphasized that while a great deal of debate surrounds what is called the secondary use of data from electronic health records, the analysis of data collected for the sake of public health itself is a primary use. It should be obvious that civil society has come to depend on such surveillance and research—and therefore that there is an obligation to conduct it.

Public health data repositories are generally created and maintained without the explicit consent of those whose information fills them. The success of public health surveillance by trusted authorities entails the conclusion that reasonable people value this service and that their consent should therefore be implied. Indeed, without such an inference, public health itself would be impossible.

It should be uncontroversial to identify appropriate uses of public health data repositories—they emerge from the very reasons the repositories were created in the first place. A use that did not involve analysis of disease for the sake of prevention and treatment (including injury and certain noncommunicable maladies such as obesity and substance abuse) will require special justification or might not be permissible at all. For instance, while it could be scientifically useful to track the location of HIV cases in a community, it would be ethically unacceptable to use that information to infer the identity of people to target for higher insurance rates or to use that information so, for instance, businesses could exclude individuals from employment.

It would also be inappropriate to allow certain individuals or groups to search such databases. Imagine if a racist organization wanted to query a database to perpetuate bias against a minority population. That said, custodians of electronic health repositories should anticipate that legitimate uses and users might encounter unintended results, as might occur when data-mining software contributes to findings that could be used for unethical purposes. This risk underscores the need for adequate mechanisms of review and governance.

Privacy and Confidentiality

One of the oldest and most important values in the health professions is often the first mentioned in enumerations of ethical issues arising in the use of health information technology. Privacy is of extraordinary importance, but it often arises in concert with other ethical issues, some of which are at least as important. In the previous section, for instance, I noted the role of patient consent for certain kinds of data uses. Privacy and informed consent are inextricably linked, and you could argue that consent is of greater importance because with it you can allow information to be shared and used widely. In any event, privacy occupies an important, if noisy, place in public debate and the law.

Foundations and Definitions

In many ways, everyone is a privacy advocate. (Do not let that label support the notion that those who apply it to themselves value privacy more than others.) People value privacy for many reasons, but the principle that governs the right to privacy is based on the following axiom: Information about an individual should (generally) be controlled by that individual. Your credit card debt, magazine subscriptions, and HIV status are for you to disclose—or not. We live our lives under the presumption that our conversations are not eavesdropped, our friends and lovers not scrutinized, our doctors and nurses able to keep a confidence. Indeed, it has been suggested that without a justified expectation of privacy, we could not live a normal life. Privacy is essential to nothing less than the way we live our lives.

The terms "privacy" and "confidentiality" are not synonymous, although they are often used as if they were interchangeable. It is best to make the following distinction: confidentiality applies to information ("the lab results are confidential"), where privacy pertains to people ("she lived a private life"). Privacy also is used to refer to people's concerns about and desires for confidentiality ("I'm worried they won't protect my privacy") and so is a broader term, often implying the other.

Health information can be exceptionally important and sensitive, and it enjoys special status in most cultures. There are several reasons for this. One is that patients are often thought of as vulnerable, and so their information deserves special status. Another is that health information is a source of bias and discrimination more frequently than other personal information.

It follows from this that there are two overarching reasons why privacy and confidentiality matter. The first relies on the duty-based approach in which individuals are entitled to control disclosure of their healthcare information no matter what the consequences or lack of consequences. That means it does not matter what the information is about—stubbed toe or schizophrenia, hair loss or HIV—the patient gets to decide because the information is about them. The second reason leads to the same conclusion but via a different route. This approach depends on consequences and includes the fact that patients are unlikely to tell their nurses or doctors the truth if privacy cannot be secured. On this account, privacy and confidentiality are very practical matters—better healthcare results from their protection. These two approaches are based on the ethical foundations reviewed in the section "Tools for Ethical Analysis." They both give the same answer: protect privacy and confidentiality by giving patients control over their information.

That control is not absolute. There are circumstances in which confidentiality, say, is less important than public health, which has duties of its own. (The threat posed by a patient with infectious tuberculosis is greater than the benefit gained by protecting his confidentiality.) Also, as you have seen, there are many circumstances in which we have good reason to presume that a rational person would permit use of personal information without explicit consent.[11] Contemporary debates over privacy and confidentiality are often shaped by arguments about privacy and competing duties and when and whether explicit consent is necessary.

 HIT PRO EXAM TIP   Note the distinction between ethical and legal reasons for protecting privacy.

HIPAA

Making credible public policy out of these ethical foundations is a large challenge. Until 2003, which was the effective date of the Privacy Rule under the Health Insurance Portability and Accountability Act (HIPAA),[12] health privacy in the United States was governed by a separate law for each state. This was widely agreed to be untenable, given the widespread transmission of health data across state lines. Most such data exchange was for insurance purposes, but it was clear that in an increasingly paperless world, something more was required to protect privacy rights related to digitized health information. While HIPAA is addressed in detail in Chapter 13, this law can illustrate some of the ethical standards that undergird the appropriate use of health information technology.

Right of Access

You have already encountered the ethical rule that individuals have the right to control their health information. Under HIPAA's Privacy Rule, all individuals have a "right of access" that includes the right to look at and get a copy of their health records. While there are exceptions to this (psychotherapy notes, for instance), the idea is that such access should be easy. One could argue that it should be very easy, but many institutions do not make it so. An institution with a functioning electronic health record should be able to make a copy on a compact disc or even e-mail an authenticated patient the record. There is no good legal or ethical reason not to do so.

The law says institutions may require that patients put their requests in writing. It even permits denials under certain circumstances, including the fear that the information is likely to harm the requester or someone else. But even in these cases, the institution must provide an opportunity to appeal.

What is interesting to note here is how difficult it can be for a law simultaneously to ensure respect for a right and to anticipate and manage future circumstances in which there might be good reasons for exceptions.

Public Health and Law Enforcement

While you have already considered ethical issues in public health informatics, it is worth underscoring that the federal Privacy Rule permits applicable institutions (covered entities under HIPAA) to divulge patient information (protected health information) to public health as well as law enforcement authorities. The reasons why this has to be the case are based on a number of values, all of which should be undisputed.

- Individual rights are not always more important than collective welfare.
- Solidarity can be as important as autonomy.
- Civil society must find ways to strike a balance between the rights of individuals and groups.

Another way of putting this is that privacy is not absolute. Indeed, public health has long thrived on the presumed consent of those it benefits. Further, many public health tasks can be accomplished without the identification of individual people. As a matter of policy, this means that those "privacy advocates" who insist that individual consent is required for all uses of personal health information are mistaken. When a reasoned or ethically optimized policy is being crafted, or is evolving, it is important that zealotry not be confused with advocacy.

HIT PRO EXAM TIP   It is and should be very difficult to justify impediments for ordinary public health work, especially when the identity of individual patients is not known.

HIPAA and Institutional Ethics

The federal Privacy Rule is imperfect in many ways. Most if not all laws could use improvement. This is just a feature of governance in open societies. What is striking about HIPAA in this regard is how often it is invoked, blamed, or cited as an impediment when in fact it is innocent. Over the years, it has been alleged that HIPAA forbids the use of e-mail containing patient information, does not allow guardians or other personal representatives to access patient information, and bans uttering patient names out loud in clinics. All are false, but it is interesting to observe how willing some people are to over- and misinterpret the law.

While a sociological analysis is probably required to determine the reasons for this, we might hypothesize it is somehow related to the stance many institutions have taken to HIPAA from the outset. That is, because it is a law, HIPAA has been seen more as a compliance issue than an ethical one. One might have hoped that privacy protection, an ancient and patient-centered value, would become an assignment for institutional ethics committees—committees whose responsibilities include drafting ethics-related policies. Instead, HIPAA policies at most institutions have been under the purview of compliance offices, risk managers, and general counsel.

One could argue that this is a sad surrender to liability fears more than a celebration of patient rights. While the inclination of institutions to embrace risk-averse policies is probably understandable, we might surmise that it would also be risk averse to signal a commitment to patient rights by adopting high-quality education programs and deploying standard ethics mechanisms to serve the goal of privacy protection in an increasingly wired and wireless world.

Special Challenges

In this section, I review some of the ethical issues that arise in concert with evolving health information technologies. These are not analyses but observations intended to make the point that professionals working in health information technology have a full and tasty plate of issues to address, study, and make part of their professional lives.

Genetics and Bioinformatics

In the future, all genetic information will be stored electronically. We will look back on an era of biobanks and blood spots as quaint, if not primitive. Moreover, genomic information will have become a standard component of the electronic health record. While "genethics" has been part of the standard bioethics curriculum for decades, comparatively little attention has been paid to issues raised when, say, data-mining software is used to analyze genetic data sets or patients themselves acquire tools to query their own genomes. Those issues include dramatically increased numbers of "incidental findings" (information acquired without intent or preparation) and challenges arising at the intersection of probabilistic data and lower-than-optimal health literacy. Institutions will need to adopt new standards and policies to govern bioinformatics research and the ways probabilistic genomic information is applied to patient care. Well-known problems related to the fact that family members share many genetic traits and risks will be amplified when all records are digitized and easily available.

Documentation

While we live under a paperless imperative, the electronic health record has already given rise to some unanticipated problems. One of these is related to documentation. Many institutions have observed the phenomenon of clinicians using—or overusing—copy-and-paste functions to write progress notes and consultation reports. This has led in some cases to a rapid and distracting bloating of the electronic record, which in turn makes it more difficult to review the record to find salient information. This of course undermines one of the core benefits of the electronic record in the first place. It also has had the effect of immortalizing errors made earlier in documenting care of a patient. The problem of appropriate use of specific functions will require thoughtful analysis and corresponding institutional policies. In the meantime, some institutions have responded by preventing the use of copy-and-paste functions.

Interactions with Industry

Health information technology is an industry-driven enterprise. While academic medical centers do research and offer education in biomedical and health informatics, hospital and practice applications are developed and made by a number of corporations. While this is similar in some respects to the pharmaceutical and medical device industries, health information technology vendors sponsor comparatively little academic research, and they are not regulated by the government. While the pharmaceutical and device industries have been the subject of a great deal of debate and commentary, health information technology vendors have for the most part not enjoyed similar deliberation, despite some controversy.[13] The questions of whether and to what extent vendors should be regulated are large, complex, and subject to intense debate. What should cause no disagreement, however, are observations about the ethical duties of any entity that develops, manufactures, and sells electronic health records and other systems. They include that there should be no restrictions on users communicating about bugs and system improvements, that various systems be available for some degree of public and head-to-head research studies, and that vendors not provide payments for referrals and endorsements. A patient-centered stance would counsel that electronic health records be vetted and analyzed with an eye to quality and safety as much as to intellectual property and other business interests.

Social Networking and the Web

As patients increasingly live online, so does the part of their lives pertaining to health and medicine. From chat rooms and social media sites to web-based advice and online diagnostic toys, the twenty-first century is reshaping the way information is assembled, shared, and used. It is also reshaping the way misinformation is assembled, shared, and used. You learned earlier that many patients are made vulnerable by their maladies. Alas, vulnerability can mutate into gullibility on the Web. I can conclude the discussion here with an unremarkable endorsement of that suite of core values mentioned at the outset. Veracity (tell the truth), transparency (don't hide what a reasonable person would need to know to make a decision), and accountability (take responsibility for your actions) are solid guideposts for those who would give or seek solace or advice in networked communities. Those who give advice have extra responsibilities; first among these is to ensure that they are competent to do so. More importantly, they have the obligation to ensure that the context and medium are appropriate. For clinicians, the online world is only sometimes and perhaps rarely a safe place to practice a patient-centered profession that relies so much on touch, trust, and honest communication.

Chapter Review

Health information technology is an exciting but too-often-neglected source of ethical issues. The necessary and now inevitable conversion of all health data to electronic media means that those issues will increase in importance—and hence that health IT professionals will have a corresponding duty to be familiar with these issues and be able to address them.

In this chapter, I reviewed the foundations of ethical reasoning, with special regard to health information technology; used the concepts of "appropriate uses" and "appropriate users" to introduce ethical challenges that arise in the use of decision-support systems and electronic health records and in research, including outcomes research; and gave an ethical overview of the importance and limitations of privacy protection.

I also provided brief overviews of several "special challenges," in part to underscore the point that ethics should be seen as an ubiquitous and practical tool for all professionals who have the opportunity to work in such an exciting and promising new field.

Questions

To test your comprehension of the chapter, answer the following questions and then check your answers against the list of correct answers at the end of the chapter.

1. Which of the following is not among or related to the sources of healthcare professionals' duties?

   A. Patient vulnerability

   B. Clinician-patient power differential

    C. HIPAA's Privacy Rule

    D. Veracity

2. Which of the following contributes to a clinician being an appropriate user of a decision-support system?

    A. MD or ARNP certification

    B. Education in use of the system

    C. Obtaining patient consent for diagnosis

    D. Waiver of liability for missed differential diagnosis

3. Which of the following is not a good ethical reason to protect privacy?

    A. HIPAA requires covered entities to protect patient privacy.

    B. Patients have a right to control access to their information.

    C. Health outcomes are improved if patients trust that their information will be safeguarded.

    D. Patients have a reasonable presumption that their information will be protected.

4. Which of the following is the best reason to analyze anonymized patient records for public health without individual consent?

    A. Patients care and know little about epidemiology.

    B. Informed consent creates an insurmountable cost burden.

    C. There is too little time to get consent in public health emergencies.

    D. Patient rights must be balanced against the common good.

5. Which of the following values is of least importance in governing online health communication?

    A. Copyright protection

    B. Accountability

    C. Transparency

    D. Trust

Answers

1. **C.** While HIPAA is an important law that codifies standards for protecting patient privacy, the law itself is not an ethical element of healthcare professionalism. The others are.

2. **B.** An appropriate user is always one trained or educated in the use of a tool.

3. **A.** While HIPAA requires privacy protection, it is a legal and not an ethical requirement. The other answers are based on ethics.

4. **D.** Privacy is not absolute, and public health, or the needs of communities, sometimes take precedence.

5. **A.** Copyright protection is of importance to those who make their intellectual property available, but unlike the others, it is not a value that should govern online health interactions.

References

1. Medical professionalism in the new millennium: A physician charter. (2004). Accessed on July 13, 2012 from www.abimfoundation.org/Professionalism/~/media/Files/Physician%20Charter.ashx.

2. Code of ethics for nurses with interpretive statements. (2001). Accessed on July 13, 2012 from http://nursingworld.org/MainMenuCategories/EthicsStandards/CodeofEthicsforNurses/Code-of-Ethics.pdf.

3. Goodman, K. W., Adams, S., Berner, E. S., Embi, P. J., Hsiung, R., Hurdle, J., Jones, D. A., Lehmann, C. U., Maulden, S., Petersen, C., Terrazas, E., and Winkelstein, P. (2012). AMIA's code of professional and ethical conduct. *Journal of the American Medical Informatics Association.* Accessed on September 9, 2012 from http://jamia.bmj.com/content/early/2012/06/24/amiajnl-2012-001035.full

4. IMIA code of ethics for health information professionals. (2002, 2011). Accessed on July 13, 2012, from www.imia-medinfo.org/new2/node/39.

5. Gert, B.; Culver, C. M.; and Clouser, K. D. (2006). *Bioethics: A systematic approach, second edition.* Oxford University Press.

6. Miller, R. A.; Schaffner, K. F.; and Meisel, A. (1985). Ethical and legal issues related to the use of computer programs in clinical medicine. *Annals of Internal Medicine; 102,* 529–536.

7. Miller, R.A. (1990). Why the standard view is standard: People, not machines, understand patients' problems. *Journal of Medicine and Philosophy, 15,* 581–591.

8. Rethinking the power and potential of personal health records. Accessed on July 14, 2012, from www.projecthealthdesign.org/home.

9. Cushman, R.; Froomkin, A. M.; Cava, A.; Abril, P.; and Goodman, K. W. (2010). Ethical, legal and social issues for personal health records and applications. *Journal of Biomedical Informatics, 43,* S51–S55.

10. Massoudi, B. L.; Goodman, K. W.; Gotham, I. J.; Holmes, J. H.; Lang, L.; Miner, K.; Potenziani, D. D.; Richards, J.; Turner, A. M.; and Fu, P. C. (2012). An informatics agenda for public health: Summarized recommendations from the 2011 AMIA PHI Conference. *Journal of the American Medical Informatics Association, 19,* 688–695.

11. Goodman, K. W. (2010). Ethics, information technology and public health: New challenges for the clinician-patient relationship. *Journal of Law, Medicine and Ethics, 38,* 58–63.

12. Health information privacy. (2012). Accessed on July 14, 2012, from www.hhs. gov/ocr/privacy/index.html.

13. Goodman, K. W.; Berner, E. S.; Dente, M. A.; Kaplan, B.; Koppel, R.; Rucker, D.; Sands, D. Z.; and Winkelstein, P. (2011). Challenges in ethics, safety, best practices, and oversight regarding HIT vendors, their customers, and patients: A report of an AMIA special task force. *Journal of the American Medical Informatics Association, 18,* 77–81.

The Role of Information Technology in Healthcare

Janet M. Marchibroda with David deBronkart*

In this chapter, you will learn how to

- Describe how healthcare information technology (IT) improves the quality, safety, and efficiency of care
- Describe the key components of the electronic health record (EHR)
- Discuss the benefits and current adoption rates of EHRs among physicians and hospitals
- Discuss barriers to EHR adoption for both physicians and hospitals
- Explain how federal programs address many of the barriers to EHR adoption
- Describe the benefits of health information exchange and current levels of adoption
- Discuss the barriers to health information exchange
- Explain how federal programs are promoting and supporting health information exchange
- Describe the different types of electronic tools used by consumers and patients to help them navigate their health and healthcare and their benefits
- Describe the barriers to adoption of consumer-facing electronic tools among both consumers and providers
- Explore how current drivers in the healthcare system are likely to impact the adoption and evolution of EHRs, health information exchange, and consumer-facing applications in the future

Concerns about rising costs and uneven quality in the U.S. healthcare system have spurred significant interest in and adoption of healthcare IT as a foundational component of efforts designed to improve health, improve healthcare, and reduce the cost of

---

* David deBronkart contributed to the section "Engaging Consumers Using Electronic Tools."

care. A considerable amount of research supports the positive impact that healthcare IT has on healthcare-related outcomes.

A recent comprehensive review of the literature indicates that 92 percent of the more than 150 articles recently published on healthcare IT reached conclusions that were positive overall, citing positive results in areas related to efficiency of care, effectiveness of care, provider satisfaction, patient safety, and patient satisfaction.[1]

Healthcare IT enables clinicians, nurses, care managers, and other providers who care for patients—as well as patients themselves—to have access to information about both the patient and what constitutes optimal care in order to support clinical decision making at the point of care and in between visits. A majority of the investment in healthcare IT in the United States to date has been made in applications that support the delivery of care by clinicians, hospitals, and other healthcare providers. These applications are ordinarily referred to as *electronic health records*.

Healthcare IT also enables the exchange of data across the settings in which patients receive care. Because of the fragmented nature of the U.S. healthcare system, information about the patient resides within the range of settings in which healthcare and services are delivered, including physician practices, hospitals, laboratories, pharmacies, health plans, and even patients themselves. Mobilizing this information through health information exchange enables those who care for patients—as well as patients themselves—to have access to important information about the patient, regardless of where it is located.

Finally, healthcare IT enables consumers and patients to more effectively manage their health and healthcare by offering online educational resources, tracking and self-monitoring tools, easy access to their health records across the range of settings where they receive care, and even secure modes of communication to connect with their clinicians between visits.

This chapter will explore the role of IT in each of these three areas: bringing information to clinicians and other care providers to support the delivery of care through the use of EHRs; through health information exchange, mobilizing information that resides across the many settings in which individuals receive care and services; and utilizing online and electronic tools to support consumers as they manage their health and healthcare.

A fourth area in which healthcare IT plays a critical role in improving the quality, safety, and cost-effectiveness of care is that which relates to the analysis of electronic data to support improvements in the health of populations. Healthcare IT enables healthcare organizations to access and analyze electronic health information to monitor performance, identify opportunities for improvement, and take actions to improve outcomes in cost, quality, and patient satisfaction.

The analysis of large electronic data sets also supports other population health goals, including accelerating research on the effectiveness of various treatments on health outcomes, monitoring the safety of medical products such as medical devices and pharmaceuticals, identifying new therapies designed to battle deadly diseases such as cancer, and monitoring and responding to public health threats. A more detailed description of these other uses of IT to improve health and healthcare at the population level are addressed in Chapters 7 and 8.

An Overview of Electronic Health Records and Their Use by Physicians and Hospitals Across the United States

Historically, electronic health records have been the cornerstone of HIT-related efforts focused on improving health and healthcare. Over the last several years, the adoption of EHRs has steadily grown but still remains fairly low. EHRs enable clinicians, hospitals, and other providers to have access to important information about the patient, as well as clinical decision support, both of which assist with the delivery of higher-quality, more cost-effective care. EHRs enable clinical alerts and reminders that help clinicians avoid drug interactions that can cause harm and reduce both gaps and duplications in care.

A review of EHRs used both in physician practices and in hospitals, current adoption rates, key challenges associated with adoption, and federal programs designed to address such challenges, is provided in the following sections.

Physician Use of Electronic Health Records

Physician use of EHRs has grown steadily in the United States over the past several years. Adoption of a "basic" EHR among office-based physicians has nearly tripled in the last five years, from 11.8 percent in 2007 to 33.9 percent in 2011.[2]

A "basic" EHR is defined as one that includes basic features such as the following:

- Patient history and demographics
- Patient problem list
- Physician clinical notes
- Comprehensive lists of medications and allergies
- Computerized orders for prescriptions
- The ability to view laboratory and imaging results electronically

Adoption of "any EMR/EHR system," which is a medical or health record system that is all or partially electronic, grew from 34.8 percent in 2007 to 57 percent in 2011.

EHR adoption among physicians varies by specialty status, physician age, and practice size. Primary-care physicians are more likely to adopt EHRs than nonprimary-care specialists, older physicians (55 and older) are less likely to adopt EHRs than their younger counterparts, and physicians in small (one to two providers) practices are less likely to adopt than those who deliver care in larger practices.[3]

Commonly cited barriers to EHR adoption among physicians include lack of access to capital to support purchase of systems; uncertainty about the return on investment; lack of capacity to evaluate, select, and install such systems; concerns that the systems will become obsolete; worries about privacy and security protections; and lack of a trained workforce to assist with implementation.[4, 5, 6]

TIP EHR user satisfaction is higher among individuals who have participated in the selection of their EHR system versus those who have not.[7]

Hospital Use of Electronic Health Records

Adoption of EHRs among hospitals has also experienced steady growth, but similar to adoption rates of physicians, adoption rates among hospitals continue to be fairly low. Eighteen percent of hospitals had a "basic" EHR system in place in 2011, up from 11.5 percent the previous year; while the percentage of hospitals that had a "comprehensive" EHR system increased from 3.6 percent in 2010 to 8.7 percent in 2011.[8]

A "basic" system is defined as full implementation of the following technologies in at least one clinical unit of the hospital:

- Computerized systems for patient demographics
- Physician notes
- Nursing assessments
- Patient problem lists
- Laboratory and radiologic reports
- Diagnostic test results
- Order entry for medications[5]

On the other hand, a "comprehensive" EHR system includes all of the functions that a basic system can perform and 14 additional functions. In addition, to meet the comprehensive definition, all functions must be present in all major clinical units in the hospitals.[5]

EHR adoption rates are not the same across all hospitals. Small, nonteaching, and rural hospitals tend to adopt EHRs more slowly than other hospitals.[7] Barriers to adoption among all hospitals are similar to those cited for physicians and are generally more pronounced in smaller or rural systems. They include lack of capital for up-front costs, concerns about the ongoing costs of maintaining and upgrading systems, physician resistance, and lack of a trained workforce to assist with implementation.[8]

 TIP Overall EHR user satisfaction is highly correlated with the length of training. At least three to five days of EHR training is necessary to achieve the highest level of overall satisfaction.[9]

Federal Programs Designed to Address Barriers to EHR Adoption

The Health Information Technology and Economic and Clinical Health (HITECH) Act of 2009 brought an unprecedented and significant amount of investment to accelerate the adoption of healthcare IT to support improvements in the quality, safety, and efficiency of care. A majority of the $30 billion investment is in the form of incentive payments through the Centers for Medicare and Medicaid Services (CMS) Medicare and Medicaid EHR Incentive Programs.[10] Informally known as *meaningful use*, the programs provide financial incentives to eligible professionals and hospitals when they use certified EHR technology in specific meaningful ways to improve quality, safety, and efficiency.

To qualify for incentive payments, eligible professionals and hospitals must meet certain "core" objectives and also meet a small number of objectives selected from a "menu" set.

Table 4-1 summarizes the core and menu objectives associated with the first stage of the CMS Medicare and Medicaid EHR Incentive Programs.

Objective	Hospitals	Eligible Professionals (EPs)
CORE OBJECTIVES		
1. Use computerized physician order entry (CPOE) for medication orders.	X	X
2. Implement drug-drug and drug-allergy interaction checks.	X	X
3. Maintain an up-to-date problem list of current and active diagnoses.	X	X
4. Generate and transmit permissible prescriptions electronically (*eprescribing*).		X
5. Maintain active medication list.	X	X
6. Maintain active medication allergy list.	X	X
7. Record demographics: preferred language, gender, race, ethnicity, date of birth, and, for hospitals, date and preliminary cause of death.	X	X
8. Record and chart changes in vital signs: height, weight, blood pressure, body mass index, growth charts for children.	X	X
9. Record smoking status for patients 13 years old or older.	X	X
10. Report clinical quality measures to CMS (or in the case of Medicaid, the states).	X	X
11. Implement one clinical decision support rule (along with ability to track compliance with that rule).	X	X
12. Provide patients with an electronic copy of their health information (including diagnostic test results, problem list, medication lists, and medication allergies, as well as discharge summary and procedures for hospitals) upon request.	X	X

Table 4-1   Core and Menu Objectives for Stage 1 CMS Medicare and Medicaid EHR Incentive Programs[11,12]

Objective	Hospitals	Eligible Professionals (EPs)
CORE OBJECTIVES		
13. Provide patients with an electronic copy of their discharge instructions at time of discharge, upon request.	X	
14. Provide clinical summaries for patients for each office visit.		X
15. Capability to exchange key clinical information (for example, problem list, medication list, medication allergies, and diagnostic test results) among providers of care and patient-authorized entities electronically.	X	X
16. Protect electronic health information created or maintained by the certified EHR technology through the implementation of appropriate technical capabilities.	X	X
MENU OBJECTIVES		
17. Implement drug formulary checks.	X	X
18. Record advance directives for patients 65 or older.	X	
19. Incorporate clinical lab test results into EHR as structured data.	X	X
20. Generate lists of patients by specific conditions to use for quality improvement, reduction of disparities, research, or outreach.	X	X
21. Send patient reminders per patient preference for preventive/follow-up care.		X
22. Provide patients with timely electronic access to their health information (including lab results, problem list, medication lists, and allergies).		X
23. Use certified EHR technology to identify patient-specific education resources and provide those resources to the patient if appropriate.	X	X
24. The EP or hospital or critical access hospital (CAH) that receives a patient from another setting of care or provider of care or believes an encounter is relevant should perform medication reconciliation.	X	X
25. The EP or hospital or CAH that transitions their patient to another setting of care or provider of care or refers their patient to another provider of care should provide a summary care record for each transition of care or referral.	X	X
26. Capability to submit electronic data to immunization registries or immunization information systems and actual submission according to applicable law and practice.	X	X

Table 4-1 Core and Menu Objectives for Stage 1 CMS Medicare and Medicaid EHR Incentive Programs[11, 12] *(continued)*

Objective	Hospitals	Eligible Professionals (EPs)
MENU OBJECTIVES		
27. Capability to submit electronic data on reportable (as required by state or local law) lab results to public health agencies and actual submission according to applicable law and practice.	X	
28. Capability to submit electronic syndromic surveillance data to public health agencies and actual submission according to applicable law and practice.	X	X

Table 4-1 Core and Menu Objectives for Stage 1 CMS Medicare and Medicaid EHR Incentive Programs[11,12] (continued)

A total of $6.2 billion has been made through the CMS Medicare and Medicaid EHR Incentive Programs through June 30, 2012, $2.2 billion of which was paid to approximately 119,000 eligible professionals and the remaining $4 billion of which was paid to about 3,400 hospitals.[13]

The remaining $2 billion in funds authorized by HITECH have been devoted to programs and activities led by the Office of the National Coordinator for Health Information Technology (ONC) to address other key barriers to the adoption and meaningful use of healthcare IT to support higher-quality, safer, more cost-effective care, including the need for implementation assistance, the need for workforce training, and the need for standards and certification processes to provide assurance (Table 4-2).

Barrier	HITECH Program	Funding Amount
Lack of financing or a business case for adoption	Medicare and Medicaid EHR Incentive Programs	Up to $27 billion[14]
Lack of capacity to evaluate, select, and implement a system	Regional Extension Center Program	$677 million[15]
Lack of a trained workforce to support implementation	Workforce Development Programs	$118 million[16]
Concerns about systems becoming obsolete Concerns about the lack of interoperability across EHR systems	Standards and Certification Program	$64 million[17]
Concerns about lack of infrastructure for exchange	State Health Information Exchange Cooperative Agreement Program	$547 million[18]
Concerns about privacy and security protections	Office of the Chief Privacy Officer[19]	n/a

Table 4-2 Ways in Which HITECH Programs Address Barriers to EHR Adoption, Meaningful Use, and Health Information Exchange

TIP IT professionals will be expected to understand the purpose and context associated with key elements of the EHR. They will also be expected to understand the requirements of meaningful use.

An Overview of Methods to Electronically Exchange Data Across Settings

The U.S. healthcare system is highly fragmented, with care and services for an individual patient being delivered across a diverse range of settings that can include primary-care clinician practices, specialists' offices, hospitals, laboratories, pharmacies, acute-care clinics, and long-term care settings. An average Medicare beneficiary has more than 15 visits annually and sees 6.4 unique physicians in a year.[20]

In addition, an individual might also capture information at home that is relevant to the health record that is used for care, such as blood pressure readings for patients with hypertension or blood glucose level readings for patients with diabetes. With the use of remote-monitoring devices and mobile technology, increasingly these readings can be transmitted automatically to the patient record and utilized by a care management team to identify trends and issues that require intervention.

High-quality, cost-effective care requires the coordination of care and sharing of information about the patient, across the many settings where care is delivered and tests are performed. Traditionally, this information has been shared using mail, phone, or fax, and in many cases, this information is not shared at all, resulting in the repeat of tests—which can be costly—or in less than optimal care. Primary-care clinicians report that missing clinical information is common, consumes time and other resources, and may adversely affect patients.[21]

The electronic sharing of information—often referred to as *health information exchange*—enables the team of doctors, nurses, and other professionals who care for an individual patient to have access to information about the patient, such as the results of lab or imaging tests performed, prescribed medications, previous diagnoses, allergies, and other information to support higher-quality, safer, effective, and evidence-based care.

While the electronic exchange of information plays a critical role in supporting higher-quality, cost-effective care, the level of health information exchange across the United States today is extremely low. Only 19 percent of hospitals are currently exchanging clinical record information electronically with providers outside of their health system.[22] Very few physicians are electronically exchanging information with other settings outside of their practices. One study indicates that 73 percent of the time, primary-care providers do not receive discharge information from hospitals within two days of their patients' discharge, and when they are sent, they are rarely shared electronically.[23] Data types considered by practicing clinicians to be very important or essential for clinical decision making associated with transitions of care include relevant imaging test results, laboratory test results, and medications.[24]

Physicians perceive benefits in health information exchange. One study indicated that 86 percent of physicians perceive that health information exchange will have a very positive or somewhat positive impact on improving the quality of patient care, and 71 percent perceive a similarly positive impact on reducing healthcare costs.[25] Studies have also shown that health information exchange does reduce costs.[26]

To date, health information exchange has been facilitated by a wide variety of publicly and privately funded health information exchange organizations. One industry study validated 228 health information exchange efforts, 67 of which were primarily funded and governed by government entities and 161 of which were primarily governed and funded by private sponsoring entities.[27] Another recent study identified 179 U.S.-based regional health information organizations, 75 of which were operational.[28] A majority of these efforts have experienced challenges with securing funding and achieving financial sustainability.

Barriers to health information exchange are well documented. The most significant barrier to exchange is the lack of a business case. The predominant method of payment in the U.S. healthcare system today provides reimbursement for the number of visits, tests, or procedures performed, as opposed to rewarding outcomes in quality or cost. As a result, there is little incentive for providers to access information that resides in another setting, to reduce duplicative tests or procedures, or otherwise to improve the quality or cost of care.[29]

Two current developments are likely to create the business case for health information exchange. Driven by significant pressures to reduce cost and improve quality, new models of care delivery and payment are now rapidly emerging, sponsored by the federal government, states, and private-sector providers and health plans. These models are taking many forms but share common attributes, including increased focus on accountability and coordination of care and payment that is increasingly based on outcomes in cost and quality as opposed to volume.[29] Achievement of the goals of these new models of care will require clinicians and other members of the care team to have access to information about the patient from the various settings in which care and services are delivered, which will necessarily be facilitated by health information exchange.

In addition, while there were limited requirements for health information exchange under the first stage of the CMS Medicare and Medicaid EHR Incentive Programs, the second stage, which is projected to go into effect in 2014, is expected to have more robust requirements for the electronic exchange of information—using standards—to support transitions of care.[30]

Other barriers include the lack of standards adoption and interoperability and lack of access to infrastructure to support exchange.[29,31] Continued concerns about privacy and security have also been cited as a key barrier.[25]

Concurrent with the release of rules for the CMS Medicare and Medicaid EHR Incentive Programs, ONC also releases federal rules on the standards and certification criteria required for the "certified EHR technology" that must be used for providers to qualify for such incentives. Rules released for stage 1 of the meaningful use program included an initial set of standards to promote the interoperability of EHR systems, including data content standards associated with laboratory test results, medications, problems, and procedures.[32] Additional standards to promote interoperability of systems and health information exchange are expected to be released as part of the final rules associated with stage 2 of meaningful use.[30]

In addition to providing financial incentives, adopting standards for interoperability, and promoting compliance with such standards through a certification program, the federal government has also taken other steps to promote health information exchange. Through the State Health Information Exchange Cooperative Agreement Program, ONC awarded approximately $547 million to 56 states, eligible territories, and qualified state-designated entities to support the development of capabilities for exchange.[18] Several initiatives have also been launched by the Department of Health and Human Services to develop new policies and clarify existing policies associated with privacy and security.[19]

As expectations regarding the use of interoperable systems and the electronic exchange of information across settings continue to grow, IT professionals will be expected to be familiar with standards that promote interoperability across systems and the various methods and infrastructure that will support health information exchange.

Engaging Consumers Using Electronic Tools

A wide range of online, electronic, and mobile tools are now available to help consumers manage their health and healthcare. Despite that the Internet plays a significant role in many other aspects of American life, including how people manage their finances, shop for goods and services, and even work, consumer usage of online and electronic applications to support their health and healthcare has yet to become mainstream. As the healthcare system itself becomes more digitized, it is anticipated that the usage of consumer-facing applications will also accelerate.

Consumer-facing tools fall into three primary categories.

- Those supporting individual patient education, self-care, and peer support
- Those supporting both the information and transaction needs associated with care delivery
- Those supporting the actual delivery of care[33]

An overview of electronic tools in each of these areas, along with current adoption rates and barriers to adoption, is explored in more detail in the following sections.

Electronic Tools Supporting Patient Education and Self-Care

The number of consumers in the United States who have used online or electronic tools to support their informational needs in healthcare is high. According to a recent survey, 80 percent of Internet users have looked online for information about any of 15 health topics such as a specific disease or treatment.[34] In 2011, 17 percent of mobile users were using their devices to look up health and medical information.[34]

Increasingly, consumers are using online and electronic tools for self-monitoring and tracking. For example, 20 percent of adults have tracked their weight, diet, exercise routine, or some other health indicators or symptoms online.[34] Forty-two percent of consumers would be interested in using a web site, program, or application to track information about their chronic illness.[35]

As the availability of and interest in social media and other applications that enable online dialogue has increased considerably, so has the use of such tools for health and healthcare. Online communities among patients and caregivers who share similar illnesses or experiences have increased in popularity. One study indicates that 4 percent of adults have posted comments, questions, or information about health or medical issues.[34] One example of a peer support and information-sharing community is Patients Like Me, an online community of more than 157,000 patients with Amyotrophic Lateral Sclerosis (ALS), Multiple Sclerosis (MS), and several other conditions, who share not only their experiences and advice with one another but also information about their health status, including reactions to various therapies. This information is helpful not only to their peers; it can also augment traditional sources of input to the effectiveness and safety of treatments and other interventions.

Electronic Tools Supporting Patient Information and Transaction Needs Associated with Care Delivery

Personal health records (PHRs) enable consumers to both input and aggregate information about themselves, including information derived from a variety of sources, including health plans and the various clinicians, hospitals, and other providers from which they receive care. PHRs have been in existence for some time, but uptake has not been significant, with current estimates ranging anywhere from 7 percent to 11 percent.[35, 36, 37]

TIP Many believe that the slow uptake of PHRs is related to the limited ability to access and download health information that resides within the EHR of the physician or hospital from which they have received care. As a result, PHRs are for the most part "empty vessels" and therefore not very useful; they must be populated manually, which is tedious and requires sustained effort. Other barriers to PHR adoption include lack of awareness of the availability of such tools, concerns about privacy and security, and limited access to such tools, which can take the form of limited access to the Internet, limited computer literacy or computer skills, or unmet technical or information support needs.[33, 35, 38]

Physician practices, hospitals, and other providers are beginning to enable patients to view—and in some cases—download information about their care from the EHR, including lab test results, images, medications prescribed, care summaries, and follow-up needed, as well as appointments. Both the current availability and the adoption of these services by providers are limited, despite increasing demand from consumers. While 57 percent of PHR users believe that reviewing test results online would be useful, only 6 percent of consumers have actually done so.[35] This low level of adoption is likely because of the lack of adoption of these services among providers.

The significant increase in the use of mobile technology generally is expected to further increase demand for health information from consumers. Fifty-two percent of consumers say that they would use a smartphone, tablet, or other handheld device to monitor their health if they were able to access their medical records and download information about their medical condition and treatments.[36]

Physicians and hospitals are also beginning to enable patients to conduct certain transactions online, including scheduling appointments and renewing prescriptions, but again, uptake among providers has been slow. While 48 percent of PHR users believe that scheduling a doctor visit online would be useful, hardly any consumers are able to do so today.[35] Similarly, while 52 percent of PHR users believe that renewing prescriptions online would be useful, only 15 percent of consumers have actually done so.[35]

Why aren't physician practices and hospitals offering consumer-facing applications if their patients see value in these tools? One of the most obvious reasons is that most physicians and hospitals have not yet adopted EHRs, which are a precursor to offering consumer-facing applications. Physicians in particular are concerned about the "business case" for such offerings, with 63 percent of physicians citing the lack of reimbursement for time spent installing and using such tools as a key barrier.[39] A majority of physicians also has concerns about being held liable for knowing all of the information contained in the PHR, as well as the level of privacy and security protections associated with these applications.[39]

The CMS Medicare and Medicaid EHR Incentive Programs currently require hospitals and clinicians to provide patients with an electronic copy of their health information.[11, 12] It is anticipated that future requirements will also likely include a patient's ability to view and download their information from the EHR.[30] Eligible professionals will also likely be required to send patients reminders for preventive and follow-up care.[30]

Use of Consumer-Facing Electronic Tools to Support Care Delivery

TIP Finally, clinicians and other healthcare providers are increasingly using online, electronic, and even mobile technology tools to support the actual delivery of care. This is taking many forms.

For example, the use of remote monitoring and telehealth to monitor and communicate with patients while in their homes is increasingly taking hold. Augmenting traditional office-based care with ongoing monitoring of patients through the use of medical devices that can check their conditions and automatically send information to the clinician or care management team—particularly for patients with chronic disease—can help identify flags or issues before they become serious and more costly to treat.

Remote monitoring has yet to take off in the United States, even though consumers and clinicians alike see value in their use. While 61 percent of consumers express interest in using a medical device that would enable them to check their conditions and send information to their doctors electronically through a computer or a cell phone,[36] only 6 percent of consumers have actually used a medical device that connects to a computer.[35] One of the primary barriers to the adoption of remote monitoring is again the predominant reimbursement model in healthcare today that rewards face-to-face visits and procedures, as opposed to virtual encounters and better outcomes.

With e-mail being one of the standard modes of communication for Internet users, *secure messaging* (e-mail between clinicians and patients using secure methods) is becoming more popular among patients, with positive results. Fifty percent of PHR users believe that e-mailing providers would be useful.[35] Research indicates that secure messaging between patients and their providers improves quality of care and outcomes.[38,40] Some clinicians worry about the volume of e-mails that would result from offering secure messaging services—an outcome that many organizations that offer such services today say is unfounded.[29]

One variation of secure messaging is the use of "reminders" for patients. Clinicians or other members of the care team can either securely e-mail or send text messages to remind the patient to come in for either a preventive measure or follow-up test that is needed, or they can remind the patient to refill a prescription. Forty-four percent of consumers believe that getting reminders for tests would be useful.[35]

While consumers perceive value in their clinicians using electronic methods of communication and research indicates that positive outcomes in quality and cost of care can result, there is very little uptake of these consumer-facing applications among clinicians today.

 TIP Many physicians are concerned about the workflow (and therefore cost and resource) impact of the asynchronous and unexpected arrival of outside information from patients.[33] There are also concerns about privacy and security protections related to such services.[39] Finally, for the most part, the current methods of reimbursement and payment in the U.S. healthcare system largely don't reward the usage of these tools or any positive outcomes in cost or quality that would result.

Looking Forward

The U.S. healthcare system is poised for significant change because of pressures associated with rising healthcare costs, uneven quality, and eroding coverage. Delivery system and payment reforms that promise to improve both the quality and the cost-effectiveness of care are rapidly emerging with leadership by both the public and private sectors. Such reforms rely on a strong information foundation that healthcare IT provides. EHRs must continue to adapt to the needs of these new models of care. The demand for robust health information exchange is expected to significantly increase. New delivery models and rewards based on outcomes in cost and quality will depend on—among other things—more activated, engaged, and informed patients, which can be supported by online and electronic tools.

Healthcare IT professionals of the future will need to be able to track rapid changes in healthcare delivery and payment and be able to adapt to address rapidly emerging demands that result from these changes. While the challenges are daunting, the opportunities are considerable. Healthcare IT has the potential of significantly advancing the transformation of the U.S. healthcare system to one that is less fragmented and more coordinated, accountable, and transparent; one that puts the patient in the center; and one that delivers higher-quality, more cost-effective care for all Americans.

Chapter Review

Information technology plays a significant role in improving the quality, safety, and efficiency of healthcare. Healthcare IT comes in many forms. This chapter described three types of healthcare IT that are predominantly used in the healthcare system today: healthcare IT utilized by clinicians, hospitals, and other providers to support the delivery of care (ordinarily referred to as *electronic health records*); methods by which health information is electronically exchanged across the settings where care and services are delivered (often referred to as *health information exchange*); and electronic tools utilized by consumers and patients to help them manage their health and healthcare.

In addition to a description of these three types of healthcare IT, the chapter provided an overview of benefits, current adoption rates, and barriers to adoption. It also described federal programs designed to address these barriers and offered tips for IT professionals.

Healthcare IT has the potential to lay the foundation for many of the activities that will support the transformation of the U.S. healthcare system to one that delivers higher-quality, safer, more cost-effective care for all Americans.

Questions

1. Which of the following is a benefit of electronic health records (EHRs)?

   A. Efficiency of care

   B. Effectiveness of care

   C. Patient satisfaction

   D. Provider satisfaction

   E. A and B

   F. All of the above

2. Which of the following is a significant driver for the use of EHRs?

   A. Rising healthcare costs

   B. Concerns about quality

   C. Concerns about coverage (access to health insurance)

   D. Concerns about inaccurate billing

   E. A and B

   F. All of the above

3. Which of the following is not a key barrier to EHR adoption among physicians?

   A. Concerns about privacy and security.

   B. Concerns about financing and ongoing business case.

   C. Concerns about the safety of healthcare IT products.

   D. Concerns about being able to evaluate, select, and implement a system.

   E. All of the above are barriers to EHR adoption among physicians.

4. Which of the following is not a key feature of a "basic" EHR system?

   A. Patient problem list.

   B. Physician clinical notes.

   C. Patient billing information.

   D. Patient history.

   E. Patient demographic information.

   F. Laboratory and imaging test results.

   G. List of medications.

   H. All of the above are key elements of a basic EHR system.

5. Which of the following is not a requirement of stage 1 of the CMS Medicare and Medicaid EHR Incentive Programs?

   A. Maintain an active medication list.

   B. Report clinical quality measures.

   C. Implement secure messaging.

   D. Record smoking status.

   E. All of the above are requirements of stage 1.

6. Which of the following is a commonly cited barrier to health information exchange?

   A. Lack of a business case for health information exchange

   B. Concerns about privacy and security

   C. Lack of an infrastructure for health information exchange

   D. A and B

   E. All of the above

7. Which of the following is demonstrated by more than 75 percent of all consumers?

   A. Have used a personal health record

   B. Have looked online for information about health topics

   C. Have used a social media site to share insights on their health or healthcare

   D. Have e-mailed their doctors

   E. A and B

   F. All of the above

8. Which of the following is not an electronic tool by which clinicians can engage consumers?

   A. Personal health record.

   B. Secure messaging.

   C. Practice management system.

   D. Physician web site and blog.

   E. All of the above represent electronic tools by which clinicians can engage consumers.

9. Which one of the following is a key barrier to physicians adopting electronic tools to support the engagement of consumers?

   A. Lack of reimbursement for time spent

   B. Concerns about privacy and security protections

   C. Concerns about liability

   D. A and B

   E. All of the above

10. Which of the following is a key barrier to consumers adopting electronic tools to connect with their clinicians and other providers?

    A. Concerns about privacy and security

    B. Inability to access a computer or the Internet

    C. Lack of electronic capability of their clinicians or other healthcare providers

    D. A and B

    E. All of the above

Answers

1. **F.** A comprehensive review of the literature indicates that healthcare IT has achieved positive results in all of the following areas: efficiency of care, effectiveness of care, provider satisfaction, patient safety, and patient satisfaction.

2. E. Concerns about rising healthcare costs and uneven quality have driven poli-cymakers to develop and implement laws that promote the use of healthcare IT, including EHRs. While there are also concerns about access to healthcare (insur-ance coverage) or fraud (inaccurate billing), EHRs have not been identified as a primary solution to these key issues.

3. C. Commonly cited barriers to EHR adoption among physicians are concerns about financing; privacy and security; and the capacity to evaluate, select, and implement a system. Concerns about the safety of healthcare IT products has not emerged as a primary barrier to adoption among physicians. On the contrary, evidence indicates that overall healthcare IT has a positive impact on safety by providing clinicians with information that helps them avoid medical errors.

4. C. A "basic" EHR is defined as one that includes basic features, such as patient history and demographics, patient problem list, physician clinical notes, comprehensive lists of medications and allergies, computerized orders for pre-scriptions, and the ability to view laboratory and imaging results electronically. Patient billing information is a common feature or component of a practice management system but not of an EHR.

5. C. Maintaining an active medication list, reporting clinical quality measures, and recording smoking status are all requirements of stage 1 for both eligible professionals and hospitals. While secure messaging is proposed to be a require-ment for eligible professionals in stage 2, it is not addressed in stage 1 of mean-ingful use.

6. E. Commonly cited barriers to health information exchange among providers include the following: lack of a business case, lack of standards adoption and interoperability, lack of access to infrastructure to support exchange, and con-cerns about privacy and security.

7. B. More than 80 percent of consumers have looked online for information about health topics. On the other hand, adoption rates for personal health records range from 7 to 11 percent. While the use of social media is gaining in popularity, currently only a small percentage of consumers (4 percent) post comments, questions, or information about their health on social media sites.

8. C. Personal health records, secure messaging, and a physician web site—which can include a blog—are all electronic tools used by clinicians to engage patients. Practice management systems, on the other hand, are primarily used for billing and other administrative purposes.

9. E. The following represent commonly cited barriers to the adoption of consumer-facing electronic tools by clinicians: lack of a business case or reimbursement for such activities, concerns about privacy and security protections, and in some cases concerns about liability.

10. **E.** Concerns about privacy and security and the inability to gain access to a computer or the Internet are all commonly cited barriers of consumers who are not using electronic tools to engage with their clinicians. Also, the lack of EHR adoption or adoption of other electronic capabilities designed to engage consumers among providers serves as a key barrier. Therefore, all of the listed options represent commonly cited barriers for consumers.

References

1. Buntin, M. B., Burke, M., Hoaglin, M., and Blumenthal, D. (2011). The benefits of health information technology: A review of the recent literature shows predominantly positive results. *Health Affairs, 31(3)*, 464–471.

2. Hsiao, C., Hing, E, Socey, T. C., and Cai, B. (2011). Electronic health record systems and intent to apply for meaningful use incentives among office-based physician practices: United States, 2011–2011. *NCHS Data Brief, 79*.

3. Decker, S. L., Jamoom, E. W., and Sisk, J. E. (2012). Physicians in nonprimary care and small practices and those age 55 and older lag in adopting electronic health record systems. Centers for Disease Control and Prevention's National Center for Health Statistics. *Health Affairs, 31(5)*, 1108–1114.

4. Boonstra, A., and Broekhuis, M. (2010). Barriers to the acceptance of electronic medical records by physicians from systematic review to taxonomy and interventions. *BMC Health Services Research, 6(10)*, 231.

5. Jha, A. K., DesRoches, C. M., Campbell, E. G., Donelan, K., Rao, S. R., Ferris, T. G., et al. (2009). Use of electronic health records in US hospitals. *New England Journal of Medicine, 360(16)*, 1628–1638.

6. Rao, S. R., DesRoches, C. M., Donelan, K., Campbell, E. G., Miralles, P. D., and Jha, A. K. (2011). Electronic health records in small physician practices: availability, use, and perceived benefits. *Journal of the American Medical Informatics Association, 18*, 271–275.

7. Edsall, R. L., and Adler, K. G. (2009). The 2009 EHR user satisfaction survey responses from 2,012 family physicians: If you're shopping for an EHR system, you might appreciate advice from a couple thousand colleagues. *Family Practice Management, 16(6)*, 10–16.

8. DesRoches, C. M., Worzala, C., Joshi, M.S., Kravolec, P. D., and Jha, A. K. (2012). Small, nonteaching, and rural hospitals continue to be slow in adopting electronic health record systems. *Health Affairs, 31(5)*, 1092–1099.

9. AmericanEHR Partners. (2011). *The correlation of training duration with EHR usability and satisfaction: Implications for meaningful use.* AmericanEHR Partners.

10. The Health Information Technology for Economic and Clinical Health (HITECH) Act, Title XIII of Division A and Title IV of Division B of the American Recovery and Reinvestment Act of 2009 (ARRA) (Pub. L. 111-5), enacted on February 17, 2009.

11. Eligible professional meaningful use core measures. (2011). Accessed on September 12, 2012, from http://www.cms.gov/Regulations-and-Guidance/ Legislation/EHRIncentivePrograms/Meaningful_Use.html.

12. Eligible hospital and critical access hospital meaningful use core measures. (2011). Accessed on September 12, 2012, from http://www.cms.gov/Regulations-and-Guidance/Legislation/EHRIncentivePrograms/Meaningful_Use.html.

13. Summary report of CMS medicare and medicaid EHR incentive programs through June 2012. (2012). Accessed on August 1, 2012, from www.cms.gov/ Regulations-and-Guidance/Legislation/EHRIncentivePrograms/Downloads/ June2012_MonthlyReport.pdf.

14. CMS Medicare and Medicaid EHR incentive programs. (2012). Accessed on August 1, 2012, from www.cms.gov/Regulations-and-Guidance/Legislation/ EHRIncentivePrograms/index.html.

15. Regional extension centers. (2012). Accessed on August 1, 2012, from http://healthit.hhs.gov/portal/server.pt/community/healthit_hhs_gov__rec_ program/1495.

16. Health ITIT workforce development program. (2012). Accessed on August 1, 2012, from http://healthit.hhs.gov/portal/server.pt?open=512&objID= 1432&mode=2.

17. Blumenthal, D. (2010). Launching HITECH. *New England Journal of Medicine, 362(5)*, 382–385.

18. State health information exchange cooperative agreement program. (2012). Accessed on August 1, 2012, from http://healthit.hhs.gov/portal/server.pt/community/ healthit_hhs_gov__state_health_information_exchange_program/1488.

19. Advancing privacy and security. (2012). Accessed on August 1, 2012, from http://healthit.hhs.gov/portal/server.pt/community/ healthit_hhs_gov__privacy_and_security/1147.

20. The clinical characteristics of Medicare beneficiaries and implications for Medicare reform. (2002). Accessed on September 12, 2012, from www .medicareadvocacy.org/news/archives/chronic-partnerpaper_clinchars.htm.

21. Smith, P., Araya-Guerra, R., Bublitz, C., Parnes, B., Dickinson, L. M., Van Vorst, R., Westfall, J. M., and Pace. W. D. (2005). Missing clinical information during primary care visits. *JAMA, 293(5)*, 565–571.

22. American Hospital Association. (2010). *AHA hospital survey*. American Hospital Association.

23. Commonwealth Fund. (2009). *Commonwealth Fund international health policy survey*. Commonwealth Fund.

24. Doctors Helping Doctors Transform Health Care and American College of Physicians. (2012). *Survey of clinicians on electronic health information needs: Interim results*. Doctors Helping Doctors Transform Health Care.

25. Wright, A., Soran, C., Jenter, C. A., Volk, L. A., Bates, D. W., and Simon, S. R. (2010). Physician attitudes toward health information exchange: results of a statewide survey. *Journal of the American Medical Informatics Association, 17*, 66–70.

26. Frisse, M., and Holmes, R.L, (2007). Estimated financial savings associated with health information exchange and ambulatory care referral. *Journal of Biomedical Informatics, 40*, S27–S32.

27. Health information exchanges: Rapid growth in an evolving market. (2011). Accessed on September 12, 2012, from https://www.klasresearch.com/Store/ReportDetail.aspx?ProductID=642.

28. Adler-Milstein, J., Bates, D. W., and Jha, A. K.. (2011). A survey of health information exchange organizations in the United States: Implications for meaningful use." *Annals of Internal Medicine, 154*, 666–671.

29. Bipartisan Policy Center. (2012). *Transforming health care: The role of health IT*. Bipartisan Policy Center.

30. U.S. Department of Health and Human Services. (2012). 45 CFR Parts 412, 413, and 495 Medicare and Medicaid programs, electronic health record incentive program—stage 2, proposed rule. *Federal Register, 77(45)*.

31. Gold, M. R., McLaughlin, C. G., Devers, K. J., Berenson, R. A., and Bovbjerg, R. R. (2012). Obtaining providers' "buy-in" and establishing effective means of information exchange will be critical to HITECH's success. *Health Affairs, 31(3)*, 514–526.

32. U.S. Department of Health and Human Services. (2010). 45 CFR Part 170 Health information technology: Initial set of standards, implementation specifications, and certification criteria for electronic health record technology, interim final rule. *Federal Register, 75(8)*, 2013–2047.

33. Ahern, D. K., Woods, S. S., Lightowler, M. C., Finley, S. W., and Houston, T. K. (2011). Promise of and potential for patient-facing technologies to enable meaningful use. *American Journal of Preventive Medicine, 40(582)*, S162–S172.

34. Pew Research Center's Internet and American Life Project. (2011). *The social life of health information: 2011*. Accessed on September 12, 2012, from http://pewinternet.org/Reports/2011/Social-Life-of-Health-Info.aspx.

35. Lake Research Partners. *Consumers and health information technology: A national survey. National Health ITIT Survey 2009–2010*. California Health Care Foundation.

36. 2011 survey of health care consumers in the United States: Key findings, strategic implications. (2011). Accessed on September 12, 2012, from http://www .deloitte.com/assets/Dcom-UnitedStates/Local%20Assets/Documents/US_CHS_ 2011ConsumerSurveyinUS_062111.pdf.

37. Markle Foundation. Markle Survey on Health in a Networked Life 2010. January 2011. Accessed from www.markle.org/health/health-networked-life.

38. Jimison, H. P., Gorman, P., Woods, S., et al. (2008). *Barriers and drivers of health information technology use for the elderly, chronically ill, and underserved*. Agency for Health Care Research and Quality.

39. Wynia, M. K., Torres, G. W., and Lemieux, J. (2011). Many physicians are willing to use patients' electronic personal health records, but doctors differ by location, gender and practice. *Health Affairs, 30(2)*, 266–273.

40. Zhou, Y. Y., Kanter, M., Wang, J. J., and Garrido, T. (2010). Improved quality at Kaiser Permanente through email between patients and physicians. *Health Affairs, 29(7)*, 1370–1375.

An Overview of Processes Associated with Healthcare Delivery Within Provider Organizations: Focus on the Ambulatory Setting

Michael Stearns

In this chapter, you will learn how to
- Be able to explain the workflow associated with scheduling a patient for a visit to an ambulatory healthcare facility
- Understand the workflow associated with the patient encounter within the electronic health record
- Be able to explain additional workflows that are associated with managing clinical data

An Overview of Key Process Associated with Healthcare Delivery in the Ambulatory Setting

Until recently, the rates of adoption of information technology by ambulatory healthcare facilities in the United States were the lowest of any industrialized nation. A survey of physicians published in 2007 reported that only 4 percent of physicians had a fully functional EHR and 13 percent had a basic system.[1] In 2011 the percentage of ambulatory physicians using any form of electronic health record rose to nearly 57 percent[2] in 2011, and that number continues to grow, in part because of the stimulus funds tied to the meaningful use of EHRs. This has created a demand for training programs that educate information technology professionals about the operational requirements of ambulatory practices tied to technology. This chapter will review the roles, workflows, and related operational requirements of ambulatory practices.

The number of physicians and other healthcare providers, including nurse practitioners and physicians assistants, varies from solo-practitioner clinics to groups of several hundred providers, but a typical ambulatory practice in the United States may have two to three providers supported by approximately nine to twelve staff members. Ambulatory practices can be roughly divided into surgical and nonsurgical specialties of medicine. Nonsurgical specialties include primary care (e.g., family medicine, internal medicine, and pediatrics) as well as a number of related specialties such as cardiology, dermatology, neurology, endocrinology, oncology, pulmonology, psychiatry, and others. Surgical specialties include general surgery, otolaryngology, orthopedic surgery, neurosurgery, cardiothoracic surgery, obstetrics and gynecology, and others. Workflows, clinical-care requirements, and documentation of the encounter tend to vary substantially depending on practice type, the EHR that is being used, and the level of sophistication of the users. This chapter will present some common workflows and clinical documentation requirements but is not meant to be all-inclusive.

Initiating a Visit with an Ambulatory Provider

Scheduling a visit with a practice has traditionally required the patient or their representative to call the office and speak with a staff member. Increasingly patients are scheduling visits through patient portals, which are electronic tools that allow patients to remotely access the clinic's scheduling software to book an appointment. In either case, the practice will have scheduling software that may be a stand-alone application or one that is integrated with other electronic tools such as a practice management system or an EHR.

Several hundred ambulatory practice scheduling tools are available in the U.S. market with a variety of capabilities and levels of integration with other software applications. The majority of the more sophisticated EHR and practice management applications have a fully integrated scheduling tool that is essentially a component of the whole system. In other cases, the scheduling software may communicate with the EHR or practice management software through an interface.

Ambulatory scheduling applications need to accommodate a number of requirements that are essential to workflow in the clinic. These include the need to create slots for different types of visits, including new patient visits, follow-up visits, and procedures. They also need to accommodate the preferences of individual providers, who may prefer different time intervals for visits of varying types (e.g., a follow-up visit with a patient with multiple complex medical conditions may take longer than a visit for a patient with single medical problem such as hypertension). The scheduling application may or may not support scheduling at multiple facilities and can be a feature that differentiates enterprise-capable EHRs from other products.

The workflow associated with scheduling a visit is fairly straightforward. If the patient is new to the clinic, in most cases they will call the clinic to schedule the visit. A receptionist or scheduling professional will then use the scheduling tool to schedule the actual visit as a new patient visit type. In some instances, the patient visit is scheduled by another clinic that may be referring the patient, and an emerging trend is allowing clinics to schedule patients in other clinics through an electronic process. A third method is through the patient portal, which has the advantage of not requiring any involvement of the clinic staff and is available when the clinic is not open.

Upon arrival at the clinic, the patient will go through a check-in process at the front desk with a member of the clinic's staff, in most cases a receptionist. When automated, a check-in module will initiate the visit process for that encounter. The tools may alert the staff member to get key information from the patient that may be demographic or clinical information. The patient will then be asked to complete forms that are most often paper-based, including their demographic information (e.g., age, gender, preferred language, race, ethnicity, address, phone numbers, marital status, and health insurance information). Some clinics have adopted kiosks that allow patients to enter this information electronically in the waiting room, and some accomplish this by allowing the patient to add or modify their demographics through patient portals or personal health records. Another merging trend is to have patients perform as much of their own data entry as possible through personal computers and mobile devices, including applications designed specifically for this purpose. Some applications will allow the patient to enter a reason for visit and other clinical information.

The patient is often asked to provide medical information during the paper or electronic intake process, which may include the reason for the visit, past medical history, allergies, medication, current symptoms, social history, and family history. If this information is obtained on paper, a clinic staff person, usually a medical assistant or a nurse, will enter the information into the electronic health record (or paper chart if the clinic is not on EHR). If the information is entered electronically by the patient, it will be available in the EHR in most cases.

 TIP Be sure that a clinically knowledgeable person reviews any clinic data entered by a patient during the scheduling process within a reasonable period of time to avoid potential delays in treating acute medical conditions such as chest discomfort.

The final step prior to the patient being seen by the provider often involves having the patient taken to a triage station or examination room. Some additional history may be obtained by a staff member with clinical training such as a medical assistant who may also obtain vital signs such as height, weight, basic metabolic index (BMI), heart rate, respiratory rate, temperature, and blood pressure. This information will be recorded on paper or entered directly into the electronic health record.

A number of EHR applications have dashboard-like tools that track the location and status of patients in the clinic, how long they have been waiting in the clinic's waiting room, what room they have been placed in, if they are actively being seen by a provider, if they are in the lab or radiology department of a clinic (when these are present), and if they have been checked out of the clinic. They also may record status information about the patient's visit, such as when the medical assistant has completed the intake process and the patient is ready to be seen by the provider. During each transition within the clinic, the appropriate staff member enters the patient's change in location or status.

 TIP It is fairly common for clinics to combine paper intake processes with electronic data entry, creating hybrid workflow models that are often inconsistent with the training and intent of the EHR designers. It may be in the best interest of the clinics to gradually move toward a higher-level usage of the EHR.

The Clinician Visit

The provider will review the clinical information that has been obtained through the check-in and triage process. In most settings, this information will be used to create or update information in what is usually referred to as the *health summary*, *face sheet*, or another similar name that typically exists as a distinct container of the electronic health record. It contains patient-specific health information that may be stored as unstructured data, structured data, or codified structured data. For the purposes of this discussion, unstructured data typically means free text that is not supported by a specific designated field. An example of this might be paragraphs of text entered into a very general category such as "History of present illness." The term "structured data" is often used for data that is entered into a specific field (e.g., last name) or for data that is stored in a codified format. An example of codified data might be a field titled "Past medical history" that contains a code that indicates the patient has a specific medical condition such as multiple sclerosis. The EHR will store the code in the database, but the graphical user interface will express the concept as free text.

Codified data aids downstream processes tied to the information needs of the patient visit, such as alerts and reminders tied to patient care (e.g., a medication contraindication), clinical decision support, population queries, research, and interoperability with other applications such as health information exchanges.

The sections of the health summary component include patient-specific information in the following categories.

The Problem List

This is often used to identify past and existing illnesses the patient has had.[2] Definitions vary, however,[3] and some providers may broaden this to include information that is relevant to patient care such as ongoing marital discord. Different specialists may have different problem lists for the same patient, reflecting their areas of expertise and focus. The problem list is a requirement for stage 1 of meaningful use, and the EHR needs to be able to represent the problem list concepts as codified data.[4] The codified data elements need to be represented either as ICD-9-CM or as SNOMED CT codes, the two terminologies that have codes that represent disease entities. The EHR application needs to allow for the problem list to be updated manually or through an automated processes via an interface to a health information exchange (HIE) or another mechanism whereby problem lists can be imported and consumed as codified data that can be used to create or maintain problem lists. The format most typically encountered at this time is the continuity of care document (CCD), but other methods may be used.

The Medication List

This consists of an active list of current medications, and some applications may allow the display of what medications the patient has taken in the past. It often includes prescription drugs and drugs that can be purchased over the counter. Besides the name of the drug, the medication list generally supports additional prescribing information, including the strength of the medication, the form (e.g., pill, tablet, liquids, inhalants, etc.), how frequently it should be taken, the amount prescribed, the route of administration, a start date, an end date when appropriate, and other information as needed (such as not to drink alcohol while taking a specific medication). Medication concepts are usually codified at the key ingredient level so that they can be used by the application to support electronic prescribing.

Electronic Prescribing Applications

An electronic prescribing application is a key component of the majority of EHRs and usually provides clinical decision support (CDS) assistance to providers. For example, it may suggest medications to use for specific conditions and recommended dosages and frequencies. CDS for medications usually requires the e-prescribing application to communicate with a third-party drug database resource. Since new medications are frequently added and others are retired, the drug database needs to be updated fairly regularly. The CDS capabilities of e-prescribing applications vary, but they may have the ability to identify a number of potential interactions and alert the provider before the medication is provided. These include alerts related to the following:

- Drug combinations that might be contraindicated
- Drugs that the patient may be allergic to
- Drugs that are contraindicated with certain diseases such as kidney disease
- Drugs that are contraindicated based on a lab value
- Drugs that are contraindicated based on the patient's age, including children and the elderly
- Warnings about the drug, related to whether it is covered by the patient's insurance plan

E-prescribing can be performed from within the health summary tool or from the medication or plan sections of the progress note. From a technical standpoint, medications must be given a concept code that can be recognized by the applications. The medication name, dose, frequency of administration, form, duration, route, and number of refills are essentially always displayed and may or may not be represented in the EHR database by codified or even structured data. Alternative medications, the associated copay, and whether the drug is formulary compliant with the patient's insurance carrier may also be displayed. In most systems, the provider is able to print, fax, or e-prescribe the medications.

The Past Medical History

In the health summary view, this section is a record of all past and current illnesses, hospitalizations, injuries, operations, and other procedures performed on the patient. It may or may not be represented by codified data. The past medical history is closely aligned with the problem list, although they differ in that the problem list is primarily a subset of the past medical history.

Allergies

This section details medication and other allergies (e.g., latex allergies). It may also provide the clinician with information about the severity and nature of the allergic reaction.

Immunization History

This is a chronological record of the patient's immunization status. It may have age-specific content and features along with the ability to order immunizations from this section of the EHR. Alternatively, the immunizations may be contained within a separate module that is not within the health summary container. The immunizations tools generally allow the provider to enter immunization type, date provided, location provided (e.g., upper arm), and lot number. The immunization tools may provide guidance and recommendations tied to the administration of immunizations.

The Family History

This section captures the medical history of relatives of the patient, emphasizing inheritable diseases. This section may or may not contain codified data and may be limited to free text entered into designated fields.

The Social History

This refers to the patient's use or nonuse of alcohol, illicit drugs, tobacco products, and related potentially harmful substances. The frequency and amount of usage are typically recorded for each component. This section also documents the patient's occupation, marital and family status, living situation, whether there is any high-risk sexual behavior (when relevant), and a number of other data elements. The information may be stored as codified data or free text.

Others

Since this is usually the first screen the clinician will review in a patient's record, a number of other items may be available on the health summary screen or presented in another way. These include the following:

- Recent lab results.
- Recent radiology results.
- Recent diagnostic study results (e.g., an EKG result).
- Recent hospitalizations.
- Pending studies.
- Studies that have been ordered and their status.
- Interventions that are needed for the patient (e.g., mammogram, colonoscopy, immunizations, etc.). This is often considered part of alerts and reminders that may be available from multiple areas of the clinical record.
- A section that addresses communications with the patient or about the patient.
- A summary of highly pertinent information about the patient.

The Clinician Visit

Workflows vary, with some providers reviewing the health summary information, reason for visit, and vital signs prior to entering the examination room, or more commonly once they enter the examination room and start interacting with the patient. At this point, the provider in a traditional visit will obtain a history, perform an examination, review any additional values, develop an assessment, and formulate a plan. The intake method when using an EHR varies considerably. Many providers will document at least a portion of the encounter while in the room with the patient. This may be done through a mobile device such as a tablet or a fixed workstation. Some providers prefer to take physical or mental notes on paper during the encounter and then enter the information at a workstation in their office, in the hallway, or in an alcove. The use of scribes who shadow providers and enter information into the EHR is another method used by some providers.

EHRs may support the ability to import prior-visit notes or portions of prior-visit notes into the EHR. If used properly, this increases the efficiency of documentation and reminds the provider to address outstanding issues from the previous visit. However, if not used properly, it tends to import information that was either not relevant or not accurate for that visit.

 TIP   The process of importing visit notes from prior visits to be used as "template" for the current visit is supported by many EHRs; however, if not used carefully, it can lead to inaccurate or even fraudulent documentation and billing. It is important that this capability be used with caution during EHR documentation.

Many electronic health record applications are based upon the guidelines published by the Centers for Medicaid and Medicare Services (CMS) in 1995[5] and 1997.[6] The guidelines define several sections of the records that are used to create a progress note or history and physical. The following sections are defined.

The Chief Complaint

This is a brief statement that identifies the primary reason for the patient visit. The definition provided by CMS is as follows: "The CC is a concise statement describing the symptom, problem, condition, diagnosis, physician recommended return, or other factor that is the reason for the encounter, usually stated in the patient's words."[7] It often includes demographic and pertinent information such as "The patient is a 44-year-old white male with a history of diabetes and hypertension who presents for blood pressure management."

The EHR will often have a section of the chart that automates the importation of the demographic information to create a portion of the sentence. The rest of the opening sentence can be created by entering free text or through the use of templates that contain drop-down menus or other methods of choosing the data elements. Often a medical assistant or other nonprovider staff member will complete this section of the note prior to the point where the provider sees the patient.

A similar approach is often used for other sections of the progress note. The EHR may or may not support codified data at this level of documentation. If it does, the codified data may be used to suggest the use of other templates for other sections of the note generation process. For example, the use of the term "hypertension" might be tied to a codified data element that represents hypertension. Templates are used by many EHRs to help with text entry. The EHR would then suggest hypertension-based templates or defaults for that to facilitate the documentation process. One of the features that differentiates EHRs is their approach to template usage, creation, and modifications, because approaches and levels of usability vary widely.

The History of Present Illness (HPI)

This is a more detailed history of the patient's presenting problem and often includes a discussion of chronic diseases when present. It is defined by CMS as follows: "The HPI is a chronological description of the development of the patient's present illness from the first sign and/or symptom or from the previous encounter to the present."[8] The documentation guidelines suggest that the providers obtain at least four of the following eight "HPI elements" regarding the presenting problem: location, duration, severity, quality, timing, context, modifying factors, and associated signs and symptoms. The HPI may or may not have the ability to capture codified data, and if it does, it may be limited to a few concepts that are needed to help with evaluation and management (E&M) coding that will explained in more detail later in this chapter. The HPI may consist of a brief paragraph or several paragraphs. All relevant subjective information is documented in this section of the record. This is an area of the record where voice recognition is particularly popular given the need for prose that has less predictability than other sections of the record.

Past, Family, and Social History (PFSH)

This section is self-explanatory and basically contains sections of the health summary described earlier reproduced in the progress note. However, in this view, the past medical history tends to include all historical data (e.g., medications, allergies, immunizations, etc.) with the exception of the family and social history, but approaches in EHRs vary. The CMS definition of the PFSH is as follows:

> The PFSH consists of a review of three areas: past history (the patient's past experiences with illnesses, operations, injuries and treatments); family history (a review of medical events in the patient's family, including diseases which may be hereditary or place the patient at risk); and social history (an age appropriate review of past and current activities).[9]

Many EHRs will pull relevant information from the health summary and place it in the corresponding section of the progress note. Some systems may require this information to be added manually. In general, the past history includes diseases, injuries, allergies, medications, hospitalizations, and other pertinent historical information other than what is contained within the family and social history sections of the health summary. Modifications to information in this section may or may not update the corresponding fields in the health summary, depending on the EHR's capabilities. The information can be captured as free text or as codified data, depending on the EHR that is being used. The addition of information may be template-driven or free text.

Review of Systems (ROS)

The ROS is typically the next section of the record and often the last section of the historical portion of the progress note. The CMS definition reads as follows: "A ROS is an inventory of body systems obtained through a series of questions seeking to identify signs and/or symptoms which the patient may be experiencing or has experienced."[10] Body systems include such items as eyes, cardiovascular, and others. Systems often allow the user to use default negatives for this section; here are some examples:

- **General**   Denies weight changes, loss of appetite, or fatigue
- **Respiratory**   Denies cough, shortness of breath, or wheezing
- **Cardiovascular**   Denies chest pain, palpitations, or swelling in extremities

The user may start with negative defaults that can be changed to positives through a drop-down menu of alternative choices stored within templates, through a more hard-coded process, or via free text modifications. Free text can also be used either alone or in conjunction with templates. The symptoms and their positive or negative value may or may not be captured as codified data. To support accurate E&M coding, the tools need to identify which ROS sections contain data and use this as one of the components to determine the overall level of service for the encounter. It is not uncommon for the patient to complete ROS information on a written intake form while they are in the waiting room, and the workflow needs to manage the process of getting this information into the electronic health record. The medical assistant or provider may take on this role. Some EHRs may allow the patient to enter their own ROS data via a kiosk, patient portal, or the personal health record. In all cases, this information will need to be reviewed by the providers. A mismatch between information captured in the HPI and the ROS is a relatively frequent occurrence that can lead to documentation errors. For example, documenting a history of chest pain in the HPI and accepting default negative including "denies chest pain" in the ROS can occur when defaults are used. For this reason, the use of codified concepts in both the HPI and the ROS may allow the system to recognize when the same concept (e.g., chest pain) is documented in both sections and alert the provider that there is a potential documentation conflict.

The Physical Examination

This section of the record documents findings related to direct observation and inspection of the patient and is normally conducted after the history is obtained. The examination typically contains an evaluation of body systems driven by the nature of presentation and the specialty of the provider.

The first section is usually the vital signs. These values may have been obtained during the triage process by a member of the clinical staff, and this data is then often pulled forward into the vital signs section of the progress note. Alternatively, the vital signs may be obtained by the provider who would then enter or modify data using various tools provided. In addition to the typical vital signs (i.e., weight, height, blood pressure, respiratory rate, BMI, temperature, and pulse), the system may also support the review of growth charts, pulse oximetry, and other information that is typically reviewed at this stage of the encounter. Some systems support interfaces with third-party vitals workstation devices that automate the recording of blood pressure, pulse, and temperature.

Following the vital signs, the provider will observe and inspect body systems and areas that are relevant to the presenting problem or reason for visit. Many EHRs will have prepopulated content that uses templates or fixed fields to document normal and abnormal findings. There are typically a fairly limited number of default normal findings that are documented per body system during a routine visit, such as the following:

> Cardiovascular Examination: Auscultation: Regular rate and rhythm, no murmurs, rub, S3 or S4. Pulses: carotid pules 2+ without bruits, radial pulses 2+, pedial pulses 2+. No peripheral cyanosis or edema noted.

Each of the previous normal findings could be replaced by one or more abnormal findings identified during the examination. In many instances, there are dozens of abnormal findings that could be documented for each normal finding. Many systems will store the abnormal findings as available choices within a template or another mechanism, allowing them to be selected during the documentation process. The tools should also allow the provider to enter free text and to remove and modify findings as appropriate.

Complex rules exist regarding how physical examination documentation is used to determine the level of service for the encounter for E&M coding purposes that are beyond the scope of this chapter but documented elsewhere.[11] In general, an EHR system that supports automated E&M coding will need to record what physician examination systems contain findings. The tools need to recognize patterns of documentation that support different levels of service, which range from "problem-focused" to "comprehensive" physical examinations. These are based upon what physical examination systems are documented and, depending on which CMS guidelines are used, how they match to specialty-specific examination types.[7] Given the complexity of the rules, the ability of an EHR to help the provider determine the level of service based on what is documented in the physical examination section of the record can have significant value. The physical examination concepts captured during documentation may be codified data elements or free text. Many systems support the use of a drawing tool that allows for freehand drawing or template anatomic images that can be drawn upon to aid documentation.

Diagnostic Test Results

Many systems allow for the incorporation of test results in the progress note. This section may reside after the HPI, before or after the physical examination, or as part of the assessment section of the encounter note, but is most often found after the physical examination because, like the physical examination, it is considered to be objective information. It allows for the manual entry or importation of laboratory results, radiology results, and results of other diagnostic studies such as electrocardiograms. The tools may also support interfaces to radiology images that are stored at another location such as the hospital via a picture archiving and communication system (PACS) interface or those stored within the EHR's database.

The Assessment

The provider utilizes this section of the record to summarize their findings and render diagnoses. They may be entered manually, or the EHR may assist them by suggesting diagnoses based on documentation to that point in the encounter. The provider may add free text manually, use templated text to add diagnoses, or use other tools to create or expand upon a discussion regarding each diagnosis. An example is provided here:

Assessment:

1. Classical Migraine: This is the most likely diagnosis at this time given the family history, age of onset, visual aura, associated nausea and photophobia, and time course. Abortive therapies are indicated at this time, and if this is not effective, prophylactic management will be considered.

The assessment is often codified so that the diagnoses can be passed forward to a billing application. The majority of clinics in the United States submit claims to payers that must first be reviewed by a billing specialist and then forwarded to a clearinghouse. This requires the use of specific codes from the assessment section of the visit tied to the diagnoses or the reason for the visit. Some systems suggest alternative diagnoses to the provider for their consideration. These may be alternative diagnoses they may want to consider or more specific diagnoses that could help with clinical documentation and reimbursement.

The Plan

The provider may elect to discuss management of the condition in the assessment or in the next section referred to as the plan. In general, the plan provides specific actions related to the treatment of the patient. The EHR may support the documentation of the plan through templates or other tools. Many of the plan items consist of orders that require subsequent action and impact workflow in the office.

Laboratory Orders

The clinician may order tests on blood, urine, fluid drained or expressed from a space, stool, or other substances, or the clinician may have obtained these during the encounter. At this point, the workflow needs to support obtaining or packaging the sample and delivering it to the laboratory for analysis. The steps will vary depending on the type of sample and whether the clinic has an in-house laboratory facility. The staff will need to be notified that a lab request is being made. In some clinics, the staff, usually a medical assistant, will obtain or package the sample and then send it to the laboratory. In other situations, the patient will be asked to travel to the laboratory. The EHR may have the capacity to generate an electronic order that can be sent to clinic staff for management of the order or via an interface directly to the laboratory. If there is no outbound ordering interface, the EHR tools may support the creation of a paper requisition that the patient will carry to the laboratory.

Radiology Orders

Some clinics, in particular orthopedic practices, routinely include radiographs as part of their workflow and have on-site radiology capabilities. The image is usually taken while the patient is in the office as a component of the visit. The workflow includes the generation of an order from the EHR, which is then conveyed via a staff member or electronically to the radiology department. The order will need to contain specific information about the radiology study that is requested. Once it has been completed, the image must be returned to the provider. In centers with digital radiology capabilities, this may be handled through the EHR. The provider would be alerted that the image was available for review. For the image to be read by the provider, minimum standards for resolution of the image should be adhered to (DICOM),[12] and this may require specific hardware and settings. The majority of clinics do not have radiology facilities on-site, and the orders are managed in a process that is similar to laboratory requisitions.

Other Tests

Other diagnostic studies and interventions that are ordered in the plan section may have similar workflows. Some studies and procedures are performed in the clinic during the visit, or they may be scheduled for a subsequent visit. For example, a patient may be scheduled for a cardiac-monitoring study in the same clinic or facility, but it cannot be performed during that visit. The order will need to be transmitted electronically to a scheduling tool and then scheduled by the staff (or the patient-driven scheduling is supported). Once the patient returns and the test has been performed, the provider who is interpreting the study will need to be alerted that the study is ready for interpretation. In many cases, this requires that an image, video, tracing, or other media be presented to the provider for digital or paper-based review. The interpreting provider will then need to generate a report through a report-generating tool if available in the EHR. A result will need to be generated in the form of a report and then transmitted to the provider who originated the order.

The clinician may also perform or schedule an outpatient procedure (e.g., a skin biopsy). This requires the plan section in the EHR to communicate the necessary information about the patient, their insurance information, and any needed details about the procedure to the person responsible for scheduling.

Medications

Prescriptions are usually generated from the plan section of the EHR using an e-prescribing tool. Even clinics that are not using an EHR often use a stand-alone e-prescribing tool. The e-prescribing requirements for meaningful use are detailed in the Final Rule for stage 1 meaningful use. (The features of an e-prescribing tool were described in the section titled "Electronic Prescribing Applications.") In addition, an e-prescribing application may also suggest medications of equal effectiveness based on cost and whether they are in a specific insurance carrier's formulary. The copay the patient has to pay when they obtain the medication may also be displayed, allowing the provider to warn the patient about the amount they will be expected to pay and potentially allowing the provider to choose an alternative drug of equal efficacy that is lower in cost to the patient.

Use Case 5-1: Using E-prescribing to Avoid Drug-Drug Contraindication

A 40-year-old male with a heart condition was prescribed a drug called Amiodarone to control his heart rhythm. While traveling, he developed a sinus infection and visited an urgent-care facility. The provider prescribed the antibiotic erythromycin for the sinus condition through an EHR with an e-prescribing tool. The e-prescribing tool alerted the provider that the use of Amiodarone and erythromycin together was contraindicated, because it could cause a potentially fatal disturbance of the patient's heart rhythm. The provider then chose a different antibiotic that was not contraindicated. For this to have occurred, the provider's EHR had to be aware that the patient was taking Amiodarone and have access to a drug-drug contraindication database.

Clinics often experience significant gains in efficiency with e-prescribing and in particular the medication refill process. Clinics usually require the patient to call the clinic when requesting a refill and place a request with a clinic staff member. This is then written down and given to the provider once the paper chart is pulled. The provider will need to review the request and create a handwritten prescription or have a staff member call the pharmacy to phone in the prescription. The patient's chart is then refilled by a staff member. With an EHR that includes a portal, many manual processes that involve ancillary staff can be eliminated. A common workflow would be for the patient to enter a medication refill request via the patient portal. This is then transmitted as an automated message to the provider who can review the request in the context of the patient's full medical record. The provider can then create a refill, send it electronically to the pharmacy, and notify the patient of this action through the patient portal. They can also manage the medication request in other ways, such as instructing the patient to come to the clinic for a visit, deny the refill request, or change the patient to a different dose or a different medication.

Immunizations

Immunizations can be ordered from the plan section, from the health summary module, or from an independent immunization module.

Patient Instructions

An important part of the plan includes information that is provided to the patient in the form of instructions and educational materials. This can be addressed through templates with preformatted text, free text, and linkages to third-party educational content that can be provided to the patient. This information is usually printed and given to the patient. The provider may also be able to send information to the patient electronically through a patient portal or a personal health record.

Referrals and Letters

The plan section is also where providers generate referrals to other providers or provide feedback to other caregivers, often in the form of a consult letter. Specialists in particular need to generate letters to referring providers. The EHR may support the ability to message electronically to other providers via an interface, or it may require the referral or consult letter to be sent via fax or printed and mailed.

Follow-up Appointments

The EHR may allow direct access to the scheduling module, allowing the patient's next visit to be scheduled by the provider, or the tools may allow for a follow-up recommendation to be generated in the plan section and then transferred to the scheduling application, if there is integration or an interface is present between the EHR and the scheduling tool.

Note Conclusion

At this point, the provider has likely completed all the documentation and generated orders and referrals. The EHR may have already identified candidate billing codes for the visit. They will usually consist of the following: disease or reason for encounter codes from the International Classification of Diseases (ICD-9-CM), procedure codes from the Current Procedural Terminology (CPT) code set, and items and services delivered during care from the Healthcare Common Procedure Coding System (HCPCS). Many EHR systems will provide coding assistance, allowing the user to review the suggested codes and making changes as needed. Once approved by the provider, the codes are then sent to the billing (practice management) application electronically. This may occur via an interface if the EHR is not a single-database EHR/practice management software application.

A specific type of coding, referred to as E&M coding and touched on in the section "The History of Present Illness (HPI)," is of particular importance because it represents the majority of revenue generated by ambulatory practices in the United States. E&M codes are a form of CPT codes. They essentially represent the level of complexity or the amount of time spent with the patient, with higher levels or reimbursement tied to more complex encounters. The rules regarding the determination of E&M codes are complex and benefit from the computational assistance provided by EHRs. The majority of providers see an increase in their coding levels and reimbursement after they start using EHRs, and this has led medical insurers to start looking at computer-assisted coding in more detail. Large fines and even criminal charges can result from overcharging government healthcare insurance carriers via inflated E&M coding in particular (Medicare, Medicaid, and others). For this reason, providers need to be fully educated on how to use E&M coding tools provided by EHRs.

To meet stage 1 meaningful use requirements, the provider will need to generate a clinical summary of the visit.[13] This summary needs to be printed and handed to the patient. This has created some workflow challenges related to the process of generating a printed document after each encounter, because the document contains HIPAA-protected information and most clinics do not have a printer in each examination room.

Transitions and Coordination of Care and Additional Workflows

An area of significant focus in healthcare is how HIT can support transitions of care between healthcare organizations, such as when the patient is being seen by multiple providers in the community, or when the patient is discharged from the hospital. There are a number of considerations tied to HIT best practices for managing information that have the potential to improve the continuity of patient care.

Document Storage and Messaging

Providers receive information from within the clinic and from outside entities via electronic messages, faxes, and paper. EHRs vary in how they manage this but may provide the ability to capture this information in an electronic form and deliver it the provider. Electronic messages from within the clinic may be managed by applications that function in ways similar to e-mail, including the ability to assign tasks to individuals. Faxes are often managed electronically, and paper records received by the clinic are scanned either before or after they are reviewed by the provider. Much of the information received from external parties needs to be stored in a patient-specific documentation storage tool that may be integrated with the EHR. This may include images, text files in multiple formats, videos, and other formats. These files are then available for review as needed.

Increasingly, information will be shared between healthcare enterprises via health information exchanges. The Direct Model[14] for health information exchange uses a format that is similar to e-mail to send secure messages between providers. Systems that are able to integrate direct messages into the standard messaging workflow will offer advantages over those that don't. Over time, messages sent via health information exchanges will be standards-based, allowing codified information generated by other EHR applications to be imported into the receiving EHR. A leading example of this is the continuity of care document, an XML-based standard that contains an expansive array or demographic, health summary, and other information about the patient. As standards mature, increasing amounts of codified clinical data will be exchanged between healthcare stakeholders, including the patient. This will present technical challenges related to system design and the preservation of data integrity.

Coordination of Care

This is a central construct of the patient-centered medical home and the accountable-care organizations and is defined as "a function that supports information sharing across providers, patients, types and levels of service, sites and time frames."[15] A relatively fully functioning EHR and HIE are required for the true coordination of care. Transitions of care, in particular discharges from hospitals and subsequent outpatient management of patients at risk for readmission, are a priority of HIT efforts. The electronic health record, health information exchanges, patient portals, and home-monitoring applications will play an essential role in facilitating interactions between healthcare providers, case managers, and the patients themselves in a manner that will allow more effective outpatient management. The amount of data that will need to be consumed by providers in order to effectively monitor patients is growing rapidly and has created concerns that it may overwhelm providers. Additional healthcare professionals, such as case managers, will likely play a greater role in U.S. healthcare.

 TIP Care coordination depends upon relatively seamless access to data across multiple sites of care. This will depend upon a greater level of interoperability between disparate HIT platforms. This is turn is tied to an increase in the level of adoption of standards, many of which are under development.

Clinical Decision Support

The most common form of clinical decision support (CDS) exists in e-prescribing tools. Applications may aid physician decision making by helping them with patient-centric management such as alerting them about when a preventative maintenance study is needed (e.g., a patient is due to have a colonoscopy) while the patient is being seen in the office. They can also aid with population management, such as running a query that demonstrates all patients who are overdue for an immunization based on established guidelines.

Report Generation

Various tools are used to generate clinical and financial reports based on data that has been entered into the system. Examples of these reports include the status of compliance with meaningful use requirements such as the clinical quality measures and general compliance with the core and menu set items. An EHR may have hundreds of preformatted financial and clinical reports that are used to assess a variety of business and clinical measures.

Order Tracking

Practices that order tests have some level of responsibility that they are performed and that the results are returned to the ordering providers. Tests results can be lost, confused with another patient's name, or misfiled before being reviewed by a provider. Order-tracking modules make sure that each test or referral that is ordered by the clinic is tracked. The practice can usually monitor all tests that have been ordered and identify the ones that are overdue, allowing them to investigate the reason.

Chapter Review

This chapter reviewed some fairly common workflows, roles, and documentation requirements related to patient care in an ambulatory setting on an EHR. Providing healthcare in ambulatory settings is dependent upon multiple workflows that vary considerably depending upon the size and the specialty of the practice and on provider preferences. The implementation of HIT in practices can result in substantial improvements in efficiency and can generate additional revenue for the practice, if the tools are used in an effective manner.

The starting point is the scheduling process, which may be performed through a traditional phone call, at the end or the prior visit, or through a patient portal. The data requirements for scheduling a patient include a tool that can capture demographic information in the form of structured data, including insurance information.

Once the patient arrives for the visit, they go through a check-in process that often requires that the patient enter clinical information on paper or via a kiosk or patient portal. This information is then used to complete the health summary portion of the patient's clinical record, including a problem list, current medications, allergies, and the past medical, family, and social history of the patient.

The next step is the clinical encounter and a fairly detailed description of how a visit note is created by the provider. The sections of the note each have unique clinical, functionality, and data requirements. The plan section is by far the most complex section from a workflow standpoint. This is where the majority of the orders are generated.

This chapter also provided a discussion of continuity of care and how the EHR and HIEs are essential for making sure that patients receive care that has continuity. Current efforts are targeting the prevention of unnecessary hospital admissions through better outpatient management of chronic medical conditions.

Questions

To test your comprehension of the chapter, answer the following questions and then check your answers against the list of correct answers at the end of the chapter.

1. Which of the following is *not* one of the methods commonly used by patients to schedule an appointment to a clinic?

   A. Patient portal

   B. In person during the prior visit

   C. Over the phone

   D. Via their personal e-mail

2. Which of the following is generally *not* considered demographic information?

   A. Age

   B. Allergies

   C. Address

   D. Insurance carrier

3. Which of the following is *not* a component of the health summary component of the EHR?

   A. The history of present illness (HPI)

   B. The problem list

   C. Allergies

   D. The medication list

4. Which of the following items is *not* true regarding the immunization record?

   A. It is used exclusively for children up to the age of 18.

   B. It contains a field for the lot number of the immunization used.

   C. It provides a chronological history of immunizations that have previously been provided.

   D. It allows for the site of administration to be documented.

5. Which of the following statements is *not* true regarding the problem list in the health summary component of an EHR?

   A. It contains currently active diseases.

   B. For meaningful use stage 1 EHR certification, the problem list items must be codified using ICD-9-CM or SNOMED CT.

   C. It contains pending orders.

   D. It can be edited.

6. Which of the following statements is *not* true regarding patient clinical data entry?

   A. Patients often fill out intake forms on paper that are later added to the EHR by a clinic staff member.

   B. Patients may access tools that allow them to enter clinical information through a patient portal, a personal health record, or a kiosk in the waiting room.

   C. Patients may enter information related to their past medical history including allergies, current medications, and the reason they are requesting a visit.

   D. Patient-entered clinical information helps improve the efficiency of the data entry process, because it allows the clinical staff to defer reviewing it until the patient arrives for the visit.

7. Which of the following statements is true regarding the social history?

   A. It contains details about the patient's family structure and living conditions.

   B. It contains demographic information such as addresses and phone numbers.

   C. It contains the patient's prior history of medical conditions.

   D. It contains the same information as the family history.

8. Which of the following statements is *not* true?

   A. The number of providers who are using EHRs in the United States in ambulatory settings was less than 20 percent in 2006 but now exceeds 50 percent.

   B. The rapid increase in adoption of EHRs and related technologies has created a strain on available resources that have the technical skills to manage EHR implementations and support.

   C. Standards that allow for seamless interoperability between healthcare organizations have been implemented throughout the United States.

   D. The current trend is to move toward greater levels of codification of clinical concepts in EHRs.

9. Which statement regarding the chief complaint section of the encounter note is *not* accurate?

   A. It may contain the reason for visit in the patient's own words.

   B. It may contain demographic information about the patient.

   C. It is often used to record a detailed history of the patient medical problems, complaints, associated signs and symptoms, and prior responses to treatment.

   D. It may be template-driven and include codified data.

10. Which statement regarding the history of present illness (HPI) is *not* accurate?

   A. Guidelines published by the Centers for Medicaid and Medicare provide specific details regarding what information should be captured in this section of the encounter note.

   B. HPI documentation may be assisted by the use of templates that provide drop-down menus (and other formats).

   C. The HPI is not used to document responses to prior treatments.

   D. The HPI is one of the sections of the record that is used to determine the overall level of service and E&M code for the visit.

11. Which of the following statements about the physical examination section of the encounter note is *not* accurate?

   A. The amount of content stored within EHR templates that record the physical examination findings is relatively low compared to other sections of the encounter note.

   B. The rules regarding how to determine the level of service (E&M) coding within EHRs based on what is documented in the physical examination are complex and benefit from computer-assisted coding tools.

   C. The information captured in the EHR varies markedly between specialties of medicine.

   D. The physical examination may contain codified data, in particular data elements that support the calculation of E&M coding.

12. Which one of the following items is *not* typically a component of the plan section of the encounter note?

   A. The assessment

   B. Medication orders

   C. Radiology orders

   D. Patient instructions

13. Which of the following statements is most accurate?

    A. Workflows within ambulatory practices tend to be relatively standard with low levels of variability between practices, regardless of their size or specialty.

    B. Practices frequently combine paper documentation processes with electronic documentation, resulting in a hybrid form of EHR implementation.

    C. Pulling notes forward from prior encounters and using them as templates for the current visit need to be performed carefully to avoid inaccurate or even fraudulent documentation.

    D. The EHR may have an interface to a PACS radiology service, but diagnostic interpretation of images should be performed on DICOM standard-compliant equipment.

14. Which of the following is *not* accurate regarding continuity of care?

    A. Continuity of care efforts focus on patient care activities that are limited to the practice site.

    B. Health information exchange is a key requirement needed for continuity of care efforts to be successful.

    C. Continuity of care efforts strive to prevent patients from being admitted to the hospital when it otherwise could have been prevented.

    D. The continuity of care document allows for key clinical information to be shared between healthcare organizations.

15. Which of the following statements is *not* accurate?

    A. Order tracking is an important consideration in the workflow of any practice, because test results that are positive and not returned to the practice or otherwise mishandled can lead to significant patient safety issues.

    B. Clinical EHR workflows may need to be customized for the practice, for the specialty, and for the level of sophistication of the users.

    C. Full EHR implementations are unlikely to result in significant changes in revenue for a practice.

    D. Mobile devices, including tablets and custom applications, are making significant inroads into clinical medicine.

Answers

1. **D.** The use of personal e-mail is generally not used to schedule patient visits for privacy and security reasons. The other three methods are used commonly, with the convenience of online scheduling through the patient portal gaining in popularity in recent years.

2. **B.** Allergies are generally not considered demographic information, which is used to capture the patient's age, race, address, contact information, insurance carrier, primary-care providers, and other relevant nonclinical information about the patient. Allergies are a component of the clinical data that is obtained on the patient, typically with a health summary module.

3. **A.** The health summary section of the EHR, which may also be called the *face sheet* or by another name, contains a problem list, allergies, past medical history, past family history, and social history among other components. It does not include the history of present illness, which is a component of the encounter note.

4. **A.** Immunizations are an important component of adult medicine, including a record of vaccinations against tetanus, meningitis, pertussis, pneumococcal pneumonia, and a number of different infectious diseases.

5. **C.** The problem list contains disease entities that need to be have codified data, as per stage 1 meaningful use requirements. It does not contain orders that are pending for the patient.

6. **D.** Patients may enter urgent symptoms that require emergent evaluations, and they may not be scheduled to be seen for several days. It is important that clinical staff review any patient-reported histories within a reasonable time frame so that no delays in recommending a intervention (e.g., telling the patient to call 911) will occur.

7. **A.** The social history records the patient's substance use, employment, social habits, family status, and living situation (e.g., lives at home with wife and two children, ages 3 and 1).

8. **C.** Standards that would allow for true interoperability are not in place in most of the United States, and this is an area of focus in HIT at this writing.

9. **C.** The history of present illness (HPI) is used to capture a detailed history from the patient and from other sources.

10. **C.** The HPI is where responses to prior treatments are typically documented.

11. **A.** The amount of clinical content needed to support the numerous normal and abnormal physical findings that may be present on any given examination is large, making the physical examination section of templates one of the more content-intensive components of an EHR application.

12. **A.** The assessment is a separate section of documentation that usually immediately precedes the plan and is where the diagnoses are recorded and discussed.

13. **A.** Workflows vary markedly between practices based on their size, specialty, level of experience with EHRs, and level of motivation of the providers.

14. **A.** Continuity of care refers to the overall management of the patient regardless of the practice setting, so it is not clinic-centric but rather healthcare community–centric.

15. C. A full implementation of an EHR tends to increase per provider revenues significantly based on improved coding accuracy, better charge capture, and improvements in efficiency.

References

1. DesRoches, C. M., et al. (2008). Electronic health records in ambulatory care: A national survey of physicians. *New England Journal of Medicine, 359*, 50–60.

2. Health information technology in the United States: Driving toward delivery system change. (2012). Accessed on July 30, 2012, from www.rwjf.org/files/research/74262.5822.hit.ex.summary.final041612.pdf.

3. 45 CFR Part 170 health information technology: Initial set of standards, implementation specifications, and certification criteria for electronic health record technology; final rule. Accessed on July 30, 2012, from www.gpo.gov/fdsys/pkg/FR-2010-07-28/pdf/2010-17210.pdf.

4. Holmes, C. (2011). The problem list beyond meaningful use. *Journal of AHIMA, 82*, 32–35

5. Department of Health and Human Services. 45 CFR Part 170, op. cit.

6. Documentation guidelines for evaluation and management services. (1995). Accessed in August, 2012, from www.cms.hhs.gov/MLN.pdf.

7. Documentation guidelines for evaluation and management services. (1997). Accessed in August, 2012, from www.cms.hhs.gov/MLN.pdf.

8. Ibid.

9. Ibid.

10. Ibid.

11. Grider, D. (2011). *The medical record auditor*. AMA Press.

12. DICOM standards. Accessed on July 30, 2012, from http://medical.nema.org/standard.html.

13. CMS meaningful use guidance, core criteria 13: Clinical summaries. Accessed on July 30, 2012, from www.cms.gov/Regulations-and-Guidance/Legislation/EHRIncentivePrograms/downloads/13_Clinical_Summaries.pdf.

14. The direct model. Accessed on July 30, 2012, from http://wiki.directproject.org/specifications+and+service+descriptions.

15. Meaningful measures of care coordination: NCVHS presentation. (2009). Accessed on July 30, 2012, from www.ncvhs.hhs.gov/091013p9.pdf.

An Overview of Processes Associated with Healthcare Payment Within Ambulatory Provider Organizations

Robert M. Tennant

In this chapter, you will learn how to
- Understand the business of a physician practice
- Identify the main ways to derive revenue
- Define the claims revenue cycle
- Recognize the standards and regulatory requirements necessary in a physician practice
- Define the steps in the claims revenue cycle
- Understand the resources necessary to maximize revenue including staff and health information technology

A physician practice is a business. For that business to continue to treat patients, it must generate revenue. The majority of this revenue is derived from contracts for professional services with government and commercial health plans and the patients themselves. However, to receive these payments, the practice must navigate a complex process known as the *claims revenue cycle*. Successful practices are those that understand the intricacies of this process, understand the intersection of government standards and requirements, utilize staff expertise, and leverage health information technology (HIT) to maximize revenue.

In recent years, much of the attention in the HIT environment has been focused on its ability to improve the clinical care provided to patients. At the same time, however, federal standardization efforts combined with practice adoption of HIT can produce significant efficiencies in the administration of patient care in physician practices. This chapter will outline the physician practice claims revenue cycle and how standards and automation are helping to streamline healthcare administration.

Foundational Standards Impacting the Claims Revenue Cycle

The movement toward automating the claims revenue cycle dates back to the inclusion of Subtitle F of the Health Insurance Portability and Accountability Act (HIPAA) of 1996. HIPAA named certain types of organizations as covered entities, including health plans, healthcare clearinghouses, and certain healthcare providers, and required them to adopt a wide range of administrative simplification standards as well as new privacy and security requirements. Of particular relevance to the claims revenue cycle, HIPAA required the issuance of regulations to create standard transactions for electronic data interchange of healthcare data. The transactions named in HIPAA that impact physician practices (and their X12N numeric designation) include the following:

- Eligibility for a Health Plan Inquiry/Response (270/271)
- Health Care Claim (837)
- Health Care Claim Status Request/Notification (276/277)
- Referral Certification and Authorization (278)
- Health Care Claim Payment/Remittance Advice (835)

 TIP If a physician practice or other covered entity conducts any one of the HIPAA transactions electronically, they must use the adopted standard and must adhere to the content and format requirements of each transaction.

ACA Administrative Simplification Provisions

The Patient Protection and Affordable Care Act (ACA) of 2010 included a number of provisions that will directly impact the claims revenue cycle. Written to improve on the standards originally mandated under HIPAA and to accelerate a number of provisions of HIPAA that were never promulgated, Section 1104 of the ACA requires the adoption and regular updating of a number of critical standards, implementation specifications, and operating rules for the electronic exchange and use of health information for the purposes of financial and administrative transactions.

Operating Rules

Although the implementation of the X12N 4010 A1 version of the HIPAA 837 claim standard in 2004 was expected to significantly improve automation of the claims revenue cycle, the design of the transaction standards permitted considerable variance in how health plans interpreted the data content requirements. Because of this variance, health plans created in excess of 1,000 "versions" of the one standard through publication of proprietary "companion" implementation guides. As a result, physician practices encountered continued challenges and additional cost in conducting each of the HIPAA electronic transactions. In 2006, the Council for Affordable Quality Healthcare (CAQH) created the Committee on Operating Rules for Information Exchange (CORE) to develop voluntary operating rules (business process standards) to help address the variation in health plan standards interpretation and to enhance the functionality of the HIPAA standards. Eligibility verification and claim status were the first two sets of operating rules developed by CORE.

NOTE These operating rules build on the existing standards to make the HIPAA transactions more predictable and consistent. CORE issued operating rules that included the identification of the rights and responsibilities of all parties in the transaction, security requirements, transmission standards and formats, response time standards, and specific data content requirements critical to practices such as establishing patient financial responsibility in real time. Due in part to their voluntary nature, these operating rules were not embraced by all HIPAA covered entities and their supporting vendors.

The ACA transforms these operating rules from voluntary to mandatory for health plans. Defining operating rules as "the necessary business rules and guidelines for the electronic exchange of information that are not defined by a standard or its implementation specifications," the ACA set specific timetables for the implementation of operating rules not just for insurance eligibility verification and claim status but for the other HIPAA standards and electronic fund transfer (EFT) as well.

NOTE The ACA requires the establishment of a standard for an electronic fund transfer transaction that is effective no later than January 1, 2014, and requires the development of a standard and single set of operating rules for electronic health claim attachments no later than January 1, 2014.

National Identifiers

HIPAA mandated the implementation of a number of national identification numbers for use in the HIPAA administrative transactions to make the claims revenue cycle more efficient. (HIPAA also mandated the development and implementation of a standardized national patient identifier. Because of privacy concerns, Congress has prohibited HHS from developing this identifier.) The current HIPAA national-identified mandates for use in the HIPAA administrative transactions include the following:

- **Employer identification number (EIN)** The EIN, issued by the Internal Revenue Service, was selected as the identifier for employers and was effective in 2002.

- **National provider identifier (NPI)** The NPI is a unique identification number for covered healthcare providers mandated for use in 2005. The law requires that all covered healthcare entities must use NPIs in all the administrative and financial transactions adopted under HIPAA. The NPI is a ten-digit number with no intelligence (i.e., the number does not contain information about the healthcare provider, such as the state in which they live or their medical specialty). The Centers for Medicare and Medicaid Services (CMS) developed the National Plan and Provider Enumeration System (NPPES) to assign standard, unique identifiers to healthcare providers.

 TIP Practices can access the NPPES to assign an NPI to a provider, maintain and update the information about the practice's providers, or locate the NPI for another provider for a referral transaction.

There are two categories of healthcare providers for NPI enumeration purposes. Type 1 providers are *individual providers* who render healthcare (e.g., physicians, dentists, and nurses). Sole proprietors and sole proprietorships are Type 1 (individual) providers. *Organization healthcare providers* (e.g., practices, hospitals, home health agencies, and ambulance companies) are considered Type 2 (organization) providers. Type 1 NPIs are assigned to providers one time regardless of whether the provider changes location or specialty. Practices typically will also have the organization itself receive a Type 2 NPI. Note that a practice may determine that its business needs require multiple Type 2 NPIs. These "subpart" Type 2 NPIs most commonly apply to practices that provide different types of healthcare or have separate physical locations where healthcare is offered.

- **Health plan identifier (HPID)** It has been long recognized that clear identification of the health plan in the claims revenue cycle is critical to reducing administrative burden for physician practices and others. In recognition of this need, HPID regulations were originally mandated in HIPAA but supporting regulations were never issued by CMS. As a result, the HPID was again mandated in Section 1104 of the ACA. On September 5, 2012, CMS published a Final Rule adopting the HPID for health plans. As with the NPI, the HPID will be assigned to health plans by the NPPES. As well, similar to the NPI subparts described above, this rule allows for Health Plans to have more than one HPID. A "controlling health plan" *must* obtain an HPID for itself and *may* obtain an HPID for a subhealth plan of the controlling health plan or direct the subhealth plan to obtain an HPID from the NPPES.

 TIP In general, if any of these separate locations conducts any HIPAA-standard transactions on its own (e.g., billing separately from the parent organization), it then must obtain and use its own Type 2 NPI.

In an effort to accommodate those entities who are not eligible for an HPID but perform certain healthcare functions (i.e., clearinghouses), CMS also adopted an Other Entity Identifier (OEID). The OEID will also be assigned by the NPPES. An "other entity" may obtain an OEID if it needs to be identified in one or more of the HIPAA electronic transactions, is not eligible for an HPID or NPI, and is not an individual.

NOTE It is hoped that implementation of the HPID and OEID will enable a higher level of automation for practices, particularly for the processing of billing and insurance-related tasks, eligibility responses from health plans, and complete descriptions of healthcare claim payments.

Practice Management System Software

Practice management system software (PMSS) is used in the physician practice to record and manage patient registration information, including demographics and insurance coverage, and to conduct patient billing and collections as well as potentially a wide variety of other operational functions. PMSS systems vary widely in their functionalities; some software is billing-specific, while other software incorporates other practices operations such as patient scheduling and registration. The most comprehensive software automates virtually all of the key practice functions and leverages the numerous HIPAA and ACA electronic transaction standards and operating rules. In addition, the more comprehensive PMSS systems can maintain large amounts of data as well as track and issue reports based on these data. Medical code sets, health plan–specific payment policies, and a list of referral physicians are typical of the types of data maintained by a PMSS.

In addition to the traditional client-server PMSS approach, practices now have another option. Application service provider (ASP) software, hosted on the vendor's web site, has become a popular option for many practices. The monthly-fee ASP model offers the benefit of not relying on the vendor to update server-based software, and in some cases the ASP approach reduces practice cost by eliminating the need for up-front costs to purchase PMSS software. These Internet-based solutions can facilitate practice access to health plan online patient eligibility verification and authorization systems and real-time claims payment systems. Security can also be enhanced, because the vendor remotely backs up all practice data on a regular basis.

TIP Some ASP-based systems have the capability of evaluating claims based on health plan contract terms, fee schedules, and payment policies, while taking into account variables that impact reimbursement, such as site-of-service differentials and edits due to services being "bundled" for payment purposes. This approach can decrease many of the expenses related to compiling and sending billing statements.

The Claims Revenue Cycle

The claims revenue cycle can be defined as all administrative and clinical functions that contribute to the capture, management, and collection of revenue for patient services. This cycle starts even before the patient arrives and ends only when all charges are accounted for. Efficiently and effectively managing this revenue cycle is a critical component of a successful physician practice.

Patient Scheduling

The first step in the claims revenue cycle is to set an appointment for the patient to be seen in the practice. While many organizations employ a manual approach involving sometimes multiple staff answering telephones, others have moved to a more automated process.

Automating patient scheduling permits the practice to take advantage of the information being provided by the patient. For example, receiving demographic and insurance information online and in advance of the appointment allows the practice to prepopulate the PMSS in order to run an insurance eligibility verification transaction and identify the patient's financial responsibility prior to the actual visit. Some PMSS products provide a direct linkage to the billing system, ensuring that all patient financial charges are captured in the system.

Integrated into the practice workflow, preregistration, preferably occurring at least a week in advance of the appointment, can be completed manually through the mailing of forms to the patient or via the practice web site, should the organization have that capability.

Patient Intake

Practices take a number of different approaches to patient intake. For new patients, typically the office will e-mail or mail a set of forms for the patient to complete prior to their first visit. Some practices have incorporated increased web site functionality and include downloadable forms on their web site for patients to print, while others have the capability for the patient to complete these forms and submit them online through the practice's web site.

These forms include demographic data, family history, previous medical history including allergies and medications, and insurance information. This is particularly true for primary-care organizations and some specialties. Established patients, depending on the length of time between visits, may also be asked to submit these forms again to ensure that their information is up-to-date.

 NOTE Medical specialties other than primary care may forgo much of the patient history if it has no relevance to the medical issue bringing the patient to the office.

The practice is also required to provide a Notice of Privacy Policies and Procedures (NPP) to all patients and have the patient sign an acknowledgment of receipt of the NPP. This NPP is to be given to patients when first seen in the practice and rewritten and redistributed to all patients upon request should there be material change to the practice's policies (i.e., adoption of an electronic health record [EHR] or participation in a local health information exchange). In addition, the practice must post the NPP in a clear and prominent location in the facility and on the organization's web site, if it has one.

Patient Identification Cards

Health plans commonly issue beneficiary identification (ID) cards that can aid in the intake process. Practices will often request the ID card each time the patient is seen by the practice to ensure that the patient has not switched health plans or has an expired card. There is a distinct lack of automation in the area of patient ID cards, with most practices copying or scanning these ID cards. Once the card is copied, practice staff then must enter the insurance data into the PMSS. This manual data entry process can lead to keystroke errors, which results in the claim being rejected by the health plan. This claim must be reworked to identify the error and resubmitted for payment.

Patient ID cards currently in use today have no mandated federal standards to rely on for format or content and most have no machine-readable elements. Many cards are inconsistently designed and feature photos, illustrations, and dark backgrounds that make legible photocopying difficult.

Use Case 6-1: Installing a Kiosk to Streamline the Intake Process

The Medical Group Management Association has identified significant costs associated with using a nonstandard, non-machine-readable patient ID card. The waste attributed to the additional time required to register the patient with a non-standard ID card at the time of service at the practice as well as the staff time spent to correct errors and resubmit claims that have been rejected because of incorrect patient demographics in practices without card readers is estimated to be more than $2.2 billion a year.[1]

While typically it is the practice patient registration staff that handles intake, more advanced practices have started installing registration kiosks as a convenient method of streamlining the intake process for both the practice and the patient. While the functionality of the kiosk varies depending on the vendor, these kiosks can often capture demographic, medical, and insurance data as well as scan identification cards and even process payments for copayments and deductibles.

NOTE The hope is that an increasing number of health plans will issue machine-readable cards to their beneficiaries. Machine-readable cards, linked to the practice's computer systems via a card reader, would lead to automatic, accurate, and cost-effective collection of patient information with the simple swipe of a magnetic stripe or scan of a bar code.

Insurance Eligibility Verification

Verifying patients' insurance eligibility and establishing patient financial responsibility are critical parts of the claims revenue cycle and, if not completed properly, can result in a significant number of claim resubmissions. For many practices, verifying patient insurance eligibility is often a manual process that can involve multiple phone calls and visits to health plan web sites. However, new standards and the related operating rules described earlier in this chapter offer the promise of a significantly streamlined insurance eligibility verification process.

Prescreening a patient's insurance eligibility will determine the patient's financial responsibility and should be completed for all patients. Some practices have the check-in staff ask the patient whether their insurance has changed since they have last been to the practice. However, should the patient forget that their employer changed health plans or if the coverage has lapsed, the result could be a denied claim. With certain health plans, Medicare being a good example, eligibility verification can be conducted on a yearly basis. The exception, of course, is if the practice will be performing a non-routine service. In these cases, even for Medicare patients, eligibility should be determined prior to every service rendered. By determining what the health plan will cover and what it will not, the practice can significantly decrease the number of denied claims because of lack of insurance coverage.

The purpose of determining in advance, or at a minimum at the time of service, insurance eligibility verification is to decrease claim denials, resubmissions, and outstanding patient balances. Once the patient has left the practice, getting those unpaid balances becomes more difficult and costs the practice more money.

It is clear that determining insurance eligibility for all of your patients who are enrolled in one type of health plan product or another adds a layer of complexity to the practice workflow. This complexity increases as the number of health plan products the practice contracts with also increases. However, the investment the practice makes in incorporating the necessary technology and staff training to conduct eligibility verification transactions, especially the leveraging of the HIPAA standards and CORE operating rules, offers a significant payoff.

For many practices, eligibility verification is conducted via the phone through a health plan's automated voice response system or via the health plan's web site. With this approach, the practice enters the patient's health plan identification number and receives the appropriate voice or web response. While this approach can be effective for a small number of patient eligibility verifications, it remains cumbersome and labor intensive.

TIP Prior to deciding to invest in the practice management system technology that has comprehensive and automated eligibility verification capability, practices should perform the following calculation. Compare the cost of the technology to the cost for the practice for the staff time required to rework and resubmit denied claims, send patients letters and follow-up communications regarding delinquent accounts, process bad-debt information, engage with one or more collection agencies, and determine how much bad debt the practice was forced to write off.

With the appropriate technology in place, practice staff has the ability to check eligibility at multiple points, including pre-arrival, check-in, and charge entry. This real-time eligibility and benefits verification functionality combined with the claims valuation engine often incorporated into the PMSS technology (or offered on the health plan's web site) permits the practice to calculate the patient's financial responsibility before or at the time of service.

Adding to the efficiency, comprehensive PMSS systems can automatically generate an estimate of the patient's out-of-pocket financial obligations after determining the health plan allowance and applying any remaining deductibles or coinsurance. Armed with this information, practice staff can advise patients of amounts due prior to procedures and collect prepayments. Because patient estimates will be more accurate, the number of patient refunds and resubmission of claims will be reduced.

TIP Not only will identifying patient financial responsibility up front capture payments efficiently and reduce the need for back-end patient collections, but it can also enhance patient satisfaction. Providing patients with service estimates based on their latest deductible, coinsurance, and benefits information improves the provider-patient relationship, while helping the group maximize cash flow and minimize payment delays.

Changes to Patient Insurance Coverage

A persistent challenge in the claims revenue cycle is the process by which a patient's insurance coverage changes. For practices to receive notification of a change in a health plan enrollee's eligibility status, the enrollee's employer must notify the health plan, which, in turn, must notify the practice. Some employer-health plan contracts stipulate a reporting often on the first or last day of the month. A problem occurs when some employers do not notify their health plans of benefit status changes for days, weeks, or even longer. A health plan, in turn, may not notify the practice until weeks after receiving this information from the employer. Further, it is not uncommon for patients who change jobs or health plans to neglect to inform the practice.

As a result, after "successfully" verifying insurance coverage, the practice provides medical services to plan beneficiaries but who are later deemed by the health plan as no longer eligible to receive health plan benefits. Claims submitted for payment will thus be denied.

Use Case 6-2: Designing an Effective Eligibility Verification Workflow

Town Center Primary Care Clinic (TCPCC) determined that insurance eligibility was a critical component of the claims revenue cycle. Critical goals of the practice include preventing the organization from providing services to ineligible health plan enrollees and minimizing denied claims and resubmissions. TCPCC implemented the following workflow process to ensure patient eligibility for services:

1. **Process the patient's insurance card** In the past, TCPCC patient intake staff photocopied every patient's insurance card (front and back) on every visit, not just new patient visits. They then moved away from this manual process and incorporated scanning capabilities (again, front and back of the card), capturing this information directly into their PMSS. Staff also ensures that the card's expiration date has not passed. With more and more of their contracted health plans now offering machine-readable patient identification cards, TCPCC purchased a swipe terminal that permits them to read and download demographic and insurance information directly into their PMSS.

NOTE Other health plans are making these cards available to patients on the plan's web site for downloading and printing. Still other health plans are e-mailing "virtual" patient identification cards for use on smartphones and other mobile devices. If possible, the practice should be able to take advantage of each of these options.

2. **Communicate with the patient** TCPCC takes the opportunity when patients call or e-mail to make appointments or when the practice confirms the appointments to inquire about the status of their insurance coverage. This alerts the practice ahead of time if there has been any change in coverage status.

3. **Correctly integrate data into the PMSS** Most importantly, TCPCC staff ensures that the patient's demographic and insurance information is correctly integrated into the PMSS. This takes additional staff time but pays off nicely for the practice with a reduced number of denied claims.

NOTE It is not uncommon for practices to experience rejected claims because of incorrect demographic or insurance information improperly transcribed for the patient identification card or a photocopy of the card. MGMA estimates that about 5 percent of rejected claims are due to errors in the demographic information or the health plan enrollee/member number.[2]

4. **Review capitation lists**   TCPCC contracts with a number of health plans under a capitation arrangement. TCPCC regularly receives capitation lists from these health plans and reviews them immediately and carefully. If the patient's name does not appear on the capitation list, TCPCC staff confirms coverage through some other eligibility verification approach.

5. **Leverage the 270/271 HIPAA transactions and supporting operating rules**   TCPCC has determined that implementing HIT and fully automating its practice patient eligibility verification process has resulted in significant administrative efficiencies. TCPCC staffs have found that whether they are generating a single eligibility transaction at the time of service or conducting a "batch" transaction the day before with multiple patients, automating the process has resulted in a significant improvement to the practice's cash flow by establishing insurance coverage and patient financial responsibility before or at the time of service. While not all the health plans that contract with TCPCC offer a standardized, real-time eligibility verification option, the practice takes full advantage of those plans that do.

The most appropriate approach to this issue is to address it effectively well in advance. Health plan contracts should clearly stipulate that the health plan is responsible for absorbing these types of losses or, at a minimum, will share the financial responsibility with the practice. In addition, eligibility verifications should be conducted for every patient. Finally, the contract should include language that describes the procedure in place and the process to contact those ineligible patients for whom the health plan will not pay and collect the outstanding balance.

Verifying patient eligibility takes significant practice staff time and effort on the front end of the process. However, utilizing a robust eligibility verification approach at this stage will result in considerable efficiency and cost savings on the back end of the process.

Medical Coding

Clinicians are paid for their professional services based on the documentation of the patient encounter. This documentation forms the basis of the two codes typically required for payment. Licensed by the American Medical Association (AMA), Current Procedural Terminology (CPT) codes describe the services and procedures performed by the clinician and are most often used as the basis for individual patient claims and provider-health plan contracts. There are three categories of CPT codes: physician procedures and services, performance management, and emerging technologies. CPT codes are five digits long, with category 1 codes numeric and category 2 and 3 codes alphanumeric with a letter in the last field.

The AMA has also developed a number of modifier codes that can be added to CPT codes to permit a better definition of the services provided by the clinician. These two-digit numeric or alpha codes are generally employed if the provider service was increased or decreased or when site-of-service on the patient (i.e., that it was the left hand that sustained the injury and was treated) identification is warranted.

 TIP The use of modifier codes is not standardized, with some health plans requiring them in certain circumstances and others refusing to pay claims that include modifier codes.

CMS created an additional set of procedure codes in 1978 known as the Healthcare Common Procedure Coding System (HCPCS). HCPCS Level 1 codes are CPT codes, and Level 2 HCPCS codes describe products, equipment, and supply codes (i.e., durable medical equipment such as crutches and ambulance services).

Created by the World Health Organization and modified for use in the United States by the Center for Health Statistics and CMS, the International Classification of Diseases, Ninth Revision, Clinical Modification (ICD-9-CM) codes are used on the claim to identify the diagnosis. Selecting the appropriate diagnosis code takes considerable expertise, and having expert coders on staff or on contract is extremely important to ensure accurate claims submission.

 NOTE On September 5, 2012, CMS published a Final Rule requiring all covered entities to use the latest revision, ICD-10-CM, in all healthcare transactions by October 1, 2014.

Moving to ICD-10-CM is expected to add considerable complexity to the billing process and require significant reengineering of practice workflow. Currently, there are more than 13,000 ICD-9-CM numeric codes divided into categories of diagnoses, moving to more than 68,000 alphanumeric codes with ICD-10-CM. To prepare for this change, physician practices will need to complete an internal review of all IT systems and workflow processes that use ICD-9-CM, upgrade or replace all software that utilize these codes, and provide ICD-10-CM training for all clinical and administrative staff impacted by this new code set.

Claims Submission

Practices employ a number of approaches to submitting and resubmitting claims for payment. Some smaller practices send health plans the CMS-1500 paper directly, while others utilize a clearinghouse for this purpose. Clearinghouses typically convert the CMS-1500 into the 5010 version of the 837 HIPAA electronic transactions standard prior to sending it to the appropriate health plan for payment. Other practices, typically larger organizations with robust HIT, have the ability to send their 837s directly to the health plans. The use of clearinghouses by practices, particularly small to medium-sized organizations, is necessitated by the lack of comprehensive PMSS in the practice and the fact that health plans have adapted proprietary interpretations of "required" and "situational" data elements on the 837 electronic claim. Clearinghouses can also offer practices additional services to assist in streamlining the claims revenue cycle.

Practices can also employ what is known as *scrubbing* software. Scrubbing software is added to PMSS and permits the practice to apply pre-adjudication edits to the claims to identify and correct any problems prior to submission. At a minimum, scrubbing software can incorporate edits derived from diagnosis and procedure code denial data provided by health plans. However, as technology has improved, the software can also incorporate medical necessity and bundling edits and health plan medical coverage and review policy. As health plan payment policies change regularly, to be most effective scrubbing software must be updated at least quarterly.

Real-Time Claims Adjudication (Negotiations Toward Settlement)

A number of health plans offer practices the option of real-time claims adjudication (RTCA), allowing for the billing of services at the time the patient is in the practice. With the appropriate software in place or access to the health plan's web site, the practice not only can bill for the service while the patient is in the office but also can receive an estimated payment and, most importantly, a detailed account of the patient's financial responsibility. At the same time, RCTA presents certain challenges for practices to implement. Charge data must be ready at the time of patient service, and practice staff must manually key in the claims data to the software or appropriate web site. From a workflow perspective, conducting RTCA is challenging because staff must focus more on "front-end" billing requirements and less on "back-end" processes.

 TIP   Because not all health plans offer this as an option and even the ones that do offer the service may not adjudicate more complex patient encounters, at this point RTCA may be best suited for submitting small numbers of "simple" claims.

Payments and Denial Management

Physician practices contract with health plans to receive payment for providing patient services. The process of receiving and processing that payment is complex even in the best-run practices, and successful management of this area of the claims revenue cycle is vital to the financial viability of the organization.

Explanation of Benefits/Remittance Advice

If the practice does not have the capability of accepting an explanation of benefits (EOB) or remittance advice (RA) from health plans in an electronic format, typically then the EOB/RA is mailed to the practice along with the check. Staff must then manually record the payment.

Although the practice may "charge" the health plan a certain amount for a patient encounter, the health plan may apply an edit or payment discount. Plans will cite a number of reasons for the reduced payment amount including that the patient portion of the bill is higher and the practice must recover the additional funds from them, that another health plan (known as a *secondary payer*) provides health insurance for the patient and payment is due from them, or that the practice–health plan contract stipulates a lower amount. Practice billing staff should enter all health plan payments and adjustments as soon as the payments come in so that secondary claims can be filed in a timely manner. For example, some married couples have coverage from both of their employers, or a Medicare recipient has a supplemental coverage. Accurate posting also provides the practice with current status on patient balances and insurance balances, which is critical in order to appropriately manage cash flow.

In some cases, the EOB/RA will not include a payment because the claim has been denied by the health plan. There are numerous potential reasons for a claim to be denied, including that the health plan has imposed a noncontractual adjustment to the claim. The problem could be either on the health plan side or on the practice side. For instance, there could have been errors in the registration process, the practice may have submitted the claim past the filing deadline, there was a lack of authorization (or appropriate referral), the service performed was not a covered benefit, or the service was deemed "not medically necessary" by the health plan.

Once the claim has been adjudicated, the health plan sends an EOB/RA back to the provider detailing what the health plan paid for and how much they paid. The 835 HIPAA transaction is the electronic version of the paper remittance advice (ERA). The 835 contains an explanation of claims payments, claims denials, and other financial information necessary for practices to reconcile patient accounts. To assist in explaining the payment amount, health plans include Claim Adjustment Reason Codes (CARCs) and Remittance Advice Remark Codes (RARCs) on the ERA. The CARCs and RARCs identify standard reasons why the payment may be different from the charge submitted by the practice. CARCs and RARCs are mandated by HIPAA, and the code definitions cannot be changed by any health plan. In general, CARC definitions tend to be generic, while RARC definitions provide more information related to adjudication of the claim. HIPAA requires that for every five CARCs displayed on the 835 ERA, at least one RARC must be returned as well to provide clearer information when claim payments are reduced or denied.

In many instances, practices have the ability to correct simple errors on the claim and resubmit or lodge a formal appeal of the claim denial. In the case of the former, the practice must implement a workflow process to identify and correct the problem and resubmit the claim for payment. Typically, these "simple" problems include such issues as the health plan subscriber identification number is incorrect or missing, the ICD-9-CM diagnosis code is not identified to the level required by the health plan, the claim contains insufficient documentation to support adjudication, or the subscriber's name used on the claim does not match the information in the health plan's system.

Denial Management Software

Denial management software can be extremely helpful for the practice to manage this portion of the claims revenue cycle. Under normal circumstances, the percentage of claims denied by health plans should be quite low. Denial management software can track statistics such as the following:

- Percentage of claims denied by health plan and resubmitted (by health plan)
- Most common reasons for denials by health plan
- Percentage and amounts of claims ultimately paid by plans and percentage written off

Once the practice has implemented denial management software and the appropriate workflow, the task for the practice is to identify the reasons for the denial, correct the individual claim issues, resubmit for payment, and also identify and correct any systemic and potential health plan–specific issues that are causing claims to be denied.

Electronic Funds Transfer

Electronic funds transfer offers an excellent opportunity for a practice to automate a manual process and achieve significant efficiencies. In many practices today, payment is received from the health plan in the mail, and administrative staff members copy the check, manually post the information, and then take time out during the workday to go to the bank to make the deposits. As the workplace has embraced direct deposit of pay checks, healthcare is now moving toward broader use of EFT, although the lack of standards and uniform business rules has slowed wide-scale adoption. The government has recently made efforts to require health plans to implement a series of standards to significantly increase the number of physician practices accepting EFT payments.

 TIP The requirement that health plans adopt EFT standards and associated operating rules is included in Section 1104 of the ACA. Standardizing this transaction will require all health plans to offer EFT, and practices should adopt PMSS systems that support EFT transactions.

Patient Collections

With some exceptions, most patients arrive at the practice with health insurance that requires some financial responsibility on the part of the patient. The amount owed by the patient varies widely from relatively low copays for primary-care visits to high-dollar deductibles for surgical procedures. In recent years, there has been significant growth in the number of patients selecting high-deductible health plan products. As discussed earlier, it is critical for the practice to establish what the patient financial responsibility is before the visit and attempt to collect that payment prior to the delivery of services. Should that not happen or should the patient financial responsibility change or not be established subsequent to the visit, the practice will have to implement a collections process.

TIP The longer these outstanding balances remain in accounts receivable, the more difficult it is for the practice to collect them. The patient collection workflow should prioritize collections based on the date of service and the amount owed by the patient.

Outstanding balance letters should be sent to the patient as quickly as possible once the balance has been established. Should these not be paid, practices will typically then call patients as the next step in the collections process. It is critical, however, that practice staff be appropriately trained and follow strict guidelines in terms of what to say, payments options to present to the patient, hours to call, and sensitivity to financial hardship issues.

TIP Patient collections is an area where practices can implement technology to automate what has typically been a manual process. Software is available that allows the organization's billing team to easily produce a standardized appeals letter that includes the pertinent details of the appealed claim.

Patient Use of the Practice Web Site

There are a number of opportunities for physician practices to incorporate the organization's web site into the claims revenue cycle and improve both cash flow and patient satisfaction.

Producing paper patient statements not only is time-consuming but costs the practice money to print and mail. E-mailing statements and permitting patients to access their statements via the practice web site are highly efficient methods of getting patients the information they need. Certain considerations are important, however. Protecting the security of the information and safeguarding the privacy of the patient should be the underlying goals for the practice. This includes either getting permission from the patient to post their statement online or permission to send them their statement through e-mail. It is important to remind patients that in most cases, the employer owns the e-mail, and the practice cannot be responsible for any disclosure of the patient's information should the employer look at the e-mail. To avoid this issue, it may be best to get a personal e-mail address from the patient.

 TIP Further enhancing cash collections, some practices have moved to online bill payment systems for their patients. More and more individuals, especially younger ones, are routinely paying bills online, and some don't even own a checkbook. While it should not be the practice's only bill payment method, offering this option to patients may decrease days in accounts receivable while at the same time can increase patient satisfaction.

Chapter Review

As you have seen, there are numerous steps and potential roadblocks on the path to payment for physician practices. The federal government has done its part by crafting a broad set of administrative simplification standards aimed at streamlining the claims revenue cycle. HIPAA, enacted in 1996, was the first of these efforts, leading to a wide array of privacy and security provisions designed to safeguard a patient's health information, national identification numbers, and the standardization of a number of critical electronic transactions such as the claim, eligibility verification, and remittance advice. A voluntary industry effort started in 2006 to enhance the usefulness of electronic transactions led to the development of "operating rules" for eligibility verification and claim status. In 2010, these operating rules and several other administrative simplification provisions were included in Section 1104 of the ACA.

From the time the patient schedules an appointment to be seen by the practice clinicians, practice staff must take steps to ensure that care is delivered effectively and that payment is received for the service. Successful practices have front-end workflow processes to ensure that patient intake and insurance eligibility verification are completed effectively. Similarly, claims submission, payment posting, and patient collections must be accomplished efficiently. Should the practice experience administrative errors caused by poor revenue cycle management, the organization runs the risk of claims rejections and a resultant cash flow disruption.

Leveraging HIT is an excellent method of automating the entire claims revenue cycle. Deploying a PMSS product that can electronically record patient demographic and insurance information, generate a real-time eligibility verification, submit claims for payment, send a claim status inquiry, capture payment information, and assist in patient collections can produce significant efficiencies for the practice. Effective use of standards and technology can greatly assist practices in navigating the complex billing and collections process.

Questions

To test your comprehension of the chapter, answer the following questions and then check your answers against the list of correct answers at the end of the chapter.

1. Which of the following national identifiers was *not* mandated by the Health Insurance Portability and Accountability Act (HIPAA) of 1996?

   A. National Employer Identifier

   B. National Provider Identifier

   C. National Clearinghouse Identifier

   D. National Health Plan Identifier

2. What legislation mandated the development of standards for the electronic funds transfer (EFT) transaction in healthcare?

   A. Americans with Disabilities Act (ADA)

   B. Health Insurance Portability and Accountability Act (HIPAA)

   C. Health Information Technology for Economic and Clinical Health (HITECH)

   D. Patient Protection and Affordable Care Act (ACA)

3. What was the entity that created the voluntary set of operating rules to enhance the existing HIPAA electronic transaction standards for eligibility verification and claim status?

   A. CMS

   B. CAQH CORE

   C. WEDI

   D. ANSI X12

4. Which of the following is *not* a potential benefit attributable to use of a standardized, machine-readable patient identification card?

   A. More efficient patient intake

   B. Faster paid claims

   C. Decreased need for nursing triage

   D. Reduced number of administrative staff

5. Which of the following does the HIPAA Privacy Rule *not* require in regards to the Notice of Privacy Policies and Procedures (NPP)?

   A. That the revised NPP be provided at the patient's request

   B. That the NPP be posted in a public area of the practice

   C. That the NPP be posted on the practice's web site, if it has one

   D. That the NPP be written in Times Roman 12-point font

6. Which of the following is *not* considered a benefit of establishing patient insurance coverage prior to the office visit?

   A. Guarantees higher payment from the health plan

   B. Establishes patient financial responsibility

   C. Leads to fewer denied claims

   D. Reduces practice outstanding debt

7. Which of the following steps is *not* considered an effective approach to dealing with changes to patient insurance coverage?

   A. Including the issue in the practice–health plan contract

   B. Verifying insurance coverage prior to the patient visit

   C. Putting in place a process to collect outstanding patient balances

   D. Relying solely on the patient to inform the practice of coverage changes

8. Which of the following steps is *not* one of the key workflow steps involved in verifying patient insurance coverage?

   A. Process the patient's insurance card

   B. Request the patient copay payment ahead of the visit

   C. Review capitation lists

   D. Communicate with the patient

9. Which organization created and maintains the Current Procedural Terminology (CPT) code set?

   A. American Medical Association

   B. American Hospital Association

   C. American Academy of Professional Coders

   D. American Health Information Management Association

10. As of 2012, what is the diagnosis code set currently used in the United States for claims submission?

    A. ICD-10-PCS

    B. ICD-10-CM

    C. ICD-9-PCS

    D. ICD-9-CM

11. The X12N standard for the electronic claim is known as what?

    A. 835

    B. 270

    C. 837

    D. 271

12. Under the law, are health plans required to pay the exact amount that the physician charges for the patient service?

    A. Yes

    B. No

13. Typically, what is *not* a step in the patient collections workflow process?

    A. Informing the health plan of the outstanding patient balance

    B. Sending a letter to the patient establishing the outstanding balance

    C. Calling the patient to discuss the outstanding balance

    D. Tracking the length of time the patient has had an outstanding balance

14. In the claims revenue cycle, what is a CARC?

    A. Claim Adjustment Refusal Code

    B. Claim Adjustment Resubmission Code

    C. Claim Adjustment Response Code

    D. Claim Adjustment Reason Code

15. Typically, what function is *not* available to the patient on a physician practice web site?

    A. Ability to pay outstanding balances

    B. Ability to review the physician's medical school transcript

    C. Ability to review the organization's Privacy Notice of Policies and Procedures (NPP)

    D. Ability to schedule an appointment

Answers

1. **C.** A National Clearinghouse Identifier was not mandated by HIPAA.

2. **D.** Section 1104 of the Patient Protection and Affordable Care Act (ACA) included the mandate to develop standards for the EFT transaction.

3. **B.** The Council for Affordable Quality Healthcare, Committee on Operating Rules for Information Exchange (CAQH CORE) created the voluntary set of operating rules.

4. **C.** A decreased need for nursing triage is not a potential benefit of a standardized, machine-readable patient identification card.

5. **D.** Although the Privacy Rule stipulates that the NPP must be written in "plain language," it does not stipulate the font type or size.

6. **A.** While establishing patient insurance coverage prior to the office visit has many advantages, it does not guarantee higher payment from the health plan.

7. **D.** Relying solely on the patient to inform the practice of coverage changes is not considered an effective approach to dealing with changes to patient insurance coverage.

8. **B.** Requesting the patient copay payment ahead of the visit typically is not one of the key workflow steps involved in verifying patient insurance coverage.

9. **A.** The American Medical Association created and maintains the Current Procedural Terminology (CPT) code set.

10. **D.** ICD-9-CM is the diagnosis code set currently used for claims submission.

11. **C.** The X12N standard for the electronic claim transaction is known as the 837.

12. **B.** No, the health plan is not required to pay the exact amount charged by the physician for the patient service.

13. **A.** Informing the health plan of the outstanding patient balance is not considered a step in the patient collections workflow process.

14. **D.** In the claims revenue cycle, a CARC is a Claim Adjustment Reason Code.

15. **B.** A physician's medical school transcript is not typically available to the patient on a physician practice web site.

References

1. Swipe it home. Accessed on September 15, 2012, from www.mgma.com/swipeithome.

2. Swipe it waste. Accessed on September 15, 2012, from www.mgma.com/swipeitwaste.

Using Healthcare IT to Measure and Improve Outcomes

Floyd P. Eisenberg

In this chapter, you will learn how to

- Understand the structure and components of a quality measure to help translate the components for implementation in electronic health records (EHRs)
- Determine whether there is sufficient precision in a quality measure definition to implement it in an EHR and obtain consistent results
- Consider clinical workflow to capture and manage data in an EHR for use in clinical decision support or quality measure reporting
- Identify evolving standards used for electronic quality measurement

Considering Automated Queries for Measurement: How to Ask Questions to an EHR

Let's get started by going through two example measures to explain the kind of detail needed to ask a question of an EHR. The EHR is primarily a database. It will provide data only if you ask in a way it can understand. And if the question is somewhat ambiguous, so will be the answer, if an answer is possible at all. To start, refer to Table 7-1 for a list of measure components.

Component	Description
Initial population	All patients who share a common set of specified characteristics. The measure can focus on all events (e.g., procedures or patient encounters) rather than individual patients. In the latter case, "population" can also refer to events. For example, the focus of the measure may be all coronary artery bypass procedures to evaluate the outcome of each. In that case, any patient with more than one procedure would be included more than once because the focus is on the procedure rather than the patient.
Denominator	May be identical to the initial population or a subset of it to further specify the purpose of the eMeasure.
Denominator exclusions	Information about the patients or events that should be removed from the eMeasure population and denominator. These are generally used to remove patients who were excluded from the research studies, and also clinical guidelines. Exclusions are used to be sure the measure evaluates only those patients for whom the information in the numerator should apply, based on the available evidence.
Numerator	The interventions (processes) that are expected or the outcome that is expected, based on the evidence, for all members of the denominator.
Denominator exceptions	Some measures remove patients or events from the denominator only if the numerator interventions or outcomes are not met. These exceptions are used to allow providers to exercise clinical judgment and make decisions about care individually for each patient in cases that do not meet the strict requirements of the guideline on which the measure is based. Denominator exceptions allow for adjustment of the calculated score for those providers with higher-risk populations. This measure component is not universally accepted by all measure developers. It is included here so you understand its purpose.
Measure population	Used only in continuous variable measures because they do not have a denominator or numerator. This component defines the patients or events that are evaluated by the measure.
Measure observations	Used only in continuous variable measures. This component describes how the individual results are to be compared. The most common comparisons are count, average (mean), and median.

Table 7-1   Quality Measure Structure

Use Case 7-1: Defining a Quality Measure, Example 1

Request: Identify all children with normal blood pressure.

Let's assume we are working for the measure developer in this case. We need to break down the question into its component parts to be sure the EHR provides the right information to calculate the result. The first question is, "What is the time period of interest?" To clarify, we can state this:

Population: All children seen during the calendar year 2012.

Now the time period is clear, but we need to be specific about which children—all of those living in the city, all of those insured by a local health plan, or all of those seen at least twice in the office practice. We will choose the last group because it is something the EHR can find for us.

Population: All children seen in the office at least twice during the calendar year 2012.

Getting a bit deeper in the review, we find that the EHR doesn't identify people as "children" or "not children." So, we need to define what we mean by the term. We generally want to use a common definition, so we will add the following:

Population: All people who are 18 or younger as of the day prior to the calendar year 2012 and who are seen in the office at least twice during the same year.

Now we are pretty sure we know those of interest to the measure. This population is our denominator, the group we will evaluate. But now we find that providers don't record blood pressure as "normal blood pressure" or "abnormal blood pressure." Rather, they measure and record every blood pressure as two values: the *systolic* (the pressure when the heart is beating) and the *diastolic* (the pressure when the heart is resting between beats). An example of a blood pressure reading, measured in millimeters of mercury (mmHg), would be recorded as 118/74; the first, higher number is the systolic reading, and the second, lower number is the diastolic reading. So, now it is important to define what level of blood pressure is considered "normal." We were asked to create the measure because there are a set of charts available based on evidence that the National Heart Lung and Blood Institute (NHLBI) published to define what is "normal."[1]

 TIP Reliable sources of evidence are those produced by government agencies and specialty organizations.

Using those charts, a provider can compare any given child's height, sex, and age to find how that child compares to other children in the United States. The result is a percentile rank. Children in the ninety-fifth percentile or higher for systolic blood pressure are considered to have *hypertension* (their systolic blood pressure is higher than 95 percent of all children). Those children ranking between the ninetieth and ninety-fifth percentiles are considered to have *prehypertension*, and all those ranking less than the ninetieth percentile are considered to have *normal* blood pressure. So, now we have a definition, and we can state our measure as follows:

Population (denominator): All people who are 18 or younger as of the day prior to the calendar year 2012 and who are seen in the office at least twice during the same year.

Numerator: All people in the population (denominator) whose systolic blood pressure is less than the ninetieth percentile based on age, sex, and height according to the NHLBI blood pressure tables.

Our measure is now specific, but there are still two missing facts that will give different results to those who try to use it. First, children seen during a calendar year have several blood pressure readings. Which reading is the one we want the EHR to report: the first, the most recent, or an average of all systolic blood pressure readings? We decide that the most recent systolic blood pressure reading is best for our measure. When we measure at the end of the year, the most recent will be the last reading during that year, whenever it happened.

Population (denominator): All people who are 18 or younger as of the day prior to the calendar year 2012 and who are seen in the office at least twice during the same year.

Numerator: All people in the population (denominator) whose most recent systolic blood pressure is less than the ninetieth percentile based on age, sex, and height according to the NHLBI blood pressure tables.

Now for the second missing fact: most providers don't record the percentile rank for systolic blood pressure when recording blood pressure values. The EHRs do have fields for systolic blood pressure, height, sex, and birth date, so all are available to compare to the NHLBI charts and find a percentile rank. However, the information will not be available as a field in the EHR unless the EHR automatically calculates it or providers routinely record it manually. The measure would need to ask for all data required (the birth date, the sex, the most recent height, and the most recent systolic blood pressure) and provide the NHLBI charts with a string of code that any EHR can read to perform the calculation for reporting. Alternatively, EHR products could provide the feature as a standard component, but since that is not a consistent EHR process, we can't rely on it for our measure. That is why many measures rely on information that can be expected in existing EHR products.

Based on the information we just reviewed, we now tell our measure developer that we have two options. The first is to encourage better standard use of EHRs and work with some vendors to include pediatric blood pressure percentile ranking because it adds value to clinical care. Our second option is to abandon the measure or look for other information that might support our needs. For this hypothetical case, we will take the first option and work with some vendors to develop best practices (evidence) and encourage other vendors and providers to follow their example.

Use Case 7-2: Defining a Quality Measure, Example 2

Request: Identify all adults who have diabetes and whose condition is controlled over time.

Let's assume we are working for the measure developer in this case like with the first case. Just like in the first case, we need to break down the measure into its component parts to be sure the EHR provides the right information to calculate the result. The first question is, "What is the time period of interest?" To clarify, we can state the following:

Population: All adults with diabetes seen during the calendar year 2012.

Now the time period is clear, but we need to be specific about which patients—all of those living in the city, all of those insured by a local health plan, or all of those seen at least twice in the office practice. So, we will choose the last group because it is something the EHR can find for us.

Population: All adults with diabetes seen in the office at least twice during the calendar year 2012.

Getting a bit deeper in the review, we find that the EHR doesn't identify people as "adults" or "not adults." So, we need to define what we mean by the term. We generally want to use a common definition, so we will add the following:

Population: All people with diabetes who are at least 18 years of age on the first day of the calendar year 2012 and who are seen in the office at least twice during the same year.

Now we are pretty sure we know those of interest to the measure. We need to be clear, though, about what we mean by "diabetes." Are we comfortable that the presence of a diagnosis on the problem list is enough to find all diabetics? Or do we also want to find all patients who are receiving medications that are used to treat diabetes so we don't miss anyone? If we do that, we have to consider excluding any patients receiving such medications for reasons other than diabetes (e.g., those with a diagnosis of polycystic ovarian syndrome). We conclude for this example that the diagnosis on a problem list is sufficient. This population is our denominator, the group in which we have interest. Now we need to define what is meant by good control. Reviewing the evidence, we find that a blood test, hemoglobin A1c (HgA1c), is a good indicator of diabetes control over a period of several months. So, we have a way to measure blood pressure control. And we find several reports about what level of HgA1c should be used to decide whether that control is *good*. So, we ask a panel of experts to convene and conclude which level should be used in the measure so we find patients who are well controlled, but we help improve care by the measure and we don't introduce possible harm, or *unintended consequences*. By setting the level too low, we could find that some providers manage their patients too strictly so they perform well on the measure but that strict management causes some patients to have significant side effects and harm from blood sugars that are too low. (Remember, any decisions we make in this example are presented only as examples for this hypothetical case.) Panels of experts will come to different conclusions than those presented here, but the example is included to show the real concerns measure developers deal with every day.

Now, based on our review, we decide not to look for a specific value of HgA1c to determine good control. Instead, we decide to look for patients who have results that most agree are out of control (HgA1 values greater than or equal to 9) and who improve over time.

Population (denominator): All people with diabetes who are at least 18 years of age on the first day of the calendar year 2012 and who are seen in the office at least twice during the same year.

Numerator: All patients in the denominator with HgA1c values >= 9 who improve their control during the measurement year.

Now we are a bit clearer, but we still haven't noted what is meant by improvement. So, we specify that improvement should be a change in the HgA1c result of at least 1. But we also need to define over what time frame that improvement should be expected. Based on the nature of the test we are using to determine control or lack of control, we conclude that there should be at least a six-month interval between the tests. That means that only patients whose first test was performed between January and June will qualify for the measure, and we realize we need to add to our denominator. We also decide (again for this example) that a second HgA1c test should be expected for all patients not in control during the measurement year.

Population (denominator): All people with diabetes who are at least 18 years of age on the first day of the calendar year 2012 and who are seen in the office at least twice during the same year and who have HgA1c results obtained in the first six months of the year with a result of >= 9.

Numerator: All patients in the denominator with HgA1c values >= 9 who have a second HgA1c result obtained at least six months after the first that occurs during the measurement year and whose HgA1c value is less than the initial value by at least 1.

This is a bit more complex than our first example. Now we need to figure out how to tell the EHR to find the two values and to calculate the difference. Providers don't routinely document change over time in any standard way, but EHRs do capture results. So, we define a measure element *delta* (change over time) and explain to the EHR from what data the change should be derived.

Population (denominator): All people with diabetes who are at least 18 years of age on the first day of the calendar year 2012 and who are seen in the office at least twice during the same year and who have HgA1c results obtained in the first six months of the year with a result of >= 9.

Numerator: All patients in the denominator with HgA1c values >= 9 who have a HgA1c delta of >=1 derived from the first HgA1c result during the measurement year and the most recent HgA1c result that was performed at least six months after the first, and both must occur during the measurement year.

Now the EHR vendor and provider are clearer about exactly what we want to be reported.

TIP   For questions about the specific elements used in a quality measure, go directly to the developer of the measure to clarify anything that seems ambiguous.

Why Measure Quality?

"If you cannot measure it, you cannot control it. If you cannot control it, you cannot manage it. If you cannot manage it, you cannot improve it."[2] But while the concept of measurement is not new,[3] the method to apply measurement to health and healthcare has evolved over the past few decades through work by many organizations (Table 7-2).

Though a goal of measurement is to help increase the consistency with which basic care is delivered, studies have shown that care provided by different organizations or providers is not the same.[8,9,10] Many have turned to measurement to provide the forcing function to standardize and consistently apply care processes that evidence strongly suggests will improve patients' health. Using consensus standards will improve the ability to evaluate and compare the quality of care provided. That is why many government programs use NQF-endorsed measures to evaluate their network of providers.

Organization	Measurement Focus
The Joint Commission[4]	Core measures of hospital quality[5]
The National Committee for Quality Assurance (NCQA)	Healthcare Effectiveness Data and Information Set (HEDIS) to evaluate care quality for people covered by those plans[6]
American Medical Association convened Physician Consortium for Performance Improvement (PCPI™)	Quality measures for clinical practice, primary care, and specialty[7]
National Quality Forum (NQF)[11]	Measure endorsement using a formal consensus development process (CDP) to carefully evaluate and endorse consensus standards, including performance measures, best practices, frameworks, and reporting guidelines[12]

Table 7-2   Some Quality Measurement Organizations

What Makes a Quality Measure Worth Measuring?

It is important to avoid measuring for the sake of measurement, that is, to avoid the inclination to measure merely because it is in vogue. Measurement should be based on an established need to change the status quo (e.g., insufficient care, too much care, unsafe care, or less than desirable outcomes) for which evidence shows that a change is effective. Evaluating evidence of processes that work requires some basic understanding of research and how such research is used to recommend guidelines for clinical practice. A research study is a process that records information (data) for a group of people to answer questions about a healthcare problem.[13] Definitions of types of studies used to evaluate evidence for measurement are available from the Agency for Healthcare Research and Quality (AHRQ) and the National Cancer Institute (NCI).[13,14]

Evidence-Based Clinical Practice Guidelines

Medical specialty societies, government agencies, and other organizations develop clinical practice guidelines intended to help providers and patients directly apply the findings of the research into the care patients receive.[16] Because clinical studies often carefully select patients for evaluation, the guidelines developed from them generally are careful to recommend treatments only to patients who are similar to those evaluated in the studies. Those patients who are similar to those in the clinical studies are generally *included*. That means a guideline based on a study of treatment for a specific disease in patients younger than 65 might apply only to patients 65 and younger. Patients older than 65 may be excluded. Criteria such as gender, age, type of disease being treated, previous treatments, and other medical conditions can be used as inclusion or exclusion criteria.[15] It has become increasingly common for clinical practice guidelines to carefully evaluate the strength of the evidence for each recommendation (based on the number and types of research studies) and to grade the recommendations. A carefully developed evaluation and grading method was developed and is maintained by the U.S. Preventive Services Task Force (USPSTF). The USPSTF assigns letter grades to its recommendations (A, B, C, D, and I). An "A" recommendation has the strongest support, and "D" is not supported; "I" is inconclusive.[16] The USPSTF further ranks the certainty (the level of evidence) as high, moderate, or low. Many medical specialty societies and other clinical guideline developers use the same or modified grading for their recommendations to help providers and patients decide how to apply the guidelines to their own care.

Clinical practice guidelines have been available for some time. A good source for established clinical practice guidelines is the Agency for Healthcare Research and Quality (AHRQ) National Guideline Clearinghouse.[17] But changing practice based on the research and the guidelines does not happen automatically. Translating research into practice can take up to two decades.[18] Even with good evidence and clinical practice guidelines, a large percentage of people in the United States were still not receiving routine preventive services in 2003.[19] For that reason, many have put their hopes in the electronic health record to help turn the tide and deliver the right care at the right time.

EHRs provide the opportunity to influence the provider's behavior at the time they interact with it to enter or retrieve information. Actions designed to provide that influence are often called *clinical decision support* (CDS). Much has been written about CDS, and you can refer to other chapters of this book and other sources for further details.[20]

What Is the Connection Between Clinical Decision Support and Quality Measurement?

It is important to note the direct connection between CDS, efforts to influence behavior at the right time within the process of care, and quality measurement that evaluates whether the expected services were provided or whether the patient's status improved as expected. For example, CDS helps to make sure a diabetic patient has a hemoglobin A1c (HbA1c) blood test to make sure their diabetes is controlled over time. After all is said and done, quality measurement evaluates whether the test was performed and whether the result shows good control of the patient's diabetes. Both rely on the same information: that the HbA1c blood test was ordered and processed by the clinical laboratory and that the result is available and in normal range. But each uses that information differently. If CDS determines the test was not performed or the result is out of range, it can be programmed to encourage the provider to order the test, or if the result is high, it can be programmed to take action to improve the patient's blood sugar control. The quality measure uses the same information to see, over time, what percentage of the provider's patients with diabetes had the test done and how many had results in normal range. CDS relies on *triggers* that initiate a rule, *input data* that the rule uses to evaluate what needs to happen, *interventions* that the rule tells the computer system to do to give the provider the *action steps* they can take to help the patient improve (Figure 7-1).

Figure 7-1

Clinical decision support requires four components: the triggers, input data, interventions, and action steps.[21]

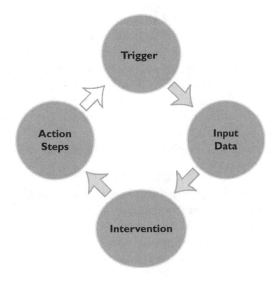

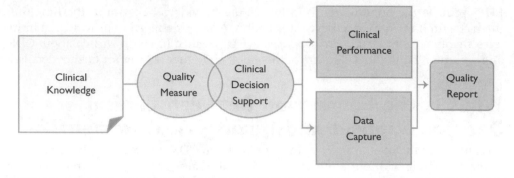

Figure 7-2 Relationship of clinical knowledge, clinical decision support, and quality measures to encourage data capture and reuse to enhance clinical performance and report on quality processes and outcomes[21]

In summary, Figure 7-2 shows the close linkage between quality measures and clinical decision support. Both are driven by the same clinical knowledge. Each requires similar data, and each plays a role in evaluating clinical performance.

What Is the Measure of a Measure?

To ensure that measures meet the needs of those who use them, it is important to manage the quality, the impact, and the value of the information they produce. Regulatory and governmental organizations require the reporting of financial and clinical patient-level data for performance measurement. Some of these programs incorporate a pay-for-performance component such that healthcare organizations and clinicians are held accountable for their performance by variation in reimbursement.[22] The Affordable Care Act allows the Centers for Medicare and Medicaid Services (CMS) to develop new models of payment for care that shares cost savings between CMS and the accountable-care organizations (ACOs). These payments are directly linked to the ACO's performance in quality measures that affect patient and caregiver experience of care, care coordination, patient safety, preventive health, and health provided for at-risk populations and the frail or elderly.[23] To ensure the measures used have the impact expected to support the ACO programs, a stringent process of review is needed. National Quality Forum (NQF) supports that need by using a formal consensus development process to endorse measures for quality performance and public reporting.[24] Criteria are summarized here, including importance to measure, scientific acceptability, usability, and feasibility:

- **Importance to measure and report** The extent to which the measure focus is important in order to make significant gains in healthcare quality (safety, timeliness, effectiveness, efficiency, equity, patient centeredness) and to improve health outcomes for a specific high-impact aspect of healthcare where there is variation in overall poor performance.

- **Scientific acceptability of the measure properties** The extent to which the results of the measure are consistent (reliable) and credible (valid) if it is implemented as specified. Scientific acceptability assessment includes reviewing reliability, validity, exclusion criteria, risk assessment strategy, scoring methods, the comparability of multiple data sources, and the methods to determine potential disparities in care provided. Also highly important is the extent to which those who will use the measure can understand the results and use them to make meaningful decisions (usability) and the extent to which the data required to compute the measure is readily available without undue burden and can be implemented (feasibility).

Endorsement evaluates the rigor of the measure. It is also important to select measures for use in individual programs that evaluate care provided. NQF convenes the Measure Application Partnership (MAP), a public-private partnership to providing input to the U.S. Department of Health and Human Services (HHS) about what performance measures it should select for public reporting and performance-based payment programs as required in the Affordable Care Act. The MAP is a comprehensive, multistakeholder group that includes input and comment from the public at large to share expertise on aspects of improving healthcare. Guided by the National Quality Strategy,[25] measures are recommended and provide input that addresses national healthcare priorities and goals, such as making care safer and ensuring that people and families are engaged as partners in their care.[26]

What Are the Types of Measures, and How Are They Different?

Measures can evaluate performance related to different aspects of health and healthcare. Several classification systems are available to describe measures. Donabedian defined three dimensions of quality that have become the backbone of how the industry defines measurement: structure, processes, and outcomes.[27]

What Are the Expectations for the EHR to Perform Measurement?

The current process for measuring quality using EHRs is evolving. Most existing measures have not been written in a format to allow direct queries to EHRs to extract data. Much of the information needed to evaluate these existing measures is based on information from claims submitted for payment or from human abstractors who review medical records in detail to know whether the measure criteria are met. Some measures use clinical data that is available because it is included in claims attachments, specifically laboratory results and pharmacy-dispensing data. Using such *clinically enriched* claims information is a step forward for measurement, but it is not able to take advantage of the potentially rich information present in the EHR. So, to implement measures that describe clinical data, the process continues to use traditional manual methods to interpret the measure to evaluate available information. This effort can include medical record abstraction, natural-language processing methods to find information from unstructured (free text) fields in the EHR, or specific fields in the EHR for clinicians to enter the data using drop-down menus or check boxes.

Adding additional fields for clinician data entry is very costly. It takes significant time and effort, it increases the likelihood of incorrect entry of information, and it is not part of the patient care workflow, so it takes time away from caring for the patient. Using check boxes further limits the value of the data since the information is an interpretation of what should be captured directly as a result of the patient interaction, in other words, the provider's statement about that interaction or confirmation. For example, checking a box that the patient's systolic blood pressure is less than 140 mmHg makes the provider interpret a result already captured and attest it is correct. Capturing the result itself from the EHR as it is initially entered is preferred since it is more accurate and less prone to error. It also comes with the benefit of knowing more information about that result (metadata) such as the method used to obtain it and the date and time it was performed.

There is some data that can be captured only using confirmation via checking the box that a process occurred. A good example is medication reconciliation. *Medication reconciliation* is the process of reviewing the patient's complete medication regimen at the time of admission, transfer, and discharge and comparing it with the regimen being considered for the new setting of care to avoid duplication, to avoid inadvertently omitting critical medications, and to prevent avoidable interactions among the medications the patient is receiving.[28] However, there is no defined set of online clicks that has been determined to automatically know that a provider has reconciled a patient's medication lists. Therefore, the provider must attest that reconciliation has been performed and is complete by using some sort of check box or signature. Even attempts to reconfigure, or "retool," measures for the EHR platform used concepts intended for a manual abstraction or provider confirmation process. And the underlying standards (discussed in the next few paragraphs) are not yet ready to directly query an EHR database. So, there is still manual intervention required to use EHR data for measurement. Figure 7-3 shows a stylized process for implementing quality measures in EHRs as it exists today.

 TIP Ideally, information collected for measures that use EHRs as a data source should include only the data captured as a result of directly caring for patients and only the data that is important to the concurrent (day-to-day) care of the patient. Any request for additional data entry merely for the purpose of administrative or measurement processes will result in dissatisfaction among providers and also reduce the time available to interact with patients.

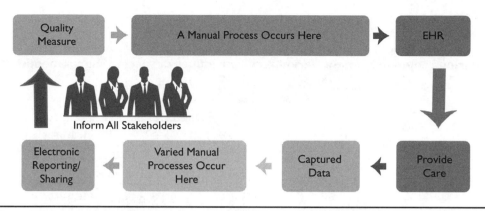

Figure 7-3 Implementing a quality measure in an EHR in mid-2012 still requires manual effort to interpret the measure and fit it into the provider's workflow in the EHR.

To resolve potential conflict between measure and clinical care requirements, measurement (i.e., queries to an electronic data source and/or electronic health record) should be defined using standard terminology and should address clinical workflow and context consistent with that used in the direct process care delivery. Clinical organizations and clinicians will be able to more clearly address quality performance through retrospective analysis and to develop clinical decision support interventions by using carefully defined, human, and electronically readable query formats.

There is much work in progress to evolve toward an automated process for measuring quality using electronic information from EHRs. The Standards and Interoperability (S&I) Framework Query Health Workgroup is working to develop standard electronic formats to ask for data directly from EHRs.[29] Much of this work is based on efforts started in 2009 with the HL7 Draft Standard for Trial Use, the Health Quality Measure Framework (HQMF), also called *eMeasure*. Working with 18 measure developers in 2010, NQF coordinated the reexpression (retooling) of more than 100 measures into eMeasures. The work was guided by the Quality Data Model (QDM) to provide standard data definitions and a standard grammar and structure to express the information required for the measure elements (Figure 7-4).[30] Much was learned from the pilot work, and a number of the reexpressed measures were used in the Health and Human Services EHR Incentive Programs for eligible providers and hospitals.[31] In addition to guiding the work of the Query Health Project, information learned from the initial retooling and implementation efforts is informing efforts to tool new measures in eMeasure format (Figure 7-5). The work also led to the development of a Measure Authoring Tool (MAT) to help measure developers better express their measures without having to learn underlying XML code.[32] The MAT is based on the QDM, and both continue to be maintained and updated. The S&I Query Health project is developing an

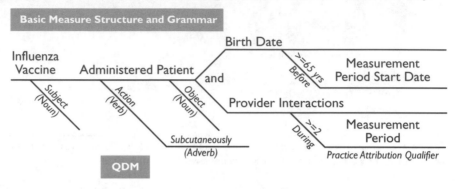

Figure 7-4 Similar to diagramming a sentence, the QDM provides grammar to allow the developer of a measure to state what is needed in a consistent way.

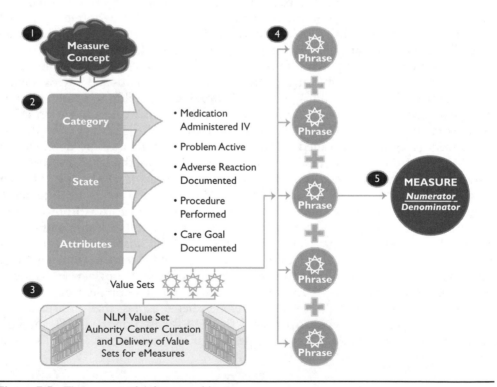

Figure 7-5 The process of defining an eMeasure

update to the HQMF Draft Standard for Trial Use (DSTU) and also an HQMF Implementation Guide to be balloted in HL7 to help improve its ability to achieve the goal of direct queries for data that already exist in EHRs. The work described is enhancing the ability to create a query to an EHR so it can search for the data expected and calculate the result. Another piece of the measurement workflow is the standard to report the results. The HL7 DSTU, Quality Reporting Document Architecture (QRDA), has been available.[33] It was recently updated with an implementation guide in May 2012, and the updates are proposed for further testing to support a standard method for reporting the results of quality measures.

 TIP   The HQMF is the standard to incorporate eMeasures into the EHR.

What Changes Are Needed to Enable Electronic Quality Measurement?

The ability to move away from measures that have been developed with the end data in mind (claims and data abstraction) and moving toward a more expansive view of what could and should be measured to improve care is a paradigm shift that measure developers and EHR vendors need to embrace. Retooling of measures developed for a different data source has the potential to expect data in an EHR for which the EHR was not designed. Such measures can be overburdened by potentially unnecessary exclusions and complex measure logic because they are based on a different paradigm of data capture. Ideally, EHRs are not designed to replicate a paper process. They should be designed and implemented in combination with efforts to improve workflow and enhance a provider's ability to provide direct patient care.

However, measure developers will need to have a sense of common EHR capabilities and be able to trust that providers consistently use the EHR structures regardless of which vendor product is implemented. For example, the presence of an up-to-date problem list in an EHR should remove the need to look for other means to determine whether a patient has a particular diagnosis (e.g., medications used to treat the condition) and allow for more population-based views of care. The presence of a longitudinal record that can trend numerical clinical results should allow measures to better evaluate care based on outcomes without adding additional variables. For example, patients with hypertension should have their blood pressure controlled regardless of the number of visits to a provider in a given year. When the claim for the visit was the only way to capture the physician's confirmation of the blood pressure result, information about visits was needed. If the measure can address numerical EHR blood pressure results directly, the visit information becomes an unnecessarily added burden to calculate.

As noted, EHR data allows greater attention to outcomes linked to evidence-based processes that can drive improvement through clinical decision support. Only processes most proximal to and with the greatest impact on patient outcomes need to be addressed. Personal health records, patient web portals, and increasingly available smartphone apps should provide important opportunities for individuals to self-report on outcomes, as well as medication use, patient experience, and decision quality. While such information may not be directly in EHRs today, it is increasingly important to address as part of the care process.

While measure developers seek to take advantage of EHR data as a rich source of information, it is not necessarily safe to assume that EHRs consistently have data structured in a way that it can be easily used. Many EHRs have evolved from systems created with the primary goal of capturing information to support claims and payment. Although important, clinical workflow was sometimes guided to support claims-related data. Newer systems are addressing claims more as a byproduct of clinical care, but even they may base the need for storing data on the clinician use cases that drove the EHR structure. It is important to think about how information is organized or modeled.

The International Health Information Terminology Standards Development Organization

The International Health Information Terminology Standards Development Organization (IHTSDO) defines two methods of modeling.[34] A model of meaning represents the underlying meaning in a way that is common to and reusable between different use cases. In contrast, a model of use structures information based on a specific intended use. If, in a hypothetical case, the intended use of a patient's blood pressure result is for a clinician to view it and make decisions, the information can be captured as text showing the systolic value over the diastolic value similar to an equation (e.g., 136/74). The data was captured and stored based on the use model that defined only a single result without the need for any specific structure. When the clinician decides it is important to follow the blood pressure over time and trend it on a graph, the EHR then needs to parse the result into its component parts and store the systolic value (136) as a number and the diastolic value (74) as a number, both of which are from the same reading. The new use model requires trending over time, and so the data is now structured. If the original modeling were based on the intended meaning, the EHR vendor would have had to provide an enhanced display, but no change in the underlying data would have been required. Many EHRs managed data input based on use requirements determined at a point in time. Similarly, quality measurement was also based on the use model of human intervention (confirmation or chart abstraction). As both EHRs and measure developers look at achieving clinical outcomes, reuse of captured data becomes increasingly important. Restructuring the process of collecting data based on its meaning will enhance the potential for reusing information and reducing the need for redundant data entry and information restructuring and will enable less cumbersome clinical care, clinical decision support, and quality measurement. In addition, the measurement infrastructure and data can itself be leveraged to encourage standardized data, coding, and tools across the healthcare continuum in a manner that has not yet been seen.

TIP   Successful structuring and reuse of data can occur through use of a standardized data model and standardized value sets.

How Are Value Sets Standardized?

Measures list data elements as criteria. To be sure those implementing the measures enter the right patients and the right information into the analysis, they must carefully explain what information from the clinical record is needed. For example, the term "blood pressure" seems specific, but blood pressure is actually a combination of two clinical findings: a *systolic* blood pressure (when the heart is contracting, or beating) and a *diastolic* blood pressure (when the heart is resting between beats). Each is measured at the same time. Blood pressure can also be taken at rest; during or after exercise; or in a lying, sitting, or standing position. Each of these qualifiers (metadata) about the blood pressure is important to understand how the finding should be used. So, a measure evaluating diastolic blood pressure to look for improvement needs to clearly indicate what is intended. There are several ways to state what is meant.

- Diastolic blood pressure (qualifier: resting; position: sitting)
- Resting diastolic blood pressure (position: sitting)
- Sitting, resting diastolic blood pressure

The first example uses a basic concept, diastolic blood pressure, and separately describes the attributes, or metadata, required—resting and sitting. It can be stated to *postcoordinate* an expression, breaking it down into its component parts, each of which has a concept in available code systems (e.g., Systematized Nomenclature of Medicine – Clinical Terms, SNOMED-CT).[35] The next two examples *precoordinate* the concept (i.e., suggest a single concept that incorporates all metadata into one code).

Traditionally, measures have used claims codes to specify which values are acceptable for each data element in their measures. This method has been successful when capturing data from claims, but it is more challenging when looking for information captured during a clinical interaction between a provider and a patient. Claims codes provide general information, but they do not allow clinicians to express what is needed to provide direct care. For example, to indicate a diagnosis of intrinsic asthma using the International Classification of Diseases, Ninth Revision, Clinical Modification (ICD-9-CM),[36] which is the coding system used for most claims in the United States, the provider would use the code 493.1. However, to indicate *persistent* asthma for which treatment is different from other types of asthma, no ICD-9-CM code is available; the provider would need to enter free text into the EHR or use a different coding system such as the International Classification of Diseases, Tenth Revision, Clinical Modification (ICD-10-CM)[37] or SNOMED-CT. ICD-10-CM will be used in billing in the next two years, but it is not currently in use in all organizations.

In another example, the provider may want to indicate a specific interaction with the patient through e-mail exchange. The coding system used for most encounter- and procedure-related claims is Clinical Procedural Terminology (CPT),[38] which includes a code for an evaluation/management visit for an established patient at different levels of intensity. To accommodate e-mail exchange, CPT added a code, but interactions between other clinicians and patients are not clearly expressed in CPT. A clinical terminology such as SNOMED-CT allows more expression of additional interactions.

As EHRs and quality measures together require more clinical data for evaluation and trending, the use of SNOMED-CT is expected to become prevalent. It is also expected that the information in the EHR will need to be mapped to claims-related code systems for billing purposes. While EHRs may capture the information at the level of detail indicated, they do not consistently store it as a postcoordinated expression. Therefore, collaboration between measure developers and EHR vendors and implementers will be important to resolve potential conflicts.

The terms, or values, used to clearly explain each data element are called a *value set*. A value set is a set of codes derived from a particular code system, or *taxonomy*.[39] For the previous example, all of the codes for diastolic blood pressure would be included in one value set.[40] Value sets are not static. The code systems from which the values are derived update on a regular basis, retiring some concepts and adding new ones. Therefore, value sets need to be maintained and versioned over time. A clear understanding of the code system used is also critical to be sure the values selected for a value set are complete and correct. To encourage greater consistency, the National Library of Medicine (NLM) has established the NLM Value Set Authority Center to provide measure developers with access to code systems that allow them to develop and share valid, complete, and reusable value sets.[41] The NLM Value Set Authority Center is expected to curate the value sets to be sure the code system is used as intended and also assist with harmonization of concepts among measure developers to avoid duplication of value sets.

Moving Forward: Retooling vs. Creating Measures de Novo Based on Data in EHRs

Moving forward will take a collaborative effort among measure developers, EHR vendors, data warehouse third-party providers, frontline clinicians, and also patients. The essential issue is to provide the appropriate meaning by asking for the information actually needed from the appropriate individual (e.g., ask for information about education provided by asking the patient if the expected information was learned, as compared to asking the provider to use a check box).

Chapter Review

This chapter discussed some of the challenges inherent in using EHRs to manage data intelligently so that data can be entered once as part of the workflow for usual patient care and reused to improve the care process concurrently with clinical decision support and retrospectively by measuring quality. The change from capturing and reporting information based on a model of use to a model of meaning is not easy, but it has the potential to significantly increase timeliness, efficiency, effectiveness, and safety while reducing redundancy. A consistent model to express information within and among systems is important to enable clear understanding. The Quality Data Model (QDM) provides such a common technological framework for defining the clinical data necessary to measure performance and accelerate improvement in patients' quality of care.[30,40] By providing a common grammar to describe the information within quality measures, the QDM enables quality measurement from a variety of electronic sources, and it is applicable to all care settings a patient is likely to interact with in a lifetime. The structure of the QDM describes a data element as the combination of a category of information, the context in which it is used (the state), and specific attributes, or metadata, that help clarify exactly what is needed to evaluate the measure.

1. Measure developers decide on the information needed for the measure.

2. The developers use the QDM grammar to describe the category and state (or context) that is acceptable to meet their needs and any related information (attributes). Examples were provided in Figure 7-4 (e.g., medication administered via IV).

3. The developers select from existing value sets or create new value sets to indicate the information they need (e.g., the specific medications) using the National Library of Medicine (NLM) Value Set Authority Center. The NLM Value Set Authority Center provides tools and curation to develop value sets and keeps them current.

4. The developers combine the newly developed data elements with their value sets into phrases that describe more detail about the information needed (e.g., medications administered within one hour before the start of a surgical procedure).

5. The developers combine the phrases into components of the measure (e.g., denominator, numerator). The QDM provides the backbone structure to help those who read the measure to understand clearly what is meant in each measure statement or phrase. The purpose of this process is to let those implementing measures look for the data that is structured in the EHR and report the same information regardless of the EHR product used in each practice or hospital.

This chapter described a combination of efforts to move toward a fully implementable query to measure the quality of care from an EHR. Efforts include a common data model (QDM), the NLM Value Set Authority Center to standardize and curate value sets, the S&I Framework Query Health Project to improve the HQMF standard to express measures as functional queries to EHRs, and HL7 work to simplify the QRDA for measure reporting. These activities will lead to infrastructure to enable the end-to-end processing of data for measurement. But change requires more than infrastructure. The most effective way to accelerate the movement to fully electronic measurement is through collaboration. Measure developers are increasingly working with EHR vendors and individual practices and hospitals to test eMeasures. Other efforts, such as the eMeasure Learning Collaborative, have the potential to address issues and share best practices related to eMeasures implementation, suggesting solutions and action plans to address these challenges.[43]

Questions

To test your comprehension of the chapter, answer the following questions and then check your answers against the list of correct answers at the end of the chapter.

1. What is a value set?

   A. A range of numbers that are normal results for laboratory tests

   B. A set of codes chosen by a measure developer to define a data element in a measure

   C. The relative strength of recommendations as supported by evidence for the interventions expected in a quality measure

   D. The combination of a measure's validity, reliability, and feasibility that describes its potential use in value-based purchasing programs

2. The chief medical officer of your organization asks you to set up a measure for his research study for all of his patients with high blood pressure whose blood pressure improves after six months, regardless of treatment given. How do you define high blood pressure?

   A. Systolic blood pressure of <120 mmHg as you found on the Web at the National Heart Lung and Blood Institute web site.

   B. Diastolic blood pressure of <80 mmHg as you found on the Web at the National Heart Lung and Blood Institute web site.

   C. Blood pressure less than the ninetieth percentile by height, age, and gender per the National Heart Lung and Blood Institute web site.

   D. You don't have enough information to proceed and ask for more clarity.

3. You are asked to measure how often doctors in your network evaluate a newborn baby's home environment for factors that might put them at risk. The factors include lead paint in the home, if the baby's mother has been screened for postpartum depression, if such depression is present whether it is under treatment, and if there are pets in the home. You cannot find specific fields in your EHR for each of these items. What actions do you take?

   A. Immediately add fields to the EHR patient demographic section for Yes/No/Not Applicable responses to lead paint in the home, mother screened for depression, if depressed mother is on treatment, and pets in the home.

B. Request input from an appropriate group of practicing clinicians to determine the workflow to capture and evaluate such information and implement a solution consistent with existing best practice upon which the majority agree.

C. Immediately add fields to the EHR patient demographic section for Yes/No/Not Applicable responses to lead paint in the home and pets in the home, and you look in the family history section of the EHR for evidence of depression in the mother.

D. Search the literature to find a screening tool shown to work for another organization and implement it directly in your EHR.

4. Which of the following is the acronym for the standard used to write an eMeasure?

A. QRDA

B. Consolidated CDA

C. HQMF

D. S&I Framework

E. QUERYHEALTH

Answers

1. **B.** A set of codes derived from a particular code system, or taxonomy, such as SNOMED-CT, ICD-9-CM, ICD-10-CM, CPT, and so on.

2. **D.** Measures require precise definition. The information provided by the chief medical officer made assumptions about which blood pressure measurement and which threshold to use to define the answer.

3. **B.** Request input from an appropriate group of practicing clinicians to determine the workflow to capture and evaluate such information and implement a solution consistent with existing best practice upon which the majority agree.

   Adding additional fields to "hardwire" a solution has the potential for causing dissatisfaction and adding additional burden to the clinician's workflow without adding substantial benefit. Using fields intended for a different purpose (e.g., family history to determine whether the child's mother is currently depressed) can lead to finding inaccurate information to support clinical decisions or measure reports. If the information is relevant to the active management of the patient's care, there is opportunity to configure the EHR and the workflow efficiently.

4. **C.** HQMF: the Healthcare Quality Measure Framework, an HL7 draft standard for trial use as of June 2012.

References

1. Blood pressure tables for children and adolescents from the fourth report on the diagnosis, evaluation and treatment of high blood pressure in children and adolescents. (2004). Accessed on June 28, 2012, from www.nhlbi.nih.gov/guidelines/hypertension/child_tbl.htm.

2. Harrington, H. J. (1991). *Business process improvement: The breakthrough strategy for total quality, productivity, and competitiveness.* McGraw-Hill.

3. History of quality. Accessed on June 28, 2012, from http://asq.org/learn-about-quality/history-of-quality/overview/overview.html.

4. The joint commission. Accessed on June 28, 2012, from www.jointcommission.org/about_us/about_the_joint_commission_main.aspx.

5. The joint commission's core measures. Accessed on June 28, 2012, from www.jointcommission.org/core_measure_sets.aspx.

6. Healthcare effectiveness data and information set. Accessed on June 28, 2012, from www.ncqa.org/tabid/59/Default.aspx.

7. AMA-convened physician consortium for performance improvement (PCPI). Accessed on June 28, 2012, from www.ama-assn.org/ama/pub/physician-resources/physician-consortium-performance-improvement.page.

8. Achieving and sustaining improved quality: Lessons from New York state and cardiac surgery. (2002). Accessed on June 28, 2012, from http://content.healthaffairs.org/content/21/4/40.long.

9. Variations in healthcare quality: Racial, ethnic, and economic disparities in medicare fee-for-service in California. (2003). Accessed on June 28, 2012, from www.chcf.org/~/media/MEDIA%20LIBRARY%20Files/PDF/C/PDF%20CareDisparitiesMedicareFFS.pdf.

10. The Dartmouth atlas of healthcare. Accessed on June 28, 2012, from www.dartmouthatlas.org.

11. National quality forum. Accessed on June 28, 2012, from www.qualityforum.org/Home.aspx.

12. Consensus development process. (2012). Accessed on June 28, 2012, from www.qualityforum.org/Measuring_Performance/Consensus_Development_Process.aspx.

13. Agency for healthcare research and quality: Glossary of terms. (2012). Accessed on June 25, 2012, from www.effectivehealthcare.ahrq.gov/glossary-of-terms/?filterletter=r.

14. Dictionary of cancer terms. (2012). Accessed on June 25, 2012, from www.cancer.gov/dictionary.

15. Field, M. J.; and Lohr, K. N. (eds). (1990). *Clinical practice guidelines: Directions for a new program.* National Academy Press.

16. U. S. Preventive Services Task Force (USPSTF) grade definitions after May 2007. (2007). Accessed on June 28, 2012, from www.uspreventiveservicestaskforce .org/uspstf/grades.htm. (Accessed June 28, 2012)

17. Agency for healthcare research and quality national guideline clearinghouse. (2012). Accessed on June 28, 2012, from http://guideline.gov/about/index.aspx.

18. Agency for healthcare research and quality: Translating research into practice (TRIP)-II. (2001). Accessed on July 11, 2012, from www.ahrq.gov/research/ trip2fac.htm.

19. The quality of healthcare delivered to adults in the United States. (2003). Accessed on July 11, 2012, from www.nejm.org/doi/full/10.1056/ NEJMsa022615.

20. A roadmap for national action on clinical decision support. (2007). Accessed on July 11, 2012, from http://jamia.bmjjournals.com/content/14/2/141.abstract. Improving outcomes with clinical decision support: An implementers guide, second edition. (2012). Accessed on June 28, 2012, from http://marketplace. himss.org/OnlineStore/ProductDetail.aspx?ProductId=3318.

21. Driving quality and performance measurement: A foundation for clinical decision support: A consensus report. (2010). Accessed on July 11, 2012, from www .qualityforum.org/Publications/2010/12/Driving_Quality_and_Performance_ Measurement_-_A_Foundation_for_Clinical_Decision_Support.aspx.

22. Agency for healthcare quality and research: Pay for performance (P4P). (2012). Accessed on July 11, 2012, from www.ahrq.gov/qual/pay4per.htm.

23. Accountable care organizations: Improving care coordination for people with medicare. (2012). Accessed on July 11, 2012, from www.healthcare.gov/news/ factsheets/2011/03/accountablecare03312011a.html.

24. National quality forum consensus development process. (2012). Accessed on July 11, 2012, from www.qualityforum.org/Measuring_Performance/ Consensus_Development_Process.aspx.

25. Report to Congress: National strategy for quality improvement in healthcare. (2011). Accessed on July 11, 2012, from www.healthcare.gov/law/resources/ reports/quality03212011a.html.

26. National quality forum measure application partnership. (2012). Accessed on June 27, 2012, from www.qualityforum.org/Setting_Priorities/Partnership/ Measure_Applications_Partnership.aspx.

27. Evaluating the quality of medical care. (2005). Accessed on July 11, 2012, from http://onlinelibrary.wiley.com/doi/10.1111/j.1468-0009.2005.00397.x/abstract.

28. Patient safety primers: Medication reconciliation. (2012). Accessed on July 11, 2012, from http://psnet.ahrq.gov/primer.aspx?primerID=1.

29. Standards and interoperability framework (S&I): Query health. (2012). Accessed on July 11, 2012, from http://wiki.siframework.org/Query+Health.

30. Quality data model update June 2012. (2012). Accessed on July 11, 2012, from www.qualityforum.org/WorkArea/linkit.aspx?LinkIdentifier=id&ItemID=71275.

31. Centers for Medicare and Medicaid Services: EHR incentive programs. (2012). Accessed on July 11, 2012, from https://www.cms.gov/Regulations-and-Guidance/Legislation/EHRIncentivePrograms/index.html?redirect=/ehrincentiveprograms/30_Meaningful_Use.asp.

32. National quality forum measure authoring tool (MAT). (2012). Accessed on July 11, 2012, from www.qualityforum.org/MAT.

33. Quality reporting document architecture (QRDA). (2012). Accessed on July 11, 2012, from www.hl7.org/special/committees/structure.

34. International health terminology standards development organization (IHTSDO) glossary, international release. (2012). Accessed on July 11, 2012, from www.ihtsdo.org/fileadmin/user_upload/doc/tig/glsct/glsct_ss_ModelOfUse.html#_c0cc3aca-4e72-40ba-af25-116e04a36fad.

35. Standardized nomenclature of medicine – clinical terms (SNOMED-CT). (2012). Accessed on July 11, 2012, from www.nlm.nih.gov/research/umls/Snomed/snomed_main.html; and International health terminology standards development organization (IHTSDO). (2012). Accessed on July 11, 2012, from www.ihtsdo.org/snomed-ct.

36. International classification of diseases, ninth revision, clinical modification (ICD-9-CM). (2011). Accessed on July 11, 2012, from www.cdc.gov/nchs/icd/icd9cm.htm.

37. International classification of diseases, tenth revision, clinical modification (ICD-10-CM). (2012). Accessed on July 11, 2012, from www.cdc.gov/nchs/icd/icd10cm.htm.

38. Current procedural terminology (CPT). (2012). Accessed on July 11, 2012, from www.ama-assn.org/ama/pub/physician-resources/solutions-managing-your-practice/coding-billing-insurance/cpt.page.

39. Value set definition and binding document. (2008). Accessed on July 11, 2012, from http://valuesets.org/wiki/index.php?title=Value_Set_Definition_and_Binding_Document.

40. Quality data model style guide. (2012). Accessed on July 11, 2012, from www.qualityforum.org/WorkArea/linkit.aspx?LinkIdentifier=id&ItemID=71276.

41. Health information technology standards – Ferguson vocabulary task force. (2012). Accessed on July 11, 2012, from http://healthit.hhs.gov/portal/server.pt?open=512&objID=1817&parentname=CommunityPage&parentid=28&mode=2&in_hi_userid=11673&cached=true.

42. eMeasure learning collaborative. (2012). Accessed on July 11, 2012, from www.qualityforum.org/Topics/HIT/eMeasure_Learning_Collaborative/eMeasure_Learning_Collaborative.aspx.

The Role of Healthcare IT in Improving Population Health

J. Marc Overhage

In this chapter, you will learn how to

- Define population health and explain how it differs from healthcare delivery.
- Describe the role of public health in managing illness outbreaks, epidemics, and pandemics.
- Identify and explain issues that affect the use of data for population health.
- Apply health data definitions and standards, as well as privacy and confidentiality issues, in typical public health scenarios.
- Identify when public health agencies can receive identifiable health information to perform public health functions without patient authorization.
- Recognize and explain how population health and clinical care needs complement each other.

We commonly think of healthcare as being focused on the prevention or diagnosis and treatment of disease in an individual, while perhaps even encompassing the maintenance of good health and wellness. Another important aspect of healthcare is population health or public health, in which care is focused on the prevention or diagnosis and treatment of an entire population of people rather than one individual at a time. Public health departments work to prevent epidemics and spread of disease, protect against environmental hazards, prevent injuries, promote and encourage healthy behaviors, respond to disasters and assist communities in recovery, and assure the quality and accessibility of health services. Accomplishing these tasks requires public health departments to monitor the health status of the population, investigate population health problems and hazards, mobilize community partners to address health problems, develop polices and plans, educate the public about health issues, and undertake various assurance activities. Some essential differences between clinical care and population health are depicted in Table 8-1.

	Clinical Care	Population Health
Scale	Individual	Population
Focus	Disease	Prevention
Approach	Treatment	Health promotion
Scale	One at a time	Millions at a time

Table 8-1 Differences Between Clinical Care and Population Health Perspectives

Many different people and organizations have a stake in population health, including public health practitioners (primarily those who work in public health departments in the United States), governments, employers, private payers, and, ultimately, all of us as individuals, since our health is, in part, determined by the health of others around us.

TIP Public health departments may provide individual patient care, but their population health functions are typically focused on populations and not on individual patients.

Despite these differences, clinical care and population health interact in many ways. For example, clinical-care providers administer many immunizations that prevent communicable diseases, and public health providers identify outbreaks of disease that may influence a provider's choice of treatment for a patient presenting with specific symptoms; a patient with fever and cough might be managed differently during an influenza outbreak than in other circumstances, for example.[1]

The American Recovery and Reinvestment Act (ARRA), passed in 2009, and the Prevention and Public Health Fund, passed in 2010 as part of the Affordable Care Act (ACA), could dramatically alter the perspective on population health in the United States over the coming years. This legislation provides significant support for population health initiatives focused on improving the population's health. The ARRA through the Health Information Technology for Economic and Clinical Health Act (HITECH) provides funding designed to stimulate the adoption of electronic health records, assure meaningful use of electronic health records, advance quality measurement, and promote health information exchange. The ACA through the Prevention and Public Health Fund provides for expanded and sustained national investment in disease prevention, wellness promotion, and public health activities. The ACA also advances the concept of accountable-care organizations (ACOs), which are provider-led organizations focused on managing the health of a population and incented to do so through new compensation models. Together these initiatives provide an opportunity to improve population health by using healthcare IT.

Public Health Reporting

To be able to improve a population's health, you have to be able to measure it. While a care provider might use a laboratory test and a thermometer to measure the health of an individual, measuring the health of a population requires different tools such as surveys, electronic surveillance, and statistical analysis methods. This is not as easy to do as it might sound. For example, we currently use more than 190 separate sources of data to track our progress against our national health goals as described in Healthy People 2020.[2] Take something as seemingly simple as knowing how many people in a population have diabetes (this number of people with a condition divided by the number of people in the population at a single point in time is called the *population prevalence*) and whether this number is growing or shrinking (the number of people to get the condition over some period of time divided by the number of people in the population is called the *incidence*). The traditional approach to measuring prevalence and incidence has been to carry out carefully constructed surveys of the populations. The Centers for Disease Control and Prevention (CDC), for example, conducts a number of such surveys. Another approach is case reporting, sometimes referred to as *active surveillance* since it requires action on the provider's part, in which care providers report selected data about patients who meet specified criteria for having notifiable conditions (conditions that public health has identified as appropriate to report) to public health departments that aggregate the data and track it to identify trends in conditions or procedures of interest. For example, public health measures immunization rates by combining data about immunizations administered through public health departments with data about immunizations from providers to create immunization registries. These databases allow public health to measure the proportion of the population that is immunized against a particular condition. One limitation of this approach is that reporting is often an extra step in a provider's care process. Data on notifiable conditions is even more difficult to obtain. Even when providers are motivated to report patients who have relevant conditions, they are often unaware of which conditions are reportable, don't think about reporting while in the midst of providing care, have difficulty remembering how to report, and so on. In addition, these reports require considerable time and expense for public health to manage. Some reports, such as birth certificates, also require validation or certification by a health professional.

 TIP Many of the case definitions provided by public health departments to guide providers on which cases to report require a diagnostic laboratory test as part of the case definition.

The use of healthcare IT in clinical care has created new possibilities for reporting. Structured and coded data captured in healthcare IT systems can be used to facilitate or automate reporting. A laboratory system or interface engine, for example, can be configured to automatically generate a report via a standards-based electronic message to public health when a result indicates a reportable condition. This approach to reporting, often referred to as *passive surveillance* because it does not require action on the provider's part, has been shown to be faster and to identify more cases than manual reporting; however, the reports may be missing some of the data elements that public health needs because the healthcare IT system doesn't have the data. A laboratory system, for example, will not contain data about whether the patient received treatment for a specific infection and so can't include this data in a report. Traditionally, public health focused on tracking conditions that had been diagnosed by care providers, but after the anthrax exposures in 2001, interest increased in tracking potential diseases in order to identify natural or human-initiated outbreaks as soon as possible. This led to using data obtained prior to a diagnosis, which is an approach referred to as *syndromic surveillance* (Figure 8-1). Until healthcare IT systems are very commonly used, public health will be forced to maintain "dual" systems.

With syndromic surveillance, a syndrome—evidence of an increasing number of patients with a specific set of symptoms or findings—is tracked with the expectation that a developing pattern of disease will be found earlier than if public health departments waited until providers identified a diagnosis causing these symptoms. This approach might prove particularly important in cases in which an unusual underlying cause might not be recognized for days or weeks. The figure illustrates that, after an exposure, the number of patients with symptoms will climb over time and then, usually, decline. The number of patients diagnosed with the condition will follow a similar pattern, but will typically lag behind the appearance of symptoms by several days.

 TIP While a variety of data such as rates of absenteeism and purchase of specific over-the-counter drugs has been used in attempts to identify disease outbreaks, using this type of data is not syndromic surveillance. Syndromic surveillance is limited to the use of data collected about patients as part of their care before a diagnosis has been established.

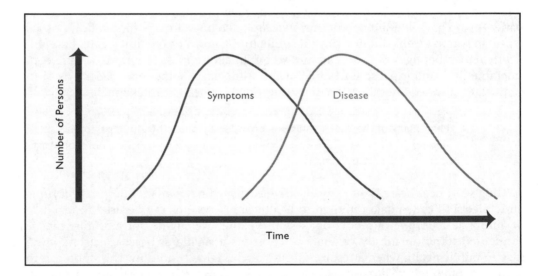

Figure 8-1 Syndromic surveillance

TIP   While it is sometimes possible for healthcare IT systems to determine which data is reportable to public health, it may not be easy. Determining whether a test result is positive (usually indicating the presence of a disease or condition), for example, can be difficult for the healthcare IT system, and in some cases it is a negative result to a test that would indicate that it should be reported.

Registries

Some of the databases used for population health purposes are referred to as *registries*. Registries typically provide information associated with a single disease, a group of related diseases, or a specific grouping of environmental contaminants. The data within registries is collected from many different sources. An immunization registry, for example, might contain data for anyone eligible to receive an immunization (which includes a large proportion of people in a population) about which immunizations they received, when, and from whom. A death registry would contain data about the date and causes of death, while a tuberculosis registry would include patients who had been diagnosed as having tuberculosis and their treatment for that condition. In most cases, the data in a registry is collected close to the time of the events recorded in the registry rather than later (or retrospectively). Some registries also include data obtained by following up with patients at specific times. Information from registries can then be used to estimate survival rates and risks for specific disease, for evaluating short- and long-term effects of environmental exposures, and for testing epidemiological hypotheses.

TIP   Be sure that you can provide a good definition of a registry.

NOTE   Many public health departments operate laboratories that perform specialized testing related to disease of particular public health interest. Some of this testing overlaps with tests performed in hospital laboratories, but some tests are highly specialized. You might want to incorporate data from these laboratories into a care provider's healthcare IT system. Ideally, the test results from these laboratories would be available in a format such as HL7 using a coding system such as LOINC, which would allow them to be incorporated into healthcare IT systems.

Health Alerts

Based on its population perspective, public health will periodically have information that it needs to communicate to providers. Examples might include requests for providers to be perform specific diagnostic testing based on patterns that public health is seeing in symptoms being reported. Another example might be to alert providers to specific treatment suggestions based on specialized testing or experience in other areas. Most of the time, these messages are not specific to individual patients but rather relevant to populations or groups of patients. Public health maintains a system called the Health Alert Network (HAN)[3] that primarily supports alerting between public health departments. In addition to publication and outreach through postings in relevant settings (for example, emergency departments), today public health may use a variety of mechanisms to reach individual providers including mail, facsimile, or e-mail. In addition, there may be benefits to using these mechanisms to create reminders in the healthcare IT system that providers can use while caring for patients in order to alert them under specific conditions. This might be particularly helpful when public health suggests structured data that would be helpful to collect for patients who meet specified criteria. While some demonstrations of this type of capability have been carried out, only limited healthcare IT systems have the ability to incorporate these types of alerts. Alerts from public health are not always well received by providers because the alerts are sometimes perceived as not being relevant to their practice; other reasons the alerts may be unwanted are limitations to scalability and targeting and alert fatigue.

Privacy and Security

Preserving the privacy and confidentiality of patients is critical. Public health agencies often provide both clinical care and public health services, and these two different functions have different privacy and security implications. When providing clinical care, public health agencies are covered entities and are subject to the same rules and requirements as other care providers. When providing public health services, different rules and requirements apply. For public health agencies to monitor the population's health, HIPAA provides exceptions for covered entities, including care providers, to disclose protected health information to public health agencies without patient authorization when the data is required or permitted by federal, state, or tribal statutes. These exceptions include the prevention and control of diseases, injuries, or disabilities; vital events such as deaths and births; issues to support public health surveillance; epidemiological investigations and interventions; and information sent to a foreign government agency that is collaborating with a public health authority (to investigate a disease outbreak, for example). There are also exceptions for the disclosure of data about people at risk for contracting or spreading a disease; workers' compensation and workplace medical surveillance; health oversight; instances of child abuse and neglect; domestic violence; neglect of the elderly or incapacitated; and data on adverse events, for product tracking, to facilitate product recalls or replacement and postmarketing surveillance reporting to pharmaceutical or device manufacturers. In cases of domestic violence, HIPAA additionally requires the covered entity to either seek agreement of the victim or make a determination that reporting is necessary to prevent serious harm to the individual or other potential victims.

TIP Public health departments are *not* covered entities under HIPAA. In some cases, parts of their activities are subject to the same privacy and security rules.

In certain limited cases such as disease surveillance, a limited data set might suffice, and covered entities might be more comfortable reporting data in this fashion. In other cases, aggregated data such as a count of the number of influenza cases seen in an emergency department in a 24-hour period might suffice. Aggregated data better protects patient confidentiality than a limited data set but can be difficult to validate and can make it much more difficult to obtain additional details about a case should they be needed. Approaches have been developed that rely on assigning an arbitrary identifier that allows the provider to link to the individual patient's data to overcome some of these limitations.

TIP While HIPAA grants broad exceptions that allow covered entities to disclose protected health information to public health, covered entities are frequently cautious and seek clear assurances that they are allowed to make these disclosures. This is particularly true when the disclosures involve conditions or data that might not traditionally have been perceived as relevant to public health.

Scope of Data

Public health functions may require almost any of the types of data that are required for clinical care including diagnoses, laboratory results, radiographic results, medications, and vital signs. The scope of data that public health might require is significantly driven by performing syndromic surveillance and the need to investigate outbreaks. In addition to these ubiquitous types of data, public health applications often benefit from geographic location data. This data is often useful in tracking the spread of disease but is available only in limited form (usually restricted to knowing the patient's home address) in most traditional healthcare IT systems. Geolocation data is increasingly available through devices such as patients' mobile phones, but this data is not yet routinely captured in healthcare IT systems.

TIP Healthcare IT systems used by providers often identify providers by using one or more IDs, and the messages they typically exchange don't include details such as name or phone number. If these messages are repurposed for use by public health, the specific provider information will often need to be added to the message.

Clinical Information Standards

In general, uses of healthcare IT for population health rely on the same clinical data standards as other uses of healthcare IT. The same terminology standards including LOINC, ICD-9CM, and RxNORM are applicable. In some cases, population health applications have driven the development of relevant standards such as the CVX vaccine's administered HL7 table.[4] Similarly, population health uses share message format standards including HL7. As for other applications of healthcare IT, public health has some unique use cases for which there are specific implementation guides that specify details appropriate to them that are different than for other use cases. Examples of use cases for which there are specific public health implementation guides include reporting vaccinations and reportable conditions.

Because public health often receives data from multiple care providers, they may have to match patients across those providers in order to avoid double counting when estimating the incidence or prevalence of conditions. They would typically employ the same approaches to patient matching as providers use in a master patient index within or between care providers.

Trends and What to Expect in the Future

Looking forward, there are a number of ways that healthcare IT is likely to evolve to better support public health. For example, you can expect that more information will flow from public health organizations to providers in the context of care such as enabling the electronic health record (EHR) system to access a patient's lifelong vaccination history and provide decision support about missing vaccinations. There may also be mechanisms that allow the list of reportable conditions to be updated to an EHR from public health automatically. Finally, similarly to the evolving need for collaboration between members of a patient's care team, public health will increasingly communicate electronically with clinical-care providers.

Methods for monitoring a population's health are undergoing a transformation as well. They are transforming from field based and descriptive to clinical, analytical, and experimental. This transition will require increased access to data about individuals in the population as well as additional data about the environment in which they live and the system in which they receive healthcare.

Chapter Review

Population health and clinical care are complementary processes. The types of data required by both are the same, but which patients they require data for are different because population health focuses on specific conditions relevant to the health of populations while clinical care focuses on one patient at a time. Data generated by providers in the course of clinical care, such as diagnoses, medication prescribed, immunizations administered, and laboratory test results, can be very useful for public health use cases, and HIPAA provides specific exemptions that allow covered entities to share specific types of data with public health. The data transmission and coding standards are essentially the same for public health applications, though there are specific implementation guides for some. Public health uses this data primarily to measure the prevalence and incidence of diseases in populations. Laboratory results generated by public health may be available to incorporate into healthcare IT and used by clinical-care providers, and you can expect that additional summary data and suggested clinical actions generated by public health will be pushed into providers' healthcare IT systems in the future.

Questions

To test your comprehension of the chapter, answer the following questions and then check your answers against the list of correct answers at the end of the chapter.

1. Public health's role in managing illness outbreaks and epidemics includes which of the following activities? (Choose all that apply.)

    A. Surveillance for disease outbreaks

    B. Identifying the source of disease outbreaks

    C. Communicating the nature of outbreaks and effective actions to address the outbreak to providers and the public

    D. Providing specialized diagnostic facilities

2. True or false. Public health departments are subject to the same privacy and security regulations as all other care providers under HIPAA.

    A. True

    B. False

3. Advantages of passive surveillance versus active surveillance include _____. (Choose all that apply.)

    A. More complete reporting of the cases that occur.

    B. The data about individual cases is more complete.

    C. More rapid reporting of cases that occur to public health.

    D. Supports reporting of data that requires certification by a health professional.

Answers

1. **A, B, C, D.** Public health performs all of the activities listed in managing outbreaks, epidemics, and pandemics. They may also assist with other tasks such as providing or facilitating access to medications or other treatments or immunizing populations in order to limit the spread of disease.

2. **B.** Public health departments often provide direct patient-care services in addition to public health services. They are required to identify those portions of their activities that are subject to the same requirements as covered entities and those that are not. HIPAA does provide a large number of specific exemptions that allow covered entities to disclose protected health information to public health departments for specific purposes under specific conditions.

3. **A, C.** Passive surveillance typically increases the number of cases identified and reduces the time from when cases occur until they are reported to public health, but the reports may be missing important data such as whether the patient has been treated for the condition. In addition, certain reports such as birth and death reports require certification by health professionals and therefore require active involvement by the provider.

References

1. Saba, V. K. & McCormick, K. A. (2011). *Essentials of nursing informatics, fifth edition*. McGraw-Hill.

2. Healthy people 2020. Accessed on August 13, 2012, from www.healthypeople .com/2020/default.aspx.

3. Health alert network (HAN). Accessed on August 13, 2012, from www.bt.cdc .gov/han.

4. HL7 standard code set for CVX (vaccines administered). Accessed on August 13, 2012, from www2a.cdc.gov/vaccines/iis/iisstandards/vaccines.asp?rpt=cvx.

Strategic Leadership and Management of Health Information Technology in Provider Organizations

John Glaser[*]

In this chapter, you will learn how to

- Understand why some organizations are very effective at using information technology
- Explain the importance of leadership and management in healthcare IT
- Align the IT strategic plan with the healthcare organization's needs and priorities
- Turn plans into action (effective execution of healthcare IT projects)
- Recognize key leadership competencies for the IT-savvy executive and clinician
- Identify the capabilities needed to be a successful healthcare CIO and understand the evolving needs of the role

Increasingly, HIT is becoming a central contributor to the strategies, objectives, and plans of healthcare providers. The ability of healthcare IT to be leveraged to improve care quality, safety, accountability, and efficiency can no longer be questioned.

However, the implementation of healthcare IT and the achievement of desired gains in care and operational performance are difficult undertakings. No amount of advice can eliminate the risks and challenges of these undertakings, but solid, strategic leadership and management of an organization's IT initiatives can help ensure the internal commitment and preparation needed for the investments to truly deliver value.

---

* Portions of this chapter were adapted from Wager, K.; Lee, F.; and Glaser, J., *Healthcare Information Systems: A Practical Approach for Healthcare Management, Second Edition*, Jossey-Bass, 2009. With permission from John Wiley and Sons.

Why Are Some Organizations Very Effective at Using Information Technology?

Some organizations are very effective at using information technology (IT) to improve their performance and their competitiveness. You can see examples in many industries, including retail, banking, transportation, insurance, and healthcare.

What do these organizations do that is different from other organizations? This question has been examined over the past several decades and continues to be explored. While different studies asked different questions, they all point to a small number of factors that distinguish those that are effective from those that are not.

The Role of Leadership

If a healthcare organization's leadership desires to use information technology to improve their care quality and reduce the costs of care, they need to take the steps necessary to ensure that their organization develops the competencies needed to implement and leverage IT effectively; for example, the organization needs to be very good at change management.

These actions are different from the steps management would take for an individual project, such as implementing an electronic health record. These actions affect many projects over many years. As an analogy, consider running. A runner's training, injury management, and diet are designed to ensure the core ability to run many marathons. This capacity development is different from developing an approach to running a specific marathon, which must consider the nature of the course, the competing runners, and the weather.

Effectiveness Factors

Several major factors are associated with effectiveness. These factors can be created and shaped by the organization's leadership.

Individuals and Leadership

It is critical that the organization possess talented, skilled, and experienced individuals. These individuals will occupy a variety of roles, such as chief executive officer (CEO), chief information officer (CIO), chief medical officer (CMO), chief nursing officer (CNO), IT staff, and user middle managers (who are the individuals whose team members will be most impacted by the technology being implemented). These leaders must understand the IT vision, communicate the vision, be able to recruit and motivate a team, and have the staying power to see the organization through several years of work with multiple significant challenges along the way.

 NOTE Implementing a major system will have more than one rough patch. These patches can be a result of some users fighting the change, insufficient process reengineering, and unstable technology. It is critical that leadership and the project team keep their cool.

Relationships

Not only must the individual players be strong, but the team must be strong. There are critical senior executive, IT executive, and project team roles that must be filled by highly competent individuals, and highly effective working relationships must exist between the individuals in these distinct roles.

Technology and Technical Infrastructure

New technologies can provide new opportunities for organizations to embark on major transformations of their activities. Leadership must develop an understanding of the capabilities of new technologies and how those capabilities could be used to further the organization's plans. The leadership must also be able to assess the relative maturity of the technology and know when to wait (if necessary) to make investments.

Innovation

The organization's (and the IT department's) culture and leadership must encourage innovation and experimentation. This encouragement needs to be practical and goal directed: a real business problem, crisis, or opportunity must exist, and the project must have budgets, political protection, and deliverables.

Evaluation of IT Opportunities

The organization will have a demand for IT investments that exceeds its financial and management resources. Comparing the value of these investments can be difficult; how do you choose between an IT investment that improves patient safety versus one that reduces care costs? Making these choices and trade-offs requires rigorous assessment processes that also enable instinct and vision to be decision factors.

Change Management

The implementation of major IT applications is always accompanied by changes in work processes and work relationships. It is very difficult to reengineer processes and help individuals adjust to the new way of working. Change management requires great skill and often takes years to accomplish.

 HIT PRO EXAM TIP Change management focuses on the human side of a HIT implementation by engaging people who are affected and addressing the complexities of human behavior. The function of change management also serves to complement project management.

Core Processes and Information Needs

IT efforts should be focused on core organizational processes and critical information needs, namely, processes and information that form the foundation of the business the organization is in. Successful organizations conduct the analyses needed to truly understand how best to use IT to improve these processes and address these information needs. Equally important is measuring whether the IT investments are resulting in the desired improvements.

IT Strategic Alignment

The alignment between the IT activities and the business challenges or opportunities must be strong. The IT plan should be tightly linked to the organization's overall strategic plan. This will be discussed in the section "Aligning the IT Strategy with the Organization's Strategy."

Strong IT Organization

The IT department must be very good at managing projects, providing IT technology guidance, understanding the organization's needs, managing a solid IT technology infrastructure, and providing excellent customer support to users.

Summary

A critical leadership role is ensuring that the organization is competent at applying IT to improve its performance. Several factors have been identified as being major contributors to competency. Leadership should assess the organization's strength in these factors and take remedial actions if necessary. An organization that is less than competent risks wasting its IT investments.

Aligning the IT Strategy with the Organization's Strategy

IT investments serve to advance organizational performance. These investments should enable the organization to reduce costs, improve service, enhance the quality of care, and, in general, achieve its strategic objectives. The goal of IT alignment and strategic planning is to ensure a strong and clear relationship between IT investment decisions and the healthcare organization's overall strategies, goals, and objectives. For example, an organization's decision to implement a computerized provider order entry (CPOE) system with clinical decision support could reflect an organizational strategy of improving the safety of patient care.

Strategic IT Planning Objectives

The IT strategic planning process has several objectives:

- To ensure that information technology plans and activities align with the plans and activities of the organization; in other words, the IT needs of each aspect of organizational strategy must be clear, and the portfolio of IT plans and activities must be able to be mapped to organizational strategies and operational needs

- To ensure that the alignment is comprehensive; that is, each aspect of strategy needs to be addressed from an IT perspective, recognizing that not all aspects of strategy have an IT component and not all components will be funded

- To identify non-IT organizational initiatives needed to ensure maximum leverage of the IT initiative (for example, process reengineering)

- To ensure that the organization has not missed a strategic IT opportunity, such as those that might result from new technologies

- To develop a tactical plan that details approved project descriptions, timetables, budgets, staffing plans, and plan risk factors

- To create a communication plan that can inform the organization of the IT initiatives that will and will not be undertaken

- To establish a political process that helps ensure the plan results have sufficient organizational support

 NOTE Linking an IT strategy to an overall organizational strategy has been difficult for decades, and it will remain difficult for years to come.

At the end of the alignment and strategic planning process, an organization should have an outline that at a high level resembles Table 9-1. With this outline, leadership can see the IT investments needed to advance each of the organization's strategies. For example, the goal of improving the quality of patient care may lead the organization to invest in databases to measure and report quality, a CPOE system, and the electronic health record (EHR).

Organizational Goal	IT Initiatives
Research and education	Patient data registry Genetics and genomics platform Grants management
Patient care: quality improvement	Quality measurement databases Computerized provider order entry Electronic health record
Patient care: sharing data across the system	Enterprise master person index Clinical data repository Common infrastructure
Patient care: nonacute services	Nursing documentation Transition of care
Financial stability	Revenue system enhancements PeopleSoft Cost accounting

Table 9-1 IT Initiatives Linked to Organizational Goals

The Process of Developing an IT Strategy

Across healthcare organizations the approaches taken to developing and managing an IT strategy are quite varied. Some organizations have well-developed, formal approaches that rely on the deliberations of multiple committees and leadership retreats. Other organizations have remarkably informal processes. A small number of medical staff and administrative leaders meet in informal conversations to define the organization's IT strategy.

In some cases, the strategy is developed during a specific time in the year, often preceding development of the annual budget. In other organizations, IT strategic planning goes on all the time and permeates a wide range of formal and informal discussions.

There is no right way to develop an IT strategy and to ensure alignment. Recognizing this variability, a normative approach to the development of IT strategy can be offered.

 NOTE With the increasing pace of change, it is very difficult to have a detailed IT strategy with a time horizon longer than two to three years.

Strategy Discussion Linkage

Organizational strategy is generally discussed in senior leadership meetings. These meetings may focus specifically on strategy, or strategy may be a regular agenda item. Regardless of their form, the organization's CIO should be present at such meetings or be kept informed of the discussion and its conclusions. If task forces and committees supplement strategy development, an IT manager should be asked to be a member. The CIO (or the IT member of a task force) should be expected to assess the IT ramifications of strategic options and to identify areas where IT can enable new approaches to carrying out the strategy.

For example, a discussion about the need to improve the organization's ability to manage chronic disease would lead to the identification of IT initiatives such as electronic health records, home-based monitoring of patients, and analytics to assess care quality and costs.

The CIO will not be the only member of the leadership team who will perform this role. Chief financial officers (CFOs), for example, will frequently identify the IT ramifications of plans to improve the revenue cycle. However, the CIO should be held accountable for ensuring the linkage does occur.

Use Case 9-1: Approving an IT Agenda

As strategy discussions proceed, the CIO must be able to summarize and critique the IT agenda that should be put in place to carry out the various aspects of the strategy. Take the case of an IT agenda that emerges from a strategy designed to improve the patient service experience in outpatient clinics. What might this particular agenda look like?

The agenda should include an overall strategic goal: improve service to outpatients. It would be further supported by stating the key problems the IT solution is intended to fix.

- Patients have to call many locations to schedule a series of appointments and services.
- The quality of the response at these locations is highly variable.
- Locations inconsistently capture necessary registration and insurance information.
- Some locations exceed capacity, whereas others are underutilized.

To combat these issues, the agenda would then suggest what the IT solution would provide.

- Common scheduling system for all locations
- A call center for "one-stop" access to all outpatient services
- Development of master schedules for common service groups, such as pre-operative testing
- Integration of scheduling system with electronic data interchange connection to payers for eligibility determination, referral authorization, and copay information
- Patient support material, such as maps and instructions, to be mailed to patients

By highlighting the IT initiatives necessary to support a provider's strategic goal, the IT agenda essentially creates a vision of the end state, after implementation.

IT Liaisons

All major departments and functions (e.g., finance, nursing, and medical staff administration) should have a senior IT staff person who serves as the function's point of contact. As these functions examine ways to address their needs (e.g., lower their costs and improve their services), the IT staff person can work with them to identify IT activities necessary to carry out their endeavors. This identification often emerges with recommendations to implement new applications that advance the performance of a function, such as a medication administration record application to improve the nursing workflow.

New Technology Review   The CIO should be asked to discuss new technologies and their possible contributions to the goals and plans of the organization. These presentations may lead to suggestions that the organization form a task force to closely examine a technology. For example, a multidisciplinary task force could be formed to examine the role of mobile devices in nursing care, materials management, and service provision to referring physicians.

Synthesis of Discussions   The CIO should be asked to synthesize the conclusions of these discussions. This synthesis will invariably be needed while developing the annual budget. And the synthesis will be a necessary component of the documentation and presentation of the organization's strategic plan. Table 9-1 presented an example of such a synthesis.

The organization should expect the process of synthesis to require debate and discussion; for example, trade-offs will need to be reviewed, priorities set, and the organization's willingness to implement embryonic technologies determined. This synthesis and prioritization process can occur in the course of leadership meetings, through the work of a committee charged to develop an initial set of recommendations, and during discussions internal to the IT management team.

After the debate has been concluded, priorities need to be established, and the IT strategy must be translated into timetables and budgets. Management will discuss various timeline scenarios, consider project interdependence, and ensure that the IT department and the organization are not overwhelmed by too many initiatives to complete all at once. The organization will use the budget estimates to determine how much IT it can afford. Often there is not enough money to pay for all the desired IT initiatives, and some initiatives with high and moderate scores will be deferred or eliminated as projects.

The final plan, including timelines and budgets, will become the basis for assessing progress throughout the year.

IT Strategic Plan Results

Once all is said and done, the alignment process should produce these results:

- An inventory of the IT initiatives that will be undertaken
- A diagram or chart that illustrates the linkage between the initiatives and the organization's strategy and goals
- An overview of the timeline and the major interdependencies between initiatives
- A high-level analysis of the budget needed to carry out these initiatives
- An assessment of any material risks to carrying out the IT agenda and a review of the strategies needed to reduce those risks

NOTE It is important to recognize the amount and level of discussion, compromise, and negotiation that goes into the strategic alignment process. Producing these results without going through the preceding thoughtful process will be of little real benefit.

Executing the Plan: Project Management

Over the course of decades and millions of projects, a set of management disciplines and processes has been developed to help ensure that projects succeed. This collected set of practices is referred to as *project management*. You can see these disciplines and processes in action in any well-run project. Excellent project management does not ensure project success; however, without such project management, the risks of failure skyrocket, particularly for large projects. The elements of project management are reviewed in the following sections. These elements are created or established after the project proposal has been approved.

Project management has several objectives:

- Clearly define the scope and goals of the project.
- Identify accountability for the successful completion of the project and associated project tasks.
- Define the processes for making project-related decisions.
- Identify the project's tasks and task sequence and interdependencies.
- Determine the resource and time requirements of the project.
- Ensure appropriate communication with relevant stakeholders about project status and issues.

Different projects require different management strategies. Projects that are pilots or experiments require less formal oversight (and are not helped by large amounts of formal oversight) than large, multiyear, multimillion-dollar undertakings. Projects carried out by two or more organizations working together will have decision-making structures different from those found in projects done by several departments in one organization.

Project Roles

Two roles are critical in the management of large projects: business sponsor and project manager.

Business Sponsor

The business sponsor is the individual who holds overall accountability for the project. The sponsor should represent the area of the organization that is the major recipient of the performance improvement that the project intends to deliver. A project to improve nursing workflow may ask the chief nursing officer to serve as business sponsor. A project that affects a large portion of the organization may have the chief executive officer as the business sponsor.

The business sponsor has several duties:

- Secures funding and needed business resources (e.g., the commitment of people's time to work on the project)
- Has final decision-making and sign-off accountability for project scope, resources, and approaches to resolving project problems
- Promotes the project internally and externally and obtains the buy-in from business constituents
- Chairs the project steering committee and is responsible for steering committee participation during the life of the project
- Helps define deliverables, objectives, scope, and success
- Helps remove business obstacles to meeting the project timeline and producing deliverables, as appropriate

Project Manager

The project manager does just that—manages the project. This person provides the day-to-day direction setting, conflict resolution, and communication needed by the project team. The project manager may be an IT staffer or a person (or function) in the business who is benefiting from the project. Among their several responsibilities, project managers do the following:

- Identify and obtain needed resources
- Deliver the project on time, on budget, and according to specification
- Communicate progress to sponsors, stakeholders, and team members
- Ensure that diligent risk monitoring is in place and appropriate risk mitigation plans have been developed
- Identify and manage the resolution of issues and problems
- Maintain the project plan
- Manage project scope

The project manager works closely with users, management, clinicians, and the business sponsor in performing these tasks. Together they set meeting agendas, manage the meetings, track project progress, communicate project status, escalate issues as appropriate, and resolve deviations and issues related to the project plan.

TIP A great project manager is an exceptionally valuable asset.

Project Committees

Managing projects of any significant size requires two major committees/teams: the project steering committee and the project team.

Project Steering Committee

The project steering committee provides overall guidance and management oversight of the project. The steering committee has the authority to resolve changes in scope that affect the budget, milestones, and deliverables. This committee is expected to resolve issues and address risks that cannot be handled by the project team. It also manages communications with the leadership of the organization and the project team.

The business sponsor should chair this committee. Its members should be representatives of the major areas of the organization that will be affected by the project and whose efforts are necessary if the project is to succeed. For example, a steering committee overseeing the implementation of a new patient accounting system might include the director of outpatient clinics, the director of the admitting department, and the medical group administrator as members. The senior IT manager should also be on this committee.

Project Team

The project team may not be called a committee, but it will meet regularly, and it does have responsibilities. The project manager chairs the project team. This team does the following:

- Manages the performance of the project work
- Resolves day-to-day project issues
- Manages and allocates resources as necessary to do the work
- Works with the steering committee, as necessary, to resolve problems; assesses potential changes in scope, timeline, or budget; and communicates the status of the project

Key Project Elements

Projects are managed through the use of several artifacts, which are covered in the following sections.

Project Charter

The *project charter* is a document that describes the purpose, scope, objectives, costs, and schedule for the project. This document also discusses the roles and responsibilities of the individuals and functions that must contribute to the project. The project charter serves three basic objectives.

- It ensures that planning assumptions or potentially ambiguous objectives are discussed and resolved (this occurs during the development of the charter).

- It prevents participants from developing different understandings of the project intent, timeline, or cost.

- It enables the project leadership to communicate as necessary with the organization about the project.

The project charter sets out these project elements:

- Project overview and objectives

- Application features and capabilities (vision of the solution)

- Project scope and limitations

- Metrics for determining project success

- Budget and overall timetable

- Project organization

- Project management strategies

Project Plan

The project charter provides an overview of the project. The *project plan* provides the details of the tasks, phases, and resources needed, by task and phase and timeline. The project plan is the tool used by the project team during the day-to-day management of the project. The project plan has several components.

- Project phases and tasks. A phase may have multiple tasks. For example, there may be a phase called *conduct analysis*, and it may involve such tasks as reviewing admitting department forms, documenting the admitting workflow, and documenting the discharge workflow.

- The sequence of phases and tasks.

- Interdependencies between phases and tasks.

- The duration of phases and tasks.

- Staff resources needed, by phase and task.

Several software tools are available that assist project managers in developing project plans. These tools enable the project manager to develop the plan, prepare plan charts and resource use by phase and task, and model the impact on the plan if timelines change or resource availability alters.

Project Plan and Charter Considerations

Developing project plans and charters requires skill and experience. Managers are often in forums (such as project steering committee meetings) where they are asked to review, critique, and approve a project plan. What should they look for in these plans?

To a large degree, the reputations of project managers precede them. If project managers have proven themselves over the course of many projects, then their plans are likely to be generally sound. If project managers are novices or have an uneven track record, their plans may require greater scrutiny. Regardless of track record, there are several cues that a project plan is as solid as one can make it at the inception of the project.

- The project charter is clear and explicit. Fuzzy objectives and vague understandings of resource needs indicate that the plan needs further discussion and development.

- The leaders of the departments and functions that will be affected by the plan or that need to devote resources to the plan have reviewed the charter and plan, their concerns have been heard and addressed, and they have publicly committed to performing the work needed in the plan.

- The project timelines have been reviewed by multiple parties for reasonableness, and these timelines have taken into consideration factors that will affect the plan—for example, key staff going on vacation or organizational energies being diverted to develop the annual budget. Additionally, any uncertainties that might exist for particular phases or tasks (e.g., if it is not fully clear how a specific task will be performed), that task timeline should have some "slack" built into it.

- The resources need to have been committed. The budget has been approved. Staff needed by the plan can be named, and their managers have taken steps to free up the staff time needed by the plan.

- The accountabilities for the plan and for each plan phase and task are explicit.

- Project risks have been comprehensively assessed, and thoughtful approaches to addressing each risk have been developed. Some examples of project risks are unproven information technology, a deterioration in the organization's financial condition, and turnover of project staff.

 TIP While project management does require detailed plans and charters, don't overdo the production of documents and plans. A project team that is skilled and works well together is much more valuable than a detailed plan.

Executing the Plan: Success Factors

Implementing systems such as the EHR and CPOE is a very complex and difficult organizational undertaking. These implementations require political mobilization of the medical and nursing staffs, the reengineering of clinical processes, significant capital commitments, the management of large-scale projects, and major changes to the information technology infrastructure.

The magnitude of this undertaking leads to a high failure rate, estimated by some to be as high as 50 percent.

Despite this failure rate, some organizations have been successful in reaping the benefits of these key technologies in improving patient care. What factors contributed to their success?

Strong Organizational Vision and Strategy

Successful organizations have developed a vision of patient care, and a strategy to achieve that vision, that is compelling, clear, and understood by the members of the organization. This vision describes the critical need for excellence in care delivery and points to clinical systems as an essential strategic contributor to the vision.

Many information system implementations do not require the bedrock of a compelling organizational vision. Clinical information systems do. These systems require the commitment and efforts of virtually all staff. These systems require deep change in operational and clinical processes and require that other investment opportunities be put off, often for several years.

For information system implementations of this significance to succeed, the organization must understand why it is implementing the system and believe that success is essential.

Talented and Committed Leadership

Clinical information system implementation and the related changes in the organization must be led by senior leadership. This leadership must come from the board and all of the senior members of the administrative and medical staffs.

These leaders must have the ability to inspire and mobilize others to get things done. They must actively engage in changing the organization. Once committed to the plan, they must have the strength to thoughtfully stay the course. These leaders must ask hard questions about the systems and their implementation. And these leaders must be pragmatic, superb practitioners of the art of the possible.

 NOTE Successful implementation of a major application is more dependent on the quality of leadership and the implementation process than it is the technology.

A Partnership Among the Clinical, Administrative, and Information Technology Staffs

Across the strata of the organization, many effective, multidisciplinary teams will be needed. These teams will design information systems, develop new ways to do the work, revise policies and procedures, craft implementation steps, develop training materials, and create approaches to resolving inevitable problems.

Team members must view their efforts as a partnership. They must illustrate the attributes of high-performance teams that are skilled, honest, dedicated, willing to compromise, and focused on the overall goal.

 HIT PRO EXAM TIP   Ensure that opinion leaders, especially within the ranks of clinical leadership, are part of the decision and implementation process. Giving these key stakeholders a degree of control over the implementation process and the design of the system is essential. Equally important is to include dissenters as part of the requirements, selection, and implementation teams.

Thoughtful Redesign of Clinical Processes

The implementation of a clinical information system should be accompanied by an examination of care processes and efforts to redesign them to reduce steps, errors, and inefficiencies. Often, the desire to make such changes leads to the decision to pursue the clinical information system.

Effecting significant changes in care processes is difficult; staff and departments can lose power, behavior change is hard, and process designers often have a limited ability to accurately envision a world that is much different from the one they inhabit.

Nonetheless, it does not serve an organization well to automate ineffective and inefficient processes.

Excellent System Implementation Skills

The implementation of complex information systems requires deep skill. These skills need to occur in a small number of critical areas.

Project management is needed to define, manage, and monitor the large number of tasks, staff, and resources that are being brought to the implementation. Good project management requires clear definitions of scope, well-reasoned delineation of tasks, astute assignment of accountability for task performance, flexibility in addressing problems and necessary modest changes in direction, and the excellent ability to identify and resolve problems.

Support is the set of activities that causes an application to "stick," meaning to become an integral part of the fabric of practice. Support includes training, responsive enhancements, ongoing communication and discussion of status and problems, and evolution of work and clinical policies and procedures.

Good to Excellent Information Technology

No information system is perfect, and users will find limitations in any clinical information system. Nonetheless, the applications need to be good enough to support the work that needs to be done. These systems must possess critical features that are required to address desired workflow and reporting needs. These systems should improve the work lives of providers rather than hinder them. In essence, the information technology infrastructure needs to be well designed and supported.

 NOTE Slow response time and uneven reliability can cripple a clinical information system implementation in a remarkably short period of time. There are few things as damaging to the credibility of an IS organization as a wounded infrastructure.

Key Leadership Capabilities of Senior Executives

Earl and Feeney (2000) assessed the characteristics and behaviors of senior leaders (in this case CEOs) who were actively engaged and successful in the strategic use of IT.[1]

These leaders were convinced that IT could and would change the organization. They placed the IT discussion high on the strategic agenda. They looked to IT to identify opportunities to make significant improvements in organizational performance, rather than viewing the IT agenda as secondary to strategy development. They devoted personal time to understanding how their industry and their organization would evolve as IT evolved. And they encouraged other members of the leadership team to do the same.

Leadership Behaviors

Five management behaviors were observed in these leaders:

- They studied rather than avoided IT. They devoted time to learning about new technologies and, through discussion and introspection, developed an understanding of the ways in which new technologies might alter organizational strategies and operations.

- They incorporated IT into their vision of the future of the organization and discussed the role of IT when communicating that vision.

- They actively engaged in IT architecture discussions and high-level decisions. They took time to evaluate major new IT proposals and their implications. They were visibly supportive of architecture standards. They established funds for exploring promising new technologies.

- They made sure that IT was closely linked to core management processes.

  - They integrated the IT discussion tightly into the overall strategy development process. This often involved setting up teams to examine aspects of the strategy and having both IT and business leaders at the table.

- They made sure IT investments were evaluated as one component of the total investment needed by a strategy. The IT investments were not relegated to a separate discussion.

- They ensured strong business sponsorship for all IT investments. Business sponsors were accountable for managing the IT initiatives and ensuring the success of the undertaking.

- They continually pressured the IT department to improve its efficiency and effectiveness and to be visionary in its thinking.

Summary

CEOs and other members of the leadership team have an extraordinary impact on the tone, values, and direction of an organization. Hence, their beliefs and daily behaviors have a significant influence on how effectively and strategically information technology is applied within an organization.

Key Leadership Capabilities of the Information Technology Leadership

The CIO plays a critical leadership role in ensuring the effective use of IT in the organization. The CIO will need to help guide the organization through the changes that will occur in the years ahead. Will these changes require an evolution of the CIO role or the skills of the CIO?

A 2009 survey of healthcare CIOs identified several characteristics, outlined in the following sections, that have enabled CIOs to be successful.[2]

Emotional Intelligence

The CIO must be able to relate to other executives, clinicians, and their staff. They must have an emotional even keel and be able to understand and appreciate the challenges faced by others.

 HIT PRO EXAM TIP   Emotional intelligence usually increases with age.

Expectation Management

The CIO has to help the organization understand what information technology, and the IT department, can do and what it can't. Organizational members must also appreciate the challenges that implementations represent.

Understanding the Business

CIOs must develop a deep understanding of the financial, operational, and clinical issues and activities of the organization and the role that information technology can play in supporting the organization. They should also have an appreciation for the broader healthcare industry.

Leadership

The CIO must be able to lead their peers and their subordinates. Leadership requires conviction, a willingness to listen, the ability to inspire, courage, and superior communication skills. The CIO should be seen as a peer by other members of the executive team.

Innate Talent

The CIO should be bright, have management aptitude, possess a solid work ethic, have excellent interpersonal skills, and be able to quickly assess complex situations.

Adaptability

The CIO must be able to adjust plans, reset expectations, alter projects, and tackle budget challenges that can be required because of changes in business direction, technology innovations and shortcomings, and realignment of business partner relationships.

Credibility and Trust

The CIO should have a track record of accomplishments. They should have very high integrity. They should be honest about mistakes and deliver on plans to correct those mistakes.

High-Quality IT Staff

The CIO must be able to recruit, energize, grow, and organize a superb IT staff.

Evolution of Leadership Capabilities

How will changes in the industry and technology affect the desired characteristics of the CIO?

The characteristics that enabled success over the past five years will be the same characteristics that enable success in the next five years. However, the performance bar will be higher for tomorrow's CIO.

Today's CIO who gets a performance letter grade of A will get a letter grade of B tomorrow. Given the financial and execution pressures, tomorrow's CIO will need to exhibit even higher levels of leadership, adaptability, and understanding of the business and expectation management.

HIT PRO EXAM TIP A successful CIO must understand the business of healthcare and be adequately skilled to face the needs of the healthcare organization of the future, including the rapid proliferation of mobile devices, clinical decision support based on genetic data, and the reimbursement changes that result from health reform.

They will need to be more effective at listening well and working with their administrative and clinical colleagues to solve problems. They will need to show greater prowess at managing and delivering on projects. Additionally, they will have to be more skilled at working with stressed colleagues and tackling complex situations. The CIO will need to increase focus on internal customers and execution with a relative de-emphasis on vendors and technology.

The role of the CIO will not experience a significant change in the content of the role, but the demands on skilled execution of the job at hand will grow exponentially as the healthcare industry continues to evolve and transform. Some organizations will add non-IT roles to the portfolio of the CIO, but these additions (e.g., materials management or human resources) are a recognition of the executive skills of the CIO incumbent rather than a broad evolution of the role.

Chapter Review

For a healthcare provider to thrive in the years ahead and achieve the level of care delivery and accountability that will become the new standard, they must implement and use a solid foundation of health information technology. A critical leadership role is ensuring that the provider is competent at applying IT to improve performance.

In this chapter, I reviewed several key factors that contribute to organizational competency. An organization that is less than competent could be at risk for squandering its IT investments.

You also learned that when embarking on an IT initiative, a necessary first step is to align the IT strategy with the organization's overall strategy to ensure a strong and clear relationship between IT investment decisions and the healthcare organization's overall strategies, goals, and objectives.

Since there is no right way to develop an IT strategy and to ensure alignment, the approaches taken to developing and managing an IT strategy are quite varied. At the conclusion of the planning process, the CIO is typically the leader who synthesizes the conclusions of these discussions. The final plan, including timelines and budgets, becomes the basis for assessing progress throughout the year.

Project management, a set of management disciplines and processes developed over time to help ensure that projects succeed, is typically practiced in any well-run project. While skilled project management does not provide a guarantee for project success, it can certainly reduce the risk of failure, particularly for large, complex IT implemen-tations.

You also learned that two roles are critical in the management of large projects: the business sponsor and the project manager. Additionally, managing projects of any significant size requires two major committees/teams: the project steering committee and the project team.

Projects are managed through the use of several artifacts, such as the project charter and project plan, which I covered in great detail. While some aspects of the plan may have some "slack" built into them, in order to gain organizational buy-in from key stakeholders, project managers are wise to ensure that a project plan is as solid as one can make it at the inception of the project.

When it comes to successfully executing the plan, there are key success factors: most notably, a strong organizational vision and strategy, supported by talented and committed leadership. You also studied the characteristics and behaviors of CEOs who were actively engaged and successful in the strategic use of IT. Because CEOs and other members of the leadership team have ultimate influence on the tone, values, and direction of an organization, their words and actions can have a significant impact on how effectively an organization responds to a strategic IT initiative.

Lastly, perhaps no other role is more critical to the success of the strategic application of health information technology than that of the CIO. Therefore, it's equally important to understand the leadership capabilities and characteristics required for success in this dynamic role. While the role of the CIO will not experience a significant change in content, skilled execution of the role is expected to increase dramatically with the mounting pressures hospitals are experiencing in the face of payment and other healthcare system reforms.

Questions

To test your comprehension of the chapter, answer the following questions and then check your answers against the list of correct answers at the end of the chapter.

1. Which of the following is *not* one of the nine factors related to an organization's effectiveness in using health information technology?

   A. Change management

   B. Multimillion-dollar budget

   C. Individuals and leadership

   D. Innovation

2. What is the key goal of IT alignment and strategic planning?

   A. To ensure a strong and clear relationship between IT investment decisions and the healthcare organization's overall strategies, goals and objectives

   B. To determine which departments require new PCs, laptops, and cell phones

   C. To ensure that each functional area of the hospital (both clinical and administrative) has a competent IT person assigned to their area

    D. To convene the organization's key stakeholders to see HIT product demos and sales presentations so that everyone can make their own purchase decisions about what technologies they'd like to implement

3. Which of the following is *not* an objective of the IT strategic planning process?

    A. To identify non-IT organizational initiatives needed to ensure maximum leverage of the IT initiative (for example, process reengineering)

    B. To establish a political process that helps ensure the plan results have sufficient organizational support

    C. To research what types of IT systems other local hospitals in the area are using

    D. To create a communication plan that will inform the organization of the IT initiatives that will and will not be undertaken

4. What is the best way to develop an IT strategy and ensure alignment?

    A. Typically, organizations that bring in a consulting firm to lead them through strategy development always have success and solid alignment across the organization.

    B. An off-site retreat, which enables the participants to get away from their daily responsibilities, produces the best end result.

    C. As long as dissenters are kept from participating in strategy development meetings, the organization will have a relatively easy time developing its strategy and ensuring alignment.

    D. There is no one right or best way to develop an IT strategy and ensure alignment.

5. Who within the leadership team should be held most accountable for synthesizing the conclusions of the IT strategy discussions and ensuring the strategy is aligned with the overall organizational strategy?

    A. The chief executive officer

    B. The chief information officer

    C. The chief financial officer

    D. The chief medical officer

6. The strategy development and synthesis process usually requires debate and discussion. What typically occurs during this phase?

    A. The organization needs to determine its willingness to implement new or unproven technologies.

    B. Trade-offs will need to be reviewed and determined.

    C. Priorities will need to be set.

    D. All of the above

7. Which of the following would *not* be considered a result of the IT strategic planning and alignment process?

   A. A thorough risk assessment related to carrying out the IT agenda

   B. The assignment of team captains for each phase of the implementation

   C. An overview of the timeline and major interdependencies between initiatives

   D. A high-level analysis of the budget required to carry out the IT initiatives

8. What do you call the set of management disciplines and processes developed over time to help ensure a project succeeds?

   A. Change management

   B. Project charter

   C. Project management

   D. Strategic planning

9. What two roles are critical in the management of large projects?

   A. CEO and CFO

   B. Business sponsor and project manager

   C. CIO and project manager

   D. CMO, who represents all the clinical departments, and CFO, who represents all the administrative areas

10. What is the main role of the project steering committee?

    A. Provides overall guidance and management oversight of the project

    B. Determines the overall IT budget

    C. Communicates project status to the entire organization

    D. Manages the performance of the project work and allocates resources as necessary

11. Which of the following is an objective of the project charter?

    A. Ensures budgetary alignment across all departments

    B. Ensures that planning assumptions or potentially ambiguous objectives are resolved

    C. Prevents participants from developing different understandings of the project intent, timeline, or cost

    D. A and C

    E. B and C

12. Which of the following is *not* a component of the project plan?

    A. Issue escalation protocol

    B. Project phases and tasks

    C. Staff resources needed

    D. Sequences, interdependencies, and duration of phases and tasks

13. Which of the following is a cue that a project plan may not be as solid as it should be?

    A. Comprehensive risk analysis has been performed.

    B. The resources needed have been committed.

    C. Accountability for each plan phase and task is explicit.

    D. Project timelines have been thoroughly reviewed for reasonableness by the CIO.

14. When it comes to implementing clinical information systems, which of the following is *not* one of the six success factors reviewed?

    A. Partnership among the clinical, administrative, and IT staffs

    B. Thoughtful redesign of administrative processes

    C. Excellent system implementation skills

    D. Strong organizational vision and strategy

15. Which of the following is *not* one of the five management behaviors observed in the senior leaders (CEOs) studied who were successful in the strategic use of IT within their organizations?

    A. They continually pressured the IT department to adopt the latest technology.

    B. They made sure that IT was closely linked to core management processes.

    C. They studied rather than avoided IT.

    D. They actively engaged in IT architecture discussions and high-level decisions.

16. Which of the following describes the evolution of the leadership capabilities of the CIO?

    A. Tomorrow's CIO will need to exhibit even higher levels of leadership, adaptability, and understanding of the business and expectation management.

    B. The role of the CIO will not experience a significant change in the content of the role, but the demands on skilled execution of the job will grow exponentially.

    C. Tomorrow's CIO will need to increase their focus on internal customers and execution with a relative de-emphasis on vendors and technology.

    D. All of the above.

Answers

1. **B.** Multimillion-dollar budget is not one of the nine factors related to an organization's effectiveness in using health information technology. The nine factors are individuals and leadership, relationships, technology and technical infrastructure, innovation, evaluation of IT opportunities, change management, core processes and information needs, IT strategic alignment, and strong IT organization.

2. **A.** The goal of IT alignment and strategic planning is to ensure a strong and clear relationship between IT investment decisions and the healthcare organization's overall strategies, goals, and objectives.

3. **C.** Researching what types of IT systems other local hospitals in the area are using is not one of the objectives of the IT strategic planning process. The key objectives include ensuring that IT plans align with the plans of the organization, ensuring the alignment is comprehensive, identifying non-IT initiatives needed to ensure maximum leverage of the IT initiative, ensuring the organization has not missed a strategic IT opportunity, developing a tactical plan, creating a communication plan, and establishing a political process to help ensure sufficient organizational support.

4. **D.** There is no one right or best way to develop an IT strategy and ensure alignment.

5. **B.** The chief information officer is accountable for synthesizing the conclusions of the IT strategy discussions and ensuring the strategy is aligned with the overall organizational strategy.

6. **D.** All of the above. As part of the debate and discussion of the strategy development and synthesis process, the organization needs to determine its willingness to implement new or unproven technologies. Additionally, trade-offs will need to be reviewed and determined, and priorities will need to be set.

7. **B.** Assigning team captains for each phase of the implementation is not a result of the IT strategic planning and alignment process. Rather, the process should produce an inventory of the IT initiatives that will be undertaken, a diagram or chart that illustrates the linkage between the initiatives and the organization's strategy and goals, an overview of the timeline and the major interdependencies between initiatives, a high-level analysis of the budget needed, and a risk assessment complete with strategies needed to reduce those risks.

8. **C.** Project management is the set of management disciplines and processes developed over time to help ensure a project succeeds.

9. **B.** Business sponsor and project manager are the two critical roles in the management of large projects.

10. **A.** The project steering committee provides overall guidance and management oversight of the project.

11. **E.** The project charter ensures that planning assumptions or potentially ambiguous objectives are resolved and prevents participants from developing different understandings of the project intent, timeline, or cost.

12. **A.** Issue escalation protocol is not a component of the project plan. The project plan's components are project phases and tasks; staff resources needed by phase and task; and the sequence, interdependencies, and duration of phases and tasks.

13. **D.** Project timelines that have been thoroughly reviewed for reasonableness by the CIO is a cue that a project plan may not be as solid as it should since project timelines should be thoroughly reviewed by *multiple parties*, not just the CIO.

14. **B.** Thoughtful redesign of administrative processes is not one of the six success factors associated with implementing clinical information systems. The success factors are strong organizational vision and strategy, talented and committed leadership, a partnership between the clinical, administrative and IT staffs, thoughtful redesign of *clinical* processes, excellent system implementation skills, and good to excellent IT.

15. **A.** That they continually pressured the IT department to adopt the latest technology is not one of the five management behaviors observed in the senior leaders (CEOs) studied who were successful in the strategic use of IT within their organizations. The five management behaviors are as follows: studied rather than avoided IT, incorporated IT into their vision of the future, actively engaged in IT architecture discussions and decisions, ensured IT was closely linked to core management processes, and continually pressured the IT department to improve its efficiency and effectiveness and to be visionary in its thinking.

16. **D.** In terms of the evolution of the leadership capabilities of the CIO, tomorrow's CIO will need to exhibit even higher levels of leadership, adaptability, and understanding of the business and expectation management. The role of the CIO will not experience a significant change in the content of the role, but the demands on skilled execution of the job will grow exponentially. Lastly, tomorrow's CIO will need to increase their focus on internal customers and execution with a relative de-emphasis on vendors and technology.

References

1. Earl, M., and Feeny, D. (2000). How to be a CEO for the Information Age. *MIT Sloan Management Review, 41(2)*, 11–23.

2. Glaser, J., and Kirby, J. (2009). Evolution of the healthcare CIO. *Healthcare Financial Management, 63(11)*, 38–41.

Communication Skills in Healthcare IT, Building Strong Teams for Successful Healthcare IT Outcomes

Liz Johnson

In this chapter, you will learn how to
- Describe the importance of communications in the healthcare IT initiatives
- Define the essential role of the customers
- Identify the components of the communication plan
- Understand the roles of federal agencies and federal regulations
- Discuss the role of social medial and mobile devices

In America's twenty-first-century healthcare system, landmark federal reform legislation enacted since 2009 is today modernizing care-delivery organizations with new health information technologies (healthcare IT) that regularly begin with the adoption of electronic health records (EHRs). Most notable of these laws are the American Recovery and Reinvestment Act (ARRA) and its Health Information Technology and Economic and Clinical Health (HITECH) Act provision, which established the Centers for Medicare and Medicaid Services' (CMS's) Meaningful Use of EHRs Incentive Programs.[1] These programs earmarked more than $19 billion in incentive payments for eligible physicians and healthcare providers who successfully meet increasingly stringent requirements for EHR implementation over the next five years.

However, the journey to successful integration of healthcare IT by providers industrywide has been fraught with challenges. Tremendous complexities exist throughout healthcare organizations working on healthcare IT reform initiatives, and these complexities create a critical need for effective communication campaigns that run throughout the life cycles of acquiring, implementing, and adopting EHRs in both inpatient and ambulatory settings. Efforts such as these, with effective communication programs in place as a core strategy, support the goal of achieving the Institute of Medicine's six aims for improvement in care-delivery quality, making it safe, equitable, effective, patient-centered, timely, and efficient.[2]

Without such communication strategies, success is far less likely. In 2002, for example, a major West Coast academic medical center heavily invested in the implementation of computerized provider order entry (CPOE) encountered significant physician resistance. In large part, the clinician unwillingness to use CPOE occurred because physicians had been insufficiently informed about and inadequately trained in the use of the clinical decision support (CDS) tool being implemented.[3] According to David Bates, MD, in a 2006 Baylor University Medical Center Proceedings paper, negative outcomes included failure to achieve leadership support or clinical buy-in from the large number of providers using the system. In the end, strong resistance from an overwhelming majority of physicians effectively derailed the entire initiative.[4]

Other provider organizations have encountered related challenges with healthcare IT implementations[5] over the past decade. Such costly, high-risk experiences—especially in an increasingly patient-centric healthcare industry—have underscored the importance of effective, cross-enterprise, patient-focused communication plans and strategies that include physicians and clinicians, administrators, IT professionals, and the C-Suite—all of whom play critical roles as new technologies are introduced. As a result, effective communication programs have quickly become a high priority for hospitals and physician practices adopting EHR and CPOE systems throughout the industry.

The purpose of this chapter, therefore, is to provide an overview of communication strategies that have proven effective in driving the implementation of EHRs to support the needs of patients, physicians, and the caregiver workforce. The chapter covers the importance of communications in healthcare IT initiatives, the customers and players, components of the communication plan, and industry considerations (roles of federal agencies, federal regulations, and the burgeoning role of mobile applications, social media, and health information exchange).

Importance of Communications in Healthcare IT Initiatives

As Georgia Tech Professor William Rouse noted in the 2008 article "Healthcare as a Complex Adaptive System: Implications for Design and Management," healthcare organizations exist as complex adaptive systems with nonlinear relationships, independent and intelligent agents, and system fragmentation.[6] While variation among them is gradually diminishing through increasing standardization of practices and systems, many provider cultures still struggle with decentralization and reliance on disparate legacy systems.[7] As a growing number of organizations across the nation elect to begin the journey of implementing EHRs in the inpatient or ambulatory setting, a cross-enterprise need arises for effective and tactical communication plans. This section provides insight on the importance of communications in healthcare IT implementation programs: in governance, the structure of a governance model, and rules for governance efforts.

Leadership and Governance

The introduction of EHRs in healthcare organizations drives transformational change in clinical and administrative workflows;[8] organizational structure (i.e., that which exists among physicians, nurses, and administrators);[9] and relationships among the frontline workers, physicians, administrators, and patients. Understanding the risks posed by the disruptive facets of organizational and process change is critical to ensuring the effective implementation of EHRs and mitigating risks of failure.[10] An essential part of risk mitigation in care-delivery reform through healthcare IT is the planning and implementing of organizational communication initiatives that help to achieve the aims of an enterprise-wide governance team.

To succeed, responsibilities for such communications initiatives should be shared among health system leaders, champions, and those charged with oversight of the implementation of healthcare IT systems, all of whom should have a role to play in governance structures whose processes are grounded in a strong communications strategy. A 2012 *Hospitals & Health Network* cover story entitled "iGovernance" summarized the importance of such an approach for transforming healthcare organizations as, "This IT governance function, guided from the top but carried out by sometimes hundreds of clinical and operations representatives, will be evermore crucial to managing the escalation of IT in healthcare delivery…." In fact, without such an informed governance process, the article states, "IT at many hospitals and healthcare systems is a haphazard endeavor that typically results in late, over-budget projects, and, ultimately, many disparate systems that don't function well together."[11]

Accountability begins at the hospital level and rises through the enterprise level. Messaging through electronic, in-person, or video media options from chief executive officers and board members of governance groups solidifies the importance of enterprise-level healthcare IT projects.[12] However, both governance structures and the communications that support them require tailoring depending on the nature of every health system. As noted by Dana Sellers, CEO of Encore Health Resources, some hospitals "aren't ready for an approach with many levels and players," and therefore, a structure that drives participation for one organization will vary in others.[11]

Governance models in healthcare organizations provide a structure that engages stakeholders to work through critical decisions and ensure that risks associated with changes in policy, technology, and workflow are mitigated to maintain or improve the quality of patient care. A strong example of such a working model is provided by my own health system: Tenet Healthcare Corporation, where I am vice president of applied clinical informatics (ACI). Tenet's nationwide, multiyear EHR implementation program, which is directed by my office, is called IMPACT: Improving Patient Care through Technology.

The mission of IMPACT is to implement a systemwide EHR and patient health record (PHR) system for all Tenet facilities and patients by 2015 while ensuring staff and physician adoption of the system throughout the process. Tenet is one of the United States' largest integrated healthcare delivery systems, employing more than 57,000 in 50 hospitals spanning 11 states from coast to coast. Figure 10-1 illustrates the structure of Tenet Healthcare's IMPACT program and the importance of communications as it has been built into the implementation of the IMPACT EHR system.

As shown here, a key to the success of Tenet's IMPACT governance is a three-tiered organizational structure that engages the corporation, regional operations, and the hospitals themselves in a coordinated effort. Another key success factor has been early commitment to key roles, including clinical informaticists, physician champions, training and communications leads, and healthcare IT leads. But binding the program together with unified, shared, and consistent messaging continues to be a foundational strategy that supports all aspects of IMPACT's execution.[13]

Barbara Hoehn, RN, MBA, summed up the importance of communications in governance in her 2010 JHIM article entitled "Clinical Information Technology Governance."[14] "Today, clinical IT is finally being universally viewed as a critical component of healthcare reform, and we are only going to get one chance to do this right," she wrote. "This means having everyone in the organization, from the Board Members to the bedside clinicians, all focused on the same plan, the same tactical initiatives, and the same outcomes."

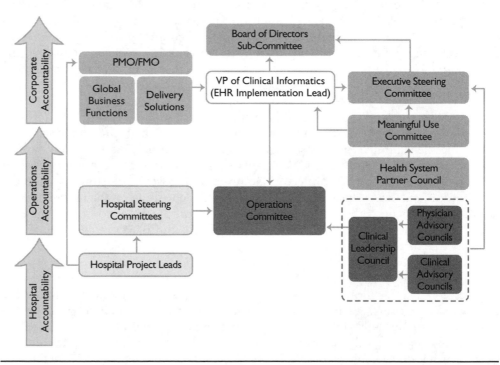

Figure 10-1   EHR implementation and oversight governance

Rules for Governance

Enabling governance committees requires a solid set of rules, since hospitals are matrixed organizations comprised of multidisciplinary staff and leaders from across a healthcare organization. A set of "rules to live by" in iGovernance is identified in Table 10-1.

The following describes each role:

1. *Hardwire the committees.* Ensure that the chair of lower-level committees be participants on the next level of committees. Their role is to bring forward recommendations and issues needing higher-level engagement for resolution.

2. *Set clear levels of successive authority.* Committee responsibilities should be well defined so members know issues they can address and issues beyond their level of authority.[14]

3. *Do real work every time.* Focus meetings on important issues in need of clinician engagement. If there are no critical items, cancel the meeting and send out status reports electronically.

4. *Form no governance before its time.* Recognize that different organizations will not be prepared to embrace a governance structure at the same time or to the same degree as others.

5. *Put someone in charge who can take a stand.* The leader of the top committee must be someone who commands respect and possesses operational authority to enact recommendations.

Focus on Customers and Players

Those who are engaged in EHR implementation initiatives should also be involved in communications associated with these multiyear programs. Figure 10-2 illustrates the spectrum of customers and players.

In the provider setting, each of these groups will have a different type of communications engagement. The media and vehicles used may be different, but the strategic focus is the same: improving the quality of patient care through strategic adoption of healthcare IT that is in turn enabled by smart communications.

1. Hardwire the committees	2. Set clear levels of successive authority	3. Do real work every time	4. Form no governance before its time	5. Put someone in charge who can take a stand

Table 10-1   Rules to Live by for Governance Participants[11]

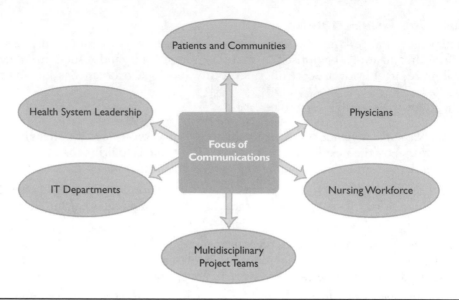

Figure 10-2 Focus of communications

Patients and Communities

In its 2001 report "Crossing the Quality Chasm: A New Health System for the 21st Century," the Institute of Medicine established the need for patient-centered communications and support as part of the six aims for improving healthcare, as noted in the introduction of this chapter.[2] Since then, patient-centric healthcare and the emergence of care-delivery models such as the patient-centered medical home (PCMH) have become central to health reform. Integral to the PCMH concept are seven joint principles established in 2007, one of which calls for a "whole-person orientation." This means each personal physician is expected to provide for all of a patient's lifetime health service needs,[15] which drives the requirement for comprehensive physician-to-patient communications and shared decision making.

Such communications are also required to support healthcare reform at the community level, as demonstrated in CMS's 2011 establishment of the Three Part Aim for the Medicare Shared Savings Program (e.g., Medicare ACO) with its focus on "better care for individuals and better health for populations."[16] In its final rule for the Medicare ACO, CMS mandated the requirement for advancing patient-centered care through accountable care organizations (ACOs), stating "an ACO shall adopt a focus on patient-centeredness that is promoted by the governing body and integrated into practice by leadership and management working with the organization's health care teams."[12]

Physicians

As discussed in the introduction of this chapter, no adoption of EHRs by health systems or practices can be expected to succeed without the endorsement and ownership of the physician community, whose working environment must inevitably sustain challenging changes to long-established workflows. Furthermore, when included from the outset of any healthcare IT transformation initiative, "physician champions" themselves can become powerful and effective communicators, assisting colleagues through healthcare IT adoption.

In fact, a government healthcare IT story recently reported that the Office of the National Coordinator for Health IT, through its regional extension centers, has recruited "physician champions" who are well on their way to becoming meaningful users of EHRs to help others in their area get over the hurdles of digitizing their medical records.[17] Therefore, not only the need for communications that support training initiatives and the management of new procedural requirements but also an understanding of the dynamics of legislated healthcare reform are important from the earliest stages of healthcare IT adoption.

However, such needs are often unmet. An April 2012 *iHealthBeat* article reported, for example, that the results of a recent survey of more than 250 hospitals and healthcare systems[18] demonstrated that significant percentages of respondent physicians had inadequate understanding of stage 1 meaningful use requirements; others cited a lack of training and change-management issues. Both statistics spotlight the continued need to directly engage physicians in healthcare IT implementations through comprehensive communications initiatives.

Nursing Workforce

For patients in both inpatient and ambulatory settings, nurses constitute the front line of patient care. But for health systems everywhere, they are also on the front line of healthcare IT reform: as pointed out by Joyce Hahn, executive director of the Nursing Alliance for Quality Care, "Nurses represent the largest potential users of electronic health records."[19] As with their physician colleagues, therefore, the role of communications is not limited to training nurses in the use of EHR systems but rather preparing them to fully engage in the design, testing, and implementation of EHRs to support improved care coordination and continuity of care. Throughout the healthcare industry, health systems CIOs are finding that "the success of large IT implementations will depend not only on the willingness of floor nurses to accept new technology, but also on the strength of the IS-nursing management connection."[20] Therefore, engaging nurses through communications both as champions and users of new healthcare IT is a strategic necessity.

An example of engagement of nursing in the process is part of the IMPACT program at Tenet. IMPACT's Nursing Advisory Team (NAT) functions as a decision-making body, and NAT's decisions will become the standard for the implementation of core clinical EHR applications. Just how these leaders are communicating their decisions has proved to be integral to promoting safe, quality patient care and improving outcomes for patients and families while supporting the Tenet Clinical Quality initiatives and the standards associated with the IMPACT program itself.[13]

> ## Use Case 10.1: Using Newsletters to Inform
>
> Many organizations use internal newsletters as a communication tool to engage the variety of project stakeholders. An issue of *The IMPACT Insider*, Tenet's weekly cross-enterprise e-newsletter for IMPACT program news, recently informed the health system's employees about how the IT department and clinical informaticists from multiple hospitals strengthened CPOE go-lives by communicating suggestions from hospitals that had already implemented CPOE to those who would soon begin such projects.[22] This has resulted in improved training processes and has better prepared Tenet's hospitals across the board for changes in the system's EHR system applications.

IT Departments and Multidisciplinary Project Teams

IT departments and project teams are responsible for meeting the challenges of new-system introductions as well as managing the continuous upgrades to existing ones. To support this work, their roles in communications efforts will involve engaging clinicians in staff positions, confirming commitments, managing change, and setting EHR deployment strategies, per "The CIO's Guide to Implementing EHRs in the HITECH Era," a 2010 paper from the College of Healthcare Information Management Executives (CHIME).[21]

Healthcare System Leadership

As noted in the section on Leadership and Governance, communications led by an executive-level steering committee, often chaired by a health system's chief executive or operating officer, represent the beginning and the end of successful healthcare IT implementation processes. The top of the organization not only establishes the size of the investment the organization is prepared to make but also communicates "the broad strategies for IT in advancing business goals and, ultimately, acting on the result of a consistently applied proposal and prioritization regimen" per the 2012 article cited earlier, "iGovernance."[11]

Building a Communications Plan

Leaders for Kaiser Permanente (KP) noted in the 2011 HIMSS Davies Award application for their KP HealthConnect EHR that they credited their communication initiatives for "creating awareness, building knowledge, managing expectations, motivating end users, and building proficiency."[23] As part of their communications plans, they included vehicles such as a central Intranet site, leadership messaging, weekly e-newsletters, regional communication tactics, and videos. Other health systems also employ e-mail updates, end-user training, superusers who function as subject-matter experts, and champions to secure buy-in for system adoption.

A 2009 article by Chad Eckes, CIO, and Edgar Staren, MD, entitled "Communication Management's Role In EHR Success," offers other ideas.[24]

- **Fact sheets, newsletters, and posters**   Collateral tailored to clinician audiences
- **Road shows**   Pre-implementation educational demos of forthcoming system capabilities
- **Town hall meetings**   Opportunities for senior leaders to hold question and answer sessions
- **Standard meeting reports**   Detailed status given of schedules, budget, risks, and progress

As noted earlier, an example newsletter is proof of how an e-newsletter can be used to communicate success stories from hospitals that have successfully implemented EHR systems. Such a vehicle is especially effective for integrated health systems whose hospitals are spread geographically across the country as part of the work to fulfill federal EHR meaningful use requirements.

Another perspective is provided by a 2005 *JHIM* article by Detlev Smaltz, PhD, FHIMSS, and his colleagues, in which they discuss the importance of project communication plans focused on stakeholder groups and meeting their needs. Table 10-2 provides a sample of this plan for three stakeholder groups.[25]

Project Phases and the Communication Functions

Healthcare IT projects often unfold over multiyear periods with pre-adoption (selection), pre-implementation, implementation (go-live), and post-implementation (outcomes) comprising the four major phases.[26] Therefore, it is important that communication plans be built and integrated within these phases, because the information needs of stakeholders will vary as projects evolve and mature. Furthermore, a variety of formal and informal communication media will be needed to reach different health-system groups, a point made in a 2009 *Journal of AHIMA* article entitled "Planning Organizational Transition to

Stakeholder	Objective	Media	Content
Executive Management	Update on cost, benefits, service quality, and milestones	• In-person meeting and briefing	• Status update and impact on outcomes
Nursing	Maintain awareness of progress; engage in design effort	• Nurse educators • Nursing leadership • Collateral • Unit meetings • Intranet website	• Project methodology • Design participation • Educational info • Outcomes impact
Medical Staff	Maintain awareness of progress; engage in design sessions	• Medical executive committee • Clinical chairs • Targeted newsletter	• Project methodology • Design participation • Educational info • Outcomes impact

Table 10-2   Sample of Healthcare IT Project Communication Plan

ICD-10-CM/PCS."[27] The article further states that because points of urgency and risks to be mitigated are also critical to key stakeholders, they should also be considered among the key elements of an effective communication strategy.

Communication Metrics

The best metrics to measure communication program effectiveness are arguably the same used to present the stories of successful healthcare IT implementations. Strong governance programs supported by a pervasive and adaptable communications strategy will have helped to drive 31 foundational, stage 1 EHR meaningful use go-lives across the country as well as 20 CPOE go-lives by the end of 2012 in a large integrated delivery network (IDN). These results were supported by weekly e-newsletters, hospital site-specific communications campaign, future state workflow localization, change readiness assessments, at-the-elbow support for providers from superusers and subject-matter experts throughout the go-live processes, physician partnering, post go-live support, and 24/7 command centers for 10 days post go-live.

Key Industry Considerations

While much of the communications focus supporting the implementation of new EHR systems and related healthcare IT is focused inside a health system, those responsible for building communication strategies must do so in the context of industry change beyond any hospital's walls. With the arrival and rapid entrenchment of the digital age over the past decade, innovations in mobile devices and social media platforms have broadened, enriching communications options to support successful healthcare IT integration. Furthermore, the actions of the federal government to ensure increasing volumes of trusted, secure health information exchange are constantly redefining how and what the healthcare industry can expect to communicate across the continuum of care in coming days, months, and years. Therefore, communications planning in support of healthcare IT initiatives must reflect the forces driving such change: an expanding world of media, the roles of federal healthcare agencies, and the adoption of regulatory standards as they are driving the evolution of health information exchange.

The Expanding World of Media

Physicians and clinicians across the industry are increasingly communicating among themselves and with their patients because of an explosion of mobile health device technology. A recent article entitled "Doctors' Tablet Use Almost Doubles in 2012" confirmed through a survey of 3,015 physicians that nearly 62 percent are using some type of tablet platform—with the dominant choice being Apple's iPad.[28] Such technologies are rapidly evolving, and clinicians are increasingly depending upon them to document patient visits, manage clinical workflows, conduct research on technical and clinical issues, and receive alerts regarding patient conditions.[29]

While the upside to this rapid increase in communication technologies is tremendous, the deployment of such devices in the marketplace may be surpassing the pace for which security precautions can keep up, as noted in a February 2012 *Forbes* article, aptly entitled "How Healthcare's Embrace of Technology Has Turned Dangerous."[30] The article acknowledged the "huge potential in helping medical providers diagnose patients more quickly and accurately, improving the patient-provider relationship, and reducing extra paperwork—and the medical errors that are sometimes caused by them." But it also called on hospitals to help "draft up an industry-wide set of best practices governing the use of mobile devices in hospital settings."

Beyond devices, new digital media vehicles encompass a multitude of healthcare-specific social media websites such as PatientsLikeMe, Sermo, and Diabetesmine that have emerged in the Health 2.0/Medicine 2.0 era as defined by Van De Belt and colleagues in their 2010 *Journal of Medical Internet Research* article.[31] Keys to enabling productive communications with today's new interactive tools recognizes that "(a) health has become more participatory... (b) data has become the new 'Intel Inside' for systems supporting the 'vital decisions' in health; and (c) a sense of 'collective intelligence' from the network would supplement traditional sources of knowledge in health decision-making" as summarized by Hesse and colleagues in their 2011 article entitled "Realizing the Promise of Web 2.0: Engaging Community Intelligence."[32]

Social media sites bring new opportunities to improve provider-to-provider communications with physician-centric channels. These include sites like Sermo and QuantiaMD, which cater only to the physician community. Other social networking sites support patient communities that bring new opportunities for marketing of services and disseminating best practices, as noted by David Nash, MD, MBA, in a May 2010 article entitled "Social Networking Impact on Patients, Doctors, and Non-profits."[33] As with mobile devices, the many positive effects to be gained from participation in social media must be considered alongside concerns for the privacy and security of protected health information. Supported by the Health Insurance Portability and Accountability Act (HIPAA) Privacy and Security Rules passed in 1996, healthcare organizations have become more vigilant in establishing rules and policies governing participation in social media. Such heightened awareness was recently noted in the April 2012 Federation of State Medical Board's Model Policy Guidelines for Appropriate Use of Media and Social Networking in Medical Practice. Even so, as these communication platforms evolve in the future, addressing issues of privacy and security will be a key concern for the industry, physicians, health systems, patients, and the healthcare reform movement as a whole.[34]

Role of Federal Healthcare Agencies

Healthcare reform during the past decade has been defined, spearheaded, and guided by federal government agencies armed with ARRA and HITECH legislation to providing funding, oversight, and industry-level guidance on the implementation and adoption of healthcare IT throughout the United States.[35] Leading the government's healthcare initiatives is the U.S. Department of Health and Human Services (HHS).[36]

Two key divisions of HHS are CMS, introduced earlier, and the Office of the National Coordinator for Health Information Technology (ONC). In addition to Medicare (the federal health insurance program for seniors) and Medicaid (the federal needs-based program), CMS oversees the Children's Health Insurance Program (CHIP), the Health Insurance Portability and Accountability Act (HIPAA), and the Clinical Laboratory Improvement Amendments (CLIA), among other services. Also, under HITECH, CMS is charged with advancing healthcare IT through implementing the EHR incentive programs, helping define meaningful use EHR technology, drafting standards for the certification of EHR technology, and updating health information privacy and security regulations under HIPAA.[37]

Much of this work is done in close conjunction with ONC and the two critically important federal advisory committees that operate under its auspices. The first of those committees is the Healthcare IT Policy Committee, which makes recommendations to ONC on the development and adoption of a nationwide health information infrastructure, including guidance on what standards for exchanging patient medical information will be required.[38] The second is the Healthcare IT Standards Committee, which focuses on recommendations from CMS, ONC, and the Healthcare IT Policy Committee on standards, implementation specifications, and certification criteria for the electronic exchange and use of patient health information (PHI).[39]

Understanding the roles of these agencies and committees—and keeping abreast of their actions—is an important responsibility for those engaged in planning and delivering communications that support healthcare IT adoption. Individually and collectively, they help drive the definition of incentive payment requirements across the three stages of EHR meaningful use. Each stage will not only create new healthcare IT performance requirements inside a given health system but also define the kinds of information exchange—in themselves forms of communication—that will be required between healthcare entities across the entire continuum of care, including those directly focused on the patient and the community. Figure 10-3 provides a snapshot of each stage's objectives.

The following are the stages in more detail:

- **Stage 1**   Beginning in 2011 as the incentives program starting point for all providers, stage 1 meaningful use consists of transferring data to EHRs and being able to share information, including electronic copies and visit summaries for patients.

- **Stage 2**   To be implemented in 2014 under the current proposed rule, stage 2 meaningful use includes new standards such as online access for patients to their health information and electronic health information exchange between providers.

- **Stage 3**   Expected to begin in 2016, stage 3 meaningful use is projected to include demonstrating that the quality of healthcare has been improved.[40]

Role of Regulatory Standards and the Evolution of Health Information Exchange

In today's era of healthcare reform, an increasing number of standards in the area of health, health information, and communications technologies are helping to guide our industry toward interoperability between independent entities and systems. The goal is to support the safe, secure, and private exchange of PHI in ever-increasing volumes to improve the quality of care.

As advised by ONC, CMS, and the HIT Policy Committee, the HIT Standards Committee is the primary federal advisory committee working to fulfill this mandate.

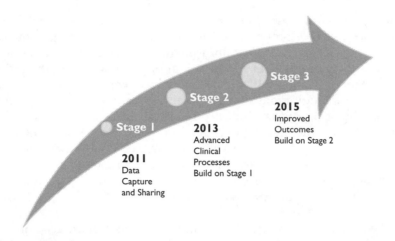

Stage 3

2015
Improved
Outcomes
Build on Stage 2

Stage 2

2013
Advanced
Clinical
Processes
Build on Stage 1

Stage 1

2011
Data
Capture
and Sharing

Figure 10-3   The three stages of EHR meaningful use

It is also a committee upon which I am proudly serving at the appointment of HHS Secretary Kathleen Sebelius. Table 10-3 summarizes the duties of this committee as provided by a 2009 Robert Wood Johnson Foundation Report, called "Health Information Technology in the US: On the Cusp of Change."[41]

The HIT Standards Committee has established over the course of its deliberations a number of important workgroups as subcommittees to the parent committee. These workgroups meet periodically to discuss their topics, present their findings at HIT Standards Committee meetings, and make recommendations to the HIT Standards Committee. Subjects defining the work of these subcommittees include clinical operations, clinical quality, privacy and security, implementation, vocabularies, the NwHIN exchange project, and a variety of other subject areas that fall under what ONC and CMS call the Power Team Summer Camp.[42]

Duties
Harmonize or updates standards for uniform and consistent implementation of standards and specifications
Conduct pilot testing of standards and specifications by the National Institute of Standards and Technology
Ensure consistency with existing standards
Provide a forum for stakeholders to engage in development of standards and implementation specifications
Establish an annual schedule to assess recommendations of HIT Policy Committee
Conduct public hearings for public input
Consider recommendations and comments from the National Committee on Vital and Health Statistics (NCVHS) in development of standards

Table 10-3   Duties of the HIT Standards Committee

Communications from these subcommittees are critical for ensuring that the current regulations and notices of proposed rule making (NPRM) are brought into the public arena. The Implementation Workgroup, which is dedicated to ensuring that what is being asked of the greater health-system and physician-practice communities is actually feasible in terms of adoption and meaningful use, employs communication tools. A strong public communications strategy is core to the work of our group, which holds hearings with broad healthcare industry representation—including health systems, physicians, EHR and other healthcare IT vendors and developers, among others—and maintains active liaison relationships with the sister HIT Policy Committee.

As a result, the Implementation Workgroup will continue to bring forward "real-world" implementation experience into the Standards Committee recommendations with special emphasis on strategies to accelerate the adoption of proposed standards or to mitigate barriers, if any.[43]

As are the meetings of the HIT Policy and Standards Committees, all workgroup meetings are held in public, and notices for each meeting appear on the ONC website and in the Federal Register.[43] Public comment is always welcome.

 CompTIA EXAM TIP Healthcare professionals and clinicians are held to a high standard when communicating via an EHR system (which the exam will also refer to as an electronic medical records, or EMR, system). This is not only because the EMR is a legal record of care delivered, but even more importantly, the completeness and quality of communication in and through the EMR can and does impact patient wellbeing and patient outcomes. HIT professionals and technicians are advised to keep this important communication standard for the EMR in mind. It can explain why healthcare professionals can be very sensitive to real or perceived problems to the smooth operating of the EMR. Empathy, sincere concern, prompt professional action, and feedback about the resolution status are called for by the HIT professional or technician when communicating about an EMR issue with a healthcare professional or clinician.

Chapter Review

ARRA, HITECH, and incentives programs supporting the meaningful use of EHRs are helping the healthcare industry make a paradigm shift in care delivery through the accelerated use of healthcare IT. CMS, ONC, and its HIT Policy and Standards Committees are driving communications at the industry level to provide all stakeholders with a common set of rules to follow for selecting, designing, implementing, and adopting EHRs. Challenges still persist, however, when effective communication plans are not developed and followed in complex healthcare IT projects that can affect physicians, nurses, administrators, and patients alike.

This chapter addressed issues regarding the importance of communications and the development of effective communication strategies in strengthening initiatives ranging from governance efforts to physician-to-patient partnerships—all as part of successful EHR implementations. Key takeaways to consider in the conclusion of this chapter include the following:

- Coordinated, cross-enterprise communications strategies are critically important parts of healthcare IT implementations, including the development of governance structures supporting the introduction and adoption of EHR systems.

- The customers and players engaged in communications include patients and communities, physicians, nurses, project teams and IT departments, and health system leadership. Remember that patient-centricity, the meaningful use program, and physician and nurse engagement are all critical points in the communication initiatives for these participants.

- Vehicles in a communications plan can include an intranet, print media, road shows, town hall meetings, and standard meetings to be used through all phases of a project, and the success of such projects can be the best measure of the communication plan's effectiveness.

- Some of the most powerful forces driving change include social media, mobile devices, and continued healthcare reforms.

- The committees of ONC, the HIT Policy and Standards Committees, and subcommittees such as the Implementation Workgroup are key drivers of national communications important to all stakeholders involved in working toward the meaningful use of EHRs.

- Tenet Healthcare's IMPACT EHR program, with its governance structure and effective communications efforts, serves as one guiding example for healthcare IT program communications.

As the healthcare industry grows increasingly interconnected through healthcare IT and other technologies, effective communication plans will remain essential parts of the process. With a commitment to the development and execution of communications strategies around the implementation of emerging healthcare IT, higher levels of ownership and commitment by professionals will help ensure the success of the U.S. healthcare reform movement in years to come.

Questions

To test your comprehension of the chapter, answer the following questions and then check your answers against the list of correct answers at the end of this section.

1. Effective communication programs support the goal of achieving the Institute of Medicine's six aims for improvement in quality care delivery. Which of the following is *not* one of the six aims?

   A. Effective

   B. Safe

   C. Noteworthy

   D. Equitable

2. What caused the lack of clinician adoption and resistance toward use of CPOE in 2001 at a major West Coast academic medical center?

   A. Insufficient funding

   B. Insufficient information and inadequate training on clinical decision support tools

   C. Lack of leadership

   D. Poor implementation

3. What is one of the characteristics of healthcare organizations existing as complex adaptive systems?

   A. Nonlinear relationships

   B. Large entities comprised of clinicians and physicians

   C. Hospitals in urban areas

   D. Healthcare organizations that care for patients with different backgrounds.

4. Which option is *not* an area where EHRs drive transformational change in healthcare organizations?

   A. Clinical and administrative workflows

   B. Organizational structure

   C. Financial systems

   D. Relationships between the frontline workers, physicians, and patients

5. What did the 2012 article entitled "iGovernance" say about the importance of IT governance for transforming healthcare organizations?

   A. It is should involve only a few executives.

   B. Priorities should be set by physicians.

   C. It should be guided from the top but carried out by sometimes hundreds of clinical and operations representatives.

   D. Financial issues should be addressed early.

6. Governance models in healthcare organizations provide a structure that engages _____ to work through critical decisions.

   A. Leaders

   B. Physicians

   C. Pharmacists

   D. Stakeholders

7. What is a key to the success of Tenet's IMPACT governance model (used as a governance example model)?

   A. Uses a three-tiered organizational structure

   B. Uses a bottom-up approach

    C. Engages multidisciplinary staff

    D. Uses technology effectively

8. What is *not* one of the rules to live by for governance committees per the "iGovernance" article?

    A. Hardwire the committees.

    B. Set clear levels of successive authority.

    C. Form no governance before its time.

    D. Have concise committee meeting agendas.

9. What type of care delivery model has been central to health reform?

    A. Specialty practices

    B. Physician hospital organizations

    C. Patient-centered medical homes

    D. Integrated delivery networks

10. Who did the regional extension centers recruit to help others get over the hurdles of digitizing their medical records?

    A. Physician champions

    B. Nurse executives

    C. Industry researchers

    D. Hospital CEOs

11. What group represents the largest potential users of electronic health records?

    A. Patients

    B. Physicians

    C. Nursing workforce

    D. Medical assistants

12. Eckes and Staren identified six examples of communication vehicles employed in EHR implementation projects. What is not one of the six?

    A. Video demonstrations

    B. Road shows

    C. Town hall meetings

    D. Newsletters and posters

13. With the arrival of the digital age, innovations in _____ have enriched communications options to support successful healthcare IT integration.

    A. Speech communications

    B. Transportation services

    C. Mobile devices and social media

    D. Fiber-optic cable

14. Social media sites improving provider-to-provider communications include
   _____.

   A. Facebook

   B. LinkedIn

   C. Sermo and QuantiaMD

   D. Twitter

15. Which subcommittee of the HIT Standards Committee is dedicated to ensuring that what is being asked of the greater health-system and physician-practice communities is actually feasible in terms of adoption and meaningful use?

   A. Operations

   B. Strategic planning

   C. Public relations

   D. Implementation

Answers

1. **C.** In the Institute of Medicine's 2001 seminal report, "Crossing the Quality Chasm: A Health System for the 21st Century," six aims for improving the quality of healthcare were identified as safe, equitable, effective, patient-centered, timely, and efficient.

2. **B.** A well-known West Coast academic medical center experienced significant resistance to its CPOE implementation, and this proved to serve as a strong lesson-learned case example for the industry on the importance of effective communications on CPOE and EHR implementation projects.

3. **A.** Healthcare organizations have been described as complex adaptive systems. Not only do they have these types of relationships, but they also have independent and intelligent agents (i.e., actors within the system who possess a high degree of autonomy and authority) and system fragmentation.

4. **D.** Financial systems are not one of the stated areas that EHRs are driving transformational change in.

5. **C.** It should be guided from the top but carried out by sometimes hundreds of clinical and operations representatives. The other answer options were not referenced in the chapter as part of an IT governance approach and not identified as such in the "iGovernance" article.

6. **D.** Governance models can require engagement of all types of stakeholders to reach critical decisions. Leaders, physicians, nurses, and pharmacists can all be types or categories of stakeholders.

7. **A.** Tenet Healthcare's governance model engages the corporation, regional operations, and their hospitals in a coordinated effort as part of the three-tiered organizational structure.

8. **D.** While having well-planned meetings is important, it was not one of the "rules to live by" for governance committees. Options A, B, and C were part of the rules to live by along with putting someone in charge who can take a stand and doing real work every time.

9. **C.** Options A, B, and D are all important types of care-delivery models, but the patient-centered medical home has been a focal point of health-reform efforts during the past decade.

10. **A.** Regional extension centers recruited physician champions to serve as role models and share best practices and lessons learned in becoming meaningful users of EHRs.

11. **C.** The nursing workforce is the single largest group of users of electronic health records.

12. **A.** Eckes and Staren's 2009 article entitled "Communication Management's Role in EHR Success" identified six communication vehicles that included fact sheets, newsletters, posters, roadshows, town hall meetings, and standard meeting reports, all of which did not include video demonstrations.

13. **C.** These two types of innovations have strengthened communication options, increasing the success of EHRs and other healthcare IT.

14. **C.** The two physician-centric social media sites referenced in the chapter for improving provider-to-provider communications are Sermo and QuantiaMD.

15. **D.** Out of six subcommittees of the ONC-HIT Standards Committee, the Implementation subcommittee has a strong public communications strategy and maintains an active liaison role with the HIT Policy Committee.

References

1. Blumenthal, D., & Tavenner, M. (2010). The "meaningful use" regulation for electronic health records. *New England Journal of Medicine, 363,* 501–504.

2. Committee on Quality of Healthcare in America. (2001). *Crossing the quality chasm: A new health system for the 21st century.* National Academies Press.

3. Bass, A. (2003). Health-care IT: A big rollout bust. *CIO Magazine.* Accessed on May 4, 2012, from www.cio.com/article/29736/Health_Care_IT_A_Big_Rollout_Bust.

4. Bates, D. W. (2006). Invited commentary: The road to implementation of the electronic health record. *Proceedings, 19,* 311–312.

5. Shortliffe, E. H. (2005). Strategic action in health information technology: Why the obvious has taken so long. *Health Affairs, 24,* 1222–1233.

6. Rouse, W. (2008). Healthcare as a complex adaptive system: Implications for design and management. *The Bridge, 38(1).*

7. Kaplan, B., & Harris-Salamone, K. D. (2009). Healthcare IT success and failure: Recommendations from literature and an AMIA workshop. *Journal of the American Medical Informatics Association, 16,* 291–299.

8. Campbell, E. M., Sittig, D. F., Ash, J. S., Guappone, K. P., & Dykstra, R. H. (2006). Types of unintended consequences related to computerized provider order entry. *Journal of the American Medical Informatics Association, 13,* 547–556.

9. Bartos, C. E., Butler, B. S., Penrod, L. E., Fridsma, D. B., & Crowley, R. S. (2008). Negative CPOE attitudes correlate with diminished power in the workplace. *AMIA Annual Symposium Proceedings,* 36–40.

10. Ash, J. S., Anderson, J. G., Gorman, P. N., Zielstorff, R. D., Norcross, N., et al. (2000). Managing change: Analysis of a hypothetical case. *Journal of the American Medical Informatics Association, 7,* 125–34.

11. Morrissey, J. iGovernance. (2012). *Hospitals & Health Networks Magazine.* Accessed on May 6, 2012, from www.hhnmag.com/hhnmag_app/jsp/ articledisplay.jsp?dcrpath=HHNMAG/Article/data/02FEB2012/0212HHN_ Coverstory&domain=HHNMAG.

12. The CIO's guide to implementing EHRs in the HITECH era. (2010). Accessed on May 4, 2012, from www.cio-chime.org/advocacy/CIOsGuideBook/CIO_Guide_ Final.pdf.

13. Johnson, E. O. (2012). IMPACT journey program briefing. Tenet Healthcare Corporation.

14. Hoehn, B. J. (2010). Clinical information technology governance. *Journal of Healthcare Information Management, 24,* 13–14.

15. Joint principles of the patient-centered medical home (2007). Accessed on May 30, 2012, from www.pcpcc.net/content/joint-principles-patient-centered-medical-home.

16. Overview and intent of Medicare Shared Savings Program. (2011). *Federal Register, 76,* 67804.

17. Physician champions' help other docs with EHR adoption. (2011). Accessed on June 1, 2012 from www.govhealthit.com/news/physician-champions-help-other-docs-ehr-adoption.

18. Providers make progress in EHR adoption, challenges remain. Accessed on May 22, 2012, from www.ihealthbeat.org/articles/2012/4/24/providers-make-progress-in-ehr-adoption-challenges-remain.aspx.

19. Nursing and meaningful use: What's the connection? (2011). Accessed on June 1, 2012, from http://championnursing.org/blog/nursing-and-meaningful-use.

20. Mitchell, M. B. (2012). The role of the CNIO in nursing optimization of the electronic medical record. Health Information Management Systems Society (HIMSS) 2012 Annual Conference Presentation.

21. The CIO's guide to implementing EHRs in the HITECH era. (2010). Accessed on May 4, 2012, from www.cio-chime.org/advocacy/CIOsGuideBook/CIO_Guide_Final.pdf.

22. Tenet Healthcare Corporation. (2013). Release process improvements announced for IMPACT's Cerner Millennium hospitals. *The IMPACT Insider Newsletter*.

23. Health Information Management Systems Society (HIMSS). (2011). *2011 Davies Enterprise Award for Kaiser Permanente*.

24. Eckes, C. A., & Staren, E. D. (2009). Communication management's role in EHR success. *HealthIT News*. Accessed on May 22, 2012, from www.healthcareitnews.com/blog/communication-management%E2%80%99s-role-ehr-success?page=0,1.

25. Smaltz, D. H., Callander, R., Turner, M., Kennamer, G., Wurtz, H., Bowen, A., & Waldrum, M. R. (2005). Making sausage—effective management of enterprise-wide clinical IT projects. *Journal of Healthcare Information Management, 19*, 48–55.

26. Rodríguez, C., & Pozzebon, M. (2011). Understanding managerial behaviour during initial steps of a clinical information system adoption. *BioMedCentral Medical Informatics & Decision Making, 11*, 42.

27. D'Amato, C., D'Andrea, R., Bronnert, J., Cook, J., Foley, M., et al. (2009). Planning organizational transition to ICD-10-CM/PCS. *Journal of the American Health Information Management Association (AHIMA), 80*, 72–77.

28. Vecchione, A. (2012). Doctors' tablet use almost doubles on 2012. *Information Week*. Accessed on May 26, 2012, from www.informationweek.com/news/healthcare/mobile-wireless/240000469.

29. Maragioglio, J. (2012). The future of mHealth: Doctors use gadgets to improve healthcare. *MobileMedia*. Accessed on May 27, 2012, from www.mobiledia.com/news/126994.html.

30. Lai, E. (2012). How healthcare's embrace of mobility has turned dangerous. *Forbes*. Accessed on May 26, 2012, at www.forbes.com/sites/sap/2012/01/05/how-healthcares-embrace-of-mobility-has-turned-dangerous.

31. Van De Belt, T. H., Engelen, L. J., Berben, S. A., & Schoonhoven, L. (2010). Definition of Health 2.0 and Medicine 2.0: A systematic review. *Journal of Medical Internet Research, 12*, 18.

32. Hesse, B. W., O'Connell, M., Augustson, E. M., Chou, W. Y., Shaikh, A. R., Rutten, L. J. (2011). Realizing the promise of Web 2.0: Engaging community intelligence. *Journal of Health Communication, 16*, 10–31.

33. Social networking impact on patients, doctors, and non-profits. (2010). Accessed on May 26, 2012, from www.kevinmd.com/blog/2010/05/social-networking-impact-patients-doctors-nonprofits.html.

34. Lewis, N. (2011). Healthcare social media sites neglect privacy protections. *Information Week*. Accessed on May 26, 2012, from www.informationweek.com/news/healthcare/patient/229218547.

35. Recent federal initiatives in health information technology. (2009). Accessed on June 3, 2012, from www.rwjf.org/pr/product.jsp?id=50308.

36. Health communications and health information technology. Accessed on May 11, 2012, from www.healthypeople.gov/2020/topicsobjectives2020/overview.aspx?topicid=18.

37. SearchHealthIT. Accessed on June 3, 2012, from http://searchhealthit.techtarget.com/definition/Centers-for-Medicare-Medicaid-Services-CMS.

38. Healthcare IT policy committee. Accessed on May 26, 2012, from http://healthit.hhs.gov/portal/server.pt/community/healthit_hhs_gov__health_it_policy_committee/1269.

39. Healthcare IT standards committee. Accessed on May 26, 2012, from http://healthit.hhs.gov/portal/server.pt/community/healthit_hhs_gov__health_it_standards_committee/1271.

40. Secretary Sebelius announces next stage for providers adopting electronic health records. (2012). Accessed on May 31, 2012, from www.hhs.gov/news/press/2012pres/02/20120224a.html.

41. Health information technology in the United States: On the cusp of change. (2009). *Robert Wood Johnson Foundation Report*, 53.

42. HIT standards committee workgroups. Accessed on June 3, 2012, from http://healthit.hhs.gov/portal/server.pt/community/healthit_hhs_gov__hit_standards_committee_workgroups/1471.

43. Implementation workgroup. Accessed on June 3, 2012, from http://healthit.hhs.gov/portal/server.pt?open=512&objID=1482&parentname=CommunityPage&parentid=2&mode=2&in_hi_userid=10741&cached=true.

PART II

Healthcare Regulatory Requirements

Donald T. Mon, Editor

Healthcare Information Technology and Healthcare Policy

Liz Johnson, Judy Murphy[*]

In this chapter you will learn how to

- Discuss the key issues driving healthcare reform in the United States
- Explain the rationale for elements of the Health Information Technology for Economic and Clinical Health (HITECH) Act in terms of the history of healthcare information technology (healthcare IT)
- Describe the history of regulation of healthcare IT in the United States
- Discuss how financial incentives for the use of healthcare IT have changed over time
- Describe the significant developments and federal initiatives that have influenced the evolution and adoption of healthcare information systems
- Describe the criteria to achieve meaningful use intended for stage 1 and stage 2
- Explain the process and value of EHR certification

On March 23, 2010, President Barack Obama signed into law the landmark Patient Protection and Affordable Care Act (PPACA). As upheld on June 28, 2012, in an historic and landmark decision by the U.S. Supreme Court, PPACA was a hard-fought federal statute that represents the sweeping healthcare-reform agenda envisioned by the Democratic 111th Congress and the Obama administration. Despite legal challenges that sought (and still seek) to reverse "Obamacare," the law was designed to ensure that all Americans have access to healthcare that is both affordable and driven by quality standards. It includes broad provisions for the improvement of healthcare delivery that were declared constitutional and, at the time of writing this chapter, will run through the end of the present decade, barring additional Congressional actions.[1]

---

[*] Adapted from Virginia K. Saba and Kathleen A. McCormick, *Essentials of Nursing Informatics, Fifth Edition*, 247–263. © 2011 by The McGraw-Hill Companies.

For the Obama administration and the nation, PPACA turned a spotlight on the ever-increasing recognition that advanced healthcare information technology (healthcare IT) is essential to support the massive amounts of electronic information exchange foundational to industry reform. In fact, the universal agreement that meaningful healthcare reform cannot be separated from the national—and arguably global—integration of healthcare IT, based on accepted, standardized, and interoperable methods of data exchange, provided the linchpin for other critically important legislation that created a glide path for PPACA.

It was such consensus that resulted in the passage into law of the American Recovery and Reinvestment Act of 2009 (ARRA) and its key HITECH provision in the early weeks of Mr. Obama's presidency. Backed with an allocation of $19.2 billion, this legislation authorized the Centers for Medicare & Medicaid Services (CMS) to provide reimbursement incentives for eligible professionals and hospitals that take steps to become "meaningful users" of certified electronic health record (EHR) technology to improve care quality and better manage care costs.[2]

At the core of the new reform initiatives, the incentivized adoption of EHRs by eligible hospitals and providers across the land will improve care quality and better manage care costs. It will also help to meet clinical and business needs, because capturing, storing, and displaying clinical information from EHRs when and where it is needed can improve individual patient care while providing aggregated, cross-patient data analysis.

EHRs will manage healthcare data and information in ways that are patient-centered, secure, and information-rich. Improved information access and availability across the continuum of care will increasingly enable both the provider and the patient to better manage each patient's health by using capabilities provided through enhanced clinical decision support and customized education materials.

In this massive transformation from disconnected, inefficient, paper-based "islands" of care delivery to a nationwide, interconnected, and interoperable system driven by EHRs and advancing healthcare IT innovation, the importance of healthcare IT professionals is difficult to overstate.[3] Major forces of reform are today fueling sharply increased demand for a larger healthcare IT workforce across the U.S. healthcare landscape. As Reed Abelson of the *New York Times* wrote in late 2011, "… health care in America has changed in ways that will not be easily undone. Provisions already put in place, like tougher oversight of health insurers…are already well cemented and popular."[4]

In a similar article *USA Today* concurred, reporting that healthcare IT job growth is being driven by the general restructuring of the healthcare industry. This includes not only the provisions created by the PPACA, but also 2009 federal stimulus funding, new government regulations, and increasing use of healthcare IT across the industry.[5]

Supporting this viewpoint, the Bureau of Labor Statistics has projected that employment growth in the healthcare IT area will increase overall by 20 percent through 2018 (Occupational Outlook Handbook, 2010–2011 Edition),[6] with some segments like network and computer systems administrators expanding by 28 percent.[7] As the population continues to age, health-related issues are expected to increase, more tests and procedures will be performed, and more data and records will require management. In addition, the need to slow the increase in healthcare costs and provide affordable and better healthcare to Americans has grown. As a result, healthcare IT professionals will be required to support physicians, nurses, allied healthcare professionals, and patients.

Information security concerns are also increasing for many healthcare organizations as managers realize that current security measures are insufficient to protect the privacy of growing volumes of patient healthcare information (PHI).[7] As a direct result, more new opportunities for computer and information management professionals will be driven by organizations upgrading their healthcare IT systems and switching to newer, faster, and more mobile networks.[8]

As a major factor in such dynamics, the growing commitment by healthcare systems and physician practices to the implementation and demonstrated meaningful use of certified EHR systems will also continue to create new opportunities for healthcare IT professionals. At the time of this writing, participation in meaningful-use stage 1 alone has accounted for well over $5 billion in Medicare and Medicaid incentives payments to nearly 94,000 hospitals and physicians. One year into the program to drive the adoption and meaningful use of certified EHRs, 42 percent of all eligible hospitals have received an incentive payment for demonstration of meaningful use. One out of every nine Medicare-eligible physicians and professionals are meaningful users of EHRs.[9]

All in all, some 50,000 qualified healthcare IT workers will be needed to meet the demands of hospitals and physicians as they move to adopt EHRs and connect to statewide health information exchanges (HIEs). In fact, the Bureau of Labor Statistics, Department of Education, and independent studies estimate a workforce shortfall over the next five years.[10] For this reason, in collaboration with the National Science Foundation, the U.S. Department of Education, and the Department of Labor, the Office of the National Coordinator for Health Information Technology (referred to as ONC) has designed the Health IT Workforce Development Program to assist in the training and assessment of qualified graduates, who will reduce the estimated healthcare IT workforce shortfall by 85 percent.

Given the critical importance of healthcare IT professionals to the future of healthcare transformation, it is important to understand the key components driving change in the industry: the primary influencers, organizations, programs, and processes that have shaped or defined polices for the integration of healthcare IT that will affect all segments of healthcare. This chapter includes the following sections, which identify and define the historic and present roles of such influencers:

- Forces of Change in Today's National Healthcare System
- Mandate for Reform: ARRA and Its HITECH Provision
- State and Regional Healthcare IT Programs
- HIT Federal Advisory Committees and Agencies
- Influencing Healthcare IT Transformation through Testimony and Comment

Forces of Change in Today's National Healthcare System

The long journey to the passage of PPACA, ARRA, and HITECH goes back several decades. In 1991, the Institute of Medicine (IOM) concluded that computerization could help to improve patient records and information management, leading to higher quality of care, in its landmark report, *The Computer-Based Patient Record: An Essential Technology for Healthcare.*[11] That was followed nearly a decade later with other groundbreaking reports calling for the use of healthcare IT to improve the efficiency, safety, and quality of the U.S. healthcare system—*To Err Is Human* in 1999[12] and *Crossing the Quality Chasm* in 2001.[13] These reports were a call to action for a paradigm shift from reliance on paper and verbal communication for managing patient care to a new era where healthcare professionals are supported by technology in their clinical decision-making.

There were also other significant forces of change. One of the earliest and most influential was the President's Information Technology Advisory Committee (PITAC).

PITAC: The Winds of Change

In 1997, the President issued an executive order that established the visionary, 24-member PITAC, which was composed of both corporate and academic leaders from across the United States. Since its inception, the committee has provided the President, Congress, and those federal agencies involved in networking and IT research and development with expert, independent advice on maintaining American preeminence in advanced information technologies. These technologies include such critical elements of the national IT infrastructure as high-performance computing, large-scale networking, cyber security, and high-assurance software and systems design.[14]

In 1999, as part of its seminal work to define how IT could drive progress in the twenty-first century, PITAC established a panel to provide guidance on how IT could be leveraged to transform healthcare and increase access to care for all citizens. Driving the panel's work was the firm conviction that the federal government's role in leading the way to healthcare reform through technology was both critical and, at the time, sorely lacking.[15]

A few years later, in a report entitled *Transforming Health Care Through Information Technology*, PITAC found that "at present, the U.S. lacks a broadly disseminated and accepted national vision for information technology in healthcare."[16] To rectify the situation, the panel strongly recommended that the Department of Health and Human Services (HHS) define a clear vision of how IT could improve the U.S. healthcare system, follow up with resources sufficient to accomplish its objectives, and appoint a senior IT person to provide strategic leadership.

President Bush's Executive Order and the Birth of the ONC

On January 20, 2004, President George W. Bush in his State of the Union address called for "… an Electronic Health Record for every American by the year 2014 … By computerizing health records, we can avoid dangerous medical mistakes, reduce costs, and improve care."[17] He went on to issue an executive order ("Incentives for the Use of Health Information Technology and Establishing the Position of the National Health Information Technology Coordinator") that has affected every healthcare entity, provider, and informatics nurse professional in the United States.[18]

The goals of the order were as follows: to establish a national healthcare IT coordinator position; to develop a nationwide interoperable healthcare IT infrastructure; and to develop, maintain, and direct implementation of a strategic plan to guide implementation of interoperable healthcare IT in both public and private sectors. The interoperable healthcare IT was seen as a means to reduce medical errors, improve quality, and produce greater value for healthcare expenditures. The same year, Dr. David Brailer was appointed as the first coordinator by Tommy Thompson, then HHS Secretary.

The Office of the National Coordinator for Health Information Technology (referred to as ONC) remains today the principal federal entity charged with coordination of nationwide efforts to implement and use the most advanced healthcare IT and the electronic exchange of healthcare information. ONC is a key player in the execution of ARRA and its HITECH provision. ONC's current coordinator is Dr. Farzad Mostashari, who was appointed by HHS Secretary Kathleen Sebelius in May 2011, succeeding Dr. David Blumenthal.

On the road to healthcare reform, many other organizations and initiatives provided the vision, leadership, and processes that paved the way toward the legislative action seen in ARRA, HITECH, and PPACA. Ensuring the translation mandated by the legislation, other groups such as ONC's HIT Policy and HIT Standards Committees are today defining and shaping the healthcare agenda on an ongoing basis.

Healthcare IT Training Programs: An Essential Element of Reform

PITAC's 2001 recommendations to President George W. Bush included a call for trained professionals who could apply healthcare IT to healthcare reform, noting that it would be necessary to "establish programs to increase the pool of biomedical research and healthcare professionals with training at the intersection of health and information technology."[19] In its findings, the report warned that the pool of professionals at the time was "remarkably small."

As discussed in this chapter's introduction, today's urgent need for healthcare IT experts is challenged by a shortage of the very professionals who are best positioned to carry transformation forward. With consensus around the essential requirement for advanced healthcare IT and the mounting pressures of shortages in healthcare IT experts and other medical professions, the U.S. government through HHS has enlisted the talent and resources of some of the nation's leading universities, community colleges, and major research centers to advance the widespread adoption and meaningful use of healthcare IT. These schools are offering a wide variety of training programs that are helping to build the depth and breadth of the healthcare IT workforce as a critical component in the transformation of American healthcare delivery.

Both on-campus and online programs in healthcare IT are available at the certificate, associate, bachelor's, and master's degree levels. Certificate programs typically require between 15 and 30 credit hours and are often designed for working professionals.[20] The American Medical Informatics Association (AMIA) created a revolutionary "10 X 10" Program in 2005, with the goal of training 10,000 healthcare professionals in applied health informatics by 2010, and became a model for certificate-based programs.[21]

Through ARRA, federal awards and grants totaling some $84 million to 16 universities and junior colleges are providing incentives for healthcare IT education to speed the growth of a new pool of healthcare IT professionals. These programs are now supporting the training and development of more than 50,000 new healthcare IT professionals, as mentioned in the chapter introduction. For more information, see "Workforce Training" in the section "Mandate for Reform: ARRA and Its HITECH Provision."

The Health Insurance Portability and Accountability Act (HIPAA): Privacy and Security

HIPAA, which passed in 1996, required HHS to develop regulations that both protect the privacy and security of electronic health information and facilitate its efficient transmission.[22] HIPAA's goals are to allow the flow of health information needed to provide and promote high-quality healthcare while protecting the public's health and well-being. Prior to HIPAA, no generally accepted set of standards or requirements for protecting health information existed in the healthcare industry. At the same time, new technologies were evolving to move the healthcare industry away from paper processes and to increase the reliance on electronic information systems to conduct a host of administrative and clinically based functions, such as providing health information, paying claims, and answering eligibility questions.[23]

To comply with the requirements of the act, HHS published what are commonly known as the HIPAA Privacy Rule and the HIPAA Security Rule. The rules apply to all health plans, healthcare clearinghouses, and to any healthcare provider that transmits health information in electronic form.

The HIPAA Privacy Rule

The HIPAA Privacy Rule, which took effect on April 14, 2003, established national standards for the protection of individually identifiable health information. As such, the rule regulates the use and disclosure of an individual's health information, referred to as *protected health information* (PHI), and sets forth standards for individuals' privacy rights to understand and control how their health information is used. The rule applies to those organizations identified as "covered entities," which include healthcare clearinghouses, employer-sponsored health plans, health insurers, and other medical service providers that engage in the transfer of PHI. PHI is defined broadly and includes any part of an individual's medical record or payment history.[24] The HIPAA Privacy and Security Rule is covered in more depth in Chapter 13 by Chris Apgar.

The HIPAA Security Rule

The HIPAA Security Rule took effect on April 21, 2003, with a compliance date of April 21, 2005, for most covered entities. The Security Rule complements the Privacy Rule; while the Privacy Rule pertains to *all* PHI, including paper and electronic records, the Security Rule deals specifically with electronic protected health information (ePHI). Still, a major goal of the Security Rule is to protect the privacy of individuals' PHI while allowing covered entities to adopt new technologies to improve the quality and efficiency of patient care. Given the diversity of the healthcare marketplace, the Security Rule is designed to be flexible and scalable so that a covered entity can implement policies, procedures, and technologies that are appropriate for the entity's particular size, organizational structure, and risks to consumers' electronic ePHI.[25]

In the years following its passage and implementation, HIPAA regulations have had a significant impact on healthcare informatics. For example, under HIPAA, patients must be permitted to review and amend their medical records. Healthcare providers have expressed concern that patients who choose to access their records could experience increased anxiety. Other studies, however, have determined that patients' access to records has already enhanced doctor-patient communications, and the risks in increasing patients' access to their records are minimal.

The passage of ARRA has expanded HIPAA's mandate to impose new privacy and security requirements. One of the greatest changes to HIPAA presently affecting the healthcare community and healthcare IT professionals are the modifications published on January 16, 2009, in the HIPAA Electronic Transaction Standards Final Rule.

As originally framed, the old ANSI X12 Standards for HIPAA transactions were to be replaced by Version 5010, which regulates the transmission of certain healthcare transactions among hospitals, physician practices, health plans, and claims clearinghouses. In addition, the old version of the National Council for Prescription Drug Program (NCPDP) standard for pharmacy and supplier transactions was to be replaced by Version D.0.[26]

As the first major change since HIPAA's implementation, the introductions of these new standards are meant to enhance business functionality, clarify ambiguities, and better define situational and required data elements. The new rules apply to all physicians, providers, and suppliers who bill Medicare carriers, fiscal intermediaries, Medicare administrative contractors (MACs), and durable medical equipment MACs for services provided to Medicare beneficiaries.[27]

When first announced, the switch to the 5010 standards was supposed to be in place on January 1, 2012. But in November 2011, CMS decided that, although it would not change the actual deadline for complying with the standards, it would not initiate enforcement action until March 31. Soon thereafter, in continued reconsideration of what it called "a number of outstanding issues and challenges impeding full implementation,"[28] CMS pushed the enforcement date to June 30, 2012.

The conversion to the HIPAA 5010 standards is seen as key to the larger switch from the ICD-9 clinical coding system to the vastly more detailed ICD-10 system[29]—ICD-10 will be required for all providers effective October 1, 2014.

EHR Certification and the Changing Role of CCHIT

With the passage of ARRA and HITECH, ONC has become the driving force behind the definition of meaningful use of EHRs and the certification of EHR systems. This new reality has changed the operating environment for the Certification Commission for Healthcare Information Technology (CCHIT), which until recent years had been the sole agency designated to certify EHR systems. The CCHIT is covered in Chapter 31.

CCHIT was founded in 2004[30] with support from three industry associations in healthcare information management and technology: the American Health Information Management Association (AHIMA), the Healthcare Information and Management Systems Society (HIMSS), and the National Alliance for Health Information Technology (NAHIT). In September 2005, HHS awarded CCHIT a contract to develop the certification criteria and inspection process for EHRs and the networks through which they interoperate. Since then, in its work to certify EHRs, CCHIT established the first comprehensive, practical definition of the capabilities that were required in such systems. The certification criteria were developed through a voluntary, consensus-based process engaging diverse stakeholders. Many healthcare IT professionals were involved in this process—helping to define the certification criteria for the hospital and ambulatory environments as well as to outline the testing processes used by CCHIT.[31]

However, in the months following the 2009 passage of ARRA, questions surfaced about CCHIT's future role. On March 2, 2010, ONC confirmed the merits of this debate when it issued a new Notice of Proposed Rulemaking (NPRM),[32] which proposed the establishment of two certification programs for the purposes of testing and certifying EHRs—one temporary and one permanent. These new programs were not limited to CCHIT. Then, on June 24, 2010, ONC published the Final Rule on the Temporary Certification Program for EHRs.

Under the temporary program, ONC authorized approved organizations, called ONC–Authorized Testing and Certification Bodies (ONC–ATCBs), to both test and certify EHRs and EHR modules, thereby assuring the availability of certified EHR technology prior to the beginning of the reporting period defined under ARRA. After the first year, the permanent certification program replaced the temporary program and now separates the responsibilities for performing testing and certification. In addition to EHR and EHR modules certification, the permanent program includes the certification of other types of heathcare IT, such as personal health records (PHRs) and health information exchange (HIE) networks.[33]

Today, six companies have earned HHS's approval as ONC–ATCBs. As listed on ONC's official website, they are Surescripts, LLC of Arlington, VA; ICS Labs of Mechanicsburg, PA; SLI Global Solutions of Denver, CO; InfoGard Laboratories, Inc. of San Luis Obispo, CA; CCHIT of Chicago, IL; and Drummond Corp. of Austin, TX.[34]

Standards and the National Health Information Network

In late 2005, HHS commissioned the Healthcare Information Technology Standards Panel (HITSP) to assist in developing a National Health Information Network (NHIN), which would create a nationwide, interoperable, private, and secure exchange of health information between EHRs.[35] The standards are covered in depth in Chapter 12.

NHIN was created to provide a set of standards that regulate the connections among providers, consumers, and others involved in supporting health and healthcare. The purpose of these standards is to enable normalized health information to follow the consumer; they are intended to make health records, laboratory results, medication information, and related medical data readily available and accessible to providers, pharmacists, and even consumers over the Internet, thereby helping to achieve the goals of the HITECH Act today. Importantly, NHIN was also dedicated to ensuring that consumers' health information remains secure and confidential in the electronic environment.

In January 2011, NHIN began to be referenced as the "Nation*wide* Health Information Network" (NwHIN). The change is intended to emphasize that NwHIN is a set of standards, services, and policies that enable secure health information exchange over the Internet. These standards are today being used by three federal initiatives: the Direct project, NwHIN exchange, and the CONNECT software project. The name change also serves notice that NwHIN continues to evolve, with the government acting as a facilitator—not a convener. In fact, its development depends on an environment of collaboration, transparency, and buy-in from the bottom up, including small as well as large physician groups and healthcare systems that are working to share patient records with other care delivery entities across the continuum of care.[36]

Interoperability

Interoperability is the ability of health information systems to work together within and across organizational boundaries to advance the effective delivery of healthcare for individuals and communities by sharing data between EHRs. For interoperability to occur, standards are required for data transport, content exchange, and vocabulary management. This is why standards development is so important—it enables the interoperability needed for regional and national health data exchange and is essential to the development of the NwHIN.

Debate exists as to how interoperability should develop relative to EHR adoption in terms of timing. Many industry leaders believe that interoperability should precede EHR use. They are convinced that the ability to share information should be designed into EHRs and that the infrastructure and industry capacity for securely networking this information should exist up front. Others argue that interoperability will follow widespread EHR adoption. This side of the debate believes that once health information becomes electronic and everyone is using EHRs, interoperability will naturally follow, because it will be easier and cheaper than manual data sharing.[37, 38]

In May 2012, ONC released to the public a request for information (RFI) on the governance of NwHIN, believing this would constitute a critical step toward enabling trusted and interoperable electronic health information exchange nationwide. As stated on its website, ONC sees a common set of "rules of the road" for privacy, security, business, and technical requirements as a means of laying the necessary foundation to enable our nation's electronic health information exchange capacity to grow. It can also help achieve the Bush and Obama administrations' vision for an electronically connected health system for the twenty-first century that delivers efficient and quality healthcare for all Americans.

The new RFI has asked for public feedback on how a governance mechanism would best provide confidence to patients that their health information is being shared appropriately and securely, reassure providers they are dealing with trusted entities when sending or receiving patient information, promote an open and competitive market for electronic health information exchange, and enable innovation to thrive.[39] At the time of this writing, this NPRM was still out for comment, with feedback from both the HIT Standards and Policy Committees included as powerful influencers of ONC's efforts to ensure a future of healthcare information exchange.

Integrating the Healthcare Enterprise

Integrating the Healthcare Enterprise (IHE) is a global initiative, now in its twelfth year, to create the framework for passing vital health information seamlessly from application to application, system to system, and setting to setting across multiple healthcare enterprises. IHE brings together healthcare IT stakeholders to demonstrate the implementation of standards for communicating patient information efficiently throughout and among healthcare enterprises by developing a framework of interoperability. Because of its proven process of collaboration, demonstration, and real-world implementation of interoperable solutions, IHE is in a unique position to significantly accelerate the process for defining, testing, and implementing standards-based interoperability among EHR systems.[40]

Nonprofit Organizations Driving Reform: AMIA and HIMSS

Among the many nonprofit organizations today advancing healthcare IT and healthcare informatics, few have had more positive impact on the industry than the American Medical Informatics Association (AMIA) and the Healthcare Information and Management Systems Society (HIMSS). Both organizations have significant numbers of healthcare IT professionals who are expert informaticists, as well as committees, task forces, and working groups that support the healthcare IT community.

AMIA

AMIA is dedicated to promoting the effective organization, analysis, management, and use of information in healthcare to support patient care, public health, teaching, research, administration, and related policy. For more than thirty years, the members of AMIA and its honorific college, the American College of Medical Informatics (ACMI), have sponsored meetings, education, policy, and research programs. The federal government frequently calls upon AMIA as a source of informed, unbiased opinions on policy issues relating to the national healthcare information infrastructure, uses and protection of personal health information, and public health considerations, among others.[41]

With an overall mission of advancing the informatics profession relating to health and disease, AMIA champions the use of healthcare information and communications technology in clinical care and research, personal health management, public health/population, and transactional science with the ultimate objective of improving health. The association is also dedicated to expanding the size and strengthening the competency of the U.S. healthcare informatics workforce and supporting the continued development of the healthcare informatics profession.

HIMSS

HIMSS was founded in 1961 and is a comprehensive healthcare-stakeholder membership organization focused exclusively on providing leadership for the optimal use of IT and management systems that will improve healthcare. A global organization with offices in Chicago; Washington, D.C.; Brussels; and Singapore; HIMSS represents over 23,000 members, 73 percent of whom work in patient-care delivery settings. HIMSS also includes corporate members and nonprofit organizations that share its mission to transform healthcare through the effective use of IT and management systems.[42]

The society was founded on the premise that an organized exchange of experience among members could promote a better understanding of the principles underlying healthcare systems and improve the skills of those who direct healthcare IT programs and the practitioners who analyze, design, or evaluate healthcare IT systems. In today's environment of rapid reform and transformation, HIMSS frames and leads healthcare public policy and industry practices through its educational programs, professional development, and advocacy initiatives designed to promote information and management systems' contributions to ensuring quality patient care.[43]

Mandate for Reform: ARRA and Its HITECH Provision

ARRA and its important HITECH provision were passed into law on February 17, 2009. Commonly referred to as the "Stimulus Bill" or "Recovery Act," the landmark legislation allocated $787 billion to stimulate the economy, including $147 billion to rescue and reform the nation's seriously ailing healthcare industry. Of these funds, $19 billion in financial incentives were earmarked for the relatively short period of five years to drive reform through the use of advanced healthcare IT and the adoption of EHRs. As noted in this chapter's introduction, the incentives were intended to help healthcare providers purchase and implement healthcare IT and EHR systems, and the HITECH Act also stipulated that clear penalties would be imposed beyond 2015 for both hospitals and physician providers who failed to adopt use of EHRs in a meaningful way. This section describes some of the key components of ARRA and HITECH.[2]

HITECH Incentives for Meaningful Use of EHRs

The majority of the HITECH funding will be used to reward hospitals and eligible providers for "meaningful use" of certified EHRs by "meaningful users" with increased Medicare and Medicaid payments. The law specifies that eligible healthcare professionals and hospitals can qualify for both programs when they adopt certified EHR technology and use it in a meaningful way. Exactly how HITECH, as administered by ONC and CMS, defines "meaningful use" is a dynamic, evolutionary process that will involve three stages: [44]

- **Stage 1**   Beginning in 2011 as the incentives-program starting point for all providers, meaningful use consists of transferring data to EHRs and being able to share information, including electronic copies and visit summaries for patients.

- **Stage 2**   Beginning in 2014, this stage of meaningful use will include new standards such as patients' online access to their health information and electronic health information exchange between providers.

- **Stage 3**   Expected to begin in 2016, meaningful use is projected to include demonstrating that the quality of healthcare has improved.[44]

Milestones in Meaningful-Use Reform

The following milestone dates and their significance to the healthcare reform movement in the United State are summarized in the following paragraphs:

December 31, 2009   CMS, with input from ONC and the HIT Policy and Standards Committees, published a proposed rule on the meaningful use of EHRs in stage 1 and began a 60-day public comment period.

July 28, 2010   After reviewing more than 2,000 comments, HHS issued the final stage 1 rule, with criteria for meeting meaningful use divided into five initiatives:[45]

- Improve quality, safety, efficiency, and reduce health disparities.

- Engage patients and families.

- Improve care coordination.

- Improve population and public health.

- Ensure adequate privacy and security protections for personal health information.

Specific objectives were written to demonstrate that EHR use would have a meaningful impact on one of the five initiatives. Under the final rule, participating providers are today working to meet 14 core (required) objectives for hospitals and 15 for providers. For both hospitals and providers, the rule sets out 10 other objectives in a "menu set" from which they must choose and comply with five. If the objectives are met during the specified year and the hospital or provider submits the appropriate measurements, then the hospitals or providers will receive the incentive payment. The hospital incentive amount is based on the Medicare and Medicaid patient volumes; the provider incentives are fixed per provider. The incentives are paid over five years, and the hospital or provider must submit measurement results annually during each of the years to continue to qualify. The objectives will mature every other year, with new criteria and standards being published in 2011, 2013, and 2015.[46]

November 30, 2011 In the launch of an initiative called "We Can't Wait," HHS and the Obama administration acknowledged the challenges of meeting stage 2 timeline requirements. Under the original requirements, eligible doctors and hospitals that begin participating in the Medicare EHR Incentive Programs in 2010 would have had to meet new standards for the program in 2013. But if they chose not to participate in the program until 2012, they could wait until 2014 to meet the same standards and still be eligible for identical incentive payments. Therefore, to encourage faster adoption, HHS's announcement cleared the way for doctors and hospitals to adopt healthcare IT in 2011 without formally meeting the new standards until 2014. These policy changes were also accompanied by greater outreach efforts to provide more information to doctors and hospitals about best practices. They also sought to help vendors whose products were straining to keep up with the changing requirements for their technologies, which allow healthcare providers to meaningfully use EHRs.[47]

February 23–24, 2012 CMS and HHS proposed the stage 2 meaningful-use criteria for providers using EHR technology and receiving stage 1 incentives payments from Medicare and Medicaid. The proposed rule, which was submitted to the public for a comment period that ended on May 7, 2012,[48] was intended to define more than the stage 2 criteria that eligible providers must meet to qualify for incentives payments. In addition, the finalized stage 2 rules also define the "payment adjustments" or penalties that (beginning in 2015) providers will face if they fail to demonstrate the meaningful use of certified EHR technology and fail to meet other program participation requirements.[44] Also as proposed, the rule identified standards and criteria for the certification of EHR technology to ensure that eligible hospitals and professionals have systems available to them that are capable of performing the functions required by both stage 1 and stage 2.[44]

What's New in Stage 2?

On August 23, 2012 the final requirements for stage 2 were published. With stage 2, HHS has expanded the meaningful use of EHR technology.[49] The final stage 2 criteria for meaningful use focuses on increasing the electronic capture of health information in a structured format, as well as increasing the exchange of clinically relevant information between providers of care at care transitions. To accomplish such objectives, the rule maintains the same core and menu structures as were used in stage 1. Eligible professionals will be required to meet (or qualify for exclusion from) 17 core objectives and 3 of 6 menu objectives or a total of 20 measures. Eligible hospitals and critical access hospitals (CAHs) must meet (or qualify for exclusion from) 16 core objectives and 3 of 6 menu objectives or a total of 19 measures.[49]

The stage 2 rule includes the following new requirements:[49]

- Changes to the denominator of computerized provider order entry (CPOE) (stage 1 optional, stage 2 required)

- Changes to the age limitations for vital signs (stage 1 optional, stage 2 required)

- Elimination of the "exchange of key clinical information" core objective from stage 1 in favor of a "transitions of care" core objective that requires electronic exchange of summary of care documents in stage 2 (effective stage 2)

- Replacing "provide patients with an electronic copy of their health information" objective with a "view online, download and transmit" core objective (effective stage 2)

The stage 2 rule also contains new objectives that have greater applicability to many specialty providers. The addition of these objectives recognizes the leadership role that many specialty providers have played in the meaningful use of healthcare IT for improving quality in the following areas:

- Making imaging results and information accessible through certified EHR technology

- Identifying and reporting cancer cases to a state cancer registry, except where prohibited, and in accordance with applicable law and practice

- Identifying and reporting specific cases to a specialized registry (other than a cancer registry), except where prohibited, and in accordance with applicable law and practice[49]

Quality Measures

One of the meaningful-use criteria for both hospitals and physicians is the requirement to report quality measures to either CMS (for Medicare) or to the states (for Medicaid). Quality measurement is considered one of the most important components of the incentive program under ARRA/HITECH, since the purpose of the healthcare IT incentives is to promote reform in the delivery, cost, and quality of healthcare in the United States. Dr. David Blumenthal, the former national coordinator of healthcare IT, emphasized this point when he said, "health IT is the means, but not the end. Getting an EHR up and running in healthcare is not the main objective behind the incentives provided by the federal government under ARRA. Improving health is. Promoting healthcare reform is."[50]

Beginning in 2014, CMS selected the set of quality measures based on several factors, including conditions that reflect national health priorities that contribute to the morbidity and mortality of Medicare patients, and that would enable the measurement of care in new dimensions, including a focus on patient/caregiver engagement. CMS also reiterated its commitment to streamlining reporting requirements across quality programs such as the Physician Quality Reporting System (PQRS), Hospital Inpatient Quality Reporting (IQR), CHIPRA, and Medicare Shared Savings (ACO) programs.

In stage 1 for providers, there were 44 measures, with a requirement to report on six of these. Beginning in 2014, providers will have to report on nine of 64 clinical quality measures that cover three of the six National Quality Strategy domains. EPs beyond their first year of participation will be able to satisfy the reporting requirements for meaningful use through successful participation in the PQRS EHR reporting option. Also, EPs who are participants in the ACO program and who meet the quality reporting requirements using certified EHR technology can use group reporting.

For hospitals, stage 1 meaningful use lists 15 measures, with a requirement to report on all of them.[51] In 2014, hospitals must report on 16 of 20 approved clinical quality measures that cover three of the six National Quality Strategy domains.

Because HHS itself was not yet ready to electronically accept quality-measure reporting in 2011, the stage 1 rule specified that hospitals and eligible providers could submit summary information on clinical quality measures to CMS through attestation. Beginning in 2014, hospitals and providers in their first year of meaningful use will continue to report quality measures through attestation; however, starting with their second year's submission, quality measures will be submitted electronically as aggregate or patient-level data.

In the final rule, CMS responded to comments they had received concerning the fact that some measures were still under development and not all had been endorsed by the National Quality Forum (NQF), the entity under contract to HHS to develop healthcare-related benchmarks. Although NQF endorsement is not required by statute, CMS stated that the expectation was that all measures critical to the program would eventually obtain NQF endorsement.[53]

ONC and Establishment of the HIT Policy and Standards Committees

To drive rapid, healthcare IT–based reform under such an aggressive plan, the HITECH legislation re-energized ONC with specific accountabilities and significant funding. It also created two new Federal Advisory Committees under its control: the HIT Policy Committee and the HIT Standards Committee. Members of the two committees are public and private stakeholders who are tasked to provide recommendations on the HIT policy framework, standards, implementation specifications, and certification criteria for the electronic exchange and use of health information.[55] Additional information regarding these two committees is provided later in this chapter, in the section "HIT Federal Advisory Committees and Agencies."

Standards and Interoperability

ARRA and the HITECH Act recognized that a key element of the widespread adoption and use of healthcare IT would be the development of uniform electronic standards that would allow various healthcare IT systems to communicate with each other, thereby interconnecting the industry.

As discussed earlier in this chapter in the sections "Standards and the National Health Information Network" and "Interoperability," ONC and its HIT Standards and Policy Committees have made considerable progress in addressing concerns over interoperability implementation through their work on a number of important standards initiatives: NwHIN, the Direct Project, and the CONNECT software project.

As part of the RFI process discussed earlier—a process that will draw public feedback on future development of NwHIN—the NwHIN Workgroup and the NwHIN Power Team are developing recommendations for extending the secure exchange of health information using NwHIN standards, services, and policies to the broadest audience possible. Further, a group of federal agencies; local, regional, and state-level health information exchange (HIE) organizations; and integrated delivery networks formerly known as the NwHIN Cooperative have been helping to develop the NwHIN standards, services, and policies and demonstrate live health information exchange through what is now called the NwHIN Exchange.[56]

ONC has coined this new name to mark the evolution of NwHIN into an independent, nonprofit, public-private partnership that includes the Department of Defense, the Social Security Administration, the Department of Veterans Affairs, CMS, and a number of nonfederal hospitals and healthcare organizations, as well as local HIEs.[56] Details of the new business model are currently being defined, with one of the most critical aspects of the planning being a sustainability plan. NwHIN will also continue to evolve as new technologies are integrated and as new partner organizations take active roles. The transition from ONC to public-private oversight should be completed by fall 2012, but the change is intended to be virtually seamless for the exchange's users.

The closely associated Direct Project, launched in March 2010, is developing standards and services required to enable secure, directed health information exchange at a more local and less complex level among trusted providers in support of both stage 1 and stage 2 meaningful-use incentive requirements (e.g., a primary-care provider sending a referral or care summary to a local specialist electronically, or a physician requesting lab tests electronically). This project will expand the existing NwHIN standards and services to enable the simple, direct, and secure transport of health information between healthcare providers at the local level and their patients. The Direct Project is *complementary* to the work of the NwHIN. Both models will be needed to support nationwide health information exchange.[57]

The CONNECT software project is a free, open-source software solution that supports health information exchange—both locally and at the national level. CONNECT uses NwHIN standards, services, and policies to make sure that HIEs are compatible with other exchanges being set up throughout the country. CONNECT is the result of a unique collaboration among federal agencies that is coordinated through the Federal Health Architecture program with ONC. Now available to any organization, CONNECT can be used to help set up HIEs and share data using nationally recognized interoperability standards. This software solution was initially developed by federal agencies to support their health-related missions.[58]

Privacy and Security

Earlier sections introduced HIPAA and its privacy and security rules as well as recent developments in the area of standards development. But it is also clear that HITECH has significantly expanded federal privacy and security laws under HIPAA. Today, HIPAA's legal scope stands as follows:[59]

- HIPAA privacy and security laws now apply directly to business associates of covered entities.

- The law defines actions that constitute a breach of patient health information (including inadvertent disclosures) and requires notification to patients if breaches occur.

- HIPAA allows patients to pay in full for a healthcare item or service and to request that the claim not be submitted to the health plan.

- Physicians are required to provide patients, upon request, an accounting of disclosures of health information made through the use of an EHR.

- The sale of a patient's health information without the patient's written authorization is prohibited, except in limited circumstances involving research or public health activities.

- Covered entities are prohibited from being paid to use patients' health information for marketing purposes without patient authorization, except limited communication to a patient about a drug currently prescribed for that patient.

- PHR vendors must notify individuals of a breach of patient health information.

- Noncovered HIPAA entities such as HIEs, Regional Health Information Organizations, e-Prescribing Gateways, and PHR vendors are required to have business associate agreements with covered entities for the electronic exchange of patient health information.

- HIPAA can now authorize increased civil monetary penalties for HIPAA violations.

- HIPAA now grants stronger authority to state attorneys general to enforce HIPAAprovisions.

For additional information, see Chapter 13.

Comparative Effectiveness Research

ARRA and HITECH increased funding by more than $1 billion for Comparative Effectiveness Research (CER) and established the Federal Coordinating Council for Comparative Effectiveness Research (FCC-CER).[60] This group is an advisory board comprised of clinical experts responsible for reducing duplication of efforts and encouraging coordination and complementary uses of resources, coordinating related health services research, and making recommendations to the President and Congress on CER infrastructure needs.

As part of this legislation, the Agency for Healthcare Research and Quality (AHRQ) received $1 billion of additional funding for CER.[60] The AHRQ's mission is to improve the quality, safety, efficiency, and effectiveness of healthcare for all Americans. As one of 12 agencies within the HHS, AHRQ supports research that helps people make more informed decisions and improves the quality of healthcare services.[61] Some of AHRQ's funding must be shared with the NIH to conduct or support CER.[60]

Additional funding ($3 billion) was also made available to the Patient-Centered Outcome Research Institute (PCORI), a nonprofit organization created by legislative authority in March 2010 to conduct research that would provide information about the best available evidence to help patients and their healthcare providers make more informed decisions. PCORI's research is intended to give patients a better understanding of the prevention, treatment, and care options available as well as the science that supports those options.[62]

Workforce Training

As discussed in the introduction to this chapter, the rapid advancement toward a more technologically enabled healthcare system is driving a growing demand for healthcare IT professionals—highly skilled healthcare IT experts who can support the provider community in the adoption and meaningful use of EHRs. To meet this demand, ONC has funded the Health IT Workforce Development Program.[63] The program's goal is to train a new workforce of healthcare IT professionals who will be ready to help providers implement EHRs to improve healthcare quality, safety, and cost effectiveness. For the program, ONC has awarded $116 million in funding for four programs as follows:

- **Community college consortia to educate healthcare information technology professionals** Five regional groups of 82 community colleges in all 50 states have $68 million in grants to develop or improve nondegree healthcare IT training programs that can be completed in six months or less. The funded community colleges were tasked to train more than 10,500 new healthcare IT professionals by 2012.

- **Assistance for university-based training** Nine grants totaling $32 million were awarded to colleges and universities to quickly establish or expand healthcare IT training programs for healthcare IT professional roles requiring training at the university level.

- **Curriculum development centers** $10 million was awarded to five universities for the development of educational materials for the community college consortia program. The materials will also be made available to other schools across the country.

- **Competency examination** A two-year, $6 million grant was awarded to fund the development of competency exams for healthcare IT professionals.[63]

NIH and NLM Grants to Support HIT Research

The passage of ARRA and the HITECH Act earmarked substantial funding in support of HIT research, in addition to programs supporting HIT training. For its part, the NIH received an infusion of funds for 2009 and 2010 as part of ARRA. NIH designated more than $200 million in these two years for a new initiative called the NIH Challenge Grants in Health and Science Research. This program supported research on topics that address specific scientific and health research challenges in biomedical and behavioral research that would benefit from significant, two-year jump-start funds. NIH funded more than 200 grants, each up to $1 million, depending on the number and quality of applications.[64]

In addition, the National Library of Medicine (NLM) offers Applied Informatics grants to health-related and scientific organizations that wish to optimize use of clinical and research information. These grants help organizations leverage the capabilities of healthcare IT to bring useful biomedical knowledge to end users by translating the findings of informatics and information science research into practice through novel or enhanced systems, incorporating them into real-life systems and service settings.[65] In April 2012, Donald A.B. Lindberg, MD, Director of the National Library of Medicine (NLM), announced that NLM had awarded 14 five-year grants totaling more than $67 million for research training in biomedical informatics, the discipline that seeks to apply computer and communications technology to improve health.

SHARP Research Grants

Alongside the NIH and NLM focus on incentivizing research, ONC also made available $60 million to support the development of Strategic Health IT Advanced Research Projects (SHARP). The SHARP program funds research focused on achieving breakthrough advances to address well-documented problems that have impeded adoption of healthcare IT and accelerating progress toward achieving nationwide meaningful use of healthcare IT in support of a high-performing, continuously learning healthcare system. ONC awarded four cooperative agreements of $15 million, with each awardee implementing a research program addressing a specific research focus area: healthcare IT security, patient-centered cognitive support, healthcare application and network architectures, and secondary use of healthcare IT data.[66]

State and Regional Healthcare IT Programs

With recognition that the regional electronic exchange of health information is essential to the successful implementation of NwHIN and to the success of national healthcare reform in general, the HITECH Act authorized and funded a State HIE Cooperative program,[67] a Beacon Community program, and a Regional HIT Extension program.[68] Taken together, these grant programs offer much-needed local and regional assistance and technical support to providers while enabling coordination and alignment within and among states. Ultimately, this will allow information to follow patients anywhere they go within the U.S. healthcare system.

State HIE Cooperative Agreement Program

The State HIE Cooperative Agreement program funded states' efforts to rapidly build capacity for exchanging health information across the healthcare system both within and across states. Awardees are responsible for increasing connectivity and enabling patient-centric information flow to improve the quality and efficiency of care. Key to this is the continual evolution and advancement of necessary governance, policies, technical services, business operations, and financing mechanisms for HIE over each state, territory, and state-designated entities' four-year performance period. This program builds on existing efforts to advance regional and state-level health information exchange while moving toward nationwide interoperability.[67]

On January 27, 2011, an additional $16 million was made available to states through ONC's new challenge grants program. This program provided funding to 14 states to encourage breakthrough innovations in targeted areas for health information exchange that can be leveraged widely to support nationwide health information exchange and interoperability.[69]

Beacon Communities

Also funded by HITECH, ONC's Beacon Community program is helping guide the way to a transformed healthcare system. The program funded more than a dozen demonstration communities that had already made progress in the adoption of healthcare IT, including EHRs and health information exchange. Beacon Communities are designed to advance new, innovative ways to improve care coordination, improve the quality of care, and slow the growth of healthcare spending.[69] Their goals are to show how healthcare IT tools and resources can contribute to communities' efforts and make breakthrough advancements in healthcare quality, safety, and efficiency, as well as in public health at the community level, demonstrating that these gains are sustainable and replicable.

In 2010, ONC awarded $250 million in grants over three years to 17 selected communities throughout the United States. Since then these communities have made inroads in the development of secure, private, and accurate systems of EHR adoption and health information exchange.[70] Each of them, with its unique population and regional context, is actively pursuing the following areas of focus:

- Building and strengthening the healthcare IT infrastructure and exchange capabilities within communities, positioning each community to pursue a new level of sustainable healthcare quality and efficiency over the coming years

- Translating investments in healthcare IT in the short run to measurable improvements in cost, quality, and population health

- Developing innovative approaches to performance measurement, technology, and care delivery to accelerate evidence generation for new approaches

Health IT Extension Program

The HITECH Act authorized a Health Information Technology Extension Program, which consists of regional extension centers (RECs) and a national health information technology research center (HITRC).[70] The regional centers offer technical assistance, guidance, and information on best practices to support and accelerate healthcare providers' efforts to become meaningful users of EHRs. The extension program established an estimated 64 regional centers, each serving a defined geographic area. To date, the regional centers have supported over 120,000 primary care providers in achieving meaningful use of EHRs and enabling nationwide health information exchange.

The extension program also established a HITRC, funded separately, to gather relevant information on effective practices and help the regional centers collaborate with one another and with relevant stakeholders to identify and share best practices in EHR adoption, effective use, and provider support.[70] The HITRC has been sharing information among the RECs for over two years, and in 2012 is going to be publicly available as a resource to all via the HealthIT.gov website.

HIT Federal Advisory Committees and Agencies

In 1972, decades before ARRA, HITECH, and PPACA, the Federal Advisory Committee Act became law and is still the legal foundation defining how federal advisory committees and agencies (FACAs) should operate.[71] As then prescribed, characteristics of such groups included openness and inclusiveness, specific authorization by either the President or the head of the overseeing agency, transparency, and clearly defined timelines for operation, termination, and renewal. In 2009, as mandated by ARRA and HITECH, ONC created two new federal advisory committees, the HIT Policy Committee and the HIT Standards Committee, in order to gain broad input on the use of healthcare IT to support healthcare reform. The National Committee on Vital and Health Statistics (NCVHS) and the National Quality Forum (NQF) are two other key groups involved in the national healthcare reform movement.

The HIT Policy Committee

The HIT Policy Committee is charged with making recommendations to ONC on a policy framework for the development and adoption of a nationwide health information infrastructure, including standards for the exchange of patient medical information.[72] Serving the committee are seven workgroups to address and make recommendations to the full committee on key reform issues such as meaningful use of EHRs, certification and adoption of EHRs, information exchange, NwHIN, the strategic plan framework, privacy and security policy, and enrollment in federal and state health and human services programs.

The HIT Standards Committee

The HIT Standards Committee is charged with making recommendations to ONC on standards, implementation specifications, and certification criteria for the electronic exchange and use of health information.[73] In harmonizing or recognizing standards and implementation specifications, the HIT Standards Committee is also tasked with providing for all associated testing by the National Institute of Standards and Technology (NIST). Serving the committee are four workgroups addressing clinical operations, clinical quality, privacy and security requirements, and implementation strategies that accelerate the adoption of proposed standards.

The National Committee on Vital and Health Statistics (NCVHS)

The NCVHS was originally established more than 60 years ago by Congress to serve as an advisory body to the HHS on health data, statistics, and national health information policy.[74] It fulfills important review and advisory functions relative to health data and statistical problems of national and international interest, stimulates or conducts studies of such problems, and makes proposals for improvement of U.S. health statistics and information systems. In 1996, NCVHS was restructured to meet expanded responsibilities under HIPAA and became a federal advisory committee. In 2009, the committee was the first to hear testimony and make recommendations to ONC on meaningful-use criteria to measure effective EHR use.

The National Quality Forum (NQF)

NQF is a nonprofit organization that aims to improve the quality of healthcare for all Americans through fulfillment of its three-part mission: to set national priorities and goals for performance improvement, to endorse national consensus standards for measuring and publicly reporting on performance, and to promote the attainment of national goals through education and outreach programs. NQF has taken the lead in defining the quality measures to qualify for the meaningful-use incentives under HITECH.[75]

Influencing HIT Transformation through Testimony and Comment

This chapter has discussed the need for healthcare IT competencies; awareness of how healthcare IT is changing the way we diagnose, treat, care for, and manage patients; as well as healthcare policies that affect healthcare practices and the global healthcare landscape. In addition, healthcare informatics professionals cannot underestimate the power of communication to bring about meaningful change in our nation's healthcare delivery system.

In 2005, the World Health Organization's Commission on the Social Determinants of Health asked, "What narrative will capture the imaginations, feelings, intellect and will of political decision-makers and the broader public and inspire them to action?"[76] Years later, the question is more important than ever to the healthcare IT professionals who stand in an unprecedented position to effect change. Public comment through the growing number of media outlets—supported by the emergence of the Internet and social media—translates theory and knowledge into meaningful activity that can drive and define local, state, and federal policy, addressing key health and social issues and improving the lives of the patients affected by them.[77]

Outlets for communications that can reach pivotal society segments and the ears of key individual influencers in healthcare reform include not only traditional media (newspapers, magazines, books) but also new mass-media formats like web-based video and blogs, Twitter, and other social media sites. Whether commenting over these outlets from organizations like HIMSS or AMIA or as an individual active in healthcare transformation, such communication can change public perceptions of current issues and help form and influence public attitudes and decisions.

The Future

Leaders in healthcare agree: the future depends on a system that will continue to innovate using healthcare IT and informatics to play instrumental roles in patient safety, change management, and quality improvement, as evidenced by quality outcomes, enhanced workflow, and user acceptance. These areas highlight the value of an informatics-trained workforce and their roles in the adoption of healthcare information technologies that deliver higher quality clinical applications across healthcare organizations.

That value can only increase as new directions and priorities emerge in healthcare. In an environment where the roles of all healthcare providers are diversifying, the informatics workforce must guide the system appropriately from positions as project managers, consultants, educators, researchers, product developers, decision support and outcomes managers, chief clinical information officers, chief information officers, advocates, policy developers, entrepreneurs, and business owners. This is especially true where the informatics workforce can contribute leadership in the effective design and use of EHR systems. To achieve our nation's healthcare reform goals, the healthcare community must leverage the sources of patient-care technologies and information management competence that the informatics workforce can provide to insure that the national investment in healthcare IT and EHRs is implemented properly and effectively over coming years.

Chapter Review

The passage of landmark healthcare reform legislation including ARRA and the HITECH Act in 2009 and PPACA in 2010—as upheld by the U.S. Supreme Court on June 28, 2012—has changed the landscape of the U.S. healthcare industry forever, perhaps more than any expert envisioned just scant years ago.

There is a growing recognition that advanced healthcare IT is both essential to support the enormous amounts of electronic information that will be collected and exchanged and foundational to industry transformation and healthcare reform. As the massive transformation from disconnected, inefficient, paper-based "islands" of care delivery to a nationwide, interconnected, and interoperable system driven by EHRs and healthcare IT innovation, the importance of an informatics-trained workforce has become increasingly evident. This workforce needs to proactively contribute to the development, use, and evaluation of information systems. They need to serve on national committees and initiatives focused on healthcare IT policy, standards and terminology development, standards harmonization, and EHR adoption. Performing their front-line roles, this workforce will have a profound impact on the quality and effectiveness of healthcare and emerge as leaders in the effective use of healthcare IT to improve the quality and efficiency of healthcare services.

Questions

To test your comprehension of the chapter, answer the following questions and then check your answers against the list of correct answers that follows the questions.

1. The Patient Protection and Affordable Care Act (PPACA) was signed into law on March 23, 2010. This law has many sections, but what does it primarily provide for?

   A. A healthcare system to match Canada

   B. A free healthcare system for all

   C. Access to affordable healthcare for all

   D. One electronic health record for all

2. What does the American Recovery and Reinvestment Act (ARRA) of 2009 and its key Health Information Technology for Economic and Clinical Health (HITECH) Act provide?

   A. Adoption of one national electronic health record

   B. Access to patient health data via the Internet

   C. Incentivized adoption of EHRs to improve quality care

   D. A national standard for providing healthcare

3. By what means does the HITECH provision of ARRA improve care quality and better manage costs?

   A. Standardizing generic prescription drugs to all

   B. Providing access to patient information through secure data exchange

   C. Providing a national identification system for every patient

   D. Providing access to more medical testing and procedures

4. The journey to passage of the PPACA began 20 years ago. Which organization concluded computerization could help improve information management and result in higher quality of care?

   A. CMS (Centers for Medicare & Medicaid Services)

   B. CDC (Centers for Disease Control and Prevention)

   C. AMA (American Medical Association)

   D. IOM (Institute of Medicine)

5. The executive order in 2004 supported computerization of health records to avoid medical mistakes and reduce costs. Which national coordinator position was created from this order?

   A. HHS (Health and Human Services)

   B. ONC (Office of the National Coordinator for HIT)

   C. HIE (Health Information Exchange)

   D. NIH (National Institutes of Health)

6. The HITECH Act provides incentives for the meaningful use of certified electronic health records. Certification criteria were developed through voluntary, consensus-based processes. Which three industry associations supported the formation of the Certification Commission for HIT (CCHIT)?

   A. ICD-10, CMS, HIMSS

   B. NIH, FDA, AHIMA

   C. AHIMA, NAHIT, HIMSS

   D. CDC, ONC, CMS

7. To share and exchange health information requires information systems to work together. What are the three elements of information exchange required for interoperability to occur?

   A. Data transport, content exchange, and vocabulary management

   B. Data modeling, infrastructure, and privacy

   C. Content exchange, security, and access

   D. Innovation, infrastructure, and patient consent

8. To achieve stage 1 meaningful use, the final criteria were divided into multiple initiatives. What are those initiatives?

   A. Improve quality, safety, and efficiency; reduce health disparities; and engage patients and their families

   B. Improve populations and public health

   C. Improve care coordination and ensure adequate privacy and security protections for personal health information

   D. All of the above

9. What is the the purpose of the Nationwide Health Information Network (NwHIN)?

   A. To provide a nationwide network infrastructure for health data

   B. To develop the standards, services, and policies for health information exchange

   C. To create a national mechanism for sharing health data

   D. To allow health information to be networked across the nation

10. What is the CONNECT software project?

    A. A free, open-source software solution that supports health information exchange

    B. A way of connecting disparate electronic health records

    C. A federal initiative complementary to the work of the NwHIN

    D. A software solution that facilitates the exchange of health information for federal agencies only

11. Which of the following is an example of how HITECH has expanded federal privacy and security laws under HIPAA?

    A. The sale of a patient's health information without the patient's written authorization is prohibited, except in limited circumstances involving research or public health activities.

    B. HIPAA allows patients to pay in full for a healthcare item or service and to request that the claim not be submitted to the health plan.

    C. Physicians are required to provide patients, upon request, an accounting of disclosures of health information made through the use of an EHR.

    D. All of the above

12. Which of the following goals is the Health IT Workforce Development Program designed to accomplish?

    A. Develop a new workforce capable of doing healthcare IT research.

    B. Create educational programs to advance the goals of using healthcare IT to drive quality care.

    C. Train a new workforce of healthcare IT professionals to help providers implement EHRs to improve healthcare quality, safety, and cost effectiveness.

    D. Develop a training program to advance the HITECH goals.

13. In which of the following areas does the SHARP program fund research?

    A. Breakthrough advances to address well-documented problems that have impeded adoption of healthcare IT

    B. Accelerating progress toward achieving nationwide meaningful use of healthcare IT

    C. Supporting a high-performing, continuously learning healthcare system

    D. All of the above

14. What are the Beacon Communities designed to accomplish?

    A. Advance new, innovative ways to improve care coordination using healthcare IT

    B. Make breakthrough advancements in healthcare quality, safety, and efficiency as well as in public health at the community level, using healthcare IT

    C. Demonstrate that any gains achieved are sustainable and replicable

    D. All of the above

15. Which of the following goals is the purpose of the regional extension centers (RECs)?

    A. Help potential meaningful users to receive incentive payments

    B. Aid providers in determining how to do health data exchange

    C. Extend the reach of healthcare IT research into all care settings

    D. Offer technical assistance and guidance on selecting and implementing EHRs

16. Which of the following options describe characteristics of federal advisory the committees?

    A. Openness; inclusiveness; transparency; and clearly defined timelines for operation, termination, and renewal

    B. Specific authorization by Congress

    C. The requirement to follow parliamentary procedures

    D. All of the above

Answers

1. **C.** PPACA was signed into law on March 23, 2010. This law has many sections but primarily provides for access to affordable healthcare for all.

2. **C.** ARRA of 2009 and its key HITECH Act provide incentivized adoption of EHRs to improve quality care.

3. **B.** The HITECH provision of ARRA improves care quality and better manages costs by providing access to patient information through secure data exchange.

4. **D.** The IOM that concluded that computerization could help improve information management and result in higher quality of care.

5. **B.** The ONC was created by executive order in 2004.

6. **C.** AHIMA, NAHIT, and HIMSS were the three industry associations supporting the formation of CCHIT.

7. **A**. Data transport, content exchange, and vocabulary management are the three elements of information exchange required for interoperability to occur.

8. **D**. To achieve stage I meaningful use, the final criteria include the following initiatives: improve quality, safety, and efficiency; reduce health disparities; engage patients and their families; improve populations and public health; improve care coordination; and ensure adequate privacy and security protections for personal health information.

9. **B**. The purpose of the Nationwide Health Information Network (NwHIN) is to develop the standards, services, and policies for health information exchange.

10. **A**. The CONNECT software project is a free, open-source software solution that supports health information exchange.

11. **D**. HITECH expands privacy and security laws under HIPAA to prohibit the sale of a patient's health information without the patient's written authorization, except in limited circumstances involving research or public health activities; allows patients to pay in full for healthcare items or services and to request that the claim not be submitted to the health plan; and requires physicians to provide patients, upon request, an accounting of disclosures of health information made through the use of an EHR.

12. **C**. The Health IT Workforce Development Program is designed to train a new workforce of healthcare IT professionals to help providers implement EHRs to improve healthcare quality, safety, and cost effectiveness.

13. **D**. The SHARP program funds research focused on breakthrough advances to address well-documented problems that have impeded adoption of healthcare IT, accelerating progress toward achieving nationwide meaningful use of healthcare IT, and supporting a high-performing, continuously learning healthcare system.

14. **D**. The Beacon Communities are designed to advance new, innovative ways to improve care coordination using healthcare IT; make breakthrough advancements in healthcare quality, safety, and efficiency, as well as in public health at the community level, using healthcare IT; and demonstrate that any gains achieved are sustainable and replicable.

15. **D**. The RECs offer technical assistance and guidance on selecting and implementing EHRs.

16. **A**. The characteristics of a federal advisory committee include openness; inclusiveness; transparency; and clearly defined timeliness for operation, termination, and renewal.

References

1. The Henry J. Kaiser Family Foundation. *Summary of new health reform law.* Accessed on May 22, 2012, from www.kff.org/healthreform/upload/8061.pdf.

2. ARRA and HITECH Act Resource Center. Accessed on Sept. 15, 2012, from http://www.first-insight.com/News_Events-ARRA-HITECHACT.html.

3. Welcome to health information technology. *Catholic University of America.* Accessed on May 22, 2012, from http://health IT.cua.edu.

4. Abelson, R., Harris, G., & Pear, R. (2011). Whatever court rules, major changes in health care likely to last. *New York Times.* Accessed on May 23, 2012), from www.nytimes.com/2011/11/15/health/policy/health-care-is-changing-despite-federal-uncertainty.html?pagewanted=all.

5. Mitchell, R. (2011). Health care jobs grow…in administration. *USA Today.* Accessed on May 23, 2012, from www.usatoday.com/money/industries/health/story/2011-11-30/health-care-creates-jobs/51506244/1.

6. Health information technology. *Catholic University of America.* Accessed on May 22, 2012, from http://hit.cua.edu.

7. U.S. Department of Labor, Bureau of Labor Statistics. *Network and Computer System Administrators Job Outlook, Occupational Outlook Handbook.* Accessed on May 22, 2012, from www.bls.gov/ooh/Computer-and-Information-Technology/Network-and-computer-systems-administrators.htm.

8. U.S. Department of Labor, Bureau of Labor Statistics. *Computer and Information Systems Managers Job Outlook, Occupational Outlook Handbook.* Accessed on May 22, 2012, from www.bls.gov/ooh/Management/Computer-and-information-systems-managers.htm.

9. Mosquera, M. (2012). CMS EHR incentive payments surpass $5B. *Government Health IT.* Accessed on May 23, 2012, from www.govhealthit.com/news/cms-ehr-incentive-payments-tip-5b.

10. Skills for the 21st century: Health information technology. *eHealth.* Accessed on May 22, 2012, from www.iowaehealth.org/documents/resource/38.pdf.

11. Dick, R., & Steen, E. (1997). IOM, Committee on Improving the Patient Record. *The computer-based patient record: An essential technology for healthcare.* National Academy Press. Accessed on June 26, 2012, from www.iom.edu/Reports/1997/The-Computer-Based-Patient-Record-An-Essential-Technology-for-Health-Care-Revised-Edition.aspx.

12. Kohn, L., Corrigan, J., & Donaldson, M.(eds.). (1999). IOM. *To err is human: Building a safer health system.* National Academy Press. Accessed on June 26, 2012, from www.nap.edu/openbook.php?isbn=0309068371.

13. IOM, Committee on Quality of Health Care in America. (2001). *Crossing the quality chasm: A new health system for the 21st century.* National Academy Press. Accessed on June 26, 2012, from www.nap.edu/catalog.php?record_id=10027.

14. National Coordination Office for Networking and Information Technology Research and Development, President's Information Technology Advisory Committee (PITAC)—Archive. Accessed on June 26, 2012, from www.nitrd.gov/Pitac/index.html.

15. President's Information Technology Advisory Committee (PITAC) Final Report: Fact Sheet. (1999). Accessed on June 26, 2012, from www.cra.org/govaffairs/advocacy/pitac_fs.pdf.

16. President's Information Technology Advisory Committee (PITAC). (2001, February). *Panel on Transforming Health Care, Transforming Health Care Through Information Technology, Report to the President.* Accessed on June 26, 2012, from www.internet2.edu/health/files/pitac-hc-9feb01.pdf.

17. Bush, G.W. (2004, January 20). State of the Union Address. Accessed on June 26, 2012, from www.americanrhetoric.com/speeches/stateoftheunion2004.htm.

18. Bush, G.W. (2004). Executive Order: Incentives for the Use of Health Information Technology and Establishing the Position of the National Health Information Technology Coordinator. Accessed on June 26, 2012, from http://edocket.access.gpo.gov/cfr_2005/janqtr/pdf/3CFR13335.pdf.

19. Online education programs in health information technology with training info. *Education Portal.com.* Accessed on June 26, 2012, from http://education-portal.com/online_education_programs_in_health_information_technology.html.

20. ONC. *HITECH and funding opportunities.* Accessed on June 26, 2012, from http://healthit.hhs.gov/portal/server.pt/community/healthit_hhs_gov__hitech_and_funding_opportunities/1310.

21. AMIA. *AMIA 10 X 10 Program: Training healthcare professionals to become informatics leaders.* Accessed on June 26, 2012, from www.amia.org/education/10x10-courses.

22. Public Law 104-191, 104th Congress. *Health Insurance Portability and Accountability Act of 1996.* Accessed on June 26, 2012, from www.cms.gov/HIPAAGenInfo/Downloads/HIPAALaw.pdf.

23. The History of HIPPA. *All things medical billing.* Accessed on May 25, 2012, from www.all-things-medical-billing.com/history-of-hipaa.html.

24. HHS. (2003, May, rev.). *Summary of the HIPAA Privacy Rule, HIPAA Compliance Assistance.* Accessed on June 26, 2012, from www.hhs.gov/ocr/privacy/hipaa/understanding/summary/privacysummary.pdf.

25. HHS. *Health information privacy: Summary of the HIPAA Security Rule.* Accessed on June 26, 2012, from www.hhs.gov/ocr/privacy/hipaa/understanding/srsummary.html.

26. What everyone should know about HIPAA version 5010. *The Record.* Accessed on May 23, 2012, from www.bcbsm.com/newsletter/therecord/record_1210/record_1210b.shtml.

27. An introductory overview of the HIPAA 5010. *Medicare Learning Network (MLN) matters.* Accessed on May 23, 2012, from www.cms.gov/Outreach-and-Education/Medicare-Learning-Network-MLN/MLNMattersArticles/downloads/se0904.pdf.

28. Robeznieks, A. (2012). CMS delays 5010 enforcement, again. *Modern Healthcare.* Accessed on May 23, 2012, from www.modernhealthcare.com/article/20120315/NEWS/303159955.

29. CMS to delay enforcement of HIPAA 5010 by 3 more months. *iHealthBeat.* Accessed on May 23, 2012, from www.ihealthbeat.org/articles/2012/3/15/cms-to-delay-enforcement-of-hipaa-5010-by-3-more-months.aspx.

30. About the Certification Commission for Health Information Technology. Accessed on June 26, 2012, from www.cchealth IT.org/about.

31. CCHIT. *About CCHIT.* Accessed on May 25, 2012, from www.cchit.org/about.

32. NPRM definition. *PC Magazine Encyclopedia.* Accessed on May 25, 2012, from www.pcmag.com/encyclopedia_term/0,1237,t=NPRM&i=48112,00.asp.

33. Summary of proposed rule certification programs for health information technology. (2010, March 9). *Premier, Inc.* Accessed on June 26, 2012, from www.premierinc.com/about/advocacy/issues/10/health IT/Premier-Summary-ONC-NPRM-EHR-Certification.pdf.

34. ONC. *ONC: Authorized testing and certification bodies.* Accessed on May 23, 2012, from http://healthit.hhs.gov/portal/server.pt?open=512&mode=2&objID=3120.

35. American National Standards Institute (ANSI). Health Information Technology Standards Panel (HITSP). *Enabling healthcare interoperability.* Accessed on June 26, 2012, from www.health ITsp.org/government.aspx.

36. Enrado, P. (2011). NHIN's evolution to NwHIN: From the ground up. *Healthcare IT News NHIN Watch.* Accessed on May 23, 2012, from www.nhinwatch.com/perspective/nhins-evolution-nwhin-ground.

37. Barr, F. (2008, November 6). Healthcare interoperability: The big debate. *eHealth Insider.* Accessed on June 26, 2012, from www.ehi.co.uk/insight/analysis/359/healthcare-interoperability:-the-big-debate.

38. Connor, D. (2007). Healthcare pros debate interoperability standards. *Network World.* Accessed on June 26, 2012, from www.networkworld.com/news/2007/022707-healthcare-pros.html.

39. ONC seeks public comment on RFI on governance of the Nationwide Health Information Network. *Health IT Buzz*. Accessed on May 23, 2012, from www.healthit.gov/buzz-blog/electronic-health-and-medical-records/nc-seeks-public-comment-governance-request-information-enable-electronic-health-information-exchange.

40. IHE: Changing the way healthcare connects. Accessed on June 26, 2012, from www.ihe.net.

41. American Medical Informatics Association (AMIA). Accessed on June 26, 2012, from https://www.amia.org.

42. Health Information Management and Systems Society (HIMSS). Accessed on June 26, 2012, from www.himss.org/ASP/aboutHimssHome.asp.

43. HIMSS Legacy Workgroup. (2007). The history of HIMSS. Accessed on June 26, 2012, from www.himss.org/content/files/HIMSS_HISTORY.pdf.

44. HHS. Secretary Sebelius announces next stage for providers adopting electronic health records. Accessed on May 24, 2012, from www.hhs.gov/news/press/2012pres/02/20120224a.html.

45. Blumenthal, D. (2010, July 13). The "meaningful use" regulation for electronic health records. *New England Journal of Medicine*. Accessed on June 26, 2012, from http://healthcarereform.nejm.org/?p=3732.

46. Geodert, J. (2010, July 13). A first look at final MU criteria. *Health Data Management*. Accessed on June 26, 2012, from www.healthdatamanagement.com/news/meaningful-use-final-rule-incentives-hitech-ehr-40624-1.html?ET=healthdatamanagement:e1346:155319a:&st=email&utm_source=editorial&utm_medium=email&utm_campaign=HDM_Daily_071610.

47. HHS. We Can't Wait: Obama Administration takes new steps to encourage doctors and hospitals to use health information technology to lower costs, improve quality, create jobs. Accessed on May 24, 2012, from www.hhs.gov/news/press/2011pres/11/20111130a.html.

48. Legal Health Information Exchange. Public comments for meaningful use stage 2 NPRM due May 7. Accessed on May 24, 2012, from www.legalhie.com/meaningful-use/public-comments-for-meaningful-use-stage-2-nprm-due-may-7.

49. CMS. CMS proposes definition of stage 2 meaningful use of certified electronic health records (EHR) technology. Accessed on May 24, 2012, from https://www.cms.gov/apps/media/press/factsheet.asp?Counter=4286&intNumPerPage=10&checkDate=&checkKey=&srchType=1&numDays=3500&srchOpt=0&srchData=&keywordType=All&chkNewsType=6&intPage=&showAll=&pYear=&year=&desc=&cboOrder=date and also https://www.cms.gov/Regulations-and-Guidance/Legislation/EHRIncentivePrograms/Stage_2.html.

50. Blumenthal, D. (2009). National HIPAA Summit in Washington, D.C., September 16, 2009.

51. CMS. Medicare and Medicaid EHR incentive program. Accessed on May 25, 2012, from https://www.cms.gov/Regulations-and-Guidance/Legislation/ EHRIncentivePrograms/downloads/MU_Stage1_ReqSummary.pdf.

52. CMS. Proposed clinical quality measures for 2014. Accessed on May 25, 2012, from https://www.cms.gov/Medicare/Quality-Initiatives-Patient-Assessment-Instruments/QualityMeasures/ProposedClinicalQualityMeasuresfor2014.html.

53. CMS posts stage 2 quality measures. *Healthcare Informatics.* Accessed on May 25, 2012, from www.healthcare-informatics.com/news-item/cms-posts-stage-2-clinical-quality-measures.

54. HIMSS: Limit clinical quality measures in stage 2. *Health Data Management.* Accessed on May 25, 2012, from www.healthdatamanagement.com/news/ ehr-electronic-health-records-meaningful-use-stage-2-44440-1.html.

55. About the HITECH Act: HITECH Act Summary. *HITECH Answers.* Accessed on June 25, 2012, from www.hitechanswers.net/about/about-the-hitech-act-of-2009.

56. National health information network soon will stand on its own. *American Medical News.* Accessed on June 25, 2012, from www.ama-assn.org/ amednews/2012/03/26/bisg0329.htm.

57. ONC. *The Direct Project.* Accessed on June 25, 2012, from http://healthit.hhs .gov/portal/server.pt?open=512&mode=2&objID=3340.

58. ONC. *The CONNECT Project.* Accessed on June 25, 2012, from http://healthit .hhs.gov/portal/server.pt?open=512&mode=2&objID=3340.

59. HHS. *Protecting the privacy of patient information, HIPPA summary: Fact sheet.* Accessed on June 26, 2012, from www.ast.org/pdf/Standards_of_Practice/ HIPPA_Summary_Fact_Sheet.pdf.

60. HHS. *Comparative effectiveness research funding.* Accessed on June 26, 2012, from www.hhs.gov/recovery/programs/cer.

61. AHRQ. *AHRQ at a glance.* Accessed on June 26, 2012, from www.ahrq.gov/ about/ataglance.htm.

62. Patient-Centered Outcomes Research Institute (PCORI). Accessed on June 18, 2012, from www.pcori.org.

63. Get the facts about health IT workforce development program. *Health IT Workforce Development Program Facts at a Glance.* Accessed on June 26, 2012, from http://healthit.hhs.gov/portal/server.pt?open=512&objID=1432&mode=2.

64. HHS. *HIH challenge grants in health and science research.* Accessed on June 27, 2012, from http://grants.nih.gov/grants/funding/challenge_award.

65. NLM's university-based biomedical informatics research training programs, *U.S. National Library of Medicine.* Accessed on June 27, 2012, from www.nlm .nih.gov/ep/GrantTrainInstitute.html.

66. ONC. *Strategic Health IT Advanced Research Projects (SHARP) Program.* Accessed on June 27, 2012, from www.nlm.nih.gov/ep/GrantTrainInstitute.html.

67. ONC. *State Health Information Exchange Cooperative Program.* Accessed on June 27, 2012, from http://healthit.hhs.gov/portal/server.pt/community/ state_health_information_exchange_cooperative_agreement_program/1336/ home/16375.

68. ONC. *Health Information Technology Extension Centers Program.* www.healthit .hhs.gov/portal/server.pt?open=512&objID=1335&mode=2.

69. ONC. *Get the facts about Beacon Community Program.* Accessed on June 27, 2012, from http://healthit.hhs.gov/portal/server.pt?open=512&objID=1805& parentname=CommunityPage&parentid=2&mode=2&cached=true.

70. ONC. *Beacon Community Program: Improving health through health information technology.* Accessed on June 27, 2012, from http://healthit.hhs.gov/portal/ server.pt?open=512&objID=1805&parentname=CommunityPage&parentid= 2&mode=2&cached=true.

71. U.S. General Services Administration. *The Federal Advisory Committee Act.* Accessed on June 27, 2012, from www.gsa.gov/portal/content/100916.

72. ONC. *The Health IT Policy Committee (a federal advisory committee).* Accessed on June 27, 2012, from http://healthit.hhs.gov/portal/server.pt?open=512&objID= 1269&parentname=CommunityPage&parentid=5&mode=2.

73. ONC. *The Health IT Standards Committee (a federal advisory committee).* Accessed on June 27, 2012, from http://healthit.hhs.gov/portal/server.pt?open= 512&objID=1271&parentname=CommunityPage&parentid=3&mode=2.

74. National Committee on Vital and Health Statistics (NCVHS), *Search Health IT.* Accessed on June 27, 2012, from http://searchhealthit.techtarget.com/ definition/National-Committee-on-Vital-and-Health-Statistics-NCVHS.

75. National Quality Forum (NQF). Accessed on June 27, 2012, from www.qualityforum.org/About_NQF/About_NQF.aspx.

76. World Health Organization Secretariat of the Commission on Social Determinants of Health, (2005 Background Report) Action on the Social Determinants of Health: Learning from previous experiences, p. 44.

77. Kaminski, J. (2007). Activism in Education Focus: Using communicative and creative technologies to weave social justice and change theory into the tapestry of nursing curriculum. Accessed on June 27, 2012, from http://econurse.org/ EthelJohns.html.

Navigating Health Data Standards and Interoperability

Joyce Sensmeier[*]

In this chapter, you will learn how to
- Discuss the need for health data standards
- Describe the standards development process and the organizations involved in it
- Delineate the importance of interoperability
- Describe current health data standards initiatives
- Explore the value of health data standards

Standards are foundational to the development, implementation, and interoperability of electronic health records (EHRs). The effectiveness of healthcare delivery is dependent on the ability of clinicians to access health information when and where it is needed. The ability to exchange health information across organizational and system boundaries, whether between multiple departments within a single institution or among a varied cast of consumers, providers, payers, and other stakeholders is essential. A harmonized set of rules and definitions, both at the level of data meaning as well as at the technical level of data exchange, is necessary to make this possible. There must also be a socio-political structure in place that recognizes the benefits of shared information and incentivizes the adoption and implementation of such standards.

[*] Adapted from Virginia K. Saba and Kathleen A. McCormick, *Essentials of Nursing Informatics, Fifth Edition*, 233–245. © 2011 by The McGraw-Hill Companies.

This chapter examines health data standards and interoperability in terms of the following topic areas:

- Need for health data standards
- Standards development process, organizations, and categories
- Knowledge representation
- Standards coordination and harmonization
- Health data standards initiatives
- Business value of health data standards

Introduction to Health Data Standards

The ability to communicate in a way that ensures the message is received and the content is understood is dependent on standards. Data standards are intended to reduce ambiguity in communication so that actions taken based on the data are consistent with the actual meaning of that data. On February 17, 2009, President Barack Obama signed the American Recovery and Reinvestment Act (ARRA) into law. Title XIII of ARRA, called the Health Information Technology for Economic and Clinical Health (HITECH) Act, allocated $19.2 billion to further promote the widespread adoption and standardization of healthcare IT. This goal is being advanced through a phased-in series of improved clinical data capture that supports more rigorous quality measurement and improvement. This transformation requires data capture and sharing, as well as advanced clinical processes, to enable improvement in health outcomes. The ultimate end state can only be achieved through the organized structure and effective use of information to support optimal decision-making and more effective care processes, thus improving health outcomes and reducing cost growth.

While current information technologies are able to move and manipulate large amounts of data, they are not as proficient in dealing with ambiguity in the structure and semantic content of that data. The term "health data standards" is generally used to describe those standards having to do with the structure and content of health information. However, it may be useful to differentiate data from information and knowledge. Data are the fundamental building blocks on which health and healthcare decisions are based. Data are collections of unstructured, discrete elements (facts) that exist outside of any particular context. When data are interpreted within a given context and given meaningful structure within that context, they become information. When information from various contexts is aggregated following a defined set of rules, it becomes knowledge and provides the basis for informed action.[1] Data standards represent both data and their transformation into information. Data analysis generates knowledge, which is the foundation of professional practice standards.

Standards are created by several methods:[2]

- A group of interested parties comes together and agrees upon a standard.
- The government sanctions a process for standards to be developed.
- Marketplace competition and technology adoption introduces a de facto standard.
- A formal consensus process is used by a standards development organization (SDO) to publish standards.

The standards development process typically begins with a use case or business need that describes a system's behavior as it responds to an external request. Technical experts then consider what methods, protocols, terminologies, or specifications are needed to address the requirements of the use case. An open and transparent consensus or balloting process is desirable to ensure that the developed standards have representative stakeholder input, which minimizes bias and encourages marketplace adoption and implementation.

Legislated, government-developed standards are able to gain widespread acceptance by virtue of their being required either by regulation or in order to participate in large, government-funded programs, such as Medicare. The healthcare IT industry is motivated to adopt and implement these standards into proprietary information systems and related products in order to be in compliance with these regulations and achieve a strong market presence. Because government-developed standards are in the public domain, usually they are made available at little or no cost and can be incorporated into any information system; however, they are often developed to support particular government initiatives and may not be as suitable for general, private sector use. Also, given the amount of bureaucratic overhead attached to the legislative and regulatory process, it is likely that maintenance of these standards may lag behind fast-paced changes in technology and the general business environment.

Standards developed by SDOs are typically consensus-based and reflect the perspectives of a wide variety of interested stakeholders. They tend to be robust and adaptable across a wide range of implementations; however, most SDOs are nonprofit organizations that rely on the commitment of dedicated volunteers to develop and maintain standards. This often limits the amount of work that can be undertaken in a certain timeframe. In addition, the consensus process can be time consuming and may result in a slow development process that does not always keep pace with technologic change. Perhaps the most problematic aspect of consensus-based standards is that there is no mechanism to ensure that they are adopted by the industry, because there is usually little infrastructure in place to actively and aggressively market them. This has resulted in the development of many technically competent standards that are never implemented.

In spite of our best efforts, standards development is not always a smooth or simple process. "Conflict may occur in the development of the standards, for example, within the confines of a technical committee designing a particular standard, where participants may disagree over the nature of the standard to be developed, or where one or more participants may take part in order to block the creation of a new standard, or by virtue of competition among supporters of several incompatible extant standards."[3] The American National Standards Institute (ANSI) is the private, nonprofit organization that administers and coordinates the U.S. voluntary standards and conformity assessment system. In this role, ANSI oversees the development and use of voluntary consensus standards by accrediting the procedures used by standards developing organizations and approving their finished documents as American National Standards.

The United States Standards Strategy[4] states that "The goal of all international standards forums should be to achieve globally relevant and internationally recognized and accepted standards that support trade and commerce while protecting the environment, health, safety, and security." There are a number of drivers in the current standards landscape that are working to accelerate health data standards adoption and implementation through innovative efforts and incentives to address this charge. The U.S. standardization system is based on the set of globally accepted principles for standards development shown in Table 12-1.

Currently, the United States has the most robust standardization system in the world, which gives the nation a competitive advantage. Unlike many other countries, the U.S. standards development system considers the views of all interested parties in a balanced way, according to the principles outlined in Table 12-1. And the openness and transparency of the system means that participants' needs can be more rapidly met through innovative, collaborative solutions.[5]

Principle	Description
Transparency	Essential information regarding standardization activities is accessible to all interested parties.
Openness	Participation is open to all affected interests.
Impartiality	No one interest dominates the process or is favored over another.
Effectiveness and relevance	Standards are relevant and effectively respond to regulatory and market needs, as well as scientific and technological developments.
Consensus	Decisions are reached through consensus among those affected.
Performance based	Standards are performance based (specifying essential characteristics rather than detailed designs) where possible.
Coherence	The process encourages coherence to avoid overlapping and conflicting standards.
Due process	Standards development accords with due process so that all views are considered and appeals are possible.
Technical assistance	Assistance is offered to developing countries in the formulation.

Table 12-1 ANSI Principles for Standards Development

Standards Categories

Four broad areas are used to categorize health data standards.[6] Health data interchange standards are used to establish a common, predictable, secure communication protocol between and among systems. Vocabulary standards consist of standardized nomenclatures and code sets used to describe clinical problems and procedures, medications, and allergies. Content standards and value sets are used to share clinical information such as clinical summaries, prescriptions, and structured electronic documents. Security standards include those standards used for authentication, access control, and transmission of health data.

Health Data Interchange Standards

Health data interchange standards primarily address the format of messages that are exchanged between computer systems, document architecture, clinical templates, the user interface, and patient data linkage.[7] To achieve data compatibility between systems, it is necessary to have prior agreement on the syntax of the messages to be exchanged. That is, the receiving system must be able to divide the incoming message into discrete data elements that reflect what the sending system wishes to communicate. The following section describes some of the major organizations involved in the development of health data interchange standards.

Accredited Standards Committee X12

Accredited Standards Committee (ASC) X12 has developed a broad range of electronic data interchange (EDI) standards to facilitate electronic business transactions. In the healthcare arena, X12N standards have been adopted as national standards for such administrative transactions as claims, enrollment, and eligibility in health plans, and first report of injury under the requirements of the Health Insurance Portability and Accountability Act (HIPAA) of 1996 Privacy and Security Rules. Due to the uniqueness of health insurance and the varying policies for protection of personal health information from country to country, these standards are primarily used in the United States. The HIPAA rules directed the Secretary of the Department of Health and Human Services (HHS) to adopt standards for transactions to enable health information to be exchanged electronically, and the Administrative Simplification Act, one of the HIPAA provisions, requires standard formats to be used for electronically submitted healthcare transactions. The ASC X12N 837 Implementation Guide has been established as the standard of compliance for claims transactions.

Institute of Electrical and Electronic Engineers

The Institute of Electrical and Electronic Engineers (IEEE) has developed a series of standards known collectively as P1073 Medical Information Bus, which support real-time, continuous, and comprehensive capture and communication of data from bedside medical devices such as those found in intensive care units, operating rooms, and emergency departments. These data include physiologic parameter measurements and device settings. IEEE standards for information technology focus on telecommunications and information exchange between systems including local and metropolitan area networks.

Current IEEE standards development activities include efforts to develop standards that support wireless technology. The IEEE 802.xx suite of wireless networking standards, supporting local and metropolitan area networks, has advanced developments in the communications market. The most widely known standard, 802.11 (commonly referred to as Wi-Fi), allows anyone with a "smart" mobile device or computer with either a plug-in card or built-in circuitry to connect to the Internet wirelessly through myriad access points installed in offices, hotels, airports, coffeehouses, convention centers, and even parks, among other locations. Many healthcare organizations are evaluating and implementing wireless solutions that support point-of-care technology.

National Electrical Manufacturers Association

The National Electrical Manufacturers Association (NEMA), in collaboration with the American College of Radiologists (ACR) and others, formed DICOM (Digital Imaging and Communications in Medicine) to develop a generic digital format and a transfer protocol for biomedical images and image-related information. DICOM enables the transfer of medical images in a multivendor environment and facilitates the development and expansion of picture archiving and communication systems (PACS). The specification is usable on any type of computer system and supports transfer over the Internet. The DICOM standard is the dominant international data interchange message format in biomedical imaging.

World Wide Web Consortium

The World Wide Web Consortium (W3C) is the main international standards organization for development of standards for the World Wide Web (abbreviated WWW or W3). W3C also publishes XML (Extensible Markup Language), which is a set of rules for encoding documents in machine-readable format. XML is most commonly used in exchanging data over the Internet. It is defined in the XML 1.0 Specification produced by the W3C and several other related specifications, all of which are available in the public domain. XML's design goals emphasize simplicity, generality, and usability over the Internet, which also makes it desirable for use in cross-enterprise health information exchange. Although XML's design focuses on documents, it is widely used for the representation of arbitrary data structures, for example in Web Services. Web Services use XML messages that follow the Simple Object Access Protocol (SOAP) standard and have been popular with the traditional enterprise. Other data exchange protocols include the REST architectural style, which was developed in parallel with the Hypertext Transfer Protocol (HTTP) used in web browsers. The largest known implementation of a system conforming to the REST architectural style is the World Wide Web.

Vocabulary Standards

A fundamental requirement for effective communication is the ability to represent concepts unambiguously for both the sender and receiver of the message. Natural human languages are incredibly rich in their ability to communicate subtle differences in the semantic content, or meaning, of messages. While there have been great advances in the ability of computers to process natural language, most communication between health information systems relies on the use of structured vocabularies, terminologies, code sets, and classification systems to represent healthcare concepts. Standardized terminologies enable data collection at the point of care; enable retrieval of data, information, and knowledge in support of clinical practice; and elicit outcomes. The following examples describe several of the major vocabulary systems.

Current Procedural Terminology

The Current Procedural Terminology (CPT) code set maintained by the American Medical Association (AMA) accurately describes medical, surgical, and diagnostic services. It is designed to communicate uniform information about medical services and procedures among physicians, coders, patients, accreditation organizations, and payers for administrative, financial, and analytical purposes. The current version is CPT 2010. In addition to descriptive terms and codes, it contains modifiers, notes, and guidelines to facilitate correct usage. While primarily used in the United States for reimbursement purposes, it has also been adopted for other data purposes.

International Statistical Classification of Diseases and Related Health Problems: Ninth Revision (ICD-9)

The International Statistical Classification of Diseases and Related Health Problems: Ninth Revision and Clinical Modifications (ICD-9-CM) is a version of a mortality and morbidity classification used since 1979 for reporting in the United States. It is widely accepted and used in the healthcare industry and has been adopted for a number of purposes including data collection, quality-of-care analysis, resource utilization, and statistical reporting. It is the basis for the diagnostic related groups (DRGs), developed for Medicare, which are used extensively in the United States for hospital reimbursement as part of the prospective payment system. While ICD-9 procedure codes are the acceptable HIPAA code set for inpatient claims, Healthcare Common Procedure Coding System/Current Procedural Terminology (HCPCS/CPT) codes are the valid set for outpatient claims.

International Statistical Classification of Diseases and Related Health Problems: Tenth Revision (ICD-10)

The International Statistical Classification of Diseases and Related Health Problems: Tenth Revision (ICD-10) is the most recent version of the ICD classification system for mortality and morbidity, and it is used worldwide. In addition to diagnostic labels, the ICD-10 also encompasses nomenclature structures. The transition from ICD-9-CM to ICD-10-CM/PCS comes with various unknowns, such as the quality of coded data, reimbursement rates, and interoperability concerns. On January 16, 2009, HHS published two final rules to adopt updated HIPAA standards that require the transition to ICD-10-CM/PCS be implemented by October, 2013.[8] Subsequently, the Department of Health and Human Services has made corrections to a recently published final rule that now sets October 1, 2014 as the ICD-10 compliance date. For those who prepare appropriately, leveraging the ICD-10 investment will allow organizations to move beyond compliance to achieve competitive advantage.[9] Moving to the new code sets will also improve efficiencies and lower administrative costs due to replacement of a dysfunctional, outdated classification system.

Nursing and Other Domain-specific Terminologies

The American Nurses Association (ANA) has spearheaded efforts to coordinate the various minimum data sets and standardized nursing terminologies. The ANA Committee for Nursing Practice Information Infrastructure (CNPII) evaluates minimum data sets and standardized terminologies to determine whether they meet specific criteria. The ANA has recognized the following nursing terminologies that support nursing practice: ABC Codes, Clinical Care Classification, International Classification of Nursing Practice, Logical Observation Identifiers Names and Codes (LOINC), North American Nursing Diagnosis Association, Nursing Interventions Classification (NIC), Nursing Outcomes Classification (NOC), Nursing Management Minimum Data Set, Nursing Minimum Data Set, Omaha System, Patient Care Data Set (retired), Perioperative Nursing Data Set, and SNOMED CT.[10] These standard terminologies enable knowledge representation of nursing content. Nurses use assessment data and nursing judgment to determine nursing diagnoses, interventions, and outcomes. These elements can be linked together using terminology standards to represent nursing knowledge.

RxNorm

RxNorm is a standardized nomenclature for clinical drugs and drug delivery devices produced by the National Library of Medicine (NLM). Because every drug information system follows somewhat different naming conventions, a standardized nomenclature is needed for the consistent exchange of information, not only between organizations but also within the same organization. For example, a hospital may use one system for ordering and another for inventory management. Still another system might be used to record dose adjustments or to check drug interactions. The goal of RxNorm is to allow various systems using different drug nomenclatures to share data efficiently at the appropriate level of abstraction. RxNorm contains the names of the prescription formulations that exist in the United States, including devices that administer the medications in a pack containing multiple clinical drugs or clinical drugs designed to be administered in a specified sequence.

Unified Medical Language System

The Unified Medical Language System (UMLS) consists of a metathesaurus—a large, multipurpose, and multilingual thesaurus—that contains millions of biomedical and health-related concepts, their synonymous names, and their relationships. There are specialized vocabularies, code sets, and classification systems for almost every practice domain in healthcare. Most of these are not compatible with one another, and much work needs to be done to achieve usable mapping and linkages between them. There have been a number of efforts to develop mapping and linkages among various code sets, classification systems, and vocabularies.

One of the most successful is the UMLS project undertaken by the NLM. The NLM supports the development, enhancement, and distribution of clinically specific vocabularies to facilitate the exchange of clinical data to improve retrieval of health information. In 1986, the NLM began an ambitious long-term project to map and link a large number of vocabularies from a number of knowledge sources to allow retrieval and integration of relevant machine-readable information. These knowledge sources include MEDCIN, a system of standardized medical terminology; MedDRA, a medical dictionary for regulatory activities terminology; and MeSH, the NLM-controlled vocabulary thesaurus used for indexing articles for PubMed.

The NLM is the central coordinating body for clinical terminology standards within HHS. The NLM works closely with the U.S. Office of the National Coordinator for Health Information Technology (ONC) to ensure NLM's efforts are aligned with the goal of the President and the HHS Secretary to achieve nationwide implementation of an interoperable health information technology infrastructure to improve the quality and efficiency of healthcare.[11]

Content Standards

Content standards relate to the data content that is transported within information exchanges. Information content standards define the structure and content organization of the electronic message/document information content. They can also define a set of content standards (messages/documents). In addition to standardizing the format of health data messages and the lexicons and value sets used in those messages, there is widespread interest in defining common sets of data for specific message types. A minimum or core data set is "a minimum set of items with uniform definitions and categories concerning a specific aspect or dimension of the healthcare system which meets the essential needs of multiple users."[12]

American Society for Testing and Materials

The American Society for Testing and Materials (ASTM) is one of the largest SDOs in the world and publishes standards covering all sectors in the economy. The ASTM Committee E31 on Healthcare Informatics has developed a wide range of standards supporting the electronic management of health information. One of these standards, the Continuity of Care Record (CCR), was developed in collaboration with the Massachusetts Medical Society, the Healthcare Information and Management Systems Society (HIMSS), the American Academy of Family Physicians, and the American Academy of Pediatrics. The CCR is a core data set of the most relevant and timely facts about a patient's healthcare. It is prepared by a practitioner at the conclusion of a healthcare encounter in order to enable the next practitioner to readily access such information. It includes a summary of the patient's health status (e.g., problems, medications, allergies) and basic information about insurance, advance directives, care documentation, and care plan recommendations. The primary use for the CCR is to provide a snapshot in time containing the pertinent clinical, demographic, and administrative data for a specific patient.

Clinical Data Interchange Standards Consortium

The Clinical Data Interchange Standards Consortium (CDISC) is a global, multidisciplinary consortium that has established standards to support the acquisition, exchange, submission, and archiving of clinical research data and metadata. CDISC develops and supports global, platform-independent data standards that enable information system interoperability to improve medical research and related areas of healthcare. One example is the Biomedical Research Integrated Domain Group (BRIDG) model, a domain-analysis model representing protocol-driven biomedical/clinical research. The BRIDG model emerged from an unprecedented collaborative effort among clinical trial experts from CDISC, the National Institutes of Health (NIH)/National Cancer Institute (NCI), the Food and Drug Administration (FDA), Health Level Seven (HL7), and other volunteers. This structured information model is being used to support development of data interchange standards and technology solutions that will enable harmonization between the biomedical/clinical research and healthcare arenas.

Health Level Seven

Health Level Seven (HL7) is a standards organization that develops standards in multiple categories including health data interchange and content. HL7 standards focus on facilitating the exchange of data to support clinical practice both within and across institutions. HL7 standards cover a broad spectrum of areas for information exchange including medical orders, clinical observations, test results, admission/transfer/discharge, document architecture, clinical templates, user interface, EHR data, and charge and billing information. A primary example of an HL7 standard is the HL7 Clinical Document Architecture (CDA) Release 2, Continuity of Care Document (CCD), which is an implementation guide for sharing Continuity of Care Record (CCR) patient summary data using the HL7 CDA document exchange model for clinical documents.

In a recent, joint standards-development effort, HL7 published the Consolidated CDA guide as "the single source for implementing the CDA documents." In creating this single implementation guide, HL7 aimed to eliminate conflicts among the previously scattered documentation and reduce ambiguity of the standard in general. This guide was produced and developed through the joint efforts of HL7, Integrating the Healthcare Enterprise (IHE), the Health Story Project, and ONC. The project was carried out within the ONC's Standards and Interoperability (S&I) Framework with a number of goals, one of which is providing a set of harmonized CDA templates for the United States. Use of the harmonized standard offers a huge step forward for interoperability through its adoption in the Health Information Technology: Standards, Implementation Specifications, and Certification Criteria for Electronic Health Record Technology, 2014 Edition.

The HL7 EHR System Functional Model and Standard defines key functions of Electronic Health Record Systems (EHR-S) to enable consistent expression of system functionality.[13] The HL7 EHR-S Functional Model, through the creation of functional profiles for care settings and realms, enables a standardized description and common understanding of functions sought or available in a given setting (e.g., intensive care, cardiology, office practice in one country or primary care in another country). HL7 has also published a Personal Health Record System (PHR-S) Functional Model. This standard includes a reference list of functions that a PHR system should use to manage and maintain a PHR.

GELLO is an HL7 standard that supports query and expression language for decision support. GELLO is based on the Object Constraint Language (OCL) developed by the Object Management Group. The GELLO language can be used to build up queries to extract and manipulate data from medical records. These criteria can be used in decision-support knowledge bases such as those designed to provide alerts and reminders, guidelines, or other decision rules. The HL7 Clinical Decision Support Work Group has developed a set of standard specifications for context-aware knowledge retrieval. The first of these specifications, entitled Context-Aware Knowledge Retrieval (Infobutton), Knowledge Request Standard, was approved in September 2010 as a normative ANSI/ISO HL7 standard. During patient care, clinicians frequently have need for information related to their clinical care activities. The Infobutton makes it easier for providers to access the information they need at the point of care. HL7 standards are widely implemented by healthcare care provider organizations worldwide, many of which have adapted the basic standards for use in their particular settings.

International Health Terminology Standards Development Organisation

The International Health Terminology Standards Development Organisation (IHTSDO) is a not-for-profit association in Denmark that develops and promotes use of SNOMED CT (Systematized Nomenclature of Medicine—Clinical Terms) to support safe and effective health information exchange. It was formed in 2006 with the purpose of developing and maintaining international health terminology systems. SNOMED CT is a comprehensive clinical terminology, originally created by the College of American Pathologists (CAP) and, as of April 2007, it is owned, maintained, and distributed by the IHTSDO. The CAP continues to support SNOMED CT operations under contract to the IHTSDO and provides SNOMED-related products and services as a licensee of the terminology. The NLM is the U.S. member of the IHTSDO and, as such, distributes SNOMED CT at no cost in accordance with the member rights and responsibilities outlined in the IHTSDO's Articles of Association. SNOMED CT is one of a suite of standards required by the HITECH Act for the electronic exchange of clinical health information in the United States to achieve meaningful use.

National Council for Prescription Drug Programs

The National Council for Prescription Drug Programs (NCPDP) develops both content and health data interchange standards for information processing in the pharmacy services sector of the healthcare industry. As an example of the impact that standardization can have, since the introduction of these standards in 1992, the retail pharmacy industry has moved to 100 percent electronic claims processing in real time. NCPCP standards are also forming the basis for electronic prescription transactions. Electronic prescription transactions are defined as EDI messages flowing between healthcare providers (i.e., pharmacy software systems and prescriber software systems) that are concerned with prescription orders. NCPDP's Telecommunication Standard Version 5.1 was named the official standard for pharmacy claims within HIPAA, and NCPDP is also named in other U.S. federal legislation titled the Medicare Prescription Drug, Improvement, and Modernization Act. Other NCPDP standards include the SCRIPT Standard for Electronic Prescribing and the Manufacturers Rebate Standard.

Security Standards

HIPAA Security Standards for the Protection of Electronic Health Information at 45 CFR part 160 and part 164, Subparts A and C, also known as the HIPAA Security Rule, were developed to protect electronic health information and implement reasonable and appropriate administrative safeguards that establish the foundation for a covered entity's security program.[14] Prior to HIPAA, no generally accepted set of security standards or general requirements for protecting health information existed in the healthcare industry. Congress passed the Administrative Simplification provisions of HIPAA to protect the privacy and security of certain health information, as well as to promote efficiency in the healthcare industry through the use of standardized electronic transactions. Subtitle D of the HITECH Act, entitled "Privacy," helps to support this goal by adopting amendments designed to strengthen the privacy and security protections of health information originally established by HIPAA.

ISO IEC 27002 2005 Standard

The ISO IEC 27002 2005 standard consists of recommended information security practices. It establishes guidelines and general principles for initiating, implementing, maintaining, and improving information security management in an organization. The objectives outlined provide general guidance on the commonly accepted goals and best practices for control objectives and controls for information security management. ISO/IEC 27002:2005 is intended as a common basis and practical guideline for developing organizational security standards and effective security management practices and helping build confidence in interorganizational activities.

Standards Coordination, Harmonization, and Interoperability

It has become clear to many public and private sector standards advocates that no one entity has the resources to create an exhaustive set of health data standards that will meet all needs. New emphasis is being placed on leveraging and harmonizing existing standards to eliminate the redundant and siloed efforts that have in the past contributed to a complex, difficult-to-navigate, health data standards environment. As described earlier in this chapter, advances are being made in the area of standards harmonization through the coming together of industry groups to accelerate and streamline the standards development and adoption process towards achievement of the desired goal—interoperability.

In addition to the various SDOs described above, the following sections provide brief descriptions of some of the major international, national, and regional organizations involved in broad-based standards coordination, harmonization, and interoperability. Since many of the health data standards issues, such as security, are not unique to the healthcare sector, this breadth of scope offers the potential for technology transfer and advancement across multiple sectors.

ONC Standards and Interoperability Framework

The ONC Standards and Interoperability (S&I) Framework is an approach adopted by ONC's Office of S&I to fulfill its charge from the HITECH Act of enabling harmonized interoperability specifications to support national health outcomes and healthcare priorities, including meaningful use and the ongoing efforts to create better care, better population health, and cost reduction through delivery improvements.[15] The S&I Framework effort has created a forum where healthcare stakeholders can focus on solving real-world interoperability challenges. Each S&I initiative tackles a critical interoperability challenge through a rigorous process that typically includes the following elements:

- Development of clinically oriented user stories and robust use cases

- Harmonization of interoperability specifications and implementation guidance

- Provision of real-world experience and implementer support through new initiatives, workgroups, and pilot projects

- Mechanisms for feedback and testing of implementations

Working in collaboration with a wide community including consumers, providers, government organizations, and other stakeholders, this process identifies real-world needs, prioritizes them, and creates explicit documentation of the use cases, functional requirements, and technical specifications for interoperability.

Health IT Standards Committee

ARRA provided for the creation of the Health IT Standards Committee under the auspices of the Federal Advisory Committee Act (FACA). The committee is charged with making recommendations to the ONC on standards, implementation specifications, and certification criteria for the electronic exchange and use of health information. In developing, harmonizing, or recognizing standards and implementation specifications, the committee also provides for the testing of the same by the National Institute for Standards and Technology (NIST). The committee has formed several workgroups comprising stakeholder representatives and subject matter experts focused on the following topic areas: clinical operations, clinical quality, privacy and security, and implementation.

International Organization for Standardization

The International Organization for Standardization (ISO) develops, harmonizes, and publishes standards internationally. ISO standards are developed, in large part, from standards brought forth by member countries, and through liaison activities with other SDOs. Often, these standards are further broadened to reflect the greater diversity of the international community. In 1998, the ISO Technical Committee (TC) 215 on Health Informatics was formed to coordinate the development of international health information standards, including data standards. Consensus on these standards influences health informatics standards adopted in the United States. This committee published the first international standard for nursing content, titled "Integration of a Reference Terminology Model for Nursing." This standard includes the development of reference terminology models for nursing diagnoses and nursing actions with relevant terminology and definitions for implementation.

Integrating the Healthcare Enterprise

Standards, while a necessary part of the interoperability solution, are not alone sufficient to fulfill the needs. Simply using a standard does not necessarily guarantee that health information exchange will occur within and across organizations and systems. Standards can be implemented in multiple ways, so implementation specifications or guides are critical to make interoperability a reality.[16] Standard implementation specifications, or profiles, are designed to provide specific configuration instructions or constraints for implementation of a particular standard or set of standards to achieve the desired interoperable result.

Integrating the Healthcare Enterprise (IHE) is an international organization that provides a detailed framework for implementing standards, filling the gaps between creating the standards and implementing them. Through its open, consensus process, IHE has published a large body of detailed specifications, called profiles, that are being implemented globally today by healthcare providers and regional health information exchanges to enable standards-based, safe, secure, and efficient health information exchange. For example, several IHE profiles are being advanced as components of the HL7 Consolidated CDA standard.

IHE maintains the Product Registry as a mechanism for registering and searching products that support IHE profiles. This registry includes IHE Integration Statements, which are documents prepared and published by vendors to describe the conformance of their products with the IHE Technical Framework. These statements identify the specific IHE capabilities a given product supports in terms of IHE actors and profiles. Users can then reference the appropriate IHE profiles in requests for proposals, thus simplifying the systems acquisition process.

Public Health Data Standards Consortium

The Public Health Data Standards Consortium (PHDSC) is a national, nonprofit, membership-based organization of federal, state, and local health agencies; professional associations; academia; public and private sector organizations; international members; and individuals. Its goal is to empower the healthcare and public health communities with healthcare information technology standards to improve individual and community health. PHDSC represents a common voice from the public health community to the national standards efforts by identifying priorities for new standards, promoting integration of health data systems, and educating the public health community about health data standards.

It is increasingly recognized that combining the strengths of standards coordination efforts can minimize siloed, duplicative efforts and lead to significant gains for the healthcare sector as a whole. As we have discussed, this melding of approaches is being achieved at the organizational, national, and international levels by the development of coordinating bodies and consortia, as well as through government-directed laws, regulations, committees, and initiatives.

Testing and Certification

To accelerate the development, use, maintenance, and adoption of health data standards across the industry, and to spur innovation, ONC is developing tools to facilitate the entire standards lifecycle and maximize re-use of concepts and components, including tools and repositories for browsing, selecting, and implementing appropriate standards. ONC is working with NIST to provide testing tools to validate that a particular implementation conforms to a set of standards and implementation specifications.

The annual IHE North American Connectathon is the healthcare IT industry's largest, face-to-face testing event where healthcare IT systems can test their ability to exchange information across organizational boundaries to demonstrate the capabilities and benefits of those systems. A technical project management team develops detailed test plans and organizes the process to maximize interoperability testing between corresponding systems from different vendors. Independent monitors observe and record test results, which are published online in the Connectathon results database.

An EHR certification process was established by ONC through which organizations can be approved as certifying entities to which vendors may submit their EHR systems for review and certification. The Health Information Technology: Standards, Implementation Specifications, and Certification Criteria for Electronic Health Record Technology, 2014 Edition; Revisions to the Permanent Certification Program for Health Information Technology (45 CFR Part 170) Final Rule, published by HHS in 2012, identifies the technical standards that must be met in the certification process and coordinates those requirements with the meaningful-use objectives.

Current Initiatives

In the current healthcare environment, health data standards and interoperability efforts are continuing to increase in importance. Now that the Supreme Court has found the Patient Protection and Affordable Care Act (PPACA) constitutional, the adoption of the Accountable Care Organization (ACO) model, bundled payments, health insurance exchanges, and value-based purchasing will likely be advanced. These efforts will include new requirements for health data standards and interoperability that will increase pressure to accelerate current initiatives.

Health Information Exchanges

Formal entities are now emerging to provide both the structure and the function for health information exchange efforts, both at independent and governmental or regional/state levels. These organizations, called health information exchanges (HIEs), are geographically or organizationally defined entities that develop and manage a set of contractual conventions and terms and also arrange for the means of electronic exchange of information.

The HITECH Act authorized the establishment of the State Health Information Exchange Cooperative Agreement Program in the United States to advance appropriate and secure health information exchange across the healthcare system. The purpose of this program is to continuously improve and expand these services to reach all healthcare providers in an effort to improve the quality and efficiency of healthcare. Cooperative agreement recipients have been funded and are advancing the necessary governance, policies, technical services, business operations, and financing mechanisms for health information exchange over a four-year performance period. This program builds from existing efforts to advance regional and state-level HIEs while moving toward nationwide health information exchange.

Nationwide Health Information Network

The Nationwide Health Information Network (NwHIN) is a set of standards, services, and policies that enable secure health information exchange over the Internet. The purpose of the NwHIN is to provide a foundation for the exchange of healthcare IT across diverse entities, within communities and across the country, to achieve the goals of the HITECH Act. This component of the national healthcare IT agenda will enable health information to follow the consumer, be available for clinical decision making, and support appropriate use of health information beyond direct patient care so as to improve population health. ONC recognizes a broad range of exchange needs for the NwHIN, from simple, local applications to more robust exchanges with federal agencies or large nationwide entities.

The Business Value of Health Data Standards

Clearly the importance of health data standards in enhancing the quality and efficiency of healthcare delivery is being recognized by national and international leadership. Reviewing the business value of defining and using data standards is critical for driving the implementation of these standards into applications and systems. Having health data standards for data exchange and information modeling will provide a mechanism against which deployed systems can be validated.[17] Reducing manual intervention will increase worker productivity and streamline operations. Defining information exchange requirements will enhance the ability to automate interaction with external partners, which in turn will decrease costs.

As an example of the importance and value of health data standards, a standardized nursing language is necessary so that nursing knowledge can be represented and communicated consistently among nurses and other healthcare providers. Identifying, defining, and capturing key data elements in a database will build a library of evidenced-based care that can be measured and validated.[18] Enhanced data collection will contribute to greater adherence to standards of care, assessment of nursing competencies, and evaluation of nursing outcomes, thus increasing the visibility of nursing interventions and improving patient care.

By using data standards to develop their emergency-department data-collection system, New York State demonstrated that it is good business practice.[19] Their project was completed on time without additional resources and generated a positive return on investment. The use of standards provided the basis for consensus between the hospital industry and the state, a robust pool of information that satisfied the users, and the structure necessary to create unambiguous data requirements and specifications.

Other economic stakeholders for healthcare IT include software vendors or suppliers, software implementers who install the software to support end user requirements, and the users who must use the software to do their work. The balance of interests among these stakeholders is necessary to promote standardization to achieve economic and organizational benefits.[20] Defining clear business measures will help motivate the advancement and adoption of interoperable healthcare IT systems, thus ensuring the desired outcomes can be achieved. Considering the value proposition for incorporating data standards into products, applications and systems should be a part of every organization's information technology strategy.

Use Case 12-1: Maintaining the Patient Story Across Transitions of Care

A significant percent—by some estimates as high as 85 percent—of the information needed to care for a patient at some point crosses enterprise boundaries. This example demonstrates how to maximize the information available to the EHR and maintain the patient story using all available channels, from unstructured, scanned documents to dictated notes enriched with an abstractor or computer-assisted and NLP coding. It applies standards and profiles for clinical document exchange published through the HL7/IHE Health Story Consolidation Project in conjunction with the ONC S&I Framework. The meaningful-use objectives that it addresses are improving quality, safety, efficiency, and reducing health disparities; and improving care coordination.

Clinical Workflow

A patient visits his primary care physician (PCP) due to fatigue, rapid weight loss, and increased thirst. The PCP conducts an exam, dictates and authenticates a progress note, pulls historical patient information for review, and consults an endocrinologist, who agrees to see the patient the next day. The PCP creates and sends a lab order and asks the patient to go for testing. The PCP dictates a referral request, which is sent to the endocrinologist along with all related historical documents. The patient visits the endocrinologist and shares hard copies of his lab results. The endocrinologist's office scans the lab results, and the endocrinologist performs a full physical examination of the patient. The endocrinologist produces a History & Physical and Referral Response letter, which is made available to the PCP and a Clinical Knowledge Exchange. The PCP electronically reviews the full patient story in preparation for patient follow-up.

Domain	Profile	Actors
IT infrastructure (ITI)	Cross-enterprise document reliable interchange (XDR)	Source, recipient
	Cross-enterprise sharing of scanned documents (XDS-SD)	Consumer, creator
Patient care coordination (PCC)	Cross-enterprise sharing of medical summaries (XDS-MS)	Consumer, creator

Table 12-2   IHE Domains and Profiles

Table 12-2 shows the IHE domain committee, profiles, and actors involved in creating the system. The following HL7 resources were used in this example:

- HL7 Clinical Document Architecture (CDA) R2 Normative Edition 2005
- HL7 Implementation Guide for CDA Release 2: IHE Health Story Consolidation, Release 1
- HL7 Implementation Guide for CDA Release 2: History & Physical
- HL7 Implementation Guide for CDA Release 2: Progress Note
- HL7 Implementation Guide for CDA Release 2: Unstructured Documents
- HL7 Patient Demographics Query (PDQ)
- HL7 greenCDA Implementation Guide
- Trifolia Workbench: Consolidation Project Edition 1.0

For more information, visit www.ihe.net/registry, www.hl7.org, and www.healthstory.com.

Chapter Review

This chapter introduced health data standards; the organizations that develop, coordinate, and harmonize them; the process by which they are developed; examples of current standards initiatives; and a discussion of the business value of health data standards. Four broad areas were described to categorize health data standards. Health data interchange standards are used to establish communication protocols between and among systems. Vocabulary standards are used to describe clinical problems and procedures, medications, and allergies. Content standards and value sets are used to share clinical information such as clinical summaries, prescriptions, and structured electronic documents. And security standards are used for authentication, access control, and transmission of health data. Organizations involved in the development, harmonization, and coordination of health data standards were described.

A discussion of the standards development process highlighted the international and socio-political context in which standards are developed and the potential impact they have on the availability and currency of standards. The increasingly significant role of the federal government in influencing the development and adoption of health data standards was discussed. Several key initiatives, including the ONC S&I Framework, regional HIEs, and the NwHIN, were highlighted. Finally, the chapter emphasized the business value and importance of health data standards and their adoption in improving the quality and efficiency of healthcare delivery and health outcomes.

Questions

To test your comprehension of the chapter, answer the following questions and then check your answers against the list of correct answers that follows the questions.

1. Title XIII of the American Recovery and Reinvestment Act (ARRA) allocated $19.2 billion to further promote the widespread adoption and standardization of health information technology (IT). What is the acronym for the act represented by Title XIII?

   A. HIPAA

   B. NwHIN

   C. ANSI

   D. HITECH

2. The term "health data standards" is generally used to describe those standards having to do with which of the following?

   A. Structure and content of health information

   B. Privacy and security rule

   C. Document architecture and network

   D. Claims, enrollment, and eligibility

3. Which of the following methods are used to create standards?

   A. A group of interested parties comes together and agrees upon a standard.

   B. The government sanctions a process for standards to be developed.

   C. Marketplace competition and technology adoption introduces a de facto standard.

   D. A formal census process is used by a standards development organization (SDO).

   E. All of the above.

4. Why is the healthcare IT industry motivated to adopt and implement legislated, government-developed standards into proprietary information systems and related products?

   A. Government-developed standards are more suitable for general, private sector use.

   B. Maintenance of government-developed standards is typically on a fast pace.

   C. Government-developed standards typically enable compliance with regulations.

   D. Bureaucratic overhead is lessened with government-developed standards.

5. Which of the following principles is *not* included in the United States Standards Strategy's globally accepted principles for standards development?

   A. Transparency

   B. Openness

   C. Consensus

   D. Complexity

6. What are the four broad areas used to categorize health data standards?

   A. Health data interchange, vocabulary, content, security

   B. Health data exchange, structured, content, security

   C. Terminology, vocabulary, content, privacy

   D. Nomenclatures, code sets, protocols, and transactions

7. Which of the following organizations is involved in the development of health data interchange standards?

   A. American Medical Association (AMA)

   B. Institute of Electrical and Electronic Engineers (IEEE)

   C. American Nurses Association (ANA)

   D. National Library of Medicine (NLM)

8. Interoperability can be more rapidly advanced through coordinated, joint standards-development efforts. Which of the following is a recent example of such an effort between HL7, IHE, the Health Story Project, and ONC?

   A. EHR-S Functional Model

   B. PHR-S Functional Model

   C. BRIDG

   D. Consolidated CDA guide

9. The HIPAA Security Rule was developed to protect electronic health information and implement reasonable, appropriate administrative safeguards. Prior to

HIPAA, which of the following security standards was in place to protect health information?

A. ISO IEC 27002 2005 Standard

B. HITECH

C. SNOMED CT

D. GELLO

E. None of the above

10. The ONC Standards and Interoperability Framework is focused on enabling harmonized interoperability specifications to support national health outcomes and healthcare priorities. Which of the following items is *not* a part of the rigorous process that is followed to address these interoperability challenges?

A. Development of clinically oriented use cases

B. Development of proprietary standards

C. Harmonization of interoperability specifications

D. Provision of real-world experience and implementer support

11. Integrating the Healthcare Enterprise (IHE) has developed a mechanism for registering and searching products that support IHE profiles. What is this mechanism called?

A. IHE Technical Framework

B. Consolidated CDA guide

C. IHE Product Registry

D. IHE Integration Statements

12. The HITECH Act has authorized the establishment of the State Health Information Exchange Cooperative Agreement Program in the United States. What is the purpose of this program?

A. Advance secure health information exchange across the healthcare system

B. Enable secure health information exchange over the Internet

C. Provide a mechanism against which deployed systems can be validated

D. Reduce manual intervention to increase worker productivity

13. Which of the following characteristics does the Nationwide Health Information Network (NwHIN) *not* include?

A. Standards

B. Services

C. Policies

D. Business operations

14. Which of the following does *not* represent a business value of health data standards?

   A. Reduced costs

   B. Decreased worker productivity

   C. Reduced manual intervention

   D. Ability to validate deployed systems

15. When New York State used data standards to develop their emergency-department data-collection system, which of the following outcomes resulted?

   A. Need for additional resources

   B. Dissatisfied users

   C. Ambiguous data requirements

   D. Positive return on investment

Answers

1. **D.** Title XIII of ARRA is called the Health Information Technology for Economic and Clinical Health Act, or HITECH.

2. **A.** Health data standards are generally used to describe those standards having to do with the structure and content of health information.

3. **E.** All of these means are options for standards development.

4. **C.** The healthcare IT industry is motivated to adopt and implement government-developed standards into proprietary information systems and related products in order to be in compliance with these regulations and achieve a strong market presence.

5. **D.** Complexity is not included in the set of globally accepted principles for standards development. The nine principles are transparency, openness, impartiality, effectiveness and relevance, consensus, performance based, coherence, due process, and technical assistance.

6. **A.** The four broad areas used to categorize health data standards are health data interchange standards (used to establish a common, predictable, secure communication protocol between and among systems); vocabulary standards (standardized nomenclatures and code sets); content standards (used to share clinical information); and security standards (used for authentication, access control, and transmission of health data).

7. **B.** The Institute of Electrical and Electronic Engineers (IEEE) has developed a series of standards that focus on telecommunications and information exchange between systems, including local and metropolitan area networks.

8. **D.** In a recent, joint standards-development effort HL7 published the Consolidated CDA guide as "the single source for implementing the CDA documents." This guide was produced and developed through the joint efforts of HL7, IHE, the Health Story Project, and ONC.

9. **E.** Prior to HIPAA, no generally accepted set of security standards or general requirements for protecting health information existed in the healthcare industry.

10. **B.** Working in collaboration with a wide community including consumers, providers, government organizations, and other stakeholders, the ONC Standards and Interoperability Framework process identifies real-world needs, prioritizes them, and creates explicit documentation of the use cases, functional requirements, and technical specifications for interoperability. Proprietary solutions are privately developed and licensed and are not the result of the ONC S&I Framework process.

11. **C.** IHE maintains the Product Registry as a mechanism for registering and searching products that support IHE profiles. The registry includes IHE Integration Statements, which are documents prepared and published by vendors that describe the conformance of their products with the IHE Technical Framework.

12. **A.** The HITECH Act authorized the establishment of the State Health Information Exchange Cooperative Agreement Program in the United States to advance appropriate and secure health information exchange across the healthcare system.

13. **D.** Business operations is not one of the characteristics of the Nationwide Health Information Network. The NwHIN is a set of standards, services, and policies that enable secure health information exchange over the Internet. The purpose of the NwHIN is to provide a foundation for the exchange of healthcare IT across diverse entities, within communities and across the country, to achieve the goals of the HITECH Act.

14. **B.** Having health data standards for data exchange and information modeling will provide a mechanism against which deployed systems can be validated. Reducing manual intervention will increase (not decrease) worker productivity and streamline operations. Defining information exchange requirements will enhance the ability to automate interaction with external partners, which will reduce costs.

15. **D.** By using data standards to develop their emergency department data collection system, New York State completed their project on time without additional resources and generated a positive return on investment. The use of standards provided the basis for consensus between the hospital industry and the state, a robust pool of information that satisfied the users, and the structure necessary to create unambiguous data requirements and specifications.

References

1. Nelson, R., Saba, V. K., & McCormick, K. A. (Eds.). (2006). *Essentials of nursing informatics, Fourth edition*. McGraw-Hill Companies.

2. Hammond, W. E. (2005). The making and adoption of health data standards. *Health Affairs, 23*,1205–1213.

3. Busch, L. (2011). *Standards: Recipes for reality.* The MIT Press.

4. ANSI (2010). The United States Standards Strategy. American National Standards Institute.

5. ANSI (2012). ANSI Response to Request for Comments on Incorporation by Reference. 1 CFR Part 51 [NARA 12-0002]. National Archives and Records Administration, Office of the Federal Register.

6. HHS. (2010). Health Information Technology: Initial Set of Standards, Implementation Specifications, and Certification Criteria for Electronic Health Record Technology; Final Rule.

7. IOM, Committee on Data Standards for Patient Safety. (2004). Patient safety: Achieving a new standard for care. Institute of Medicine.

8. HIMSS. (2012). HIMSS ICD-10 Playbook Version 2. Accessed from www.himss .org/ASP/topics_icd10playbook.asp.

9. Bowman, S. (2008). Why ICD-10 is worth the trouble. *Journal of AHIMA, 79,* 24–29.

10. Rutherford, M. A. (2008). Standardized nursing language: What does it mean for nursing practice? *Online Journal of Issues in Nursing, 13.*

11. Health information technology and health data standards at NLM. (2010). Accessed from www.nlm.nih.gov/healthit.html.

12. Health Information Policy Council. (1983). Background paper: Uniform minimum health data sets (unpublished). USDHHS.

13. Health Level 7. (2007). EHR TC Electronic Health Record-System Functional Model, Release 1 February 2007. Health Level Seven.

14. CMS. (2007). HIPAA Security Series: Security 101 for Covered Entities, 2,1–11. Centers for Medicare and Medicaid Services.

15. Standards and Interoperability Framework. (2012). Accessed from www.siframework.org/index.html.

16. Sensmeier, J. (2010). The impact of standards and certification on EHR systems. *Foundations of Nursing Informatics, HIMSS10,* Atlanta, GA.

17. Loshin, D. (2004). The business value of data standards. *DM Review,14,* 20.

18. Rutherford, M. A. (2008). Standardized nursing language: What does it mean for nursing practice? *Online Journal of Issues in Nursing, 13.*

19. Davis, B. (2004). Return-on-investment for using data standards: A case study of New York State's data system. Accessed from www.phdsc.org/standards/pdfs/ROI4UDS.pdf.

20. Marshall, G. (2009). The standards value chain. *Journal of AHIMA, October 9,* 58–65.

Additional Study

The field of health data standards is a very dynamic one, with existing standards undergoing revision and new standards being developed. The best way to learn about specific standards activities is to get involved in the process. All of the organizations discussed in this chapter provide opportunities to be involved with activities that support standards development, coordination, and implementation. Listed below are the World Wide Web addresses for each organization. Most sites describe current available activities and publications, and many have links to other related sites.

Accredited Standards Committee (ASC) X12. www.wpc.edi.com.

American Medical Association (AMA). www.ama-assn.org.

American National Standards Institute (ANSI). www.ansi.org.

American Nurses Association (ANA). www.nursingworld.org.

American Society for Testing and Materials (ASTM). www.astm.org.

Clinical Data Interchange Standards Consortium (CDISC). www.cdisc.org.

Digital Imaging Communication in Medicine Standards Committee (DICOM). www.nema.org.

Health Level Seven (HL7). www.hl7.org.

Institute of Electrical and Electronic Engineers (IEEE). www.ieee.org.

Integrating the Healthcare Enterprise (IHE). www.ihe.net.

IHE (2011). IHE Product Registry. http://product-registry.ihe.net.

International Health Terminology Standards Development Organisation (IHTSDO). www.ihtsdo.org.

International Organization for Standardization (ISO). www.iso.org.

International Statistical Classification of Diseases and Related Health Problems (ICD-9, ICD-9CM, ICD-10). www.cdc.gov/nchswww.

National Committee on Vital and Health Statistics (NCVHS). http://aspe.os.dhhs .gov/ncvhs.

National Council for Prescription Drug Programs (NCPDP). www.ncpdp.org.

National Electrical Manufacturers Association (NEMA). www.nema.org.

National Institute of Standards and Technology (NIST). www.nist.gov/index.html.

National Library of Medicine (NLM). www.nlm.nih.gov/healthit.html.

Office of the National Coordinator for Health Information Technology (ONC). www.hhs.gov/healthit.

Public Health Data Standards Consortium (PHDSC). www.phdsc.org.

RxNorm. www.nlm.nih.gov/research/umls/rxnorm.

Unified Medical Language System (UMLS). www.nlm.nih.gov/research/umls.

World Wide Web Consortium (W3C). www.w3.org.

Regulatory Aspects of Healthcare IT: Legal Best Practices and Requirements

Chris Apgar

In this chapter, you will learn how to

- Understand, in an introductory way, the legal requirements that healthcare IT (HIT) professionals need to be aware of as they transition to the HIT industry
- Define business associate, covered entity, privacy, security, and protected health information
- Identify legal documentation requirements—what needs to be "baked in" or included in application development to meet legal requirements
- Understand the use of business associate contracts, creation of limited data sets, and requirements related to the reduction of legal risk as HIT professionals work with healthcare organizations and vendor partners
- Describe the implications for healthcare IT on the necessary requirements to assure privacy and security for electronic healthcare information

Introduction to the Healthcare Legal Environment

The healthcare regulatory environment is ever-changing and requires frequent monitoring to stay ahead of regulatory deadlines. The most significant change in healthcare law as it relates to privacy, security, and the exchange of administrative health data (e.g., claims, remittance advices, eligibility determinations, etc.) was the Health Insurance Portability and Accountability Act (HIPAA) of 1996 administrative simplification provisions.[1] Since its passage, privacy- and security-related requirements have expanded because of the passage of other federal and state laws.

This chapter focuses primarily on the legal requirements related to the HIPAA Privacy Rule, the HIPAA Security Rule (45 CFR Parts 160 and 164), and the Health Information Technology for Economic and Clinical Health (HITECH) Act (PL 111-5, Division A, Title XIII, Subpart D).[2] It is important to keep in mind that the HIPAA administrative simplification provisions address more than privacy and security. HIPAA established standards around how healthcare administrative data is transmitted and defined national identifiers for employers, healthcare providers, and some health plans.

HIT professionals must thoroughly understand the transaction, code-set, and national-identifier rules and related transaction and code sets specifications when developing claims adjudication systems, online administrative transactions, and other applications related to nonclinical data exchange. Most HIPAA legal requirements, such as business associate contracts, fall under the umbrella of privacy and security—hence the focus on privacy and security in this chapter. It is important to remember that other requirements may apply to the development, enhancement, and maintenance of healthcare-related applications even when they don't require the execution of specific legal documents.

Congress and state legislative assemblies continue to pass statutes that may impact the legal side of the healthcare regulatory equation. Also, federal and state agencies periodically revise administrative rules and issue guidance to the healthcare industry. These changes often impact the legal requirements healthcare organizations are subject to. It is important to be aware of those changes and adapt them appropriately.

HIPAA and HITECH Act Overview

The purpose of this chapter is to summarize the requirements of the HIPAA administrative simplification provisions, Privacy and Security Rules, HITECH Act requirements, and what rules take precedence when state laws differ from HIPAA and HITECH. The listed requirements can be referred to when reviewing existing privacy and security programs and regulatory compliance.

Covered entities are required to adhere to the complete HIPAA Privacy and Security Rules as modified by the HITECH Act. A *covered entity* can be a health plan (public or private), a healthcare provider who exchanges (directly or indirectly) HIPAA-covered transactions, or a healthcare clearinghouse. Covered entities can be both covered entities and business associates. Covered entities are subject generally to the statutory provisions and the rule provisions, but many covered entities are not subject to all provisions of the rules. As an example, there are specific requirements included that only health plans must follow, others that only healthcare providers must follow, and another set of provisions that only healthcare clearinghouses are required to adhere to.

Business associates are required to adhere to the use and disclosure provisions of the HIPAA Privacy Rule and the complete HIPAA Security Rule (HITECH Act requirement). A *business associate* is a third party that uses and discloses protected health information on behalf of a covered entity. Examples of business associates include billing agencies, electronic health record (EHR) vendors, third-party administrators, health information organizations (HIOs), and accountable-care organizations (ACOs).

Protected health information (PHI) is individually identifiable health information that can be used to identify an individual and that individual's past, present, or future medical condition (acute and mental health). It is made up of specific identifiers listed in the HIPAA administrative simplification provisions rules. PHI includes demographic data in addition to healthcare-related data.

If questions arise regarding the summary, covered entities and business associates are encouraged to refer back to the final rules, the HITECH Act, other applicable state and federal privacy and security laws, and/or contact legal counsel. This document is not intended to represent legal advice.

Legal Documents Review

HIPAA and the HITECH Act include requirements related to the construction of several legal documents. One of the most significant legal documents referenced is the business associate contract. A business associate contract is a legally binding contract which spells out the privacy and security standards that business associates and their third party vendors are required to implement and adhere to. If the contract is between two private entities, it takes the form of a contract and the required provisions are outlined in the HIPAA Privacy and Security Rules. If it is between public or governmental entities, it may take the form of a memo of understanding (MOU), administrative rules, or an inter-agency agreement. The HITECH Act now requires business associates and covered entities enter into "contracts or other written arrangements (e.g., MOUs, administrative rules or inter-agency agreements)."

The HIPAA Privacy Rule also includes requirements related to the construction of authorization forms, the Notice of Privacy Practices, among others. Other legal documents may be generated by covered entities that may be needed to implement requirements outlined in the HIPAA Privacy and Security Rules, such as consent forms, amendment request forms, and requests for a copy of an individual's designated record set (DRS; medical record or claims record).

HIPAA Administrative Simplification Provisions

45 CFR Part 1603 can be described as the general rules or requirements that are detailed in the HIPAA Enforcement Rule, the Transactions and Code Sets Rule, the National Identifiers Rules, the Privacy Rule, the Security Rule, and the interim final Breach Notification Rule. Part 160 includes general definitions, describes when state law preempts HIPAA, federal audit authority, and other general provisions that form what amounts to the "rules of the road" that apply to Part 160 and the remaining administrative simplification provisions.

State Law Preemption: 45 CFR 160.203

The provisions of the HIPAA Privacy Rule are preempted when state law is more stringent than the provisions of the Privacy Rule. "More stringent" is defined as providing greater protection of an individual's PHI or providing an individual greater access to their PHI.

If state law is contrary to HIPAA and is not more stringent, HIPAA preempts state law. *Contrary* is defined as a condition that would make it impossible for a covered entity to comply with HIPAA and state law. Certain state laws that allow collection of PHI for specific purposes, such as for public health or health oversight, are not preempted by HIPAA. If the Secretary of HHS determines that a state law is contrary to HIPAA, before the law can be effective it must be approved as an exception to HIPAA. Certain state laws, such as the monitoring and collection of PHI related to controlled substances, must be approved by the Secretary of HHS prior to the collection of PHI by states. Even when exemption has been granted, the Secretary may later revoke such exemption.

Complaints to the Secretary: 45 CFR 160.306

Complaints may be filed with the Secretary (delegated to the Office of Civil Rights, OCR) regarding noncompliance with the Privacy Rule and the Security Rule. Complaints must be filed within 180 days from the date the complainant knew or should have known about the violation. This includes business associate complaints related to covered entity noncompliance with the HIPAA Privacy and Security Rules. If the complaint alleges willful neglect or suspected willful neglect, OCR is required to investigate.

Compliance Reviews: 45 CFR 160.308

OCR (for privacy and security) and the Centers for Medicare and Medicaid Services (CMS; for transactions, code sets, and national identifiers) shall conduct compliance reviews to determine whether covered entities and, where applicable, business associates are complying with the HIPAA administrative simplification provisions.

Record Keeping and Access: 45 CFR 160.310

Covered entities and business associates are required to maintain records relating to their compliance with the HIPAA Privacy and Security Rules (business associates are required only to demonstrate compliance with the use and disclosure provisions of the HIPAA Privacy Rule) and make such records available to OCR for the purpose of demonstrating compliance in the event of a compliance review or to assist with a compliance investigation.

HIPAA Privacy Rule

45 CFR Part 164, Subpart E3 is better known as the HIPAA Privacy Rule. Subpart E defines the privacy requirements covered entities must adhere to. Especially important are the sections that outline the requirements related to the use and disclosure of protected health information, individual privacy rights, and administrative requirements related to privacy. Business associates are now required to adhere to the use and disclosure provisions of Subpart E pursuant to the HITECH Act.

Healthcare Operations: 45 CFR 164.501

Covered entities may use and disclose PHI for the purpose of healthcare operations. Healthcare operations include quality assessments, case-management grievance resolution, underwriting, provider credentialing, contacting providers and patients regarding alternative treatment, etc.

Organized Health Care Arrangement: 45 CFR 164.501

Covered entities may enter into an agreement to operate under an umbrella arrangement that simplifies the process of recordkeeping, distribution of required documentation to the patient, etc. This means the covered entities entering into an organized health care arrangement (OHCA) must adopt joint privacy policies, procedures, and practices; adopt a joint notice of privacy practices that is distributed to patients; and document the relationship between covered entities that make up the OHCA.

Uses and Disclosures of PHI: 45 CFR 164.502(a)

Covered entities and business associates are permitted to disclose PHI to an individual; for treatment, payment, and healthcare operations; when authorized by the patient/member or authorized representative; to friends and family (as long as the patient/member is allowed the opportunity to object to such release); and disclose certain portions of an individual's PHI in the facility directory. Covered entities and business associates are required to disclose PHI to an individual with limited exceptions, to OCR, and as required or allowed by law.

Minimum Necessary: 45 CFR 164.502(b)

Covered entities and business associates are required to disclose only the minimum amount of PHI necessary to satisfy the reason for which the PHI is disclosed. The minimum necessary standard does not apply for treatment, when required by law, when disclosed to OCR, for disclosures related to an individual or the individual's personal representative authorizations, and when disclosed pursuant to provisions of the HIPAA Privacy Rule to comply with the Privacy Rule. The PHI required to generate a HIPAA-covered transaction is considered to have met the minimum necessary standard.

Agreed Upon Restrictions to Disclosure: 45 CFR 164.502(c)

A covered entity can, but is not required to, agree to disclosure restrictions as requested by the patient/member. Covered entities are required to honor any restriction request if the request is to restrict disclosure to the patient's health plan for purposes of payment or healthcare operations when the patient paid for care, healthcare services, or supplies (such as durable medical equipment) "out of pocket" in full at the time services are rendered. Business associates are required to adhere to any restrictions granted by covered entities.

Disclosure of De-identified Information: 45 CFR 164.502(d)

There are no restrictions regarding the disclosure of de-identified PHI.

Release of PHI to Business Associates: 45 CFR 164.502(e)

Covered entities must adhere to minimum necessary standards when disclosing PHI to business associates except for the release of PHI for the purposes of treatment. Business associates must adhere to minimum necessary standards when disclosing PHI to third-party vendors who use and disclose PHI on behalf of the business associate.

Further disclosures are described for the release of PHI for deceased individuals, whistleblowers, hybrid entities such as health plans and clearinghouses, and affiliates of covered entities.

Business Associate Contracts: 45 CFR 164.504(e)

Covered entities and business associates are mutually responsible for entering into formal contracts or other written agreements that clearly define a business associate's relationship with a covered entity and what PHI will be used and disclosed between a covered entity and business associate. Business associate contracts (private) or other written arrangement (government) must require the business associate to comply with the HIPAA Privacy Rule. Covered entities are required to reasonably ensure that business associates adhere to the provisions of the HIPAA Privacy Rule. In addition to the requirements included in the contract or other written arrangement as defined pursuant to 45 CFR 164.314(a), the contract must specify that the business associate

- Comply with the use and disclosure provisions of the HIPAA Privacy Rule
- Assist the covered entity in providing individuals a copy or the ability to view their medical/claims record
- Amend or assist in amending records as requested by the covered entity
- Restrict access to an individual's record or parts of their record at the request of the covered entity
- Report any suspected violations of the HIPAA Privacy Rule on the part of the covered entity to the covered entity and, if not cured within a reasonable period of time, report the violation to OCR

Group Health Plans: 45 CFR 164.504(f)

Covered entities are required to disclose only the minimum amount of PHI necessary to assist in-group health plan operations. The plan document needs to clearly state when and what PHI is disclosed and for what purpose. The group health plan, as specified in the plan document, needs to reasonably ensure that appropriate safeguards are in place so that PHI is not disclosed outside of the group health plan (this includes to other workforce members of covered entities who are not assigned tasks related to the management of the group health plan).

Covered Entities with Multiple Functions: 45 CFR 164.504(g)

Covered entities that perform multiple functions (provider, health plan, healthcare clearinghouse) need to ensure that PHI exchanged between the multiple functions is appropriate and meets minimum necessary requirements.

Consent: 45 CFR 164.506

A covered entity is not required to obtain an individual's consent prior to sharing PHI for treatment, payment, or healthcare operations. The covered entity may ask but not require the individual to provide consent prior to providing treatment or enrollment in a health plan. The covered entity is required to inform the individual in plain language of the purpose of consent, the right of the individual to request a restriction to release PHI, that a covered entity is not required to honor requests for restriction of release, and that such restrictions, if honored, may be revoked upon notice to the individual. Consent applies only to release of PHI for treatment, payment, and healthcare operations.

Authorization Requirements: 45 CFR 164.508

Unless specifically allowed pursuant to the HIPAA Privacy Rule, disclosures of PHI are not allowed without specific authorization of the individual. This includes psychotherapy notes. A valid authorization needs to be specific and limited by time or event. Authorization is required for the use of PHI for research purposes unless an institutional review board (IRB) or privacy board approves the use of PHI for research without authorization. A covered entity may not condition treatment on providing authorization unless the treatment is related to research (45 CFR 164.512(i)). Also, a covered entity cannot condition health-plan enrollment on providing authorization unless authorization is required for underwriting purposes. The individual may revoke authorizations, but such revocation does not apply to the use and disclosure of PHI prior to such revocation.

Further rules are written related to covered entities using PHI for marketing purposes. The use of PHI for the purpose of research must clearly define the purpose of such release. An individual can object under HIPAA to the publication of their PHI in a facility directory.

Release Without Consent or Authorization: 45 CFR 164.512

A covered entity is permitted to release PHI without consent or authorization for the following purposes:

- To a public health authority
- To a public authority for child abuse or neglect reasons
- If the person is subject to the Food and Drug Administration (FDA) rules for tracking recalls of prescription medication, reporting adverse events resulting from certain forms of treatment, etc.
- If an individual presents for treatment of a communicable disease
- Reporting a medical incident related to a work-site injury

Release is also covered to permit disclosure of PHI in the event of domestic violence and when a personal representative is suspected of abusing or neglecting a patient. Covered entities are also allowed to release PHI for judicial and administrative proceedings when court documents specifically authorize such release. This is also true for the release of PHI to law enforcement authorities in identifying certain wounds or related injuries.

Healthcare Oversight Activities: 45 CFR 164.512(d)

Covered entities are authorized to release PHI for healthcare oversight activities to the following entities:

- The healthcare system
- Government benefit programs
- Entities subject to government oversight activities
- Entities subject to civil laws where such release is necessary to determine compliance with civil laws

Release of PHI for Research Without Authorization: 45 CFR 164.512(i)

PHI may be released for research purposes without authorization from the individual if such is approved by an institutional review board prior to release of PHI.

Avert a Serious Threat to Safety: 45 CFR 164.512(j)

A covered entity may release PHI if, in the professional judgment of the covered entity, such release will prevent a serious threat to public safety or to the safety of another.

Disclosure for Specialized Government Functions: 45 CFR 164.512(k)

A covered entity may release PHI for the following purposes:

- Military activity
- Medical suitability determinations (State Department)
- National security or intelligence activity
- Correctional institutions or law enforcement custodial situations
- Protective services for the President and others
- Covered entities that are governmental programs providing public benefits

Workers' Compensation: 45 CFR 164.512(l)

Covered entities may disclose PHI to workers' compensation programs for the purpose of meeting workers' compensation activities. Workers' compensation is specifically exempted from coverage under the Privacy Rule.

Limited Data Set: 45 CFR 164.514(e)

Covered entities may use or disclose a limited data set if the covered entity enters into a data-use agreement with the limited-data-set recipient. A limited data set includes PHI but excludes the following identifiers of the individual or the individual's relatives, employers, or household members:

- Name
- Postal address information, other than town or city, state, and zip code
- Telephone numbers
- Medical-record numbers
- Health plan beneficiary numbers
- Account numbers
- Certificate/license numbers
- Vehicle identifiers and serial numbers including license-plate numbers
- Web addresses
- Internet protocol (IP) address numbers
- Device identifiers and serial numbers
- Full-face photographic images and any comparable images
- Biometric identifiers, including finger and voice prints

Covered entities may use or disclose a limited data set only for the purposes of research, public health, or healthcare operations. Covered entities are not in compliance with this provision if covered entities knew of an activity or practice of the limited-data-set recipient that constituted a material breach or violation of the data-use agreement, unless the covered entity took reasonable steps to cure the breach or end the violation.

The HITECH Act required covered entities to disclose a limited data set instead of adhering to the minimum necessary standard if feasible until OCR formally defines "minimum necessary." At this time, OCR has not defined "minimum necessary."

HIPAA defines ways in which a covered entity may use certain PHI for fundraising purposes and underwriting.

Notice of Privacy Practices: 45 CFR 164.520

A provider must present a notice of privacy practices to a patient during first encounter and make every effort to obtain written verification from the patient that the notice of privacy practices was presented to the patient. Health plans are required to mail notices of privacy practices to participating members. Health plans are not required to obtain written verification from members that they received a copy of the notice. Covered entities are required to notify individuals when significant changes are made to the notice.

Also, covered entities are required to notify individuals once every three years of the availability of the notice. See 164.520(b) for detailed instructions regarding what needs to be included in a notice of privacy practices. If the covered entity maintains a web site, the notice must be prominently posted on the web site. Covered entities participating in an organized healthcare arrangement may issue a joint notice of privacy practices.

Restriction Requests: 45 CFR 164.522(a)

A covered entity must allow individuals an opportunity to request a restriction of the release of PHI for treatment, payment, and healthcare operations. The covered entity is not required to honor any requests for restriction, but if the covered entity does honor a request for restrictions of release of PHI, the covered entity has a responsibility to ensure such restrictions are implemented and adhered to. A covered entity may terminate restrictions by providing notice to the individual but must honor any granted restrictions related to the release of PHI made prior to providing notice to the individual. Covered entities are required to honor any restriction requests if they relate to treatment, services, and related medical costs when the individual pays "out of pocket" for all costs at time of service and requests that the covered entity not disclose information about the treatment, service, and related medical costs to the individual's health plan for payment or healthcare operations.

Confidential Communications: 45 CFR 164.522(b)

A covered entity must accommodate any reasonable requests for alternate forms of communication with an individual.

Access to Protected Health Information: 45 CFR 164.524

A covered entity must allow an individual access to the PHI contained in their designated record set, with the following exceptions:

- Psychotherapy notes
- Information collected in preparation for a civil or criminal proceeding
- Information (laboratory results) specifically identified under Clinical Laboratory Improvement Amendments (CLIA) or specifically exempted from CLIA

Covered entities may deny an individual's access to their PHI in the following cases, and such denial is not reviewable or open to appeal by the individual:

- Access is deniable on the basis of the preceding exceptions.
- PHI is generated by a correctional institution or on behalf of the correctional institution.
- PHI is collected for research purposes and the individual previously agreed to a denial of access while the research is being conducted.
- Such PHI is protected by the Privacy Act.
- Information is provided by a third party where a request for the protection of confidentiality of release was granted.

The individual has the right to appeal to a qualified medical professional the denial of release of their PHI for the following purposes:

- An authorized healthcare professional has determined that release would be harmful to the individual or others.

- The PHI makes reference to another individual.

- An authorized healthcare professional has determined that release to a personal healthcare representative would be harmful to the represented individual or others.

The covered entity has 30 days to provide access to an individual's designated record set. The time line for release of information may be extended for up to 60 days if the records are not readily available. The covered entity must make the designated record set available for review for free but may charge a reasonable fee for copies of the designated record set. If the covered entity denies the individual access to part of their designated record set, the covered entity must notify the individual in writing and inform the individual if they have a right of appeal and, if so, how to appeal the denial decision.

Accounting of Disclosures: 45 CFR 164.528

A covered entity must make available to the individual an accounting of disclosures of PHI if disclosure is made for purposes other than treatment, payment, healthcare operations, or it has been specifically authorized by the individual. This includes accounting for inadvertent or inappropriate disclosures of PHI, but it does not include accounting for incidental disclosures of PHI.

An inadvertent disclosure is not the same as incidental disclosure. A good example of inadvertent disclosure would be exposing a member of a covered entity's workforce to PHI, to which that individual did not have a reason to be exposed based on his or her job duties. This would be the case if a fax document was not picked up from the fax machine in a secure area of a covered entity's facility and another employee viewed patient information that did not pertain to his or her job. Incidental disclosures are disclosures of PHI that occur during the normal course of care or health plan operations. As an example, incidental disclosure of PHI would include one patient overhearing a conversation between a physician and another patient in another bed in a semi-private room in a hospital.

 TIP   A PHI-disclosure record must be maintained for six years. The covered entity has 60 days to provide an accounting of disclosures if requested by an individual.

The HITECH Act required publication of rules that would require covered entities with EHRs to account for any disclosure of PHI made from EHRs for any reason. At this time no rule has been finalized. Until the rule is finalized, EHR disclosure accounting is not required.

Privacy Official: 45 CFR 164.530(a)

A covered entity must appoint a privacy official who is responsible for overseeing the covered entity's privacy program and compliance with the Privacy Rule.

Workforce Training: 45 CFR 164.530(b)

A covered entity must provide privacy training to the workforce. The workforce includes employees, temporary employees, volunteers, and contracted employees.

Standard Safeguards: 45 CFR 164.530(c)

A covered entity must implement policies, procedures, and practices that reasonably ensure administrative, technical, and physical security of all PHI regardless of the form in which the PHI is stored.

Complaint Process: 45 CFR 164.530(d)

A covered entity must establish a process allowing an individual an opportunity to file a complaint about a covered entity's privacy policies, procedures, and practices.

Sanctions: 45 CFR 164.530(e)

A covered entity must provide for workforce sanctions in the event the Privacy Rule or a covered entity's privacy policies, procedures, or practices are violated.

Mitigation: 45 CFR 164.530(f)

A covered entity is required to take all reasonable action to mitigate damages in the event PHI is inadvertently or inappropriately released or accessed by an unauthorized third-party individual or entity.

Waiver of Rights: 45 CFR 164.530(h)

A covered entity is prohibited from requiring an individual to waive their rights under the Privacy Rule as a condition of treatment, payment, healthcare operations, or enrollment in a health plan.

Privacy Policies and Procedures: 45 CFR 164.530(i)

Covered entities are required to develop and implement privacy policies and procedures that fully implement the requirements of the Privacy Rule. Covered entities are required to periodically review and update privacy policies and procedures to accommodate changes in business practices and law. Covered entities are also required to update and distribute their notice of privacy practices if changes in policy and procedure materially impact the provisions of the notice.

HIPAA Security Rule (45 CFR Part 164, Subpart C)

Covered entities and business associates are required to comply with all standards. If an implementation specification is required, covered entities and business associates must comply with the implementation specification. If the implementation specification is addressable, covered entities and business associates must implement the specification as spelled out in the rule, implement a safeguard that is the equivalent of the specification, or clearly document why the specification will not be adopted. The primary reason for not adopting an implementation specification cannot be cost. The following codes are used for the implementation specifications described in the sections that follow:

- **Required (R)**   The implementation specification must be implemented/ adhered to.

- **Addressable (A)**   Based on the risk analysis, "addressable" means the covered entity or business associate must implement/adhere to the implementation specification, implement/adhere to an equivalent security safeguard, or document why the implementation specification will not be implemented/adhered to (the reason cannot be solely based on the cost of implementation/adoption).

Security Management Process: 45 CFR 164.308(a)

This is the first administrative safeguards standard. The standard requires the implementation of policies and procedures to prevent, detect, contain, and correct security violations.

- **Risk analysis (R)**   Need to complete a risk analysis periodically to assess security risks to the organization (appropriate practice risk analysis should be conducted annually or whenever major system or business changes occur).

- **Risk management (R)**   Need to establish a risk-management program that adequately implements the risk assessment findings; evaluates security incidents as they occur, taking appropriate mitigating action; and reasonably ensures ongoing compliance with the HIPAA Security Rule.

- **Sanction policy (R)**   Need to implement policies and practices that provide for sanctions of the workforce in the event of security violations (workforce includes employees, temporary employees, volunteers, and contracted employees).

- **Information system activity review (R)**   Software applications, network servers, etc. need to be configured to create audit trails that track activities involving electronic protected health information (ePHI)—such as data modification, creation, deletion, etc.

Assigned Security Responsibility: 45 CFR 164.308(a)

A security official (officer) needs to be appointed.

Workforce Security: 45 CFR 164.308(a)

This standard requires the implementation of policies and procedures to reasonably ensure that all covered entity and business associate workforce members have appropriate access to electronic PHI, and to prevent PHI access to workforce members who should not have access.

- **Authorization and/or supervision (A)**   Processes/policies need to be implemented that provide for appropriate workforce supervision when accessing ePHI. Also, policies/practices need to be implemented that provide for system/application access controls.

- **Workforce clearance procedure (A)**   Need to implement policies that reasonably ensure workforce access to ePHI is appropriate.

- **Termination procedures (A)**   Policies/procedures need to be implemented that reasonably ensure workforce access to ePHI is terminated when the workforce member is terminated.

Information Access Management: 45 CFR 164.308(a)

The next standard requires the implementation of policies and procedures related to authorization of access to electronic PHI.

- **Access authorization (A)**   Policies/procedures need to be implemented that govern authorization to access ePHI.

- **Access establishment and modification (A)**   Policies/procedures need to be implemented that outline how access to ePHI is granted and modified to meet minimum necessary requirements.

Security Awareness and Training: 45 CFR 164.308(a)(5)

The full workforce needs to be provided security awareness training and training on security policies, procedures, and practices.

- **Security reminders (A)**   Periodic security reminders need to be distributed to all workforce members.

- **Protection from malicious software (A)**   Anti-malware (e.g., anti-virus, anti-spyware, etc.) software needs to be acquired, regularly updated, and utilized to reasonably ensure viruses, worms, Trojans, and spyware do not infect the network, software applications, hardware, email, and portable media.

- **Log-in monitoring (A)**   An audit trail needs to be created that records when a workforce member logs on to the network or a software application (generally the purpose is to audit for multiple unsuccessful login attempts and reasonably ensure that workforce members and/or third-party individuals or entities are not accessing applications, data, etc. during nonwork hours where appropriate).

- **Password management (A)**   Policies/procedures need to be implemented that assist in proper password management (i.e., creation, periodic changes, etc.). This means the operating system and software applications need to accommodate the use of a password that is unique to each user/workforce member (it is advisable to determine whether multifactor authentication is required to provide greater protection when accessing especially sensitive data, using a laptop that stores PHI and is transported outside the organization, etc.).

Security Incident Procedures: 45 CFR 164.308(a)(6)

Covered entities and business associates are required to implement policies and procedures to address security incidents. Security incidents are more than breaches of PHI. Examples of security incidents that do not involve the breach of PHI include unsuccessful attempts to breach a firewall, transmission of un-encrypted PHI, and a denial of service attack that shuts down a covered entity's network.

- **Response and reporting (R)**   Policies/procedures need to be implemented that define actions to be taken in the event of a security incident (e.g., suspected inappropriate access, data breach, suspected identity theft, etc.). This means audit trails need to be present to assist in investigating security incidents. Also, the incident response team needs to be prepared to investigate suspected or known incidents, mitigate as necessary, and recommend implementation of stronger security controls as necessary (appropriate practice requires inclusion of privacy incident investigation, mitigation, and follow-up action).

Contingency Plan: 45 CFR 164.308(a)(7)

This standard requires implementation of policies and procedures that define how a covered entity or business associate will respond to an emergency or other disaster that could damage systems that store and utilize electronic PHI.

- **Data backup plan (R)**   Need to implement data-backup and recovery processes that provide for the backing up of ePHI and proper recovery processes so the data can be recovered if data is corrupted or lost.

- **Disaster recovery plan (R)**   Disaster recovery plans need to be developed that clearly outline how critical data is to be recovered in the event of a disaster. Plans need to be thorough. Plans also need to address business/clinical, physical, and technical recovery.

- **Emergency mode operation plan (business continuity plan) (R)**   Plans need to be implemented that allow access to critical ePHI in the event of a disaster and while operating in an emergency mode. This also means allowances need to be made to accommodate access to ePHI in the event of an emergency or when the authorized user is not available and access to the data is critical to continued operation. Plans also need to address mission-critical business/clinical, physical, and technical activities/requirements.

- **Testing and revision procedure (A)**   Need to implement policies/procedures that define periodic testing activity for the disaster recovery plan and the emergency mode operations plan.

- **Applications and data criticality analysis (A)**   Data needs to be analyzed to determine whether it is critical and addressed as such in the disaster recovery plan and the emergency mode operation plan.

Evaluation: 45 CFR 164.308(a)(8) (R)

Periodic technical and nontechnical evaluations need to be conducted to reasonably ensure compliance with the provisions of the HIPAA Security Rule (appropriate practice requires inclusion of an evaluation of compliance with the HIPAA Privacy Rule).

Business Associate Contracts and Other Arrangement: 45 CFR 164.308(b)

This standard requires a covered entity to obtain satisfactory assurances from business associates that they will comply with the requirements of the HIPAA Security Rule. It also requires due diligence on the covered entity's part. Business associates are also required to obtain satisfactory assurance from third party vendors that those vendors will adhere to the requirements of the HIPAA Security Rule.

- **Written contract or other arrangement (R)**   Covered entities and business associates are equally responsible to ensure both parties enter into written contracts (private) or other arrangements (government) where the business associates' outside covered entities have access to covered entities' ePHI and perform business activities for covered entities (use and disclose PHI on behalf of covered entities). This does not include treatment, payment, and healthcare operations performed by other covered entities related to their normal operations.

General Breach Description Notification Requirements: 45 CFR 164.404

Covered entities have an obligation to notify individuals of the breach. The definition of a breach and the notification requirements are as follows:

- A breach is considered to be discovered as of the first day the breach is discovered or should reasonably have been discovered.

- Notifications must be made "without unreasonable delay" but no later than 60 calendar days after the breach discovery by the covered entity or business associate to the covered entity.

- The covered entity or business associate has the burden of demonstrating that notifications were made in a "timely" manner. "Timely" means individuals are notified or, if it involves a business associate, the covered entity as soon as feasible or no later than 60 calendar days from the date the breach was discovered or should have been discovered. This includes retaining appropriate documentation related to breach notification.

Methods of Notification: 45 CFR 164.404

Notice must be provided to the individual using the following form:

- It is the responsibility of the covered entity to notify affected individuals even if the breach was reported to the covered entity by the business associate, unless agreed to in advance between the covered entity and the business associate. Even if it is agreed in advance, the covered entity is ultimately responsible if the business associate fails to notify individuals in a timely fashion.

- Written notification by first-class mail to the individual (or the next of kin of the individual if the individual is deceased) at the last known address or, if e-mail is the specified notification preference of the individual, by e-mail. There may be several individual notifications if additional information about the breach becomes available after the first notice is sent.

- If there is insufficient or out-of-date contact information (including phone number, e-mail address, or available contact information) that prevents direct individual notification, a substitute notice is required.

- The substitute notice is required if there are ten or more individuals where there is insufficient or out-of-date contact information. The substitute notice includes conspicuous posting of the breach for 90 days on the home page of the web site of the covered entity or notice in major print or broadcast media, including major media in geographic areas where the individuals affected by the breach likely reside.

- Media and/or web notices need to include a toll-free phone number that is active for no less than 90 days so that the individual can call to learn whether the individual's unsecured PHI was or potentially was a part of the breach.

- If the notice is made through the media, the notice must be made to well-known media outlets in the state or jurisdiction. Also, if the breach involved more than 500 residents of a given state or jurisdiction, media announcement is required (45 CFR 164.406).

Notification Content

The breach notice must include the following items:

- A brief description of what happened, including the date of the breach and the date of the discovery of the breach, if known

- A description of the types of PHI breached or inappropriately disclosed (e.g., full name, Social Security number, date of birth, home address, account number, health condition, etc.)

- The steps individuals should take to protect themselves from potential harm resulting from the breach

- A brief description of what the covered entity is doing to investigate the breach, mitigate losses, and protect against further breaches

- Covered entity contact information (must include a toll-free number, e-mail address, web site, or postal address)

Notification Delay for Law Enforcement Purposes: 45 CFR 164.412

If a law-enforcement official determines that required notification would impede a criminal investigation or cause damage to national security, notification shall be delayed for the period defined by law enforcement.

Specific Covered Entity Requirements: 45 CFR 164.404

In the event of a breach, a covered entity that stores, uses, or discloses unsecured PHI is required to notify each individual whose unsecured PHI has been, or is reasonably believed to have been, breached or inappropriately accessed by an individual or entity (includes internal and external breaches/inappropriate disclosure) within 60 days.

Covered entities are required to notify OCR within 60 days of when the breach was discovered or should have been discovered if it involves 500 or more individuals (45 CFR 164.408). This notice is required immediately following the discovery of the breach. If the breach involved fewer than 500 individuals, the covered entity is required to maintain a breach log (this is in addition to disclosure accounting; breaches and inappropriate disclosures already must be recorded in any patient or individual disclosure accounting). The breach log must be reported to OCR within 60 days from the end of the calendar year. OCR maintains a list on its web site that lists all covered entities who have reported a breach involving 500 individuals or more.

Specific Business Associate Requirements: 45 CFR 164.410

In the event of a breach, a business associate that stores, uses, or discloses unsecured PHI is required to notify the covered entity of the breach. The notice needs to include the identification of each individual whose unsecured PHI has been, or is reasonably believed to have been, breached or inappropriately accessed (includes internal and external breaches/inappropriate disclosure) and sufficient detailed information to accommodate the covered entity's individual notification requirements.

HIPAA Enforcement Interim Final Rule

The HIPAA Enforcement Rule was augmented when the Enforcement Interim Final Rule became effective. The final rule is expected to be published in Q3 or Q4 of 2012. The purpose of the interim final rule was to define "willful neglect" and to move to the HITECH Act related increases in civil penalties that covered entities and business associates may be required to pay in the event of a HIPAA rule violation.

Willful neglect is defined as cases in which the entity knew of a violation of the HIPAA rules or should have known. This means willful neglect may be found and lead to much higher civil penalties or monetary settlements when noncompliance is related to ignorance or incomplete knowledge of the compliance requirements.

The HITECH Act included language that significantly changed the level of civil penalties that could be levied against covered entities and now business associates. The categories of civil penalties were expanded and associated penalties increased.

TIP For example, while the civil penalties were previously tiered by the type of violation, OCR may now levy up to $50,000 for *any* level of violation, with a maximum of $1.5 million per calendar year for the same type of violation. Prior to the effective date of the HIPAA Enforcement Interim Final Rule, the maximum civil penalty for any violation was $100 per incident and up to $25,000 per calendar year for the same type of violation.

OCR may also reach a monetary settlement with covered entities and business associates rather than levying what could be much higher civil penalties. Since 2011, OCR has imposed civil penalties and reached monetary settlements with several covered entities.

State attorneys general were granted the authority to file suit in federal court if the attorney general considers a violation to have harmed individuals in that state. This does not prevent further or concurrent action on the part of OCR. Several state attorneys general have filed suit against covered entities and business associates since February 2010, when the power to file suit was effective.

The HITECH Act also mandated that OCR conduct regular compliance audits of covered entities and business associates. The OCR audit program was launched November 2011 with a pilot audit of 30 covered entities. The full audit program was launched June 2012. OCR has announced that the audit program will continue into the future, but no business associates will be audited during calendar year 2012. The audit program does not replace other enforcement—such as breach investigations by OCR, complaint investigations by OCR, and other compliance-related investigations that may be conducted by other federal agencies and reported to OCR if the other federal agency believes an entity is not in compliance with HIPAA.

State Privacy Laws

It was noted in the section "HIPAA Administrative Simplification Provisions" that if state law is more stringent than HIPAA, state law preempts HIPAA. Most states have enacted laws that are more stringent than the HIPAA Privacy Rule. These laws generally govern the release of certain types of PHI. Such laws generally require specific authorization prior to release of certain types of PHI, among which are the following:

- Mental health
- HIV/AIDS and sexually transmitted diseases
- Reproductive
- Genetic
- Alcohol and chemical dependency[4]
- Minors

State Security Laws

Most states have passed breach-notification laws, some much more stringent than others. Unlike the HIPAA Breach Notification Interim Final Rule, state breach laws must be followed by a much larger number of entities, from healthcare to financial to retail. Also, most state breach laws do not require notification if, say, an individual's name and health information is breached. The laws focus more on financial information that may, if breached, lead to financial-identity theft—such as the breach of an individual's name and Social Security number. It's important to determine which state breach laws apply and adhere to them, along with associated information security requirements.

Chapter Review

HIPAA, HITECH, and state law require the execution of specific legal documents that include patient authorization forms, court orders, and specific contracts, such as a business associate contract. Some of these documents existed prior to HIPAA, and some are creatures of HIPAA. It is important that healthcare organizations (covered entities, business associates, vendors marketing products that will be used to store, manipulate, and disclose PHI), and those working in the healthcare field understand what legal documents are required and when they are required.

These documents are important from a regulatory perspective—not adhering to HIPAA can lead to violations, sanctions, and civil penalties imposed by HHS. Also, if proper legal documentation is not executed and maintained, it can lead to civil suits and damage to an organization's or company's brand and reputation. HIPAA does not allow the filing of a civil suit for "private right of action." This means an individual or entity cannot file a lawsuit against another individual or entity because they violated the HPAA statute and rules. It is important to note, however, that several states have enacted legislation that does allow for private right of action under state law. In addition, lawsuits can be filed if the individual or entity believes they have been harmed because of certain actions or inaction on the part of another individual or entity. An entity may not be sued because it violated HIPAA, but it can be sued if the lack of compliance leads to damage or perceived harm to another.

Legal documents also include policies, risk analysis reports, incident response reports, training documentation, and other regulatory required documents needed to comply with HIPAA and other federal and state laws. Lack of required documentation or documentation that is inaccurate or not current represents one of the most significant regulatory risks to healthcare entities. For example, policies need to be current, accurate, and enforceable. Proper and timely execution of required legal documents is critical to avoid regulatory, legal, and other risks. The document requirements may change over time, so it is important to regularly review and update or amend these documents as needed. For example, the HITECH Act significantly changed how business associates are treated—they are now directly required to adhere to certain HIPAA rules. Prior to HITECH, business associates were required to adhere to HIPAA but not directly—only through contract with covered entities. This change resulted in the need to amend existing business associate contracts and update business associate contract templates.

Questions

To test your comprehension of the chapter, answer the following questions and then check your answers against the list of correct answers that follows the questions.

1. From a regulatory perspective, what are the differences between what a business associate is required to adhere to when it comes to the HIPAA rules and what a covered entity must adhere to?

   A. There are no differences.

   B. The business associate is required to adhere to the HIPAA Privacy and Security Rules, but the covered entity is not required to adhere to either.

   C. The business associate is required to adhere to the use and disclosure provisions of the HIPAA Privacy Rule and the full Security Rule, and the covered entity is required to adhere to the Privacy and Security Rules and the other HIPAA administrative simplification rules.

   D. Neither is required to adhere to HIPAA rules.

2. What enforcement action can the Office for Civil Rights (OCR) take if a covered entity violates provisions of HIPAA's administrative simplification rules?

   A. OCR has no enforcement authority.

   B. OCR may levy up to $50,000 for any level of violation with a maximum of $1.5 million per calendar year for the same type of violation.

   C. The penalty depends on the severity of the disclosure.

   D. OCR can impose however great a fine a court of law allows.

3. What are the privacy rights afforded patients pursuant to the HIPAA Privacy Rule (45 CFR Parts 160 and 164)?

   A. The maximum rights of quality, efficiency, and effectiveness.

   B. Patients must be informed of disclosed PHI other than for treatment, payment, and healthcare operations.

   C. There are no rights afforded to patients.

   D. These are security provisions that do not protect patient privacy.

4. A state law that is more stringent than the HIPAA Privacy Rule preempts HIPAA. What does stringent mean?

   A. Stringent is defined as providing greater protection of an individual's PHI or providing an individual greater access to their PHI.

   B. Stringent is defined as covering more serious disclosures.

      C. Stringent means allowing more enforcement.

      D. Stringent is more rigorous audits.

5. What are the document creation and retention requirements for covered entities?

      A. Covered entities are required to create and retain for six years all disclosures, complaints, mitigations, compliance reviews, and EHR audit reports.

      B. All document retention requirements are for one year only.

      C. Covered entities are required to retain all elements of PHI information indefinitely.

      D. Covered entities are required to retain disclosures to research, quality, hospital plans, organizations, and providers for six years.

6. True or false: All healthcare providers in the United States are considered to be covered entities.

      A. True

      B. False

Answers

1. **C.** The business associate is required to adhere to the use and disclosure provisions of the HIPAA Privacy Rule and the complete Security Rule, and the covered entity is required to adhere to the Privacy and Security Rules as well as the remaining HIPAA administrative simplification rules.

2. **B.** OCR may levy up to $50,000 for any level of violation with a maximum of $1.5 million per calendar year for the same type of violation.

3. **B.** Patients must be informed of disclosed PHI other than for treatment, payment, and healthcare operations.

4. **A.** Stringent is defined as providing greater protection of an individual's PHI or providing an individual greater access to their PHI.

5. **A.** Covered entities are required to create and retain for six years all disclosures, complaints, mitigations, compliance reviews, and EHR audit reports.

6. **B.** All healthcare providers are not covered entities. A healthcare provider is only a HIPAA covered entity if the provider transmits HIPAA covered transactions.

References

1. Public Law 104-191, 104th Congress. *Health Insurance Portability and Accountability Act of 1996*. Section 1, Title II, Subpart F (HIPAA administrative simplification provisions).

2. Public Law 111-5, 111th Congress. *American Recovery and Reinvestment Act of 2009*. Division A, Title XIII, Subpart D (ARRA/HITECH privacy, security, and enforcement provisions).

3. Public Law 104-191, 104th Congress. *Health Insurance Portability and Accountability Act of 1996*. 45 CFR Parts 160 and 164 (HIPAA privacy, security, and enforcement rules).

4. Ibid. 42 CFR Part 2 (alcohol and chemical dependency privacy rule).

NOTE The legal documents referenced in this chapter are available from Apgar & Associates, LLC. More information is available at www.apgarandassoc.com.

The Electronic Health Record as Evidence

Kimberly A. Baldwin-Stried Reich

In this chapter, you will learn how to
- Discuss the sources and structure of law within the United States
- Delineate the differences between federal, state, and local courts
- Describe the process of the discovery and admissibility of the electronic record as evidence into a court of law
- Consider the role the technology plays as the underpinning of the nation's evolving healthcare information infrastructure

A law is defined as "any system of regulations to govern the conduct of the people of a community, society or nation, in response to the need for regularity, consistency and justice based upon collective human experience."[1] A regulation is defined as a set of "requirements the government imposes on private firms and individuals to achieve government's purposes."[2] The healthcare industry is one of the most (if not *the* most) highly regulated industries that exists within the United States today. Healthcare regulations cover a broad range—ensuring quality, facilitating the government's role as purchaser of care, and establishing a nationwide infrastructure to facilitate the use and exchange of electronic health information. They include the policy, standards, implementation specifications, and certification criteria established through the enactment of the Health Information Technology for Economic and Clinical Health (HITECH) Act.

Sources and Structure of Law

U.S. laws establish the standards of behavior, the means by which standards are enforced, and the mechanism to guide conduct. There are four primary sources of law within the U.S. legal system:

- Federal and state constitutions
- Federal and state statutes

- Decisions and rules of administrative agencies
- Decisions of the courts

The Constitution

The U.S. Constitution was signed on September 17, 1787, at the Constitutional Convention in Philadelphia, presided over by George Washington. The U.S. Constitution is also known as the "Supreme Law of the Land." The Delegates of the Constitutional Convention devised a plan for a stronger federal government and established the executive, legislative, and judicial branches of U.S. government along with a system of checks and balances to ensure that no single branch would have too much power. The most famous limits on federal power were established in the Bill of Rights (the first 10 amendments), which guarantee basic individual protections such as freedom of speech and religion. These amendments were ratified and became part of the Constitution in 1791. The Ninth and Fourteenth Amendments to the Constitution contain provisions that limit both state and federal governmental powers and recognize an individual's "right to privacy," a concept that is pervasive in the healthcare industry today.[3]

An individual's right to privacy is rooted in the 1886 case *Boyd v. United States*. In *Boyd*, the court utilized provisions in both the Fourth and Fifth Amendments to the Constitution, claiming that, in certain cases, the two amendments sub-textually protected the privacies of individuals from governmental intrusion..."[4] However, it wasn't until 1965 in the landmark decision *Griswold v. Connecticut* that the United States Supreme Court recognized an individual's right to privacy. The first 10 amendments (the Bill of Rights) were ratified in 1791, and since then 17 more have been ratified so that we now have a total of 27 constitutional amendments.[5] The right to privacy continues to be a topic of debate and concern among healthcare providers, payers, and consumers.

Statutes

A statute is another major source of law. A statute is defined as "a federal or state written law enacted by the Congress or state legislature, respectively. Local statutes or laws are usually called 'ordinances.'"[6] The U.S. Congress is the only legislative body with powers delegated to it by the Constitution, but those powers have been interpreted broadly. State legislatures have all powers not denied them by the U.S. Constitution, by federal laws enacted under the authority of the federal government, or by their state constitutions. Local legislative bodies have only those powers granted by the state.[7]

Federal law supersedes when there is a conflict between federal and state law. In some special circumstances, "federal law may preempt an entire area of law, so that state law is superseded even if it is not in direct conflict."[8]

The enactment of the Health Insurance Portability and Accountability Act (HIPAA) established a complex and comprehensive federal scheme for the privacy and security of protected health information. While it has been established that federal law takes precedence in conflicts between federal and state law, HIPAA contains provisions that determine when HIPAA will preempt state law in matters relating to privacy and security. Generally, the more stringent rule—federal or state—is the law that will apply in matters related to the protection of health information.

State law supersedes when there is a conflict between state and local governmental code. In some special circumstances, "state law may preempt an entire area of law, so that local law is superseded even if it is not in direct conflict."[9]

Administrative Agencies

The rules and decisions set forth by administrative agencies are other sources of law. Administrative agencies are established under Article 1, Section 1 of the Constitution, which states that "[A]ll legislative Powers herein granted shall be vested in a Congress of the United States."[10] The legislature has delegated to numerous administrative agencies the power through Article 1, Section 8, Clause 18, "...to make all Laws which shall be necessary and proper for carrying into Execution the foregoing Powers, and all other Powers vested by this Constitution in the Government of the United States, or in any Department or Officer thereof."[11] A summary of the powers and authorities of the administrative agencies are outlined in the sections that follow.

The Department of Health and Human Services[12]

The Department of Health and Human Services (HHS) represents almost a quarter of all federal outlays. It administers more grant dollars than all other federal agencies combined. HHS's Medicare program is the nation's largest health insurer, handling more than 1 billion claims per year. Medicare and Medicaid together provide health-care insurance for one in four Americans.

HHS works closely with state and local governments, and many HHS-funded services are provided at the local level by state or county agencies or through private-sector grantees. The department's programs are administered by 11 operating divisions, including eight agencies in the U.S. Public Health Service and three human services agencies. The department includes more than 300 programs, covering a wide spectrum of activities. In addition to the services they deliver, the HHS programs provide for equitable treatment of beneficiaries nationwide, and they enable the collection of national health and other data.

The Food and Drug Administration[13]

The Food and Drug Administration (FDA) has the following responsibilities:

- Protecting the public's health by assuring that foods are safe, wholesome, sanitary, and properly labeled, and that human and veterinary drugs, vaccines, other biological products, and medical devices intended for human use are safe and effective
- Protecting the public from electronic product radiation
- Assuring that cosmetics and dietary supplements are safe and properly labeled
- Regulating tobacco products

- Advancing the public's health by helping to speed product innovations
- Helping the public get the accurate, science-based information they need to use medicines, devices, and foods to improve their health

The FDA's responsibilities extend to all 50 states, the District of Columbia, Puerto Rico, Guam, the Virgin Islands, American Samoa, and other U.S. territories and possessions.

The Internal Revenue Service[14]

The Internal Revenue Service (IRS) is organized to carry out the responsibilities of the secretary of the Department of the Treasury under section 7801 of the Internal Revenue Code. The secretary has full authority to administer and enforce the internal revenue laws and has the power to create an agency to enforce these laws. The IRS was created based on this legislative grant. Section 7803 of the Internal Revenue Code provides for the appointment of a commissioner of internal revenue to administer and supervise the execution and application of the internal revenue laws.

On June 28, 2012, the U.S. Supreme Court ruled on several key issues affecting the Patient Protection and Affordable Care Act (PPACA)[15] in *National Federation of Independent Business, et al. v. Sebelius, et al.*[16] The Court ruled that the "individual mandate" to require individuals to purchase health insurance was constitutional. However, the Court also ruled that the provision that would permit the secretary of HHS to withdraw all of the Medicaid funding provided to a state if that state chooses not to expand Medicaid to certain thresholds set forth in the act was unconstitutional.

Beginning in 2014, the IRS will serve as the administrative agency responsible for providing the administrative oversight and review in collection of all taxes and penalties to be assessed on individuals who do not have health insurance in accordance with the Supreme Court decision on June 28, 2012.

The National Labor Relations Board[17]

The National Labor Relations Board (NLRB) is an independent federal agency that protects the rights of private sector employees to join together, with or without a union, to improve their wages and working conditions. The NLRB seeks to achieve consistency in its decision by following positions it established in previous matters. The NLRB conducts the following five major activities in the performance of its duties:

- **Conduct elections** NLRB provides the legal framework for private-sector employees to organize bargaining units in their workplace or dissolve their labor unions through a decertification election.
- **Investigate charges** Employees, union representatives, and employers who believe that their rights under the National Labor Relations Act have been violated may file charges alleging unfair labor practices at their nearest NLRB regional office.

- **Facilitate settlements** When a charge is determined to have merit, the NLRB encourages parties to resolve cases by settlement rather than litigation whenever possible.

- **Decide cases** On the adjudicative side of the NLRB are 40 administrative law judges and a board whose five members are appointed by the president and confirmed by the Senate.

- **Enforce orders** Most parties voluntarily comply with orders of the board. When they do not, the agency's general counsel must seek enforcement in the U.S. Courts of Appeals. Parties to cases also may seek review of unfavorable decisions in the federal courts.

Court Decisions

The fourth source of U.S. law arises from judicial decisions, also known as case law (discussed in further detail below). Today, many of the legal rules and principles applied by U.S. courts are rooted in the traditional unwritten law of England, based on custom and usage known as "common law." Today, "almost all common law has been enacted into statutes with modern variations by all the states except Louisiana, which is still influenced by the Napoleonic Code. In some states the principles of Common Law are so basic they are applied without reference to statute."[18] In the process of deciding an individual case, the courts interpret regulations and statutes in accordance with the relevant federal or state constitution. The court will create and establish the "common law" when it decides cases that are not controlled by regulations, statutes, or by a constitution.

The courts are responsible for making determinations as to whether specific regulations or statutes are in violation of the Constitution. The case of *Marbury v. Madison* established that all legislation and regulations must be consistent with the Constitution and that the courts hold inherent powers to declare legislation invalid when it is unconstitutional.[19] Some state courts have established specific sets of rules for interpretation of conflicting regulations and statutes.

Administrative agencies also have discretion as to how regulations or statutes are applied—and disagreements over the application of a specific regulation or statute can and do arise frequently. While the decision of an administrative agency can be appealed to the courts, the courts generally defer decisions to the relevant administrative agency and will limit their review of the matter unless the following conditions were not met:

- Delegation of the matter to the administrative agency was constitutional.

- The administrative agency acted within its authority and followed proper procedures.

- The agency acted with a substantial basis and acted without discrimination or arbitrariness.

Case Law

Case law is defined as "reported decisions of appeals courts and other courts which make new interpretations of the law and, therefore, can be cited as precedents. These interpretations are distinguished from 'statutory law,' which are the statutes and codes (laws) enacted by legislative bodies; 'regulatory law,' which are regulations required by agencies based on statutes; and in some states, the common law, which is the generally accepted law carried down from England. The rulings in trials and hearings which are not appealed and not reported are not case law and, therefore, not precedent or new interpretations."[20] The term "common law" is often used interchangeably with case law. Due care should be used when using the terms "common law" and "case law" interchangeably, because "common law" refers to traditional unwritten law of England, while "case law" refers to the laws that were established by judicial decision.

U.S. Governmental Organization and Function

The three branches of the government—legislative, executive, and judicial—are responsible for carrying out the governmental powers and functions. Each of the three branches of government has a different primary function. Outlined below is a summary of the primary functions of each of the three branches of the U.S government:

- **Legislative branch**[21]   The legislative branch is the law-making branch of government, made up of the Senate, the House of Representatives, and agencies that support Congress. The primary function of the legislative branch is to enact laws.

- **Executive branch**[22]   The president is the head of the executive branch of the government, which includes many departments and agencies. The primary function of the executive branch is to enforce and administer the law.

- **Judicial branch**[23]   The judicial branch is made up of the Supreme Court, lower courts, special courts, and court support organizations. The primary function of the judicial branch is to adjudicate and resolve disputes in accordance with the law.

The three branches of government operate under a concept known as the separation of powers. Under this concept, as established by the framers of the Constitution, no branch of the government shall have more power or control than the other two branches in the exercise of its functions and activities.

Structure and Function of the U.S. Court System

The U.S. court system is divided administratively into two separate systems: the federal district courts and the state courts. Each court system operates independently of the executive and legislative branches of government. The federal court system is set forth in Article III, Section 1 of the Constitution, which states that "[T]he judicial Power of the United States, shall be vested in one supreme Court, and in such inferior Courts as the Congress may from time to time ordain and establish. The Judges, both of the supreme and inferior Courts, shall hold their Offices during good Behaviour, and shall, at stated Times, receive for their Services, a Compensation, which shall not be diminished during their Continuance in Office."[24] While both the federal and state court systems are responsible for hearing certain types of cases, neither system is completely independent of the other, and the systems do interact on occasion.

Federal Court System[25]

The federal court system is comprised of 92 district courts with at least one bench in each of the 50 states, as well as benches in Puerto Rico and the District of Columbia. There are a total of 1 to 20 judges in each district. District court judges are appointed by the president and serve for life. Cases handled by federal district court include: cases involving violation of federal law and/or allegations of Constitutional violations; cases directly involving a state or federal government; maritime disputes; and/or cases involving foreign governments, citizens of foreign countries, or in which citizens of two or more different states are involved.

The courts of appeals are directly above the federal district court. The court of appeals system is comprised of 11 judicial circuit courts throughout the United States, plus one court of appeals in the District of Columbia. There are a total of 6 to 27 judges in the courts of appeals. In addition to hearing appeals for their respective federal district courts, the courts of appeals also have jurisdiction to hear cases involving a challenge to an order of a federal regulatory agency.

The Supreme Court is located in Washington, D.C. and is also known as "The Highest Court in the Land." It is the only court that is explicitly mandated by the Constitution. The Supreme Court is comprised of one chief justice and eight associate justices. The Supreme Court may hear cases from a state appellate court on federal or constitutional matters. The Supreme Court has the authority to decline to review most cases and maintains final jurisdiction over all cases it hears.

State Court System[26]

The state court system is large and diverse. Currently, there are more than 1,000 various types of state courts and judges. State courts, which are also referred to as local courts, include magistrate court, municipal court, justice of the peace court, police court, traffic court, and county court. These courts are called the inferior courts. The more serious cases are heard in a superior court, also sometimes known as state district court, circuit court, or by a number of other names. The majority of healthcare medical malpractice cases are heard in the state superior court system.

State superior, district, or circuit courts are generally organized by counties, hear appeals from the inferior courts, and have original jurisdiction over major civil suits and serious crimes. Most of the nation's jury trials occur in state superior court. The highest state court is usually called the appellate court, state court of appeals, or state Supreme Court and generally hears appeals from the state superior courts and, in some instances, has original jurisdiction over particularly important cases. A number of the larger states, such as New York, may also have intermediate appellate courts between the superior courts and the state's highest court. Additionally, a state may also have a wide variety of special tribunals, usually on the inferior court level, including divorce court, mental health court, housing court, juvenile court, family court, small-claims court, and probate court.

The Patient's Medical Record

The patient's medical record, whether in paper or electronic form, contains vital clinical information to support the diagnosis and justify the care and treatment rendered to the patient. This information includes the patient's medical history, physical examination results, radiology and laboratory reports, diagnoses and treatment plans, as well as orders and notes from doctors, nurses, and other healthcare professionals. The quality and integrity of the information contained in the patient's medical record is essential for clinical, legal, and fiscal purposes, for correct and prompt diagnosis and treatment of the patient's condition, and for continuity of care.

Although the primary use of the patient's medical record is to serve as a tool for the planning and communication of the patient's treatment and care, it also serves as a secondary source of information for other uses. It provides support and documentation for insurance claims, legal matters, professional quality and peer-review activities of prescribed treatments and medications, and the education and training of health professionals. Medical records also contain useful statistical and research information for public health and resource-management planning purposes. They contain data for clinical studies, evaluation and management of the costs associated with treatment, and the assessment of population health.

EHR Standards for Records Management and Evidentiary Support

Electronic health records (EHRs) are a complex and evolving ecosystem. As such, the Health Level Seven (HL7) standards development organization (SDO) has developed an EHR system profile known as the Records Management and Evidentiary Support Functional Profile (RM-ES FP).[27] This profile serves as a framework for the functions and conformance criteria for EHR systems to follow in the design and implementation of an EHR system for healthcare organizations. On a regular and ongoing basis, an HL7 volunteer workgroup meets to review and discuss EHR conformance criteria for the RM-ES profile. The HL7 RM-ES workgroup charter is as follows:[28]

To provide expertise to the EHR work group, other standards groups and the healthcare industry on records management, compliance, and data/record integrity for EHR systems and related to EHR governance to support the use of medical records for clinical care and decision-making, business, legal and disclosure purposes.

The RM-ES functional profile is based on the premise that an "EHR system must be able to create, receive, maintain, use, and manage the disposition of records related to the business activities and transactions for an organization … the RM-ES profile identifies EHR system functions as critical for maintaining a legally sound health record."[29] Given this purpose, it is a good idea to regularly review this profile to see whether requirements for the EHR to serve as the health record for legal, business, and disclosure purposes have been updated.

A copy of the Release 1.0 HL7 RM-ES functional profile can be reviewed at http://wiki .hl7.org/images/6/6a/Functional_Profile_-_Legal_EHR.pdf. The RM-ES workgroup will begin its work on Release 2 of the RM-ES profile in the third quarter of 2012. The progress of the workgroup can be followed on the HL7 wiki.

The Role and Use of the Medical Record in Litigation

As previously discussed, one of the important secondary uses of the medical record is to provide support and documentation for legal matters. Irrespective of its form (paper or electronic) or location, the patient's medical record also serves as an important form of evidence that is often used in the litigation process. Yet the process by which medical records are discovered and admitted into evidence is evolving as rapidly as our nation's health information infrastructure. Vast and significant differences exist between the role and use of paper versus electronic health records (EHR) as evidence in a court a law. The remainder of this chapter will focus on the legal process of discovery and the role of the EHR as evidence in a court of law.

Paper-based Medical Records vs. Electronic Health Records (EHRs) in Discovery

Prior to the digital era, medical records were stored and existed in a single form—paper. Paper-based medical records are vastly different from digital media. Paper is static. A standard piece of paper weighs about 4.5 ounces, with 100 sheets weighing about 1 pound. You can see it, touch it, file it into physical folders, and easily discard it. Information is generally handwritten or typed into paper-based medical records using ink-based media. EHR systems, on the other hand, are not static like paper. Unlike paper, EHR systems contain both structured and unstructured data elements, which are virtually weightless and electronically record information through the use of a machine into the patient's medical record.[30] Not all of the electronic information contained in EHR systems can be seen by the naked eye, touched, filed, or easily discarded. An illustration of some of these differences can be found in Figure 14-1.

Prior to the digital age, the process for the discovery of relevant information from paper-based medical record systems was pretty straightforward and often very time-consuming. The discovery process often began the moment a subpoena or some other legal notice was served upon the organization. In most circumstances, the medical records director, acting as the "keeper of the record" (or records custodian), was responsible for signing an affidavit attesting that all of the paper-based medical records being produced for litigation were "true and correct copies of the original medical record" after the records were copied, bates-stamped, and produced for litigation.

Difference	Description
Volume and reproducibility issues	• EHRs exist in substantially greater volumes. • Electronic information can be replicated automatically. • Paper does not need a device such as a computer to be read. • EHRs must conform to HIPAA standards for transmission of PHI.
Dynamic content and nature of electronic data	• EHRs are easier to change than paper. • The content of electronic information can change without human intervention. • The transmission and transfer of EHR data are not fixed in final form.
Metadata	• EHRs contain metadata; paper does not. • System, application, and/or user metadata are not readily apparent. • Metadata adds a new set of retention and preservation obligations.
Lifespan/persistence of electronic data	• EHRs are much harder to dispose of; paper can be shredded and easily discarded. • Electronic data are not easily deleted.
EHRs and information exchange environment	• EHRs and exchanged data may be incomprehensible when separated from their environment. • Migrating from a legacy system to an EHR system involves a significantly different process—no more imaging of documents.
Search and retrieval of electronic data	• Electronic data may reside in numerous locations. • Paper documents are usually consolidated and maintained in a single file folder. • EHRs and the exchange environment may obscure the origin, completeness, or accuracy of the information.
EHRs and electronic exchange data are electronic evidence that must be authenticated and reviewed prior to submission into a court of law. A discovery plan for EHR data must be made early on in litigation.	

Figure 14-1 Synopsis of Differences Between Paper-based Medical Records and EHRs. Reprinted with permission from the American Health Information Management Association. © 2012 by the American Health Information Management Association.

Enactment of the HITECH Act resulted in today's widespread adoption of EHRs and the design and build of our nation's health information infrastructure of tomorrow. As in any other industry, EHRs and tomorrow's health information infrastructure will bring about both benefits and risks to our nation's healthcare system. The following sections summarize the cited benefits and risks of EHR adoption and the ability to exchange health information electronically.[31]

EHR Benefits

- **Available in emergency**   Providers are able to more easily access life-saving information about your health history to make decisions when you are in an accident or unable to speak for yourself.

- **Protected in disasters**   Your protected health information is safely stored and will not be destroyed in the event you or your loved ones are affected by a disaster. Unlike paper-based medical records, which can easily be destroyed by flood or fire, health information stored in electronic form can easily be transmitted or exchanged with healthcare providers in a time of need.

- **Improved care/reduced medical errors**   Your healthcare providers will have greater access to important information they need about the care and medications you may have received from other providers. As a result, your healthcare providers will be able to make better and more informed decisions about you and your treatment plan. For example, when you can't remember what medications you are taking, the electronic exchange of health information will provide valuable information about your medical conditions and the medications you are taking so that your providers can avoid prescribing medications that may be harmful to you.

- **Tracking for protection**   EHRs coupled with the ability to exchange health information provides an electronic mechanism to record and track the individuals who access a patient's medical record. The types of information that may be tracked and recorded include the identity and job type of the individual accessing the medical record, the date and time accessed, the reason for access, and the types of information accessed. Automated tracking is a much more efficient and effective means to enforce HIPAA privacy and security laws as compared to manual systems maintained by paper-based medical record systems.

- **Increased safety/reduced duplication**   According to the *Journal of the American Medical Association (JAMA)*, "The most important contributor to the high cost of US health care … is overutilization. Overutilization can take 2 forms: higher volumes, such as more office visits, hospitalizations, tests, procedures, and prescriptions than are appropriate or more costly specialists, tests, procedures, and prescriptions than are appropriate … medical malpractice laws and the resultant defensive medicine also contribute to overutilization."[32] EHRs and the electronic exchange of health information are valuable tools to improve patient safety and drive down healthcare costs by reducing unnecessary or potentially harmful tests (e.g., reducing the patient's exposure to radiation by eliminating unnecessary x-rays).

EHR Risks

- **Identity theft**   Identify theft is defined as "the practice of using someone else's 'personally identifiable information' (PII) to receive goods, obtain services, or conduct business."[33] As with any other industry (such as the banking industry), the mechanisms to protect the security of health information are not foolproof. Identity theft and security breaches occur in both paper-based record-keeping systems as well as electronic systems. However, while a breach of a paper-based system may affect only a single individual, many individuals may be affected when EHR systems are compromised.

- **Errors**   EHRs and the ability to exchange information electronically play an important role in helping to improve the quality and efficiency of patient care. However, when information is incorrectly entered, recorded, or exchanged between providers, a medical error may result as a result of a provider's reliance upon the information. Unlike paper-based systems, EHRs and the electronic information exchange provide a mechanism for reviewing and verifying the integrity of data prior to entry or exchange.

- **Hackers**   As is the case in all other industries that rely on the use of technology to conduct business transactions, there is an inherent risk that the firewalls and security codes of an EHR system may be broken into by a data hacker.

Despite the benefits and technological advancements provided by EHRs and the ability to exchange health information electronically, the process by which healthcare organizations and providers respond to regulatory investigations or litigation is still in its infancy.

Yesterday's best-practice standards for paper-based medical-record filing systems—such as record terminal-digit filing systems, many of which are still in use today[34]—are becoming obsolete and wholly inadequate in an environment in which health information is captured, stored, and maintained in an electronic form.

Evolving caselaw provides further examples of the benefits as well as risks of EHR adoption. For example, in April 2012, Advocate Lutheran General paid $8.25 million to Fritzie and Cameron Burkett of Chicago to settle their wrongful death suit against the hospital. Following an investigation, the hospital determined that a "data entry error was made in the formulation of the IV solution. The dosage of sodium for an IV bag from an order had been incorrectly entered into the machine that mixes IV solutions."[35]

The benefits and risks associated with EHR adoption, evolving case law, and recent amendments for the Federal Rules of Civil Procedure (FRCP)[36] are now converging and overlapping with one another in the design and build of our nation's health information infrastructure. This convergence of laws, rules, and regulations is resulting in the following:

1. A mandate to make changes to the process by which relevant information is discovered and produced for healthcare litigation.

2. A need to establish new HIT standards, systems, and approaches for the discovery and production of electronically stored health information.

Discovery and Admissibility of the EHR

As discussed earlier, the patient's medical record plays a key role in regulatory investigations and litigation. The patient's medical-record information is important to all kinds of healthcare matters such as personal injury claims, disability claims, workers' compensation cases, and medical malpractice lawsuits. Patients through their attorneys will typically seek to discover "any and all records" that may be relevant to their matter, including (but not limited to) patient medical records, peer-review records, incident reports, and/or other types of records that may contain information about the care and treatment of the patient.

Whether a record that is requested for litigation is actually discoverable or will be admitted as evidence during the course of a trial may significantly affect the outcome of a lawsuit. Therefore, it is important to distinguish between the discoverability vs. the admissibility of a record as evidence into a court of law. Following is a summary of the differences between discovery and admissibility:

- **Discovery** Discovery is defined as "the entire efforts of a party to a lawsuit and his/her/its attorneys to obtain information before trial through demands for production of documents, depositions of parties and potential witnesses, written interrogatories (questions and answers written under oath), written requests for admissions of fact, examination of the scene and the petitions and motions employed to enforce discovery rights. The theory of broad rights of discovery is that all parties will go to trial with as much knowledge as possible and that neither party should be able to keep secrets from the other (except for constitutional protection against self-incrimination)."[37] Often much of the fight between the two sides in a suit takes place during the discovery period.

- **Admissibility** Admissibility denotes "evidence which the trial judge finds is useful in helping the trier of fact (a jury if there is a jury, otherwise the judge), and which cannot be objected to on the basis that it is irrelevant, immaterial, or violates the rules against hearsay and other objections. Sometimes the evidence a person tries to introduce has little relevant value (usually called probative value) in determining some fact, or prejudice from the jury's shock at gory details may outweigh that probative value. In criminal cases the courts tend to be more restrictive on letting the jury hear such details for fear they will result in 'undue prejudice.' Thus, the jury may only hear a sanitized version of the facts in prosecutions involving violence."[38]

The Federal Rules of Evidence (FRE)[39]

The Federal Rules of Evidence (FRE) are civil code that generally governs civil and criminal proceeding in U.S. courts and bankruptcy courts and before U.S. magistrates to the extent and with the exceptions stated in the rules. The FRE are designed to secure judicial fairness, eliminate unjustifiable expense and delay, and promote the growth and development of the law of evidence.

The FRE have the force of statute, and the courts interpret them as they would any other statute. The Supreme Court promulgates the FRE, and they are amended from time to time by Congress—such as in 2008, when FRE 502 was enacted to provide limitations on the waiver of attorney-client privilege and work product protection.[40] This amendment in large part was a result of the recognition that the discovery and disclosure of electronically stored information is a far more complicated process than paper-based discovery, and today's digital era mandates the need for provisions that could protect attorney-client and work product privileges in the event of the inadvertent production of electronically stored information.

Medical Records as Hearsay

Hearsay is defined as "second-hand evidence in which the witness is not telling what he/she knows personally, but what others have said to him/her."[41] Under traditional rules of evidence, medical records are considered to be hearsay by a court of law. Hearsay is generally not admissible as evidence into a court of law, because the person who made the original statement is not available to be cross-examined. EHR systems and the electronic exchange of health information sometimes add more challenges to the hearsay rule because of the distinction between electronically stored information that was generated by the computer versus information that was entered by a user into a computer system. That said, "The courts have acknowledged the distinction between computer-generated and computer-stored information. 'If the system made the statement it is "computer-generated." If a person inputs a statement into the system that then preserves a record of it, it is "computer stored" evidence.'"[42]

Exceptions to the Hearsay Rule

Although medical records are considered to be hearsay in the eyes of the court, they generally are admitted as evidence on other grounds. The most common way in which medical records are admitted as evidence into a court of law is through FRE 803. This rule is titled "Exceptions to the rule against hearsay - regardless of whether the declarant is available as a witness." This rule is also sometimes called the "business records exception." Outlined below are items which are not excluded by the rule against hearsay, regardless of whether the declarant is available as a witness:[43]

- **Present sense impression** A statement describing or explaining an event or condition, made while or immediately after the declarant perceived it.

- **Excited utterance** A statement relating to a startling event or condition, made while the declarant was under the stress of the excitement that it caused.

- **Then-existing mental, emotional, or physical condition** A statement of the declarant's then-existing state of mind (such as motive, intent, or plan) or emotional, sensory, or physical condition (such as mental feeling, pain, or bodily health), but not including a statement of memory or belief to prove the fact remembered or believed unless it relates to the validity or terms of the declarant's will.

- **Statement made for medical diagnosis or treatment**   A statement that is made for—and is reasonably pertinent to—medical diagnosis or treatment and describes medical history, past or present symptoms or sensations, their inception, or their general cause.

- **Recorded recollection**   A record that is on a matter the witness once knew about but now cannot recall well enough to testify fully and accurately, was made or adopted by the witness when the matter was fresh in the witness's memory, and accurately reflects the witness's knowledge. If admitted, the record may be read into evidence but may be received as an exhibit only if offered by an adverse party.

- **Records of a regularly conducted activity**   A record of an act, event, condition, opinion, or diagnosis that is admissible when it meets all of the following conditions:

  - The record was made at or near the time by—or from information transmitted by—someone with knowledge.

  - The record was kept in the course of a regularly conducted activity of a business, organization, occupation, or calling, whether or not for profit.

  - Making the record was a regular practice of that activity.

  - All these conditions are shown by the testimony of the custodian or another qualified witness, or by a certification that complies with Rule 902 or with a statute permitting certification.

  - Neither the source of information nor the method or circumstances of preparation indicate a lack of trustworthiness.

Some states contain provisions that also make medical records admissible under the hearsay exception for public or official records. Medical records are also admissible in most states under workers' compensation laws.

Physician-Patient Privilege

In certain circumstances, patients or healthcare providers may wish to safeguard protected health information from discovery by asserting a physician-patient relationship, thus shielding the protected health information from discovery. Nearly all states maintain statutes that protect the communications of a physician-patient relationship from disclosure in judicial or quasi-judicial proceedings under certain circumstances. The purpose of the physician-patient privilege doctrine is to encourage the patient to discuss and disclose all information for care and treatment.[44]

Other Healthcare Records and Documentation

Aside from medical records, in today's digital era there are virtually countless other types of records and documentation that a patient, healthcare provider, or organization may wish to remain confidential. However, in the face of impending litigation these records may also contain relevant information that is necessary for one party or the other to prove its case. Table 14-1 lists some examples of these records.

Healthcare Record	Generally Maintained By
Peer-review activities, including meeting minutes, records, and reports	Healthcare organizations, providers, and EHR systems
Incident reports and risk-management data	Healthcare organizations and EHR systems
Patient complaints	Providers, healthcare organizations, and EHR systems
Patient safety data	Providers, healthcare organizations, and EHR systems
Utilization-management and profiling data	Providers, healthcare organizations, and EHR systems
Case-management records	Providers, healthcare organizations, health plans, and EHR systems
Clinical documentation improvement communication records	Providers, healthcare organizations, and EHR systems
Quality-improvement records, including meeting minutes and reports	Providers, healthcare organizations, and EHR systems
Morbidity and mortality records, including meeting minutes and reports	Healthcare organizations and EHR systems
Surgical case review reports	Healthcare organizations and EHR systems
Operating-room records, such as logs and call schedules	Healthcare organizations and EHR systems
Infection-control committee records, including meeting minutes and reports	Healthcare organizations and EHR systems
Grand round presentations	Providers and healthcare organizations
Survey reports and recommendations from the Joint Commission	The Joint Commission and the healthcare organization
State inspection reports and recommendations	The state and the healthcare organization
Credentialing committee records, including meeting minutes and reports	Healthcare organizations and EHR systems
Licensing applications	The licensing agency and the healthcare organization
HIPAA audit and system-access logs	EHR systems and patients
Clinical pathways and care protocols	Providers and healthcare organizations
Patient ombudsman records	Healthcare organizations
Continuing-education and training programs and materials for providers and staff	Providers and healthcare organizations
Policy and procedure manuals	Providers and healthcare organizations

Table 14-1   Examples of Healthcare Records That May Contain Litigation-Relevant Information

Healthcare Record	Generally Maintained By
Databases	Providers; healthcare organizations; patients; EHR, PHR, and other clinical biomedical systems
System metadata	EHR and clinical biomedical system data
System ephemeral data	EHR and clinical biomedical system data
Clinical-decision-support system protocols	Healthcare organizations, providers, EHR systems
Personal health records (PHRs)	Patients, providers, third-party service providers, healthcare organizations, and EHR systems
Texts and instant messages	Providers, patients, staff, healthcare organizational and personal devices (such as laptop computers, smart phones, tablet computers), and third-party service providers
Voicemail records	Providers, patients, staff, and healthcare organizations (personal and organization voicemail files, as relevant)
E-mail records	Providers, patients, staff, and healthcare organizations (personal and organizational e-mail files, as relevant)
Records from social media web sites, including Facebook, LinkedIn, Twitter, Yammer, YouTube, etc.	Healthcare organizations, providers, patients, and third-party service providers

Table 14-1   Examples of Healthcare Records That May Contain Litigation-Relevant Information
(continued)

Generally, any of these various types of records are discoverable unless they are protected from discovery by state statute. Each of the states maintains their own rules for making determinations as to how and what records will fall within an exception to the hearsay rule. The state statutes vary widely and are too numerous to discuss here.

With regard to healthcare, there are two types of documents that are often requested and have a well-established history regarding discovery and admissibility and are worth noting further.

Records of Peer-Review Activities

In accordance with various federal, state, regulatory, and accrediting requirements, healthcare organizations are required to establish and maintain systematic and ongoing programs to review, monitor, and evaluate the quality of patient care provided. Thus, all healthcare organizations maintain records and reports of the peer-review activities conducted within the organization. The potential value peer-review records have to a patient and an attorney suing the organization for medical malpractice is clear. Consequently, the demand for access to the records from peer review has created a substantial body of law that varies widely by state and jurisdiction.

Even if they are not protected from discovery by state statute, the activities of peer review may be determined to be inadmissible as evidence under the hearsay rule. The first step, then, in determining whether the records of the organization's peer-review activities are discoverable or admissible into a court of law is to examine state statutory and case law for an understanding of how the statutes were applied by the court. Although the application of laws governing discovery and admissibility varies widely and significantly, the following general questions should be considered by all healthcare organizations and providers in the review and analysis of the application of peer-review privilege:

- **Under what authority are the requested records being sought?** Some states declare peer-review records as confidential or privileged, while others may protect peer-review records from subpoena, discovery, or disclosure.

- **Are there other federal or state laws that might create a privilege over the documents being requested?** With some exceptions, federal laws protect the peer-review activities when the information has been provided to a qualified quality-improvement organization.[45]

- **Whose and what communications and information are protected?** The process and states vary widely here. Some states limit peer-review protection to physicians. Others designate the minutes and other reports as confidential but allow for independent discovery of information that was prepared and provided to the committee. Other states disallow as confidential any records created as the request of a peer-review committee.

- **What specific committees within the organization are considered protected?** Some state statutes protect the activities of medical-staff committees, while others protect only select committees such as peer review, quality improvement, and/or utilization review.

- **Who is seeking the records from peer-review activities?** Certain states allow physicians to access peer-review records when challenging peer-review activities.

- **What is the subject of the communication?** Generally speaking, most states require that for a peer-review record to be protected, it must be the subject of a quality review of patient care.

Incident Reports

According to the Agency for Healthcare Research and Quality (AHRQ), "Incident reporting in medicine takes many forms."[46] In general, however, an incident report is a record that is completed by a staff member or provider to record the details, circumstances, and/or witnesses to an unusual or untoward event that occurs within the healthcare facility to a patient, visitor, or family member. The purpose of the incident report is to document the exact details of the unusual or harmful event as soon as possible after the event, while the details of the occurrence are fresh in the minds of those who witnessed the event. Incident reports are useful tools for making decisions regarding liability issues that may stem from the event.

As a general rule, incident reports are protected from discovery. Even if they are not protected from discovery by state statute, the incident reports may be determined to be inadmissible as evidence under the hearsay rule. Incident reports serve not only to document the details, circumstances, and witnesses to an unusual event but also to alert defense counsel or insurers about potential liability issues that may arise at a future date. As is the case with records of peer-review activities, the first step in determining whether the records of the organization's incident reports are discoverable or admissible is to examine state statutory and case law for an understanding of how the statutes were applied by the court.

Similar to records of peer-review activities, incident reports hold significant evidentiary value to individuals and attorneys who are suing the organization for damages that may have occurred to them as a result of the untoward event. Therefore, the scope and application of any privilege that may protect incident reports from discovery is highly dependent on state law; the allegations contained in the lawsuit; and the nature, scope, and duties of the individual(s) responsible for reviewing the incident report, investigating the circumstances, and developing the report surrounding the event.

The Federal Rules of Civil Procedure (FRCP)[47]

The Federal Rules of Civil Procedure (FRCP) are a body of procedural regulations promulgated by the Supreme Court under 8 U.S.C. § 2072 (the "Rules Enabling Act"). The FRCP govern all civil actions in U.S. district courts and are designed to regulate judicial process and the manner by which cases are tried in a court of law.

Scope and Procedure for the E-Discovery Process

The scope and procedure for the process of discovery of information that may be relevant to litigation is contained in Rule 26 of the FRCP (Duty to Disclose; General Provisions Governing Discovery), which states:

"Unless otherwise limited by court order, the scope of discovery is as follows: Parties may obtain discovery regarding any non-privileged matter that is relevant to any party's claim or defense—including the existence, description, nature, custody, condition, and location of any documents or other tangible things and the identity and location of persons who know of any discoverable matter. For good cause, the court may order discovery of any matter relevant to the subject matter involved in the action. Relevant information need not be admissible at the trial if the discovery appears reasonably calculated to lead to the discovery of admissible evidence. All discovery is subject to the limitations imposed by Rule 26(b)(C)."[48]

Like the FRE, the FRCP are amended periodically by Congress. They underwent significant changes in 2006 and 2010 to address issues related to the discovery of electronically stored information in federal district courts.[49,50] The key 2006 FRCP amendments are summarized in Table 14-2.

2006 FRCP Amendments	Synopsis of Revisions/Change(s)
Rule 16(b)(5) and (6)	• The scheduling order entered under this rule includes provisions for disclosure or discovery of electronically stored information (ESI) and permits the parties to reach agreements for asserting claims of privilege or protection as trial-preparation material after production.
Rule 26(a)	• "Inventory, description and location of ESI" now states that initial disclosures during the meet and confer include a "copy of, or a description by category and location" of, relevant ESI. This "inventory" of ESI will also serve to help organizations that seek protection from burdensome e-discovery costs under Rule 26(b).
Rule 26(a)	• Rule was amended so the term "electronically stored information" has the same broad meaning as in Rule 34(a).
Rule 26(b)	• Scope of discovery now states that the scheduling order must include "provisions for disclosure or discovery of electronically stored information."
Rule 26(b)	• Created a two-tiered approach to the production of electronically stored information, making a distinction between information that is reasonably accessible and that which is not. Under the new rule, a responding party need not produce electronically stored information from sources that it identifies as not reasonably accessible because of undue burden or cost. If the requesting party moves to compel discovery of such information, the responding party must show that the information is not reasonably accessible because of undue burden or cost. Once that showing is made, a court may order discovery only for good cause, subject to the provisions of the current Rule 26(b)(i), (ii), and (iii). • Establishment of the two-tiered system seeks to provide a balanced, equitable approach in effort to resolve the unique problem presented by electronically stored information that is often located in a variety of places of varying accessibility—strongly favoring the production of relevant information from more easily accessible sources where possible.
Rule 26(b)(C)	• Establishes a balance between the costs and potential benefits of discovery. The committee notes expressly state: "The limitations of Rule 26(b)(C) continue to apply to all discovery of electronically stored information, including that stored on reasonably accessible electronic sources."
Rule 26(b)(5)	• Sets forth a procedure through which a party who has inadvertently produced trial preparation material or privileged information may nonetheless assert a protective claim to that material. The rule provides that once the party seeking to establish the privilege or work product claim notifies the receiving parties of the claim and the grounds for it, the receiving parties must return, sequester, or destroy the specified information.

Table 14-2   Summary of the Key 2006 FRCP Amendments

2006 FRCP Amendments	Synopsis of Revisions/Change(s)
Rule 26(b)(5)(A)	• Provides a procedure for a party that has withheld information on the basis of privilege or protection as trial-preparation material to make the claim so that the requesting party can decide whether to contest the claim and the court can resolve the dispute.
Rule 26(b)(5)(B)	• Provides a procedure for a party to assert a claim of privilege or trial-preparation material protection after information is produced in discovery in the action and, if the claim is contested, permit any party that received the information to present the matter to the court for resolution (i.e. "claw-back" provisions). Rule 26(b)(5)(B) is designed to work in tandem with Rule 26(f).
Rule 26(f)	• Established a requirement that the parties "meet and confer" early on in litigation to review and address issues related to the discovery of ESI. Rule 26(f) is designed to work in tandem with Rule 26(b)(5)(B).
Rule 34(a)	• Formally recognized electronically stored information (ESI) as a record and provides a mechanism by which a reviewing party has a right to "test or sample" ESI.
Rules 34(b) and 34(b)(ii)	• Amended to determine how ESI should be produced. The rule states that it is the requesting party—not the responding party—that requests "the form or forms in which electronically stored information is to be produced." • Rule 34(b)(ii) further states that if the request does not detail the form(s) of production, the responding party must produce it "in a form or forms in which it is ordinarily maintained or in a form or forms that are reasonably usable."
Rule 37(b)	• Authorizes the court to impose sanctions on a party for failure to comply with a discovery order. This provision gives courts the authority to sanction parties that destroy documents in direct violation of a discovery order.
Rule 37(e)	• Incorporated a "safe-harbor" limit on sanctions for the loss of ESI as a result of the routine operation of computer systems. This safe harbor prohibits courts from sanctioning parties who fail to produce documents "as a result of the routine, good-faith operation of an electronic information system."
Rule 37(f)	• Precludes federal courts from imposing discovery sanctions against a party for failing to produce electronically stored information that was lost as a result of the routine, good-faith operation of an electronic information system.
Rule 45	• Amended to conform to provisions for subpoenas to changes in other discovery rules, largely related to discovery of electronically stored information. Allows for the discovery of ESI from nonparties.
FORM 35 Report of the Parties' Planning Meeting	• Parties must develop and share their discovery plans with the court early in litigation—generally within the first 99 days of the case.

Table 14-2 Summary of the Key 2006 FRCP Amendments *(continued)*

Since the date of their enactment on December 1, 2006, the amendments to the FRCP have served as the structural foundation by which our nation's legal system is transitioning from paper-based discovery to electronic discovery. In 2010, the FRCP were amended once again—most notable was the revamping of Rule 26 because (a) it has significant impact on disclosures related to expert witnesses, and (b) a new rule—26(a)(C)—was added, which requires that expert witnesses disclose the subject matter of their testimony and summarize the facts and opinions to which they will testify at trial. The 2010 amendments are working to provide further clarity and direction for the legal industry in its transition from paper-based to digital discovery.[51] The key 2010 FRCP amendments are summarized in Table 14-3.

2010 FRCP Amendments	Synopsis of Revisions/Change(s)
Rule 8(c)	• Amended to delete "discharge in bankruptcy" from the list of affirmative defenses that must be asserted in a responsive pleading. This amendment conforms to Rule 8 of 11 U.S.C. § 524(a)'s requirement that a discharge in bankruptcy voids a judgment (to the extent the debtor's personal liability is a discharged debt).
Rule 26	• A new section was added to Rule 26, along with several amended sections that relate to reports from expert witnesses.
	• Rule 26(a)(C) applies to witnesses who do not provide a written report. The new rule applies to witnesses (a) who are not retained or specially employed to provide expert testimony or (b) whose duties as an employee of a party do not regularly involve giving expert testimony. Expert witnesses of these types (e.g., treating physicians or government accident inspectors) are required to disclose the subject matter of their testimony and summarize the facts and opinions to which they will testify at trial, but they are not required to submit a standard expert report.
Rule 26(b)(4)(B)	• For witnesses who must provide a written report under amended Rule 26(a)(B), the rule was further amended so that only facts or data considered by the witness in forming the expert opinion are discoverable. Prior to this amendment, testifying experts were required to disclose data or other information they considered even if the witness did not rely on or consider the information.
	• Rule 26(b)(4)(B) was amended to explicitly protect draft expert reports from disclosure. This change eliminates the need for parties to create their own agreements to protect drafts or, conversely, for the parties and the court to deal with disputes over whether these reports are discoverable.
Rule 26(b)(4)(C)	• Amended to protect all communications between counsel and testifying experts, except for communications related to the expert's compensation, facts or data provided by the lawyer that the expert considered in forming the opinions, and assumptions provided to the expert by the lawyer that the expert relied upon in forming an opinion.

Table 14-3   Summary of the Key 2010 FRCP Amendments

2010 FRCP Amendments	Synopsis of Revisions/Change(s)
Rule 56	• A complete rewrite and reorganization of Rule 56. The amendments address procedural issues related to summary judgment, including requiring a party asserting that a fact cannot be genuinely disputed to provide a "pinpoint citation" to the record; permitting submission of unsworn written declaration under penalty of perjury as a substitute for an affidavit; setting timeframes for submissions of motions; acknowledging a court's options, when a fact has not been properly supported by a party or responded to by an opposing party, to consider the fact undisputed, to grant summary judgment, or to afford a party the opportunity to amend; and clarifying a court's option to enter partial summary judgment.
FORM 52	• Amended for "technical and conforming" purposes. Serves as a template form for Report of the Parties' Rule 26 Planning Meeting. Adds provisions for disclosure on (a) the way that ESI will be handled in discovery or disclosure and (b) any agreements between the parties related to claims of privilege or work-product protection.

Table 14-3   Summary of the Key 2010 FRCP Amendments *(continued)*

Despite the 2006 and 2010 amendments, legal counsel and judges still struggle with issues associated with ESI and the discovery of information in today's digital era. It is not surprising, then, to understand how and why the 2006 and the 2010 FRCP amendments, coupled with widespread adoption of EHRs, are mandating the need for new HIT standards and approaches to support discovery of health information from EHR systems.

Furthermore, the 2010 amendments to Rule 26 demonstrate the important role expert witnesses have in both litigation and regulatory investigations. In addition, the Committee on Rules of Practice and Procedure of the Judicial Conference recognized that changes to the discovery process are necessary to reduce the costs and burdens associated with the time-wasting practices attorneys and experts undertake to avoid creating a discoverable expert record.

Duty to Preserve Relevant Evidence

Zubulake I–V[52] are a series of precedent-setting decisions handed down by Judge Shira Scheindlin from the Southern District of New York (S.D.N.Y.) that deal with the preservation and discovery of relevant evidence. In 2002, Laura Zubulake sued her employer, UBS Warburg, LLC, in federal district court for gender discrimination.[53] Zubulake was ultimately awarded a judgment against UBS Warburg of $29.2 million.[54,55]

The *Zubulake* decisions are precedent setting because significant portions of Judge Scheindlin's decisions were adopted in 2006 into the revised FRCP Rule 26. In addition, at the conclusion of the case the court established that organizations and their attorneys are responsible for implementing processes to effectively manage, disclose, and produce electronically stored information.

The *Zubulake IV*[56] opinion discusses when the duty to preserve ESI begins. Judge Scheindlin specifically stated as follows:

> The obligation to preserve evidence arises when the party has notice that the evidence is relevant to litigation or when a party should have known that the evidence may be relevant to future litigation.

In this case, the court held that the duty to preserve began at the latest on August 16, 2001, when Laura Zubulake filed her EEOC charge, but since the relevant people at UBS anticipated litigation in April 2001, the duty to preserve evidence essentially began at that time.

The *Zubulake I–V* opinions have relevance and significance to the healthcare industry. They suggest it is incumbent on all parties who may be involved in litigation to maintain, preserve, and protect electronically stored evidentiary material that is relevant and in anticipation of a lawsuit. In these opinions, the trial court addressed not only the duty to preserve evidence, such as emails and other electronically stored data, but also the duty to avoid spoliation of evidence. According to Judge Scheindlin, at the point when one "reasonably anticipates litigation," a prospective party to litigation has an affirmative duty to suspend its routine document retention and destruction policies and instruct employees to preserve any information that may be considered evidence in the case."[57]

With regard to courts' enforcement of the duty to preserve relevant information for a regulatory investigation, in 2010 The Sedona Conference published an updated commentary entitled *The Sedona Conference Commentary on Legal Holds: The Trigger and the Process,*[58] which states as follows:

> In enforcing the duty to preserve through spoliation sanctions, courts primarily rely upon their inherent powers, although Rule 37 also plays a limited role where a court order has been violated. A party that violates a preservation order or an order to compel production, or otherwise fails to preserve and produce information, may be exposed to a range of sanctions.

Preservation obligations may also be acknowledged and enforced because of statutes or regulations that are deemed to apply under the circumstances at issue. See *Byrnie v. Town of Cromwell Board of Education* ("Several courts have held that the destruction of evidence in violation of a regulation that requires its retention can give rise to an inference of spoliation."). Criminal penalties at the federal and state level may also be invoked in specific cases within the coverage of those laws. See, e.g., 18 U.S.C. § 1519 (Sarbanes-Oxley Act § 802).

Although the *Zubulake* decisions and the legal hold commentary from The Sedona Conference principally apply to cases heard in federal court, the guidance and experience from these examples can have a significant impact in the state courts, where a majority of healthcare cases are heard.

State court judges will rely upon these and a variety of other resources in making decisions related to discovery and preservation. Following are some examples of the resources available to state court judges:

- Discovery rules developed by state courts

- *Navigating the Hazards of E-Discovery: A Manual for Judges in State Courts Across the Nation* (produced by the Institute for the Advancement of the American Legal System (IAALS))[59]

- *Guidelines for State Trial Courts Regarding Discovery of Electronically Stored Information* (produced by the Conference on Chief Justices (CCJ))[60]

- *The Sedona Principles: Best Practices Recommendations and Principles for Addressing Electronic Document Production* (produced by The Sedona Conference)[61]

- *Managing Discovery of Electronically Stored Information: A Pocket Guide for Judges* (written by Rothstein, Hedges, and Wiggins of the Federal Judicial Center)[62]

- Committee on Rules of Practice and Procedures of the Judicial Conference of the United States[63]

- *Standards Relating to Civil Discovery* (produced by the American Bar Association (ABA))[64]

- *Uniform Rules Relating to the Discovery of Electronically Stored Information* (produced by the National Conference of Commissioners on Uniform State Laws (NCCUSL))[65]

- Seventh Circuit Electronic Discovery Pilot Program[66]

The first step, then, in determining whether the organization has a duty to preserve evidence in the face of threatened or impending litigation is to examine state statutory and case law for an understanding of how the statutes were applied by the court.

Establishing Legal Holds

As both the *Zubulake* opinions and The Sedona Conference commentary on preservation obligations provide, "The duty to preserve requires a party to identify, locate, and maintain information and tangible evidence that is relevant to specific and identifiable litigation. It typically arises from the common law duty to avoid spoliation of relevant evidence for use at trial and is not explicitly defined in the Federal Rules of Civil Procedure."[67]

At face value, the concept of when to preserve evidence and establish a legal hold is simple. "Once the organization reasonably anticipates litigation, all relevant information must be preserved."[68] However, as illustrated in Figure 14-2, although the legal hold is a simple concept, it is a complex process.

There are significant differences between paper-based medical records and electronically stored records and the process by which records and information are sequestered and managed in the face of a regulatory investigation or threatened or impending litigation. In the paper era, a legal hold process was reasonably straightforward—all relevant paper records were sequestered and locked into a file cabinet, where access was manually controlled and monitored.

In the digital realm, however, the legal process is not as simple and straightforward. The challenges lie not only in the dynamic and invisible nature of ESI but also in understanding who is responsible and when, where, and how to secure all relevant electronically stored information. Information that may be relevant to a regulatory investigation or litigation will exist in numerous locations and in various forms and formats (including paper). Unless the exact nature of the complaint or issue is known, it may be virtually impossible to secure all relevant electronically stored information at the time litigation is known or can be "reasonably anticipated." To complicate matters, "many of today's EHR systems lack the capacity to establish a basic legal hold."[69]

All healthcare organizations and providers have a duty, then (if they have not already done so), to begin working with their legal counsel to establish and develop their own internal litigation response plans. A component of such plans should include the identification of specific events or occurrences known as "litigation triggers," in which the organization or provider immediately identifies, preserves, and places a legal hold on all information (paper and electronic) that may be relevant to a regulatory investigation. Once an organization or provider has established a legal hold, a process should also be in place for ongoing review and monitoring of the status of the legal hold. Table 14-4 lists some examples of healthcare litigation triggers.

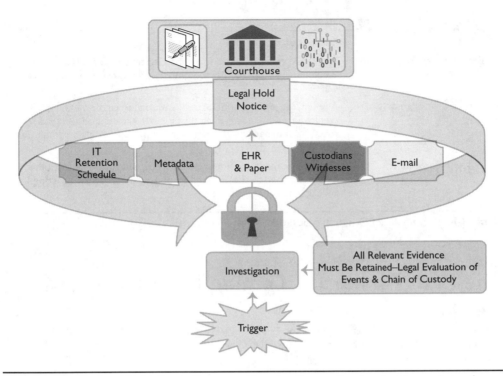

Figure 14-2 The Legal Hold: Simple Concept—Complex Process. Reprinted with permission from the American Health Information Management Association. © 2012 by the American Health Information Management Association.

Healthcare Litigation Trigger	Description
Incident reports and risk-management data	Accidents, falls, or other unusual events or losses occurring on the property resulting in the serious physical or psychological injury, harm, or loss to a patient, visitor, employee, or physician
Patient or visitor complaints	Credible threats from patients, family members, or visitors about the quality of care received or some other unusual or untoward event resulting in harm to person or property
Birth injuries	Newborns who suffer from injury or disfigurement as result of complications from delivery
Patient safety data	Injuries or harm to patients from medical devices, equipment failures, medication errors, or medical malpractice
Sentinel events	Process variations that require immediate investigation and response because the event carried significant risk of death or serious physical or psychological injury

Table 14-4 Examples of Healthcare Litigation Triggers

Healthcare Litigation Trigger	Description
Labor/employment disputes	Any legal notice received from the Department of Labor, Equal Employment Opportunity Commission, Workers' Compensation Carrier, etc.
Untoward or adverse events	Any untoward or unanticipated death occurring to a patient, visitor, employee, or physician. Examples include accidents, adverse drug reaction, improper medication administration, needle stick injuries, etc.
Employee complaints	Complaints made by employees to compliance hotline or human resources about issues related to patient care, regulatory compliance, labor, management, etc.

Table 14-4   Examples of Healthcare Litigation Triggers *(continued)*

The Path Forward: A Coming Together of Laws, Rules, and Regulations

The enactment of the American Recovery and Reinvestment Act (ARRA)[70] and the Patient Protection and Affordable Care Act (PPACA)[71] are bringing about an unprecedented sea change within the U.S. healthcare delivery system today.

The American Recovery and Reinvestment Act (ARRA)

ARRA makes possible two important infrastructure changes to the healthcare delivery system: (1) the widespread adoption of electronic health record (EHR) systems and (2) the establishment of the Nationwide Health Information Network (NwHIN).

The ARRA and PPACA landmark legislative efforts, coupled with the December 2010 report from the President's Council of Advisors on Science and Technology (PCAST) titled "Realizing the Full Potential of Health Information Technology to Improve Healthcare for Americans: The Path Forward,"[72] provide visibility and direction as to what the healthcare information infrastructure will look like and how it will operate.

The PCAST report maintains that NwHIN will serve to improve healthcare quality, reduce costs, and provide stronger patient privacy approaches as compared to today's current systems. The PCAST report also serves as a call to action and roadmap for the development of a "universal exchange language" and focus in 2013 and 2015 by the ONC and CMS on the development of meaningful-use guidelines to support the comprehensive ability to exchange health information.[73]

The vision outlined in the PCAST report as well as the ARRA, PPACA, HIPAA, and HITECH laws are now converging and overlapping with new and emerging regulations such as the FRCP amendments and the American Health Benefit Exchange (AHBE) care delivery. This is illustrated in Figure 14-3.

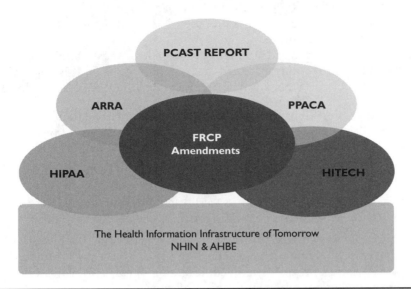

Figure 14-3 The Convergence of the FRCP with ARRA and PPACA. Reprinted with permission from the American Health Information Management Association. © 2012 by the American Health Information Management Association.

Health Information Technology for Economic and Clinical Health (HITECH) Act[74]

On January 8, 2009, in a speech at George Mason University, President-elect Barack Obama described the future of electronic health records (EHRs) and the electronic exchange of health information:

> To improve the quality of our health care while lowering its costs, we will make the immediate investments necessary to ensure that within five years, all of America's medical records are computerized. This will cut waste, eliminate red tape, and reduce the need to repeat expensive medical tests. But it just won't save billions of dollars and thousands of jobs—it will save lives by reducing the deadly but preventable medical errors that pervade our health care system.

On February 17, 2009, several weeks following that speech, the HITECH Act was signed into law as part of ARRA.

Approximately $31.2 billion was allocated by the Congressional Budget Office (CBO) to accelerate the adoption of EHR systems, with the assumption that the program will save an estimated $12 billion over a ten-year period, resulting in a net cost to the federal government of $19.2 billion.

The HITECH Act was enacted "to help save lives, lower costs, and improve the processes by which information is managed and communicated."[75] It is comprised of the following four major goals that advance the use of health information technology:[76]

- **Government oversight** Requires that the government take a leadership role in the establishment and development of standards to allow and promote nation-wide electronic data exchange to improve patient quality and care coordination

- **Investment in health information technology (HIT) infrastructure** Provided for a $19.2 billion net investment in health information technology along with Medicare and Medicaid incentives to substantially and rapidly increase EHR adoption to 90 percent for physicians and 70 percent for hospitals by 2019

- **Savings** Generated an estimated $12 billion in savings over a ten-year period, with additional savings to be generated in the healthcare sector through improvements in the quality and coordination of care and reductions in medical errors and inappropriate utilization of services

- **Establishment and enforcement of stricter federal privacy and security laws** Created new and enhanced privacy and security provisions to protect individually identifiable health information from misuse, along with breach-notification requirements for unsecured protected health information, with substantially increased penalties for noncompliance

As stated above, the HITECH Act substantially expanded the HIPAA Privacy and Security Rules and increased the penalties for violations of HIPAA. The expanded HIPAA Privacy Rule requirements established in the HITECH Act are summarized below:

- Provided that HIPAA privacy and security requirements apply directly to business associates

- Mandated federal security breach reporting requirements for HIPAA-covered entities and their business associates

- Created new privacy requirements for HIPAA-covered entities and their business associates, including new accounting requirements for EHRs, restrictions on marketing and fundraising, and other developments

- Established new criminal and civil penalties for noncompliance and new enforcement responsibilities

Security Breach Reporting Requirements

Section 13402 of the HITECH Act also established a new federal security breach reporting requirement for HIPAA-covered entities (CEs) and their business associates (BAs).[77] This section requires a covered entity that "accesses, maintains, retains, modifies, records, stores, destroys, or otherwise holds, uses, or discloses unsecured protected health information" to "notify each individual whose unsecured protected health information has been, or is reasonably believed by the covered entity to have been, accessed, acquired, or disclosed as a result of such breach."[78]

EHR Adoption within the United States[79]

In a 2012 report entitled *Health Information Technology in the United States: Driving Toward Delivery System Change,*[80] jointly published by the Robert Wood Johnson Foundation, Mathematica Policy Research, and the Harvard School of Public Health, researchers concluded that as of 2011, the adoption of basic electronic medical records (EMRs) or electronic health records (EHRs) varied greatly and significantly between the 50 states, as depicted in Figure 14-4.

Initial HITECH healthcare information infrastructure spending began in 2009 and increased considerably in 2010 and 2011 as EHR adoption rates began to increase by both physicians and hospitals throughout the country, as reported in this study.[81]

| State | Percentage | | State | Percentage | |
	Any System	Basic System		Any System	Basic System
United States	57.0	33.9	Missouri	57.0	32.9
Alabama	47.3	25.8	Montana	62.3	38.3
Alaska	59.2	29.5	Nebraska	58.5	35.6
Arizona	66.7	37.0	Nevada	52.5	23.0 †
Arkansas	51.2	24.5	New Hampshire	68.1 §	38.1
California	58.6	40.4	New Jersey	41.8 †	16.3 †
Colorado	65.8	36.0	New Mexico	54.1	27.8
Connecticut	61.9	31.5	New York	55.3	34.6
Delaware	59.5	36.5	North Carolina	58.0	31.1
D.C.	65.3	21.2 †	North Dakota	84.0 §	57.9 §
Florida	48.5	28.4	Ohio	58.9	31.6
Georgia	58.3	31.1	Oklahoma	54.7	28.2
Hawaii	71.0 §	46.8 §	Oregon	75.1 §	54.5 §
Idaho	52.6	24.5 †	Pennsylvania	50.6	27.3
Illinois	53.7	28.2	Rhode Island	43.8 †	29.2
Indiana	57.7	34.3	South Carolina	53.4	19.5 †
Iowa	73.1 §	48.6 §	South Dakota	55.4	41.2
Kansas	61.2	30.9	Tennessee	48.2	28.6
Kentucky	46.0	28.5	Texas	52.4	33.9
Louisiana	39.5 †	15.9 †	Utah	80.8 §	49.3 §
Maine	62.5	33.3	Vermont	66.8 §	35.7
Maryland	52.7	30.6	Virginia	59.5	29.1
Massachusetts	71.2 §	43.6	Washington	75.3 §	54.6 §
Michigan	51.9	29.5	West Virginia	52.9	28.2
Minnesota	77.6 §	60.9 §	Wisconsin	75.8 §	59.9 §
Mississippi	54.3	19.9 †	Wyoming	50.6	27.2

Source: Hsiao CJ, Hing E, Socey TC, Cai B. Electronic Health Record Systems and Intent to Apply for Meaningful Use Incentive Among Office-Based Physician Practices, 2001–2011. NCHS Data Brief, no. 79. Hyattsville, MD: National Center for Health Statistics, 2011.

† Significantly lower than national average (p<0.05).
§ Significantly higher than national average (p<0.05).
NOTE: EMR/EHR is electronic medical record/electronic health record.

Figure 14-4 Percentages of Office-Based Physicians Using Any EMR/EHR Having a Basic System by State as of 2011. © 2012. Robert Wood Johnson Foundation. Used with permission from the Robert Wood Johnson Foundation.

Health Information Technology in the United States: Driving Toward Delivery System Change is a four-chapter report that provides an overview of the status of EHR adoption in the United States, along with insights from the immediate past national coordinator for health information technology, David Blumenthal, about the effect technology will have on the healthcare delivery system and the progress made to date in the design and build of the nation's healthcare information infrastructure of tomorrow. The following paragraphs on EHR adoption by physicians (see Figure 14-5) and hospitals (see Figure 14-6) contain key statistical findings and graphical excerpts from that report.

Physicians

"Physicians reporting use of any EHR reached 57 percent in 2011, a substantial increase from 17 percent in 2002, while adoption of at least a basic system grew from 12 percent to 34 percent over the same time period. The rate of adoption of at least a basic EHR system increased more quickly among primary care physicians, younger physicians, practices of three or more physicians, and those in the Northeast region of the United States."[82]

"In 2011, 52 percent of all physicians indicated that they intended to apply for meaningful use incentives; however, only 10.5 percent reported both an intention to apply and an ability to meet the required functionalities."[83]

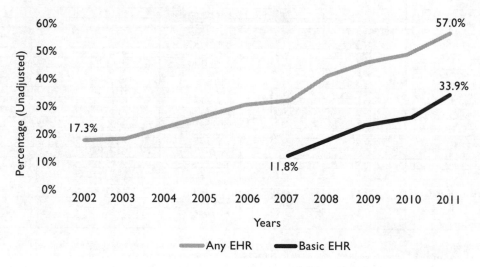

*Basic EHR defined as patient problem, medication, and allergy lists, history, and demographics; physician clinical notes; e-prescribing; and ability to view lab and imaging results electronically.

Figure 14-5 Percentage of Office-Based Physicians with EMR/EHR Systems: United States 2002–2011. © 2012. Robert Wood Johnson Foundation. Used with permission from the Robert Wood Johnson Foundation.

Hospitals

"Basic and comprehensive EHR adoption in U.S. hospitals has increased substantially between 2010 and 2011, with basic EHR adoption increasing from 11.5 percent to 18 percent and comprehensive EHR rising from 3.6 percent to 8.7 percent."[84]

"Adoption of at least a basic EHR increased more rapidly among the following groups of hospitals, as compared to their counterparts: larger organizations, teaching hospitals, and those located in an urban area."[85]

The Nationwide Health Information Network (NwHIN)[86]

The nationwide health information network (NwHIN) is defined as a "set of standards, services and policies that enable secure health information exchange over the Internet."[87] The ONC maintains that with broad implementation, the secure exchange of health information using nationwide health information network standards, services, and policies will help improve the quality and efficiency of healthcare for all Americans.

"The NwHIN will provide a foundation for the exchange of health information across diverse entities, within communities and across the country, helping to achieve the goals of the HITECH Act. This critical part of the national health IT agenda will enable health information to follow the consumer, be available for clinical decision making, and support appropriate use of healthcare information beyond direct patient care so as to improve population health."[88]

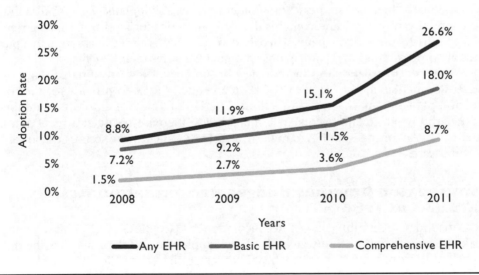

Figure 14-6 Changes in Adoption of Basic and Comprehensive EHRs in U.S. Hospitals: United States 2008–2011. © 2012. Robert Wood Johnson Foundation. Used with permission from the Robert Wood Johnson Foundation.

Since 2010, a group of federal agencies, local, regional, and state-level health information exchange organizations (HIOs) and integrated delivery networks, formerly known as the NwHIN Cooperative, has been helping to develop the network standards, services, and policies. Today, these organizations are demonstrating live health information exchange through the Nationwide Health Information Network Exchange.[89] The evolution of the NwHIN will be driven by not only by emerging technology, users, uses, and policies, but also through the enactment of new laws, rules, and regulations that will govern the use and exchange of electronically stored information.

As a result, the design and build of our nation's health information infrastructure requires that HIT professionals possess working knowledge of the laws, rules, and regulations governing the secure exchange of electronically stored information, as well as the discovery and admissibility of EHRs into a court of law. Given the nature and complexity of how EHR systems work, it is also conceivable that one day healthcare e-discovery will become its own unique job skill, and IT and health information management professionals will work alongside attorneys serving as expert witnesses who can explain where, how, and why an EHR or the electronic exchange did or did not contribute to improving a patient's quality of care.[90]

The Employee Retirement Income Security Act (ERISA)

The Employee Retirement Income Security Act (ERISA) of 1974 is a federal law that establishes the minimum standards for retirement and health benefit plans in private industry.[91] ERISA covers retirement, health, and other welfare benefit plans (e.g., life, disability, and apprenticeship plans) and contains detailed provisions for reporting to the government and disclosure to participants. There also are provisions aimed at assuring that plan funds are protected and that participants who qualify receive their benefits.

ERISA was also expanded to include new health laws. The Consolidated Omnibus Budget Reconciliation Act (COBRA) of 1986 amended ERISA to provide for the continuation of healthcare coverage (for a limited period of time) for employees and their beneficiaries when certain events arise that would otherwise result in a reduction in benefits. HIPAA amended ERISA to make healthcare coverage more secure and portable for employees.

Consolidated Omnibus Budget Reconciliation Act (COBRA) of 1986[92]

The Consolidated Omnibus Budget Reconciliation Act (COBRA) of 1986[93] is a groundbreaking law in that it not only gives displaced employees and their families the right to choose to continue their group health coverage in certain circumstances where their coverage under their health plan would normally end, but it also established the Emergency Medical Treatment and Active Labor Act (EMTALA),[94] which guarantees all individuals are afforded nondiscriminatory access to emergency care and to the healthcare system.

COBRA gives employees and their eligible dependents the right to remain in their employer's group coverage when they would otherwise lose coverage because of certain qualifying events. COBRA coverage is available for limited time periods, and the member must pay the full cost of the coverage plus an administrative fee. The member and/or dependent can increase or decrease their level of coverage. For example, the member can add dependents or elect coverage he or she did not have before.

COBRA and HIPAA Notices

Employers are required by federal regulation to notify all employees and dependents enrolling in their health plan of the federal provisions of the COBRA and HIPAA laws. The COBRA and HIPAA notifications are intended to inform employees of their rights and obligations under federal law and must be distributed to all new employees and their dependents. The initial COBRA notification and HIPAA notifications must be addressed and mailed to the employee and dependents to the address furnished by the employee within 90 days of enrollment.

Health Insurance Portability and Accountability Act (HIPAA)[95]

Ten years following enactment of the COBRA health insurance and EMTALA laws, on August 21, 1996, HIPAA, also known as Public Law 104-191, was signed into law as an amendment to the Internal Revenue Code of 1986 under COBRA. Sections 261 through 264 of HIPAA require the secretary of HHS to publicize standards for the electronic exchange, privacy, and security of health information. These standards collectively are known as the HIPAA Administrative Simplification provisions and are comprised of the following four parts:[96]

- Electronic transactions and code sets standards requirements
- Privacy requirements
- Security requirements
- National Identifier requirements

The HIPAA Administrative Simplification provisions now serve as the underlying framework and foundation for how all healthcare business transactions are conducted today. Each of the four parts is summarized below.

Electronic Transactions and Code Sets

Under HIPAA, electronic transactions involve the electronic exchange of information between two parties for a specific purpose. As put forth in the HIPAA regulations, the secretary of HHS adopted certain standard transactions for electronic data interchange (EDI) of healthcare data, along with a requirement that employers and providers process all transactions utilizing a unique identifier. Electronically changed data include claims and encounter information, payment and remittance advice, claims status, eligibility, enrollment and disenrollment, referrals and authorizations, coordination of benefits, and premium payment.

Under HIPAA, if a covered entity conducts one of the adopted transactions electronically, they must use the adopted standard—either from the Accredited Standards Committee X12 (ASC X12) or the National Council for Prescription Drug Programs (NCPDP), for certain pharmacy transactions. Covered entities must adhere to the content and format requirements of each transaction. HHS also adopted the following specific code sets for diagnoses, procedures, and drugs to be used in all healthcare transactions (electronic or paper-based): the Healthcare Common Procedure Coding System (HCPCS) for ancillary services/procedures, Current Procedural Terminology (CPT) for physicians procedures, Current Dental Terminology (CDT) for dental procedures, International Classification of Disease Revisions 9 and 10 (ICD-9, ICD-10) for diagnosis and hospital inpatient procedures, and the National Drug Code (NDC).

HIPAA Privacy Rule

"The *Standards for Privacy of Individually Identifiable Health Information* ('Privacy Rule') establishes, for the first time, a set of national standards for the protection of certain health information."[97] One of the major goals of the HIPAA Privacy Rule is "to assure that individuals' health information is properly protected while allowing the flow of health information needed to provide and promote high quality health care and to protect the public's health and well being."[98] The Privacy Rule was designed in this way to strike a balance between ensuring the important uses and disclosures of information and protecting an individual's right to privacy in seeking medical care and treatment.

HIPAA Security Rule

The HIPAA Security Rule is found in 45 CFR Part 160 Subparts A and C of Part 164. The HIPAA Security Rule established national standards to protect individuals' electronic personal health information that is created, received, used, or maintained by a covered entity while requiring that appropriate administrative, physical, and technical safeguards be put in place to ensure the confidentiality, integrity, and security of electronic protected health information.[99]

HIPAA National Identifier Requirements

The national provider identifier (NPI) is a unique identification number for all healthcare providers. In a health information exchange between HIPPA covered entities, the NPI essentially identifies which specific providers were involved in the care of the patient for that HIE transaction. The NPI is a unique ten-digit number that covered healthcare providers, health plans, and healthcare clearinghouses utilize for all electronic administrative and financial transactions. It is also intelligence-free, meaning that the numbers do not carry other information about healthcare providers, such as the state in which they live or their medical specialty. The NPI must be used in lieu of legacy provider identifiers in the HIPAA standards transactions. HIPAA requires that covered providers share their NPI with other providers, health plans, clearinghouses, and any entity that may need it for billing purposes.

The Patient Protection and Affordable Care Act (PPACA)

PPACA, conversely, is bringing about reforms in healthcare coverage, including (1) a mandate that all individuals maintain a minimal level of health insurance coverage, (2) the establishment of a prohibition against lifetime benefit limits, (3) coverage for preexisting health conditions for children, and (4) creation of the state-run American Health Benefit Exchanges (AHBE) program.

American Health Benefit Exchanges (AHBEs)

Just as the process by which healthcare organizations and providers respond to regulatory investigations or litigation is in its infancy, so too is the AHBE. Effective January 1, 2014, PPACA enables small employers and low- to moderate-income individuals to purchase affordable healthcare coverage through the establishment of state-based exchanges through AHBE. The secretary of HHS has broad authority to establish standards and regulations to implement the statutory requirements related to the state-based exchange.

To comply with PPACA, each state that elects to establish an exchange must adopt the federal standards in law and rule, and have in effect a state law or regulation that implements these standards.[100] If a state elects not to establish an exchange, PPACA requires HHS to establish and operate one in that state. This also applies in the event that HHS determines on review that state efforts to establish an exchange have not made sufficient progress to be fully operational by January 1, 2014. Figure 14-7 depicts the exchange options available to the states.

Exchange Options for States		
State-based exchange	**State partnership exchange**	**Federally-facilited exchange**
State operates all exchange activities; however, state may use federal government services for the following activities: • Premium tax credit and cost sharing reduction • Exemptions • Risk adjustment program • Reinsurance program	State operates activities for: • Plan management • Consumer assistance • Both	HHS operates; however, state may elect to perform or can use federal government services for the following activities: • Reinsurance program • Medicaid and CHIP eligibility: assessment or determination*

* Coordinate with Medicaid and CHIP Services (CMCS) on decisions and protocols

Figure 14-7 Exchange Options for States. Reprinted with permission from the National Conference of State Legislatures. © National Conference of State Legislatures.

Section 1302(b) of PPACA directs the secretary of HHS to specify the essential health benefits (EHBs) to be provided in the essential health benefits package that qualified health plans (QHPs) will be required to cover effective January 1, 2014.[101]

The secretary of HHS shall ensure that the scope of the essential health benefits is equal to the scope of benefits provided under a typical employer plan, as determined by the secretary. In order to do this, the secretary of the Department of Labor is responsible for conducting a survey of employer-sponsored coverage to determine the benefits typically covered by employers, including multiemployer plans, and providing a report on such a survey to HHS. The EHBs specified under PPACA Section 1302(b) are listed below:[102]

- Ambulatory patient services
- Rehabilitative and habilitative services and devices
- Emergency services
- Laboratory services
- Hospitalization
- Preventive and wellness services and chronic disease
- Maternity and newborn care
- Management
- Mental health and substance use disorder services, including behavioral health treatment
- Pediatric services, including oral and vision care
- Prescription drugs

According to CMS, the number of uninsured individuals in the United States is estimated to be reduced from 57 million to 23 million by 2019, as a result of the AHBEs.[103] The National Association of Insurance Commissioners (NAIC) and other stakeholders are working in close cooperation with HHS to establish and develop the standards for the AHBEs in order to realize that significant reduction.

On November 22, 2010, NAIC adopted a final version of the American Health Benefit Exchange Model Act (Model Act) for this purpose.[104] The Model Act contains definitions and guidance for general requirements and duties of the exchanges, but it does not provide specific options for governance. By 2014, the states are responsible for implementing what will ultimately become the final set of standards along with the insurance market reforms established in PPACA. If HHS determines before 2013 that a state will not have an operational exchange model by 2014 or will not be able to implement the required set of standards, HHS is required to establish and operate an exchange within the state. States operating an exchange before 2010 will be presumed to meet the standards, unless they are found to be out of compliance.

The Office of Personnel Management (OPM) is responsible for administering the states' health insurance exchange program, also known as multi-state plans (MSPs). The overriding principles and priorities that will guide federal funding and technical support are summarized as follows:[105]

- **Establishing a state-based exchange**   A planning process must drive state actions, by legislation or other means, to establish an exchange entity that meets the PPACA requirements. In the states that choose, now or at a later point in the process, not to establish an exchange, HHS will work with the state to establish the exchange.

- **Promoting efficiency**   Exchanges should be structured to have enough flexibility to respond to the local market conditions and take action to facilitate competition among plans on price and quality.

- **Avoiding adverse selection**   The OPM's authority to negotiate the terms and conditions of multi-state plans could result in MSPs susceptible to adverse selection. Adverse selection is a "phenomenon that is endemic to insurance of any kind, including health insurance. It occurs whenever people make insurance purchasing decisions based upon their own knowledge of their insurability or likelihood of making a claim on the insurance coverage in question."[106] For example, the OPM could create a lower benefit plan that results in disproportionately healthy enrollment whereas an MSP with extensive benefits might attract a sicker population. A successful exchange will avoid adverse selection. The states have been given the flexibility to provide consistent regulations inside and outside of the exchange to prevent adverse selection and HHS plans to work with states to maximize that flexibility.

- **Streamlined access and continuity of care**   States will be required to evaluate and determine eligibility for applicants in Medicaid, the Children's Health Insurance Program (CHIP), and other programs.

- **Public outreach and stakeholder involvement**   Exchanges will be responsible for an aggressive and multi-faceted outreach to inform the public of their services and coverage options.

- **Public accountability and transparency**   Exchanges will be required to provide public reports on their activities and additional reports using standardized data reporting on price, quality, benefits, consumer choice, and other factors that will help evaluate performance. They will also be responsible for providing the public with information on the performance of plans and automated comparison functions to inform consumer choice.

- **Financial accountability**   The exchanges will implement policies to prevent waste, fraud, and abuse; streamline enrollment; minimize acquisition expenses; and promote financial integrity.

The Emergence of Integrated Care Delivery Models

Although the Supreme Court found the provision that would permit HHS to withdraw all of the Medicaid funding provided to a state if that state chooses not to expand Medicaid to certain thresholds set forth in PPACA to be unconstitutional, PPACA nonetheless has laid forth the foundation for the establishment of new and evolving healthcare delivery models.

Accountable Care Organizations (ACOs)

On October 20, 2011, CMS finalized a new set of rules under PPACA designed to help physicians, hospitals, and other healthcare providers better coordinate care for Medicare patients through networks called accountable care organizations (ACOs). ACOs are groups of doctors, hospitals, and other healthcare providers who come together voluntarily to give coordinated, high-quality care to their Medicare patients.[107]

Patient-Centered Medical Homes (PCMHs)

Along with ACOs, the PPACA also provides support for the establishment of yet another evolving healthcare delivery model known at the patient-centered medical home (PCMH). The PCMH is a healthcare setting that facilitates partnerships between individual patients and their personal physicians, and when appropriate, the patient's family.

The AHRQ defines a medical home not as a place but as "a model of the organization of primary care that delivers the core functions of primary health care."[108] The PCMH model emphasizes the creation of a strong primary care foundation for the healthcare system, while the ACO model emphasizes the alignment of incentives and accountability for providers across the continuum of care.[109]

Technology: The Underpinning of the Nation's Health Information Infrastructure

The ACO and PCMH models as well as the future development of the AHBE are dependent on the effective use of EHR technology and the ability to exchange information electronically. Evidence of this can be found in one of the overriding principles and priorities guiding federal funding and technical support for the AHBE, which states as follows, "In order to be successful IT systems must be upgraded as well as other systems to support this process."[110]

As such, both the ARRA and PPACA laws set forth the rules, regulations, and legal bases in which these evolving structures will operate. Health information technology is the most promising tool providers and health plans have to conduct the sophisticated analytics and predictive modeling technologies—especially those focused on optimizing care management and quality reporting—that will be key to the future success of our nation's evolving care-delivery models in improving patient care and reducing cost.

The Rise of E-Discovery in Healthcare

According to a 2012 study by Kalorama Information, sales of EHR systems grew by 14.2 percent to reach a total of $17.9 billion in 2011.[111] Following in lockstep with EHR advancement is the electronic discovery marketplace. Currently, the discovery of electronically stored information is a $20-billion industry,[112] with sales of software products alone projected to reach $1.2 billion dollars by 2014.[113]

The discovery of electronically stored information is growing and evolving almost as rapidly as our healthcare information infrastructure.[114] This has been due in large part to the enactment of the 2006 and 2010 FRCP amendments, as well as the steady adoption of e-discovery rules in state courts. To date, roughly two-thirds of the state courts have established some form of e-discovery rules, with over 30 states adopting rules based largely on the 2006 FRCP amendments. For 2012, experts predict "the e-discovery market will remain interesting and dynamic."[115] Issues related to social media and managing information and e-discovery in the cloud will involve an application of a new technology-assisted review (TAR) technique called "predictive coding" for the identification and culling of potentially relevant information for litigation.

As a result, the changes to both the discovery process and the healthcare information infrastructure are now catching the attention of both the medical and legal professions. According to defense attorney Catherine J. Flynn, "electronic medical records can overwhelm—and often change—the course of a medical liability lawsuit."[116] As a result, due to the explosive growth in both the e-discovery marketplace and widespread adoption of EHRs, information technology with a focus on health e-discovery may become its own unique job skill.

Therefore, information technology (IT) and health information management (HIM) professionals will have vital roles in helping legal and compliance professionals preserve, search, cull, and produce information that may be relevant to litigation or regulatory investigations. They may also potentially serve as expert witnesses in litigation and regulatory investigations in helping attorneys and the courts assess and interpret the quality and integrity of the ICD, CPT, SNOMED, and LOINC (Logical Observation Identifiers Names and Codes) coded information contained in the patient's medical record.

Chapter Review

The ARRA and PPACA laws are overlapping and converging with the FRCP, HIPAA, and the HITECH Act to establish the health information and benefit exchanges of tomorrow. As a result, the healthcare industry has reached a critical junction in the design and build of our nation's health information infrastructure of tomorrow. It is important then, that all healthcare professionals understand the structure and sources of law in the United States and that the EHR serves not only as an important tool for providers in care delivery, but also as evidence that may be used in a court of law or to aid in a regulatory investigation.

Questions

To test your comprehension of the chapter, answer the following questions and then check your answers against the list of correct answers that follows the questions.

1. Which of the following is *not* one of the four primary sources of law within the United States legal system?

   A. Congress

   B. Federal and state statutes

   C. Decisions of the courts

   D. Federal and state constitutions

   E. Decisions and rules of administrative agencies

2. When does the duty to preserve relevant information for a regulatory investigation or litigation begin?

   A. When a legal hold notice is served upon the organization by the court

   B. When a subpoena is served upon the organization by the court

   C. When risk management notifies departments or individuals of their duty to preserve information

   D. At the time the organization knows or reasonably should know of its obligation to preserve information

   E. In accordance with the EHR system's retention and destruction schedule

3. Which of the following is *not* one of the four goals of the HITECH Act?

   A. Savings

   B. Investment in HIT infrastructure

   C. Government oversight

   D. Establishment and enforcement of stricter federal privacy and security laws

   E. Establishment of the AHBE

4. On June 28, 2012, the Supreme Court of the United States ruled that the individual mandate was constitutional. Which body of law is the Supreme Court referring to in this decision?

   A. HITECH

   B. PPACA

   C. HIPPA

   D. COBRA

   E. ERISA

5. Which of the following is *not* a cited benefit of EHR adoption?

    A. Increased safety/reduced duplication

    B. Available in an emergency

    C. Savings

    D. Tracking for protection

    E. Protected in disasters

6. Which of the following is *not* a cited risk of EHR adoption?

    A. Hackers

    B. Errors

    C. Identify theft

    D. Data loss

Answers

1. **A.** Congress is not one of the four primary sources of law. The four primary sources of law in the United States are federal and state constitutions, federal and state statutes, decisions and rules of administrative agencies, and decisions of the courts (also known as case law).

2. **D.** As the *Zubulake IV* decision states, "The obligation to preserve evidence arises when the party has notice that the evidence is relevant to litigation or when a party should have known that the evidence may be relevant to future litigation."

3. **E.** The establishment of the AHBE is not one of the four goals of the HITECH Act. The four main goals of the HITECH Act are government oversight, investment in HIT infrastructure, savings, and the establishment and enforcement of stricter federal privacy and security laws.

4. **B.** PPACA. The Supreme Court upheld the constitutionality of the "individual mandate" as a tax, and it found the provision that would permit the HHS secretary to withdraw all of the Medicaid funding provided to a state if that state chooses not to expand Medicaid to certain thresholds set forth in the Act to be unconstitutional.

5. **C.** Although EHRs have the potential to drive down healthcare costs and increase savings through increased safety and reduced duplication, that benefit was not specifically cited in the study, "Health Information Exchange and Health Information Technology Benefits and Risks."

6. **D.** Although data loss threats are very real through the use of EHRs, that risk was not specifically cited in the study, "Health Information Exchange and Health Information Technology Benefits and Risks."

References

1. Law.com definition of law. Accessed 7/20/2012 from http://dictionary.law.com/Default.aspx?selected=1111.

2. Litan, R. *The concise encyclopedia of economics: Regulation.* Accessed 7/20/2012 from http://econlib.org/library/Enc/Regulation.html.

3. Tutrani, N. (November 20, 2010). *The "right to privacy" and its constitutional evolution: The Ninth and Fourteenth Amendments,* p. 3. Accessed 7/22/2012 from www.regent.edu/admin/stusrv/writingcenter/docs/APSA7thedSamplePaper%28PoliticalScienceStudentWriter%27sManual%29.pdf.

4. Ibid.

5. Ratification of constitutional amendments. Accessed 7/22/2012 from www.usconstitution.net/constamrat.html.

6. Law.com definition of statute. Accessed 7/22/2012 from http://dictionary.law.com/Default.aspx?selected=2010.

7. Roach, W., Hoban, R., Broccolo, B., Roth, A., & Blanchard, T. (2006). *Medical records and the law, Fourth edition,* pp. 6–7. Jones and Bartlett Publishers, Inc.

8. Ibid., p. 7.

9. Ibid.

10. U.S. Constitution, Article 1, Section 1. Accessed 7/21/2012 from www.house.gov/house/Constitution/Constitution.html.

11. U.S. Constitution, Article 1, Section 8, Clause 18. Accessed 7/21/2012 from www.house.gov/house/Constitution/Constitution.html.

12. HHS web site. Accessed 7/21/2012 from www.hhs.gov.

13. FDA web site. Accessed 7/21/2012 from www.fda.gov.

14. IRS web site. Accessed 7/21/2012 from www.irs.gov.

15. *Patient Protection and Affordable Care Act.* Accessed 7/20/2012 from www.govtrack.us/congress/bills/111/hr3590/text.

16. *National Federation of Independent Business, et al. v. Sebelius, et al.* 132 S. Ct. 1133 (June 28, 2012). Accessed 7/21/2012 from www.supremecourt.gov/opinions/11pdf/11-210d4e9.pdf.

17. NLRB web site. Accessed 7/21/2012 from www.nlrb.gov.

18. Law.com definition of common law. Accessed 7/21/2012 from http://dictionary.law.com/Default.aspx?selected=248.

19. *Marbury v. Madison,* 5 U.S. (1 Cranch) 137 (1803).

20. Law.com definition of case law. Accessed 7/21/2012 from http://dictionary.law.com/Default.aspx?selected=148.

21. USA.gov web site. Accessed 7/21/2012 from www.usa.gov/Agencies/Federal/Legislative.shtml.

22. USA.gov web site. Accessed 7/21/2012 from www.usa.gov/Agencies/Federal/Executive.shtml.

23. USA.gov web site. Accessed 7/21/2012 from www.usa.gov/Agencies/Federal/Judicial.shtml.

24. U.S. Constitution, Article III, Section 1. Accessed 7/21/2012 from www.house.gov/house/Constitution/Constitution.html.

25. Federal Courts Resources. Accessed 7/21/2012 from www.uscourts.gov/FederalCourts.aspx.

26. State Court Resources. Accessed 7/21/2012 from www.uscourts.gov/EducationalResources/FederalCourtBasics/CourtStructure/UnderstandingFederalAndStateCourts.aspx.

27. HL7 International web site. Accessed 7/21/2012 from www.hl7.org.

28. HL7 EHR RM-ES Workgroup web site. Accessed 7/23/2012 from http://wiki.hl7.org/index.php?title=EHR_RM-ES#EHR_RM-ES_Resources.

29. Baldwin-Stried Reich, K., Ball, K., Dougherty, M., & Hedges, R. (2012). *E-discovery and electronic records,* p. 31. AHIMA Press.

30. Definition of differences between structured vs. unstructured data. Accessed 7/30/12 from www.coolinterview.com/interview/51736.

31. Health Information Security and Privacy Collaboration, Consumer Education and Engagement Collaborative of Colorado, Georgia, Kansas, Massachusetts, New York, Oregon, Washington, and West Virginia. (March 31, 2009). Health information exchange and health information technology benefits and risks. Accessed 7/30/12 from http://healthit.hhs.gov.

32. Emanuel, E. & Fuchs, V. (2008). The perfect storm of overutilization. *Journal of the American Medical Association, 299,* 2789–2791.

33. Definition of identity theft. Accessed 7/20/12 from http://idtheft.about.com/od/glossary/g/IDT-Definition.htm.

34. Rajakumar, M. Number and filing system. *Vision 2020 e-Resource.* Accessed 7/30/12 from http://laico.org/v2020resource/files/NumberandFilingsystem.html.

35. Vitello, Barbara. Lutheran General to pay $8.25 million in baby's death. *Daily Herald,* April 5, 2012. http://www.dailyherald.com/article/20120405/news/704059806.

36. Amendments to Federal Rules of Civil Procedure. Accessed 7/30/2012 from www.supremecourt.gov/orders/courtorders/frcv10.pdf.

37. Law.com definition of discovery. Accessed 7/30/12 from http://dictionary.law
.com/Default.aspx?selected=530.

38. Law.com definition of admissible evidence. Accessed 7/30/12 from http://
dictionary.law.com/Default.aspx?selected=2339.

39. The Federal Rules of Evidence. Accessed 7/30/12 from www.uscourts.gov/
uscourts/RulesAndPolicies/rules/2010%20Rules/Evidence.pdf.

40. Federal Rule of Evidence 502. Accessed 7/30/12 from http://federalevidence
.com/rules-of-evidence#Rule502.

41. Law.com definition of hearsay. Accessed 7/30/12 from http://dictionary.law
.com/Default.aspx?selected=858.

42. Baldwin-Stried Reich, K., Ball, K., Dougherty, M., & Hedges, R. (2012).
E-discovery and electronic records, p. 162. AHIMA Press.

43. Federal Rule of Evidence 803. Accessed 7/30/12 from www.law.cornell.edu/
rules/fre/rule_803#rule_902_11.

44. Wakefield, W. E. Annotation, *Physician-Patient Privilege Extending to Patient's
Medical or Hospital Records.* 10 A.L.R. 4th 552.

45. 42 U.S.C. Section 1320c-9. Accessed 7/30/12 from www.law.cornell.edu/
uscode/text/42/1320c-9.

46. Wald, H. & Shojania, K. G. AHRQ. Incident reporting. Accessed 7/30/12 from
www.ahrq.gov/clinic/ptsafety/chap4.htm.

47. FRCP web site. Accessed 7/30/12 from www.federalrulesofcivilprocedure.com/.

48. FRCP 26. Accessed 7/30/12 from www.law.cornell.edu/rules/frcp/rule_26.

49. 2006 FRCP Amendments. Accessed 7/30/12 from www.uscourts.gov/uscourts/
RulesAndPolicies/rules/EDiscovery_w_Notes.pdf.

50. 2010 FRCP Amendments. Accessed 7/30/12 from www.supremecourt.gov/
orders/courtorders/frcv10.pdf.

51. 2010 FRCP Amendments. Accessed 7/30/12 from www.uscourts.gov/uscourts/
RulesAndPolicies/rules/Supreme%20Court%202009/BK-Clean-Rules.pdf.

52. *Zubulake v. UBS Warburg, LLC.* 217 F.R.D. 309 (S.D.N.Y. 2003) (*Zubulake I*).
Zubulake v. UBS Warburg, LLC. 2003 U.S. Dist. LEXIS 7940 (S.D.N.Y. May 13,
2003) (*Zubulake II*). *Zubulake v. UBS Warburg, LLC.* 216 F.R.D. 280 (S.D.N.Y.
2003) (*Zubulake III*). *Zubulake v. UBS Warburg, LLC.* 220 F.R.D. 212 (S.D.N.Y.
2003) (*Zubulake IV*). *Zubulake v. UBS Warburg, LLC.* 229 F.R.D. 422 (S.D.N.Y.
2004) (*Zubulake V*).

53. *Zubulake v. UBS Warburg, LLC.* 217 F.R.D. 309 (S.D.N.Y. 2003) (*Zubulake I*).
Zubulake v. UBS Warburg, LLC. 2003 U.S. Dist. LEXIS 7940 (S.D.N.Y. May 13,
2003) (*Zubulake II*). *Zubulake v. UBS Warburg, LLC.* 216 F.R.D. 280 (S.D.N.Y.
2003) (*Zubulake III*). *Zubulake v. UBS Warburg, LLC.* 220 F.R.D. 212 (S.D.N.Y.

2003) (*Zubulake IV*). *Zubulake v. UBS Warburg, LLC.* 229 F.R.D. 422 (S.D.N.Y. 2004) (*Zubulake V*), *Supra*, Note 1.

54. *Zubulake v. UBS Warburg, LLC.* 229 F.R.D. 422 (S.D.N.Y. 2004) (*Zubulake V*).

55. Porter, Eduardo. UBS ordered to pay $29 million in sex bias lawsuit. *New York Times*, April 7, 2005. Accessed 8/3/12 from http://www.nytimes.com/2005/04/07/business/07bias.html

56. *Zubulake v. UBS Warburg, LLC.* 220 F.R.D. 212 (S.D.N.Y. 2003) (*Zubulake IV*), pp. 3–4. Accessed 8/3/12 from www.ediscoverylawalert.com/uploads/file/Zubulake%20v_%20UBS%20Warburg%20LLC.pdf.

57. *Zubulake V, Supra*, p. 22 footnote. Accessed 8/3/12 from http://discoveryresources.dreamhosters.com/wp-content/uploads/2008/05/zubulakev.pdf.

58. The Sedona Conference. (2010). *The Sedona Conference commentary on legal holds: The trigger and the process*, p. 268. A project of The Sedona Conference Working Group on Electronic Document Retention and Production (WG1). Accessed 8/3/12 from https://www.google.com/search?q=The+Sedona+Conference+Legal+Hold+Commentary&ie=utf-8&oe=utf-8&aq=t&rls=org.mozilla:en-US:official&client=firefox-a.

59. Institute for the Advancement of the American Legal System (IAALS). *Navigating the hazards of e-discovery: A manual for judges in state courts across the nation, Second edition.* Accessed 8/8/12 from http://iaals.du.edu/images/wygwam/documents/publications/Navigating_eDiscovery_2nd_Edition.pdf.

60. Conference of Chief Justices (CCJ). (2006). *Guidelines for state trial courts regarding discovery of electronically stored information.* National Center for State Courts.

61. The Sedona Conference. (June 2007). *The Sedona principles: Best practices recommendations and principles for addressing electronic document production.* A project of The Sedona Conference Working Group on Electronic Document Retention and Production (WG1). Accessed 8/8/12 from http://sos.mt.gov/Records/committees/erim_resources/A%20-%20Sedona%20Principles%20Second%20Edition.pdf.

62. Rothstein, B.J., Hedges, R.J., & Wiggins, E.C. (2012). *Managing discovery of electronic information: A pocket guide for judges, Second edition.* Federal Judicial Center (FJC). Accessed 8/8/12 from www.fjc.gov/public/pdf.nsf/lookup/eldscpkt2d_eb.pdf/$file/eldscpkt2d_eb.pdf.

63. Committee on rules of practice and procedures of the Judicial Conference of the United States, report to standing committee, Civil Rules Advisory Committee. (June 2–3, 2011). Accessed 8/8/12 from www.uscourts.gov/uscourts/RulesAndPolicies/rules/Agenda%20Books/Standing/ST2011-06.pdf.

64. American Bar Association (ABA). (August 2004). *Standards relating to civil discovery.* Accessed 8/8/12 from www.americanbar.org/content/dam/aba/migrated/litigation/standards/docs/103b_standards.authcheckdam.pdf.

65. National Conference of Commissioners on Uniform State Laws (NCCUSL). (2007). *Uniform rules relating to the discovery of electronically stored information.* Uniform Law Commission. Accessed 8/8/12 from www.nycourts.gov/ji/commercial-litigation/PDFs/4.b.%20NCCUSL%20Uniform%20Rules.pdf.

66. Seventh Circuit Electronic Discovery Pilot Program, Phase I and II. Accessed 8/8/12 from www.discoverypilot.com/.

67. The Sedona Conference. (2010). *The Sedona Conference commentary on legal holds: The trigger and the process*, p. 267. A project of The Sedona Conference Working Group on Electronic Document Retention and Production (WG1). Accessed 8/3/12 from https://www.google.com/search?q=The+Sedona+Conference+Legal +Hold+Commentary&ie=utf-8&oe=utf-8&aq=t&rls=org.mozilla :en-US:official&client=firefox-a.

68. Baldwin-Stried Reich, K., Ball, K., Dougherty, M., & Hedges, R. (2012). *E-discovery and electronic records*, p. 82. AHIMA Press.

69. Ibid., p. 83.

70. Public Law 111-5, 111th Congress. *American Recovery and Reinvestment Act of 2009*. Accessed from www.gpo.gov/fdsys/pkg/PLAW-111publ5/pdf/PLAW-111publ5.pdf.

71. Public Law 111-148, 111th Congress. *Patient Protection and Affordable Care Act.* Accessed from www.gpo.gov/fdsys/pkg/PLAW-111publ148/pdf/PLAW-111publ148.pdf.

72. President's Council of Advisors on Science and Technology (PCAST). (December 2010). Realizing the full potential of health information technology to improve healthcare for Americans: The path forward. Accessed 8/8/12 from www.whitehouse.gov/sites/default/files/microsites/ostp/pcast-health-it-report .pdf.

73. Ibid., p. 19. Accessed 8/8/12 from www.whitehouse.gov/sites/default/files/microsites/ostp/pcast-health-it-report.pdf.

74. Public Law 111-5, 111th Congress. *American Recovery and Reinvestment Act of 2009*, Title XIII: Health Information Technology Section 13001. Accessed 8/8/12 from www.hhs.gov/ocr/privacy/hipaa/understanding/coveredentities/hitechact.pdf.

75. Baldwin-Stried Reich, K., Ball, K., Dougherty, M., & Hedges, R. (2012). *E-discovery and electronic records*, p. 4. AHIMA Press.

76. Baldwin-Stried Reich, K. (2010). "E-discovery in healthcare: 2010 and beyond." *Loyola University School of Law, Annals of Health Law, Special Edition, 19*, 175. Accessed from www.ncbi.nlm.nih.gov/pubmed/21495567.

77. Public Law 111-5, 111th Congress. *American Recovery and Reinvestment Act of 2009*. 42 USC 17932 Section 13402, Notification in the case of a breach. Accessed 8/8/12 from www.hhs.gov/ocr/privacy/hipaa/understanding/coveredentities/hitechact.pdf.

78. Ibid.

79. Robert Wood Johnson Foundation, Mathematica Policy Research, Harvard School of Public Health. (2012). *Health information technology in the United States: Driving toward delivery system change.* Accessed 8/4/12 from www.rwjf.org/files/research/74262.5822.hit.full.rpt.final.041612.pdf.

80. Ibid. Accessed 8/8/12 from www.rwjf.org/files/research/74262.5822.hit.full.rpt.final.041612.pdf.

81. http://www.rwjf.org/files/research/74262.5822.hit.ex.summary.final041612.pdf.

82. Ibid., Executive summary. Accessed 8/4/12 from www.rwjf.org/files/research/74262.5822.hit.ex.summary.final041612.pdf.

83. Ibid., p. 3. Accessed from www.rwjf.org/files/research/74262.5822.hit.ex.summary.final041612.pdf.

84. Ibid.

85. Ibid.

86. Ibid.

87. Nationwide Health Information Network: Overview. Accessed 8/5/12 from http://healthit.hhs.gov/portal/server.pt?open=512&objID=1142&parentname=CommunityPage&parentid=4&mode=2.

88. Nationwide Health Information Network (NwHIN) definition. Accessed 8/3/12 from http://searchhealthit.techtarget.com/definition/Nationwide-Health-Information-Network-NHIN.

89. HHS. Definition of the Nationwide Health Information Network. Accessed 8/5/12 from http://healthit.hhs.gov/portal/server.pt?open=512&objID=1142&parentname=CommunityPage&parentid=4&mode=2.

90. Ibid.

91. Baldwin-Stried Reich, K. (May 2012). Trends in e-discovery: Four cases provide a glimpse of healthcare litigation's future. *Journal of AHIMA, 83,* 44–46. Accessed 7/30/12 from http://privacyandsecurityupdate.org/?p=481.

92. 29 U.S.C. Employee Retirement Income Security Income Program PL 112-90. Accessed 8/10/12 from http://uscode.house.gov/download/pls/29C18.txt.

93. Federal Register Part V. (May 26, 2004). 29 CFR Part 2590 Healthcare Continuation Coverage, Final Rule. Accessed 8/11/2012 from www.dol.gov/ebsa/regs/fedreg/final/2004011796.pdf.

94. Consolidated Omnibus Budget Reconciliation Act (COBRA) of 1986 Fact Sheet. Accessed 8/13/12 from www.dol.gov/ebsa/newsroom/fscobra.html.

95. Zibulewsky, Joseph. (October 2001). The Emergency Medical Treatment and Active Labor Act (EMTLA). *Proceedings (Baylor University Medical Center), 14,* 339–346. Accessed 8/13/12 from www.ncbi.nlm.nih.gov/pmc/articles/PMC1305897/.

96. HHS, OCR. HIPAA Administrative Simplification Regulation Text. Accessed 8/8/12 from www.hhs.gov/ocr/privacy/hipaa/administrative/privacyrule/adminsimpregtext.pdf.

97. CMS HIPAA 101 Informational Series. Accessed 8/17/12 from www.cms.gov/Regulations-and-Guidance/HIPAA-Administrative-Simplification/EducationMaterials/downloads/HIPAA101-1.pdf.

98. CMS HIPAA Privacy Brief. Accessed 8/17/12 from www.hhs.gov/ocr/privacy/hipaa/understanding/summary/privacysummary.pdf.

99. Ibid.

100. CMS HIPAA Security Rule Summary. Accessed 8/17/12 from www.hhs.gov/ocr/privacy/hipaa/administrative/securityrule/index.html.

101. NCSL – Section 1: Affordable Care Act Exchange Basics. Accessed 8/6/12 from www.ncsl.org/issues-research/health/american-health-benefit-exchanges.aspx#acabasic.

102. Rules and Regulations. (March 27, 2012). *Federal Register, 77.* Accessed 8/6/12 from www.gpo.gov/fdsys/pkg/FR-2012-03-27/pdf/2012-6125.pdf.

103. Center for Consumer Information and Insurance Oversight. (December 16, 2011). Essential health benefits bulletin. Accessed 8/6/12 from http://cciio.cms.gov/resources/files/Files2/12162011/essential_health_benefits_bulletin.pdf.

104. Foster, Richard S. (April 22, 2010). CMS memo. Accessed from www.cms.gov/ActuarialStudies/Downloads/PPACA_2010-04-22.pdf.

105. American Health Benefit Exchange Model Act, 11/22/10. Accessed 8/6/12 from www.naic.org/documents/committees_b_exchanges_adopted_health_benefit_exchanges.pdf.

106. NCSL NAIC American Health Benefit Exchange Model Act, Principles and Priorities. Accessed 8/8/12 from www.ncsl.org/issues-research/health/american-health-benefit-exchanges.aspx#p_and_p.

107. Adverse Selection Issues and Health Insurance Exchanges Under the Affordable Care Act. Adopted by the Exchanges (B) Subgroup. 6/17/11. Accessed 9/26/12 from http://states.naic.org/documents/committees_b_110622_adverse_selection.pdf

108. Definition of ACO. Accessed 8/2/12 from www.cms.gov/Medicare/Medicare-Fee-for-Service-Payment/ACO/index.html?redirect=/ACO/.

109. AHRQ. Definition of PCMH. Accessed 8/2/12 from http://pcmh.ahrq.gov/portal/server.pt/community/pcmh__home/1483/PCMH_Defining%20the%20PCMH_v2.

110. Rittenhouse, D. R., Shortell, S.M., & Fisher, E.S. (December 10, 2009). Primary care and accountable care: Two essential elements of delivery-system reform. *New England Journal of Medicine, 361*, 2301–2303.

111. NCSL. Overriding principles and priorities guiding federal funding and technical support. Accessed 8/6/12 from www.ncsl.org/issues-research/health/american-health-benefit-exchanges.aspx#p_and_p.

112. Kalorama Information. (March 13, 2012). EMR 2012: The market for electronic records. Accessed 8/17/12 from www.healthdatamanagement.com/news/ehr-electronic-health-records-meaningful-use-kalorama-44184-1.html.

113. Adrogué, S. & Baker, C. (February 6, 2012). The evolution and explosion of e-discovery will continue in 2012. *Law Technology News* (LTN). Accessed 8/17/12 from http://www.law.com/jsp/lawtechnologynews/PubArticleLTN.jsp?id=1202541317297&slreturn=20120717222613.

114. The Radicati Group, Inc. (October 11, 2010). Press release announcing "eDiscovery Market, 2010–2014" study. Accessed 8/17/12 from www.marketwire.com/press-release/The-Radicati-Group-Releases-eDiscovery-Market-2010-2014-Study-1332596.htm.

115. Baldwin-Stried Reich, K. (May 3, 2012). Testimony provided to Illinois Health Information Exchange (ILHIE) Data Privacy and Security Committee. Accessed 8/17/12 from www2.illinois.gov/gov/HIE/Documents/Kimberly_BaldwinStried_Reich_ILHIE_DataPrivacySecurityTestimony_May_3_2012_FINAL.pdf.

116. Buckles, G., Murphy, B., Tomlinson, M., & Velasco, J. (December 15, 2011). E-discovery trends: 2011 year in review & forecasting 2012. *eDiscovery Journal*. Accessed 8/17/12 from http://ediscoveryjournal.com/reports/?mode=edj-reports&id=1.

117. Gallegos, A. (March 5, 2012). Legal risks of going paperless. Accessed from www.ama-assn.org/amednews/2012/03/05/prsa0305.htm.

PART III

Healthcare Business Operations

Michael Beller, Editor

Core HIT Functionality

Thomas Payne

In this chapter, you will learn how to
- Describe an electronic medical record (EMR) and what it is used for
- Describe the functionality of an EMR
- Explain how EMRs are likely to change in the future
- Understand how various healthcare information systems interact with EMRs

An electronic medical record is a computing system that contains individuals' medical records and provides rich functionality to support the delivery of care in a healthcare entity. The EMR replaces the existing method of maintaining paper medical records and broadens the scope of medical recordkeeping because it goes beyond this to include many other functions and features that were not possible using paper. However, the EMR does share the same medical legal requirements for documenting and delivering healthcare as paper records.

Most people in the healthcare industry use the terms "EMR" and "electronic health record (EHR)" interchangeably; in this chapter, I will use the term "EMR." It is important to point out that some people make the distinction that EHR represents the record of the patient over many episodes of care in many different locations over the course of their life. In this way, an EHR can be viewed as different from an EMR, which is usually a representation of the record generated and collected in one individual clinic, hospital, or healthcare organization.

I used the term "system" in the definition of EMR because an EMR is not a single computing program but rather comprises many different computing applications and databases linked together to meet the needs of the delivery of healthcare. An EMR is more complex than a single computer program because of these different components and their need to synchronize with each other. For example, there are connections to external systems such as the laboratory, connections to devices and terminal servers used to deliver functionality to the point of care, and many other components. Elsewhere in this book you'll learn more about the complexity of health information technology systems including EMRs. This chapter will concentrate on the specific functionality of EMRs.

In small practices, if there is a clinical EMR, there may also be a practice management system used for registration and scheduling and perhaps a common or separate billing system. In hospitals, there may be dozens of computing systems beyond the EMR. These are interconnected with a network, sometimes using an interface engine. A master patient index and admission/discharge/transfer system may be a separate system or integrated with the EMR. You can find a broader description of clinical computing system architecture elsewhere.[1]

EMR Functionality

Fundamentally, the EMR is the place where everyone involved in a patient's care records and accesses information about the patient. As you have learned, the EMR is much more than a repository: you use its functionality to deliver care. The breadth of EMR functionality varies, but a report from the Institute of Medicine provides additional detail on which this chapter is based.[2]

Health Information and Data

A basic requirement of an EMR is the ability to store notes and review results such as laboratory, radiology, and other testing results. Managing this functionality is more challenging than it might seem because there is so much medical information relevant to a person's health that clinicians are at risk for missing important information if systems are difficult to navigate or don't contain the entire medical history.[3] Therefore, the display, summarization of patient information, and methods to draw attention to important data are extremely critical to the delivery of care. Without thoughtfully designed methods to store, manage, and display information, the EMR does not serve the needs of the patient well because the information needed is not available in the right place at the right time.

Results Review

Summarization, tables, display of normal ranges and highlighting if results are outside of those ranges, and many other features are important to the success, safety, and efficient use of the EMR. Some data, such as numeric results of a complete blood count, may be amenable to being displayed in a spreadsheet-like format with the ability to view and graph trends. Other results such as microbiology may be best seen and understood in textual reports. Important considerations are whether, and how, to indicate results that are pending but not yet available and how to show microbiology results from specimens that were obtained a week ago but now have results. Figure 15-1 shows an example of a patient information summary screen from an EMR which gives a global picture of the patient's data in summary form, and Figure 15-2 shows an example of a results flow sheet from an EMR which provides trended information on a patient's laboratory results.

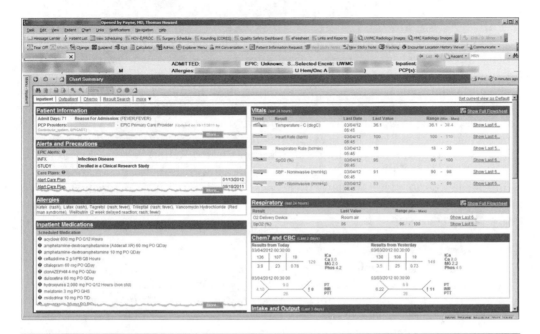

Figure 15-1 Example of a summary screen from an EMR. Reprinted with permission from Cerner Corporation. © 2012 Cerner Corporation. All rights reserved.

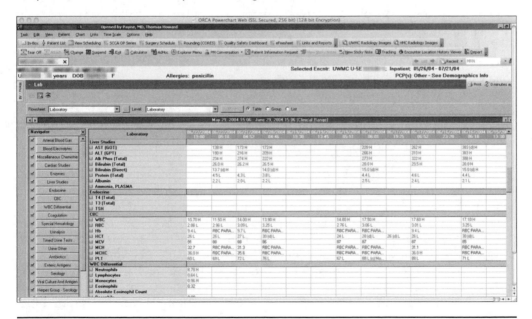

Figure 15-2 Example of a results flow sheet from an EMR. Reprinted with permission from Cerner Corporation. © 2012 Cerner Corporation. All rights reserved.

Results Management

A seemingly basic yet important function of an EMR is results management. In addition to storing and displaying data, most EMRs use a message box (sometimes referred to as an *inbasket* or *inbox*). This functionality draws attention to results that the user may have particular interest in seeing. For example, if the clinician ordered a hematocrit, results of the hematocrit would come back to the user in this part of the EMR. This saves the user the trouble of remembering the test was ordered and finding the results in the chart of the patient. The user can look in the message box to find this result and, if necessary, compare it to previous results for the same patient. The message box is also where notes created by another clinician after a clinic visit or hospitalization can be sent for the user to review. Because there are so many results and documents to review in the course of a busy day, the design, efficiency, and speed of the message box are very important to clinicians.

Documentation

Documentation is one of the most fundamental aspects of the medical record. *Documentation* refers to the notes created during or after an office visit, daily progress notes, procedure notes after an operation or other procedure, discharge summaries for a hospitalized patient, and many other types of notes to document care provided to the patient. Documentation is important because it allows all of the people involved in a person's care to understand what has happened during previous visits and understand what the plans for future care are. If the patient was found to have cancer, there may be a note by an oncologist who recommends a course of care such as chemotherapy, which is carried out in a series of visits. Each of these visits may have a note that describes progress and response to therapy including complications. Over time these documents represent the story of the patient's health, disease, and treatment along with the details that are needed for good care.

Documentation is also extremely important because it is one of the primary mechanisms used for clinician and facility reimbursement for care provided in the United States. It is also an important source of information about the quality of care that was delivered. In short, documentation of patient care is one of the key elements of the EMR.

Some health professionals—for example, hospital registered nurses—may document using forms or a spreadsheet-like format into which patient vital signs, intake and output, or values quantifying a patient's pain level or other measures may be entered. These numeric, or "structured," data fields represent a valuable form of documentation that supplements narrative text, because they make it easy to see trends over time and to quickly ascertain whether treatment goals are being met. Other professional disciplines may also use a table format for their documentation, such as respiratory therapists and physical therapists. One of the values of an EMR is that everyone involved in the patient's care can see the perspective and observations of colleagues from other professions.

EMRs should permit the collection of documents in the record to be read quickly, organized, and sometimes summarized. Equally, or even more importantly, are EMR tools for creating notes. Since the act of documenting care represents a large percentage of the workday for physicians and other healthcare professionals, the speed, efficiency, and clarity of the documents created using them are very important elements of EMR functionality. Methods for documenting care include using traditional dictation and transcription, typing with a keyboard, using voice recognition software, using a template where the user can "point and click" to build a note via a mouse to choose pre-defined options, and combinations of all of these methods. Many EMRs also facilitate the incorporation within the note of previously documented information such as allergies, medications, problems, and other discrete elements of the medical record. The EMR also needs to assist in the life cycle of the documents within it.[4] Notes may start in draft form, permitting review by the author and, in academic settings, by those who may be overseeing care such as an attending physician working with a medical student or resident. This approach allows signing and authentication of the document, adding addenda if necessary, and then permitting the final document to be communicated electronically or by other means to those whom may need to see it. In short, functionality to document care is one of the most important functional requirements of an EMR.

Order Entry and Management

Entering, managing, and communicating orders are other key features of an EMR. In its simplest form, order entry functionality permits an order to be electronically entered and transmitted to the service or person who will fulfill the order. In reality, the process is usually more complex. The term "ordering conversation" has been used to describe the give-and-take between the ordering clinician and the order recipient, and it is also an excellent opportunity for applying clinical decision support.[5] The electronic entry of orders by the ordering clinician is referred to as *computerized practitioner order entry* (CPOE). The definition of CPOE is that the person requesting the order also enters that order electronically. This distinguishes CPOE from the more common scenario where orders are written on paper and entered into the computer system by a clerk or other assistant. CPOE is one of the most complex and difficult elements of an EMR to design and to implement for many reasons.

- Most clinicians are used to the paper-based process where others clarify and enter complex orders.
- There is a high volume of orders written throughout the care of the patient.
- There is a wide diversity of the orders.
- Order accuracy is critically important (right order on the right patient).

Entering orders for cancer chemotherapy drugs is a good example of this complexity and helps highlight the risks of CPOE if not used correctly. Chemotherapy drugs can cure cancer; however, the margin of error is small, and any amount greater than the recommended dose can be highly toxic. The difference between helping and harming the patient is in part related to the dose given. If an error is made in selecting the appropriate dose, there can be serious implications for the patient.

Medication reconciliation is a hot topic in EMR functionality because it is so important yet can be so time-consuming. The term "medication reconciliation" refers to the review of the list of medications a patient is taking before and after a transition, such as admission to the hospital, at the time of a clinic visit, or at the time of transfer from one level of care in the hospital to another. It is tricky because there may be many medications, and the clinician (usually the physician) has to decide to continue or stop each medication and also confirm with the patient that the lists accurately reflect what is being taken. So, a lot of information is absorbed and acted on in a short time. How long this takes and how logical it is to use the functionality for medication reconciliation is an important factor in whether the clinician is happy with the EMR.

 TIP CPOE highlights one of the very important criteria for successfully implementing EMRs: how long it takes to use the EMR is of paramount importance to clinicians. Many clinicians count the number of "clicks" it takes to place an order, and their satisfaction is directly related to that number. If it takes too long or too many clicks to enter an order, write a note, review data, or perform any other function, then clinician acceptance and adoption of the EMR will be impacted. It is extremely difficult to design systems that are safe, accurate, and also fast to use. CPOE functionality is a great example of this challenge.

After orders are written, they are normally immediately available electronically to the laboratory, pharmacy, radiology department, bedside nurse, or other receiving service so that the order can be carried out. There are often additional actions required by the order recipient to clarify or select an alternate order from the original. This is one of the reasons that clinical decision support has the potential to be so helpful, because that feedback or those alternate orders can be suggested at the time the order is being written or immediately thereafter.

Decision Support[6,7]

This brings me to the topic of decision support. One of the core benefits of CPOE is ensuring patients are not prescribed medications they are allergic to. With CPOE, if there is an allergy to the medication ordered, the clinician can make a correction to the order and select an alternative medication. This can be done with only a minimal delay in treatment. While there are often later stages of the order entry process where the error might be caught (pharmacy or nursing), decision support at the point of order entry facilitates a more efficient process that is less reliant on downstream clinicians who then have to communicate with the ordering provider. Decision support serves an important role to prevent mistakes from happening.[8] More generally, decision support can influence the decision making that leads to orders. For example, if there is a constellation of findings and laboratory results that suggest a certain syndrome, that syndrome can be brought to the attention of the clinician so that it can be considered or further investigated. Other examples of decision support are pop-up reminders to prompt for the delivery of preventive care such as immunizations, cancer screening, laboratory tests to monitor drug treatment, and many other needed interventions. Clinical decision support is even broader than this. A template for writing a note can be thought of as a form of decision support because the template might include prompts to gather information when taking the history from patient. Links to external references that can supplement the clinician's knowledge of a condition is another form of decision support.[9] Clinical decision support is a very broad topic and is one that has received considerable attention in the medical informatics community. It is also a key element of EMR design and can be found in many areas of functionality of the EMR.

Electronic Communication

Healthcare is rarely delivered by one single person but by people working together in teams. The interaction and communication among the people working together to support a patient are extremely important. When the patient receives less than optimal care, the cause can often be traced to a problem or breakdown in communication. How an EMR handles the creation and routing of electronic communication is yet another key component of an EMR. (This includes communication with the patient—more on this in the following section.)

Communication can be supported in a variety of ways. There may be features to send messages that are analogous to electronic mail but securely within the confines of the EMR. This permits one person on the care team to send a secure message to another. Other communication tools include the ability for a patient or a referring physician to use web-based access to review results or reports. Usually when a web application is used, there are provisions for the clinician who ordered the test to offer comments on the results or reports they interpret such as "These are improved from last time" or "We need to discuss these results. Please make an appointment."

Use Case 15-1: Improving Medical Care in an Emergency Situation

This use case provides a "real-life" example of how EMRs can directly support and improve medical care in an emergency situation.

A 47-year-old male was brought to a medical center by helicopter after extraction from a car after a high-speed motor vehicle accident. Paramedics on the scene and during transport had access to his medical history through a radio link with an emergency room physician who accessed the patient's EMR. Knowledge that the accident victim had received a bone marrow transplant for lymphoma three years ago, including which medications he was allergic to, permitted in-field treatment and allowed him to be safely given blood products appropriate for his needs soon after he arrived in the emergency room. Information on who had treated him and where, his surgical history, and other information was immediately available through the EMR. Decision support through CPOE alerted clinicians to prescribe safely when minutes were critical. Notes written during and after resuscitation in the emergency room and his computed tomography (CT) scan images were available 30 minutes later to surgeons in the operating room. The patient's EMR record stacked the odds in his favor. After recovery, the entire record was available to his surgeon and oncologist in the clinic.

Administrative Processes

There are considerable administrative burdens related to the delivery of care including billing, tracking insurance coverage, auditing the record, and many other requirements. Each of these is a complex area and may be handled by separate modules or software apart from the EMR. However, the EMR should be able to support these requirements and others. For example, in the United States, payment for care includes a professional fee charged by the physician or other practitioner and a facility charge. Both have well-documented requirements, regulations, and laws that govern them. The EMR needs to support these requirements so that appropriate reimbursement can be received. These include, but are not limited to, tracking appointments and encounters, keeping up with insurance coverage changes, completing documentation, generating reports needed for measuring and improving quality, and meeting regulatory requirements. Both facilities and clinicians run the risk of audits and other legal actions if the EMR does not support their charges.

Population Management

While patients are usually seen one at a time, considerable care and education can be delivered more efficiently to a collective group of patients. The practice team or physician may have the responsibility to manage the care of a collection (or population) of individuals. A population may be defined by the practice that serves them or by a condition they share, such as diabetes mellitus. The ability to view and manage the defined population of patients and see how the plan of care has been adhered to by each of them is becomingly increasingly important. Some but not all EMRs support population management to various degrees.

Providing population management includes tools such as registries (lists of patient with common characteristics and tools to manage their care), plans of care, the ability to query to see who has a condition or might be taking a certain medication and needs intervention, and finally teams organized to deliver care.[10] As methods of reimbursement for healthcare change, it is likely that practitioners will be at risk for the care of groups of patients and that reimbursement will be tied to this rather than solely linked to the delivery of service for one patient at a time.

Support of the Patient/Person

It is widely understood that the true owner of the information contained in the electronic record is the person. Healthcare institutions are custodians of the EMR, and every person has a right to view their own record. With paper-based charts, the challenge has been the cumbersome sharing of, and associated expense of copying for, both patients and other clinicians to have access to the record. EMR features can help address this. For example, using a secure web link, patients can be permitted to view certain sections of the medical record such as results and to send messages to their care team. More broadly, there may be functionality to permit the patient to schedule appointments; read about their condition from a credible source; be reminded of tasks, tests, or other activities that are important to their health; and receive support from peers or others with the same condition. Social networking features are new to EMRs but hold promise just as they do in other aspects of our society. I do not discuss personal health records in this chapter, but you are encouraged to learn more about them.[11]

There are varying views and questions regarding how patients should be involved with their own record.

- Should patients view the entire record in real time as it is created?
- Should the creation of a progress note be a cooperative process?
- Who besides the patient could or should have access or contribute?

These, and many others, are the important questions that are being investigated. Many feel that the record is the property of the patient, and creation of the permanent record should include the patient. There is interesting research about a first step toward this goal, which is to permit the patient access to see parts of the record just as the doctor does. While this seems to be common sense, in reality making it simple for patients to see their own record is somewhat controversial. Support of the patient by the EMR is an area that is growing rapidly.

Other Health Information Technology Systems Commonly Used Within Healthcare Organizations

Though the EMR is the central healthcare IT system used in most healthcare organizations, frequently many other systems that interact with the EMR are also used to support the organization, particularly in hospitals and large organizations.

The *admission, discharge, transfer (ADT) system* tracks the location and movement of patients within an organization and communicates with the EMR and departmental systems, conveying information on bed, hospital ward location, care team, attending physician, and other information. They may be separate systems connected to the EMR using HL7 interfaces or may be integrated with the EMR and with the registration system.

The master patient index (MPI) may also be a separate system or integrated with ADT, with registration, or with the EMR. The MPI serves the critical role of establishing the identity of the person within the healthcare IT system, including and especially the EMR. Names, name spelling, and electronic identifiers used in the EMRs and departmental systems may vary, but it is critical that all data be tied to the correct individual to avoid duplicate records for the same person or erroneously including results for two people in one record.

Departmental systems often exist for radiology, the clinical laboratory, pathology, and many other departments. The departments, also known as *ancillaries* or *essential services*, are often very large and complex with information management needs met by one or more specialized departmental systems. For example, in radiology there may be a *radiology information system (RIS)* to manage scheduling, imaging reports and other operations, and a *picture archiving and communication system (PACS)* to manage images. The laboratory may have separate systems for chemistry, hematology, microbiology, and other roles or a single laboratory system for all of these and more. Most pharmacies depend heavily on automation; *pharmacy systems* may be further divided between inpatient pharmacy, retail (or outpatient pharmacy), inventory tracking, and other systems, or the organization may have a single pharmacy system to meet all of these needs. The financial and quality function of a healthcare organization likely has its own computing systems for assigning codes to a hospital stay and submitting both facility and professional fees to payers. *Decision support system (DSS)* applies to a wide variety of functionality to aid in business, strategic, clinical, quality, and research decision making. With growth in healthcare IT, DSS systems are growing rapidly.

There may be many other systems within a healthcare organization. The overall design and architecture of healthcare IT systems are for this reason extremely important so that information can be communicated between them as needed, their functionality is fully leveraged, and organizational and national standards are maintained for the data they contain. The architecture of organizational healthcare IT is described elsewhere in this book.

 CompTIA EXAM TIP The concept of patient tracking at first blush seems almost silly. Don't healthcare professionals know where their patients are at all times? You would be surprised. In today's fast paced and multifaceted ambulatory and emergency settings, and even some inpatient settings, patients move from room to room, are sent to receive a diagnostic image, or need to be quickly found by a technician or phlebotomist. For example, the ADT (Admission, Discharge, Transfer) module of an EHR tells us Ms. Jones is on 4SE in room 321 bed 2, but patient tracking software can tell us that right now she is in the radiology department for her CT. That detail of tracking information can be invaluable for nurses and other staff. Other ways patient tracking software can help is by assisting the healthcare worker to determine things such as room availability, patient checked-in or registration status, treatments ordered, why the patient is waiting excessively, and more. This class of software facilitates decreased waiting times in emergency rooms and other desirable healthcare organization efficiency outcomes.

Frequently Asked Questions

The following are answers to frequently asked questions.

What Does CPOE (and CPOM) Stand For?

CPOE stands for computerized practitioner (or provider) order entry. The *p* stands for practitioner or provider rather than just physician, because licensed practitioners, nurses, and pharmacists can also enter orders. Another acronym occasionally used is CPOM, where the *m* stands for management, not just entry, of orders. Actions such as modifying, suspending, and discontinuing orders are often as important and more complex and challenging than order entry.

When a Pop-up Alert Is Overridden, Does That Mean It Wasn't Useful?

Many studies have shown that override rates for pop-up alerts during CPOE are particularly high. However, just because an alert is overridden or ignored doesn't mean the alert didn't help the ordering practitioner. Although the order may not be canceled or changed because of the alert, the practitioner may elect to more carefully monitor the patient or to take actions that otherwise would not have occurred. So, override rates don't tell the whole story.

Are There Limits to a "Best-of-Breed" Strategy?

Rarely will an organization buy all clinical and financial systems from one supplier, and most organizations rely on interfaces to connect multiple systems. However, most experts recommend that at a minimum the CPOE pharmacy and medication administration systems share a single platform from the same vendor, at least for inpatient care. Sometimes referred to as the *medication process*, medication order entry, pharmacy verification, and nursing administration are so closely linked and interdependent that multiple interfaced systems present significant challenges and risks.

Roles and Professional Background of People Working in Healthcare Organizations

There are many healthcare professional roles active in even a moderately sized hospital or a large physician office practice. The following are just a few key professional roles with brief descriptions of each role.

Physicians

Physicians are doctors of medicine (MD) or osteopathy (DO) who have graduated from medical school. Following medical school, they almost always serve as an intern for an additional year and then as a resident for two years or longer beyond internship. (The first year of residency is often referred to as the *internship*.) Medical doctors must be licensed to practice, and many of them take additional exams for board certification. They may also be authorized to prescribe controlled substances such as narcotics. They need to have privileges to practice in the hospital, and the privileges are tied to their training and experience. Physicians often specialize in their training to become family practitioners, internal medicine physicians (internists), obstetricians, surgeons (general, orthopedic, cardiovascular, urology, and many others), or one of numerous other specialties. (Don't confuse internist with intern—the former is a specialist in internal medicine, while the latter is someone in the first year of residency.)

Registered Nurses

Nurses are graduates of a nursing school who have been granted the degree RN. They may also have a bachelor's or master's degree in nursing. Nurses serve in a wide variety of roles, including providing bedside care in the hospital, quality manager, clinical unit supervision, triage and advice, and other forms of direct patient care. They may have additional degrees to become an advance practice nurse such as an ARNP, permitting them to practice in a role similar to that of physicians including having prescriptive authority.

Physician Assistants

Physician assistants (PAs) practice in association with physicians and in general serve to extend the services that the physician delivers. They may be fairly independent with periodic oversight, or they may work in very close connection with a physician (e.g., the operating room working with an orthopedic surgeon). As is the case of ARNPs, they may have prescriptive authority and are important members of the care delivery team of a hospital, clinic, or other healthcare organization.

Medical Assistants

Medical assistants (MAs) have received specific training to help with many tasks within a clinic or hospital. They are frequently the first clinical person patients encounter in the healthcare system and are often tasked with collecting and documenting vital signs, allergies, and other basic information needed for patient care, as well as providing patients with information or facilitating patient flow. They work closely with registered nurses, physicians, and others in the clinic or hospital. They do not have prescriptive authority and typically don't have the degree of training nurses and physicians have.

Unique Considerations of Academic Roles

Those who support healthcare IT in academic settings face challenges that are not as prominent outside academia.

- The most obvious is that training is a continuous process in every discipline—medicine, nursing, pharmacy, and many other healthcare fields. Training programs must be part of regular clinic and hospital operations, and support systems that complement training must also be tailored to this constantly changing workforce. The various roles within an academic environment have different licensing, prescribing, and documentation privileges. EMRs must support this wide variety of roles, which change over time.

- Academic practice includes research: the cycle of posing questions, receiving approval to conduct trials, applying for funding, and carrying out the research study. EMRs must support research both directly (for example, by flagging orders and notes to be sent to different research payers and informing users that a patient is involved in a research study) and indirectly (for example, by supporting use of data extracted from clinical systems and EMRs to be used by investigators who have received institutional review board approval to do so).

Research about informatics is now common in academic settings. In fact, much of what we know about the benefits, risks, and "unintended consequences" of healthcare IT comes from academic informatics programs. As has been the case for other new fields, it is by studying the use of healthcare IT and patient outcomes attributable to it that you can learn what it can and cannot be expected to do. You need to retain an open mind about healthcare IT in the early stages of use and in the years to come.

Chapter Review

EMRs are more than just replacements of paper medical records. They permit viewing, summarizing, and creating key data used in the care of patients, and they permit the delivery of care through the entry of orders and in other ways. Their functionality and ease of use helps determine the safety, efficiency, and ease of patient care. Thus, they are critically important elements in modern healthcare. They are no longer the domain of just doctors and nurses: nearly everyone on a care team, including the patient, participates in creating and using the EMR. Understanding how they work, their strengths, and future enhancements is key to success in clinical informatics.

Questions

1. Patients are legally entitled to see test results, discharge summaries, and operative notes but not the text of physician progress notes unless the physician agrees.

   A. True

   B. False

2. Which of the following is considered by the Institute of Medicine to be functionality in an electronic health record?

   A. Results management

   B. Population health management

   C. Administrative support

   D. Communication tools

   E. All of the above

3. Though nurse practitioners and physicians assistants are active members of the healthcare team in many organizations, the Health Insurance Portability and Accountability Act (HIPAA) of 1996 does not permit them to write prescriptions.

   A. True

   B. False

4. Why is proper documentation in an EMR important?

   A. It helps the insurance company know how to charge the patient.

   B. It lets the patient know what care they received in an emergency department.

   C. It allows all of the people involved in a person's care to understand what has happened during previous visits and see what the plans for future care are.

   D. It provides the family of a patient access to a family member's medical record so that they can better care for their family member.

5. The electronic entry of orders by the ordering clinician is referred to as which of the following?

   A. Online entry system (OES)

   B. Computerized practitioner order entry (CPOE)

   C. Computerized ordering (CO)

   D. Medication ordering system (MOS)

6. What does medication reconciliation refer to?

   A. A pharmacist substituting a generic medication for a brand-name medication when filling a doctor's order

   B. The hospital and insurance agency agreeing on a fair price to charge patients for a medication

   C. The review of the list of medications a patient is taking before and after a transition, such as admission to the hospital

   D. Letting patients decide which medications they want to take

7. What critical role does the master patient index (MPI) serve?

   A. Establishing the identity of the person within the healthcare IT system, including and especially the EMR

   B. Tracking the location and movement of patients within an organization and communicating with the EMR

   C. Letting the nurses and physicians know which patients they are responsible for at the start of their shift

   D. None of the above

8. When a pop-up alert is overridden, it means it wasn't useful.

   A. True

   B. False

Answers

1. **B.** Patients can see their entire medical record.

2. **E.** Results management, population health management, administrative support, and communication tools are all considered to be key functions of an EMR.

3. **B.** False. Nurse practitioners and physician assistants are permitted to write prescriptions.

4. **C.** Proper documentation in an EMR is important because it allows all of the people involved in a person's care to understand what has happened during previous visits and see what the plans for future care are.

5. **B.** The electronic entry of orders by the ordering clinician is referred to as computerized practitioner order entry (CPOE).

6. **C.** Medication reconciliation refers to the review of the list of medications a patient is taking before and after a transition, such as admission to the hospital.

7. **A.** The master patient index (MPI) serves the critical role of establishing the identity of the person within the healthcare IT system, including and especially the EMR.

8. **B.** False. Just because an alert is overridden or ignored doesn't mean the alert didn't help the ordering practitioner.

References

1. Payne, T. H. (2008). Practical guide to clinical computing systems: Design, operations, and infrastructure. Elsevier.

2. National Research Council. (2003). Key capabilities of an electronic health record system: Letter report. National Academies Press.

3. Schiff, G. D., & Bates, D. W. (2010). Can electronic clinical documentation help prevent diagnostic errors? *New England Journal of Medicine, 362*, 1066–1069.

4. Payne, T. H., & Graham, G. (2006). Managing the life cycle of electronic clinical documents. *Journal of the American Medical Informatics Association, 13*, 438–445.

5. Bates, D. W., Leape, L. L., Cullen, D. J., Laird, N., et al. (1998). Effect of computerized physician order entry and a team intervention on prevention of serious medication errors. *Journal of the American Medical Informatics Association, 280*, 1311–1316.

6. Bates, D. W., Kuperman, G. J., et al. (2003). Ten rules for effective clinical decision support. *Journal of the American Medical Informatics Association, 10*, 523.

7. Lyman, J. A., Cohn, W. F., Bloomrosen, M., & Detmer, D. E. (2010). Clinical decision support: Progress and opportunities. *Journal of the American Medical Informatics Association, 17*, 487–492.

8. Kuperman, G. J., Bobb, A., Payne, T. H., Avery, A. J., Gandhi, T. K., Burns, G., Classen, D. C., & Bates, D. W. (2007). Medication-related clinical decision support in computerized provider order entry systems: A review. *Journal of the American Medical Informatics Association, 14*, 29–40.

9. Cimino, J. (2008). Infobuttons: Anticipatory passive decision support. *American Medical Informatics Association Annual Symposium Proceedings*, 1203–1204.

10. Wagner, E. H., Austin, B. T., & Von Korff, M. (1996). Organizing care for patients with chronic illness. *Milbank Quarterly, 74,* 511–544.

11. Steinbrook, R. (2008). Personally controlled online health data: The next big thing in medical care? *New England Journal of Medicine, 358,* 1653–1656.

Human Factors in Healthcare IT

Andre Kushniruk, Elizabeth Borycki

In this chapter, you will learn how to

- Describe the importance of how people interact with computers and how that relates to healthcare IT
- Differentiate human factors from human–computer interaction
- Factor in human cognition while assisting in the design of healthcare information systems
- Implement the principles of good user interface design in healthcare IT
- Describe what usability is and why it is important in healthcare IT
- Employ usability engineering methods in designing and implementing healthcare IT
- Ensure health information systems operate safely

A wide variety of health information systems and healthcare information technology have been developed that promise to streamline and modernize healthcare. These systems include electronic health record systems (EHRs), clinical decision support systems (CDSSs), and other systems designed for use by health consumers and patients for storing and accessing their own health information such as personal health records (PHRs). However, despite the great potential of these advances, acceptance of HIT systems by end users has been problematic.[1] Issues related to users finding some systems difficult to use and the need for increasing user input in the design of HIT systems have been identified as barriers to the widespread adoption of HIT systems by physicians, nurses, and other healthcare professionals. Problems encountered by users of HIT systems related to poor usability have been cited as contributing to the failure of a number of HIT projects and initiatives.[2] On the other hand, designing HIT systems that are user friendly and truly support healthcare workers and their work will lead to greater adoption of HIT systems and improved healthcare processes. This chapter will discuss some practical approaches and methods for improving the ease of use of HIT systems.

Around the world, and currently in particular in the United States, there is a move toward widespread adoption of EHRs and related information technologies. These systems allow physicians to electronically store and retrieve patient data, document care, place orders, and access computerized decision support in the form of automated reminders and alerts about patient conditions. The ultimate goal is to electronically link individual physicians and health professionals to local, regional, and national patient data repositories. With that purpose in mind, the HITECH program was created as a component of the 2009 American Recovery and Reinvestment Act to provide financial incentives to physicians for using these systems in a clinically meaningful way, commonly called *meaningful use*.[3] One expectation is that the incentives will lead to an increased use of EHRs and other HIT-related technologies by health professionals. Adoption of EHRs by end users is highly dependent upon how easy such systems are to use and how well the technology supports and facilitates the work activities of the healthcare professionals. Additionally, it has become increasingly clear there is wide variation in how different types of user interfaces (UIs) affect a clinician's workflow, activities, and decision making. In this chapter, we will discuss a range of human factors related to designing better and more effective HIT systems from the perspective of the end user. The field of usability engineering will be introduced, and practical methods for ensuring that EHR systems are useful, usable, and safe will be described.

Human Factors and Human–Computer Interaction in Healthcare

Human factors is the field of study focused on understanding the human elements of *systems*, where *systems* may be defined as software, medical devices, computer technology, and organizations.[4] The objective of studying human factors in healthcare is to optimize overall system performance and improve healthcare processes and outcomes. Two main areas covered by human factors are cognitive ergonomics, which deals with mental processes of participants in systems, and physical ergonomics, which deals with the physical activity within a system and the physical arrangement of the system.[4] *Human–computer interaction* (HCI) is a subdiscipline of human factors focusing on understanding how humans use computers to design systems that align with and support human information-processing activities.[5] HCI looks specifically at the user's interaction with a system, such as the keyboard or a touch screen, as well as how the interaction fits within the user's larger work context. Also important are the multitude of cognitive and social experiences that surround the use of an information system or technology. The four major components of HCI are

- The user of the technology
- The task or job the user is trying to carry out via the technology
- The particular context of use of the technology
- The technology itself

Each of these components can be further analyzed and broken down for improvement and for optimization. In healthcare there are multiple users of a given system that vary widely in their expectations, from physician to pharmacist to nurse. A given role can then be further defined by the focus of the clinician—general practice versus surgical specialty physicians. The task or job each user carries out using the technology covers a wide spectrum, from recording basic patient data to viewing and making clinical choices based on recommendations from a decision support system about a patient's treatment. The context in which technology is used might vary from the routine to complex or urgent situations and conditions that may involve more than one user or participant. Finally, healthcare technology itself may range from desktop applications for entering and retrieving patient data to mobile devices and "telehealth" applications used in remote patient monitoring. The four components of HCI listed earlier are useful in considering which aspects of user interactions within healthcare systems might need to be improved, modified, or redesigned in order to optimize the user experience. An underlying goal of HCI is to consider all four dimensions to improve HIT and healthcare systems so that users can carry out tasks safely, effectively, efficiently, and enjoyably.

User Interface Design and Human Cognition

The *user interface* is the component of a HIT system that communicates with a given clinician, healthcare worker, or healthcare consumer as they connect with that technology. The objective of user interaction with HIT systems is typically to carry out healthcare-related work tasks, where patient information can be manipulated, accessed, or created to support clinical decision making and work activities. Anyone using healthcare technology does so in the context of performing tasks related to their role that involve access to, manipulation of, or creation of data. From this perspective, HCI involves shared information processing between the machine and the end user. Given that dynamic, an understanding of human cognition and what users can and can't be expected to do using HIT systems, in a variety of contexts (i.e., emergent versus nonemergent), underlies the success or failure of the user-HIT interface. For example, an important aspect of human cognition that can be applied to improving user interactions with systems includes understanding the limitations of human ability to process large amounts of complex data. Strategies for reducing *cognitive load* (i.e., the amount of perception, attention, and thinking required to understand something) associated with task performance and improving the quality and relevance of information displayed on computers to end users are needed in order to ensure the effectiveness and efficiency of HIT systems.

Importance of Considering Cognitive Psychology

To understand how to design, develop, and implement effective healthcare IT, an understanding of key areas of cognitive psychology is relevant.[6] *Cognitive psychology* is the field that studies human reasoning and information processing (information seeking and decision making), including studies of perception, attention, memory, learning, and skill development. For example, studies of how clinicians gain experience and expertise in their area of work are relevant for designing user interfaces that better match the information processing of end users in that work area. Further, understanding the limitations of human memory has led user interface experts to develop simple heuristics "rules of thumb" that can be used to help guide the design of user interfaces and computer screens for HIT. For example, studies in cognitive psychology indicate that people can generally remember seven discrete pieces of information, plus or minus two, with seven-digit telephone numbers a good example.[5] This has led to the recommendation that the number of items in a computer menu follow that same guideline. In addition, studies of users learning how to use HIT have particular relevance to improving the adoption of complex HIT applications. A number of reports have shown that some applications are difficult to use and time-consuming to learn and master in real-world healthcare settings. Work in characterizing and finding ways of reducing the amount of time and effort to learn how to use such systems has considerable importance in deploying HIT systems, where users may be faced with the need to learn how to use multiple varied information systems and HIT in complex and stressed environments. Knowledge gleaned from the study of perception and attention is also highly relevant for HIT and has led to the following development guidelines about how to display information to users on a computer screen:

- Present information in a logical and meaningful way.
- Provide attention-getting visual cues, and highlight important or critical information.
- Help users focus their attention on important information.
- Make information needed in decision making easy to find and process.
- Avoid overloading the user with large amounts of irrelevant information.

Approaches to Cognition and HCI

The field of HCI has been influenced by two primary models of how humans interact with information technology and how they carry out tasks using computer systems. In the 1960s and 1970s, the concept of the human as the "information processor" borrowed from advances in computer science and used the metaphor of computer systems to describe human attention, information processing, and reasoning. For example, psychologists working in the area of HCI borrowed concepts such as "memory stores" and "processing units" from computer science in order to describe how humans think and process information. Five areas of focus as a result of this work are

- Describing the computer user's goals
- Describing how their goals were translated into intentions to carry out a task using computer systems

- Describing how user intensions became plans for executing an action using a computer system

- Describing how computer operations are actually performed by the user

- Describing how users interpret feedback from the computer system once the action has been completed[7]

Using the method of studying user interactions, it is then possible to understand where users are having problems in using a complex healthcare information system. Examples include the user having problems translating their intentions into computer actions by typing in the right command and having trouble interpreting error messages returned by the system as feedback to the user. While this model has been useful in analyzing HCI at a detailed level, it has been criticized for focusing only on the individual user interacting with an individual computer system in isolation, not as part of the rich and complex social context of healthcare work. As a result, more recent approaches to modeling HCI have appeared that focus on "distributed cognition" where information processing is shared among a number of people and systems in order to carry out real tasks in real social settings.[6] In an operating room, analyzing and understanding how to use a new surgical information system requires a thorough understanding of all the participants in the procedure, their roles, and their interactions with the system. Although understanding how one individual user interacts with such a system is important, it does not provide a complete picture of how the system interfaces with the activities of all the participants, including the patient. Interactions between the information-processing roles of the doctor, the patient, and the computer system used by the doctor are all important in understanding the impact of EHRs on the physician-patient relationship (see Use Case 16-1).[8] Considering work activity as a distributed process provides a broader framework for understanding where HIT matches user needs and provides support for the goal of completing complex healthcare activities involving multiple participants. Somewhat unique to healthcare, it is important to note that many work tasks are complex, are often time sensitive, and may involve considerable uncertainty and urgency. *Work domain analysis* is an approach used to analyze technology in these complex situations and has proven to be an effective starting point in characterizing the impact of HIT. This approach involves answering the following questions:

- Who are the classes of users in the design and testing of HIT?

- What are the tasks each class of user carries out using a technology?

- Are there situational aspects of doing the task, and did the designer consider that the task might involve time constraints or urgency?

- What are the potential problems users might encounter when using the HIT, and how can they be fixed?

All of these questions should be considered both before and after a HIT application has been implemented in a hospital or clinic.

Use Case 16-1: Observing Users Interacting with an EHR System

Observing users interacting with a system has become widely used to understand the impact of HIT on human cognition and work processes. In one such study of the introduction of a new EHR in a diabetes clinic, the vendor of the system wanted to know how the design of the system, including the way its computer screens were organized and what information it displayed to the user, would affect the interaction of the physician with the patient. This was a key consideration because the EHR was intended to be used by the physician while interviewing the patient.[8] In this study, the physician's interaction with the system was recorded while interviewing a "simulated patient" (a study collaborator who played the part of a patient). One observation of the study noted that physicians using the EHR struggled with finding the screens containing the questions they wanted to ask the patient and documenting the response. A number of physicians eventually dropped out of the study and did not adopt the system. Of those who remained, some changed their patient interviewing strategy and style and became "screen driven," asking questions based on the order of information on the screens. When interviewed about their use of the EHR, these physicians were not consciously aware that the design of the system and the layout of information had led to changes in the way they interacted with patients. The vendor used the study results to improve and streamline user training with specific examples of how to use the system while interacting with the patient.

Technological Advances in HIT and User Interfaces

A key component or dimension of HCI is the *human dimension*—or cognition, knowledge, skills, and understanding of the user interacting with a computer. The technology itself is another important consideration of HCI in healthcare. The design and build of computer-user interfaces have advanced significantly over the past several decades and continue to evolve and improve rapidly. The typical user interaction with healthcare computer systems up until the 1970s involved command-line interactions recalled from memory and entered on a keyboard to create and edit patient files and access data from laboratory and pharmacy systems. The subsequent development of graphical user interfaces (GUIs) greatly improved user interaction with those systems, and by the 1980s, those same enhancements appeared in personal and work computers. This major breakthrough in the design of user interfaces essentially extended the use of computers from only highly computer-literate end users to the larger population of work professionals and eventually the general public. The Apple Macintosh introduced the concepts of a mouse, icons, and direct manipulation of objects on the computer screen versus typing a variety of commands with only a keyboard. Operating systems such as Mac OS and Microsoft Windows replicated the office examples of files, folders, calendars, and spreadsheets on the computer desktop and allowed easy manipulation via keyboard and mouse. The use of this metaphor simplified user interactions with systems and allowed users to more rapidly learn how to use computer systems.[5] The World Wide Web introduced the hyperlink concept, providing links to text, images, and other media via a mouse click on the screen. In healthcare IT, these advances in organizing and displaying information on computer screens for end users have had a major impact on healthcare information system interactions and on the type of user interfaces that HIT has developed. With the introduction of the graphical user interface in other industries, EHR vendors have all evolved from the difficult-to-use command line such as Microsoft DOS to more user-friendly GUI-based systems using Microsoft Windows and Apple OS.[5] Improvements in the EHR user interfaces now facilitate easy access to and entry of information in a variety of source systems such as laboratory, radiology, and pharmacy. Internet or web technologies have also enhanced EHR development beyond Windows and Apple operating systems to take advantage of those capabilities.

Mobile devices such as smartphones and tablet computers, the increased use of the Web, and social media applications such as Facebook and Twitter have started a new trend in the development of collaborative/cooperative user interfaces designed to support the distributed work activities of multiple users, both health professionals and more recently patients. One example of this is the web site PatientsLikeMe (www.patientslikeme.com). Now users may be

- Located in the same place at the same time
- Geographically apart but still communicating at the same time (using video or web conferencing to discuss a patient case)
- Communicating asynchronously from different locations at different points in time (using secure e-mail to communicate with the patient or another colleague)

User interfaces are becoming increasingly important in areas such as telehealth and distance medical consultations and are providing new types of interactions that may involve multiple synchronous or asynchronous users interacting to carry out a complex task from different locations such as conducting remote patient consultations using video conferencing. Skills and expertise in this area of HCI will become increasingly important as software/hardware for supporting collaborative healthcare activities becomes more prevalent.[9]

Input and Output Devices and the Visualization of Healthcare Data

Along with the advances in operating systems and user interfaces, improvements continue to be made in the development of more effective input and output devices for

HIT. Additionally, advances in the visualization of health data are taking place, such as designing new ways for representing complex health data, supporting analysis of patient trends by health professionals, and understanding aggregated patient, health professional, and organizational data from many sources. Principles for the display of health information on computer screens include grouping information in a clinically meaningful way, avoiding overload and simplifying access to critical patient data by limiting what is presented, and standardizing information displays where possible.[5]

A variety of different approaches, styles, and technologies have been developed to support the input of health data into computer systems. Keyboards are still the most common way of entering healthcare data into a computer system, with other devices now seeing increased use. These include the computer mouse, trackballs, electronic pens, and handwriting recognition and touch screens. Voice recognition technology, as part of the EHR capturing spoken information in certain sections, is also seeing increased adoption. Each of these approaches has advantages and disadvantages, and their usefulness varies considerably depending on the context of their use in different healthcare settings. Touch screens may be useful for allowing patients to enter data in a physician's waiting room, while in infection-prone areas of a hospital they may not be recommended. Voice recognition (VR) has been useful in physicians' private offices dictating narrative portions of a patient's history in the EHR and patient referral letters. All VR systems work best when the user has had some initial training "teaching" the program their speech patterns and how to best use the technology. Increasingly, with the use of networked speech files accessible from any computer and more accurate microphones, acute-care settings are now leveraging the same tools.

When considering data entry options, there are a wide variety of approaches, including using online forms that take direct data entry through the use of specific fields, using question-and-answer dialogs that prompt the user, selecting options from drop-down and other menus, directly manipulating objects on the screen using pointing devices such as a mouse, and using voice recognition, as described earlier. Across all methods, data entered in the EHR by clinicians varies widely from complete free text entered via a keyboard to very structured data where options are limited to well-defined terms and phrases the user can select from. Free-text examples include comments about how a medication might be used and the narrative in clinician notes where the patient's own words are captured. Allergies, medications, and other patient histories are more commonly captured using structured vocabularies with some options for text entry as well. Most EHRs try to find a balance of data entry methods that facilitate complete and adequate documentation but don't limit or prevent the user from performing the task in a timely fashion in the way they documented prior to using a computer. Furthermore, clinical data may be entered into fields of systems such as EHRs as free-form text (text typed in a text box in an unrestricted way) or alternatively as semistructured data (where the format of data entered is somewhat structured by the computer system) or completely structured or coded data (where the user must select only from the options displayed to them by the system, for example, select from a list of medical diagnoses). For example, some EHRs will allow data on a patient's history of present illness to be entered as free text with no restrictions imposed by the computer system on what the user types. However, as electronic information in computer systems becomes more widely shared, structured or coded data using standard medical terms will be needed.[10] For example, in systems employing coded data input, a physician might enter into a text box a diagnosis of "diabetes," which will result in a menu listing agreed-upon forms of diabetes, such as "diabetes I" and "diabetes II," from which the user must select. This approach allows for the selection of coded and structured data that is sharable and understandable across systems and end users. However, some users may feel that the approach restricts their ability to express themselves and that, if not carefully selected, the choices offered by the system do not fully match their information needs or the particular medical or healthcare terminology or vocabulary they use. An anecdotal complaint from clinicians who use electronic tools to document their notes and from those who receive copies of those notes is that each one looks similar, contains more data than is needed, and doesn't tell the story compared to dictated or handwritten notes that were more common prior to electronic records. This tension between free-text entry and coded data entry still exists, and some recent work has been conducted in developing user interfaces for healthcare that automatically extract coded standardized medical terms from free text.[11]

The visualization of healthcare has also become an important area of research and development. There are many ways of visualizing health data, ranging from textual data to graphical displays including charts and histograms to three-dimensional images. Workstations capable of integrating complex images with text and graphics are becoming more common, and multimedia capabilities are becoming more standard in healthcare user interfaces. Experimental approaches to data visualization have led to user interfaces that use 3D graphics to reconstruct views of the body and to allow for remote robotically controlled surgeries and other medical procedures. One such system, known as the DaVinci system, has allowed for surgery at a micro level, where the surgeon operates using a computer display that allows for fine-tuned control of miniaturized surgical instruments that is less invasive than traditional surgeries and that has greatly improved medical outcomes.[12]

Other trends in the area of input and display of healthcare data are related to the concepts of ubiquitous and pervasive computing. *Ubiquitous computing* in healthcare refers to user interfaces that are mostly "invisible" and that the user may be largely unaware of. Examples include wearable computing, such as giving patients wired electronic shirts containing sensors that can detect cardiac problems and automatically alert healthcare professionals of impending heart-related events, often outside the normal acute-care environment. The move to pervasive healthcare includes the possibility for interaction with HIT throughout our daily lives.[13] Examples of pervasive health include use of mobile healthcare applications such as "mHealth" that allow healthcare professionals, patients, and the general public to access the latest evidence-based health information using cell phones, smartphones, tablets, and other devices. According to recent studies and reports, this trend will continue,[13] and in many countries the use of mobile devices for accessing the Internet and for text messaging has surpassed the use of desktop computing models. In the area of healthcare, many new HIT applications are being developed for supporting the promotion of health and for linking health professionals and patients through a range of innovative mobile applications. From an HCI perspective, increased use of mHealth affords new opportunities for communicating and receiving health information from a wider range of settings than previously possible.

Finally, work in the area of developing customizable and adaptive user interfaces to HIT applications is also promising. A criticism of many healthcare user interfaces and systems voiced by end users has been their perceived inflexibility, given the wide range of types of healthcare users and the even wider range of contexts in which they use HIT. Along these lines, work in developing customizable and adaptable user interfaces and the broader information systems holds considerable promise.

Approaches to Developing User Interfaces in Healthcare

Recommended approaches to the development of user interfaces for HIT include considering the design of user interfaces within the context of a "holistic" systems approach, where user input into the design and implementation is considered along the continuum from initial conception of interface metaphor to development, testing, and implementation.[5] User-centered design of HIT involves the following principles:

- Focus early on the users' needs and work situations.
- Conduct a task analysis where the details of the users' information needs and environment are identified.
- Carry out continual testing and evaluation of systems with users.
- Design iteratively, whereby there are cycles of development and testing with end users.

Along these lines, rapid prototyping of complex HIT user interfaces is recommended. The process begins with sharing early mock-ups (typically sketches or computer drawings of planned user interfaces) with potential end users, to obtain specific feedback to improve interface design, features offered, and potential alterations or revisions to the interface. As the system and user interface evolve during HIT development, continual user input and feedback through continual user testing are recommended.[5] In later stages, the testing of prototypes (partially working early versions of a system or user interface) and emerging user interfaces with end users may involve conventional methods, such as periodically holding focus groups with potential users (where groups of users are shown prototypes or early system versions and asked to react to and comment about) or individual interviews with future users about the design to obtain their feedback. Methods from the emerging area of usability engineering will be described in detail in the next section of this chapter.

Methods of Usability Engineering

Early stages in the development of healthcare user interfaces for HIT include the creation of an initial product description and description of the context of use of the system or user interface. Here, the capabilities of the system from the end user's perspective and the requirements of the end user are defined. It is at this stage that a number of engineering method requirements can be employed. This may involve conducting walk-throughs or observations of settings in which the technology is or will be deployed. One method that has been used is known as *shadowing*, where one or more healthcare professionals are followed during a normal day to see how they perform their work, how HIT fits (or could fit) into their practice, and where problems and errors occur with current workflow and tools. A wide range of methods can be used at this stage to obtain information about users and their work, including ethnographic observational study of the work environment, time-motion studies (where the times to complete healthcare tasks with or without HIT are recorded), and interviews with health professionals about their information-processing needs. At this stage, analyses can be conducted to describe how users carry out their healthcare-related tasks and where HIT could be inserted to improve their work processes.[5] This analysis may involve observing users as they carry out real or simulated tasks of increasing complexity using HIT, including those related to managing medications: medication dispensing, patient and order verification and administration, and complex intravenous therapies.

After completing studies of end users in their work environments as described ear-lier, initial user interface designs and specifications are created. Similar to the previous analogies of files and folders and how those have been replicated in basic personal computing, medical analogies such as rooms can be employed to streamline and opti-mize workflow using other user interface options. This approach has been used in hos-pital bed scheduling systems, where users can click different "rooms" displayed on the computer screen and visually increase their size to focus on a particular patient bed. Decisions also need to be made about the following aspects of user interface design:

- Determining the functionality of the interface and what users will be allowed to do
- Designing the layout and sequence of computer screens that users will see
- Specifying the style of interaction with the user
- Selecting an appropriate prototyping and user interface programming tool
- Planning and scheduling continual iterative user testing

While there are a number of guiding principles that have been used for both the design and testing of healthcare information systems, several of which will be described in the next section on usability engineering, it should be noted that a recurring theme in the design and development of applications such as EHRs has been a lack of agreed-upon national or industry user interfaces standards for these types of systems. A vendor may choose one type of user metaphor and lay out screen sequences and organize patient information in a way that may be quite different from another vendor, thus making it difficult for users of multiple different electronic records to remember how to use each system. Attempts at developing standards for use in the design and implemen-tation of healthcare IT user interfaces are underway, such as the Common User Interface (CUI) project of the National Health Services (NHS) in the United Kingdom, which is in collaboration with Microsoft. Its work has led to a number of nationally endorsed guidelines and recommendations for displaying health information data in an EHR in a way that is more intuitive and friendly for the user and less likely to lead to error.

Ongoing user interface review/improvement is important as technology and healthcare evolve. As described earlier, user-centered design recommends continual user input and feedback as the user interface is being developed and as soon as possible after a stable version of the user interface is available. Along these lines, an approach to the design and implementation of healthcare IT has emerged known as *participatory design*, whereby users are more closely involved in the development of healthcare user interfaces, in effect serving as "user consultants" and active participants and members of the design and implementation team, providing their expertise on what would, or would not, work from the user's perspective. Along these lines, proponents of "socio-technical design" argue that consideration of the social impact of systems, such as the effects of a new system on physician or nurse work practices and social interactions, is as important as obtaining technical requirements.[15] They further argue that lack of consideration of socio-technical issues will likely lead to lack of system acceptance and, ultimately, system failure, which has been shown to be the case in the literature regarding HIT successes and failure.

Usability of Healthcare IT

In response to the increasing complexity of user interfaces and systems, the field of usability engineering emerged in the early 1990s. The methods that have emerged from usability engineering have been applied to improve HCI in a wide range of fields, including HIT. The usability of an information system can be defined as a measure of its ease of use by human users. Usability is a concept that can be considered as a measure of how easy it is to use an information system, how efficient and effective the system is, and how easy it is to learn to use the system.[5] In addition, usability, broadly defined, also considers the safety of healthcare IT (how safe it is to use a healthcare system) as well as the concept of user enjoyment (how enjoyable it is to use a system). Good usability is important in HIT, because some earlier systems have been rejected by end users because of poor usability. In recent years, usability has become a major issue in HIT; it has become important to avoid designing systems that are difficult to use and hard to learn and that could potentially lead to inadvertent inefficiencies and medical error.

The two main approaches in usability engineering are usability testing and usability inspection.[16] Usability testing involves evaluating the usability of user interfaces, prototypes, or fully operational systems by observing representative end users as they interact with the system or user interface in the study to carry out representative tasks. For example, usability testing of an EHR might involve observing physicians interacting with a new EHR as they enter or retrieve patient data. Users are typically video recorded as they interact with the system (see Figure 16-1), and the computer screens are captured (which can be done with low-cost screen recording software). While carrying out tasks during usability testing, the users observed are often asked to "think aloud" or verbalize their thoughts while using the system to carry out tasks.[17]

HIT PRO EXAM TIP   *Usability* refers to the ease of use of a system in terms of efficiency, effectiveness, enjoyment, learnability, and safety.

The data collected from usability testing sessions, such as video recordings of users interacting with a system (including audio recordings of user verbalizations and computer screen recordings), can be played back and analyzed to identify the following:

- User problems in interacting with the system under study
- Potential inefficiencies in the user-system interaction and user interface
- Potential impact on user workflow and work activities
- Recommendations for improving the user interface and underlying system functionality[17]

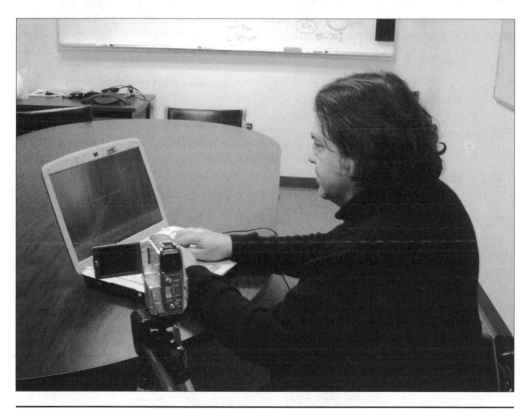

Figure 16-1   Health professional being video recorded while carrying out tasks using an EHR during a usability testing session

Usability testing has been found to be critically important in designing, implementing, deploying, and customizing HIT systems in order to ensure they are efficient, effective, enjoyable to use, easy to learn, and safe to use. Furthermore, the approach can be applied across the entire systems development life cycle (SDLC) of healthcare information systems, as illustrated in Figure 16-2. The SDLC provides a timeline or life cycle for considering when and where HIT may be evaluated and improved applying usability testing.

In the early planning stages of the SDLC usability, testing can be applied to test early system designs and user interface ideas using mock-ups or sketches of potential system ideas or screen layouts that can then be shown to users for feedback. This method can also be used to help make selections among different possible candidate systems in situations where an organization, such as a hospital, is deciding among several commercial systems. In this case, potential candidate systems can be required to undergo usability testing, with information from the testing used to help decide on a system to buy. Moving to the requirements-gathering phase of the SDLC, usability testing can be used to gain information about deficiencies with systems currently in place. Also, during requirements gathering, mock-ups can be shown to potential end users to obtain feedback and refined requirements from end users. During the design phase of healthcare IT products, usability testing can be used to obtain user feedback and input in response to partially working user interfaces in iterative cycles of user testing with the results from the usability testing back to system redesign. Once a healthcare IT system is ready for implementation, the usability testing approach can be also used to obtain information about the need for potential refinement of the system or user interface and any potential safety issues once it is to be released in a healthcare setting. Finally, once the system has been widely deployed, usability testing can be employed to determine whether the system needs to be modified, customized, or even replaced in order to continue to meet users' information and work needs.

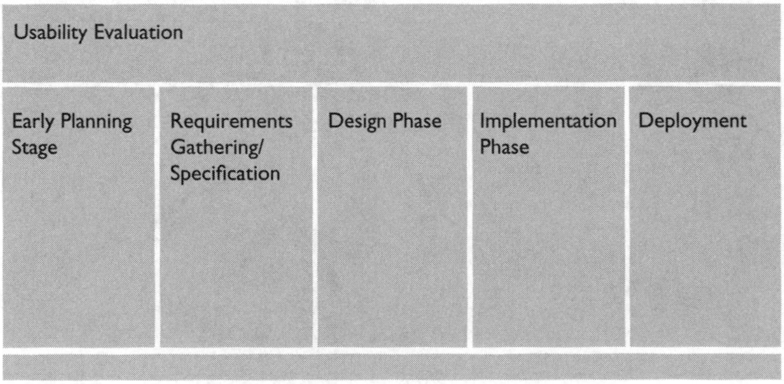

Figure 16-2 Usability evaluation in relation to the SDLC

Another main approach to conducting usability evaluations of healthcare IT is known as *usability inspection*.[18] Usability inspection methods differ from usability testing in that end users are not observed using the system under study, as in usability testing, but rather this approach involves having one or more trained usability inspectors "step through" or inspect a healthcare information system. In doing these inspections, one approach is to compare the user interface against a set of principles or heuristics for good interface design in order to identify violations of the principles or heuristics. A popular and widely used set of heuristics used in this analysis was developed by Jacob Nielsen and has been widely used in the design and evaluation of healthcare IT systems.[16] The following list summarizes the heuristics:

- Visibility of system status
  - The status of the system should be apparent to the user.
  - Example: The users should know whether patient information that was entered by them was successfully saved in the EHR.
- Match between the system and the real world
  - The terminology in the system should match that of the user.
  - Example: The medical terminology used in an EHR should match the terms that physicians using the system use in their work.
- User control and freedom
  - Systems should support undo and redo operations.
  - Example: When learning how to use an EHR, the user can explore the system's functions and features without worrying about making changes that can't be revoked.
- Consistency and standards
  - The interface should be consistent throughout.
  - Example: Differing modules in an EHR should use consistent formatting and labels.
- Error prevention
  - System should help users prevent errors.
  - Example: An alert should pop up when a physician writes an order for a medication the patient is allergic to when using a physician order entry system.
- Recognition rather than recall
  - Users should not have to remember things.
  - Example: Users should be able to select a medication from a list rather than trying to remember the medication formats accepted by the system.

- Flexibility and efficiency of use
  - The interface should accommodate the needs of the user.
  - Example: An EHR should support nurse and physician views of relevant patient information.
- Aesthetic and minimalist design
  - Simple and minimalist interfaces are often easiest to use.
  - Example: The main screens on an EHR may be simple with the option of going to more advanced screens with more options.
- Help users recognize, diagnose, and recover from errors
  - The system should help users recognize and fix errors.
  - Example: If the user misses a field on a data entry form, then that field is highlighted in red, and a message is provided to the user that highlighted fields are missing information.
- Help documentation
  - System should provide adequate help and documentation.
  - Example: If the user of an EHR needs help in using the technology, there should be online help available for them to refer to.
- Chunking
  - Information should be chunked appropriately in packets of seven plus or minus two.
  - Example: A menu containing options for using an EHR should not contain more than nine items (otherwise, it should be broken up into more than one menu).
- Style
  - Prominent and important information should appear at the top of the screen.
  - Example: Drug allergy information should appear at the top of the screen.

Results from conducting heuristic evaluations typically consist of a summary of the number and type of violations of usability heuristics identified in the analysis. This information is then fed back into the system and user interface customization and redesign process to improve the user interface and system.[19] For a comprehensive set of usability guidelines providing detailed guidance on development of web-based applications, refer to the excellent article, "Research-Based Web Design and Usability Guidelines" (www.usability.gov/guidelines).[20]

A second form of usability inspection is known as the *cognitive walk-through*.[18] In conducting a cognitive walk-through, the analyst considers the profile of potential end users: what is the level of computer expertise of the typical user, and what is their prior experience with this type of HIT? This method first involves specifying a task to be analyzed using a healthcare IT system, such as entering medications into a medication list in an EHR system. The analyst then systematically steps through the user interface to carry out the specified task. In doing so, the analyst notes and records the following:

- User goals (entering a medication)
- User steps (recording exactly what the user types or clicks)
- The system's responses to each user step
- Potential user problems in carrying out the task specified

Table 16-1 gives an example of a cognitive walk-through. The results can be used to identify the following:

- Inefficient sequences requiring too many user steps
- Inappropriate or hard-to-understand system feedback
- Potential usability problems
- Problems in achieving goals required to complete a healthcare-related task using the HIT system under study

In general, conducting usability inspections of healthcare IT is faster and may be conducted at a lower cost than doing usability testing, which involves setting up observations of real users of a healthcare IT system. However, it should be noted that usability inspection, although it is a powerful method for predicting user errors, cannot fully predict what users will actually do when faced with HIT in the hospital or clinical setting. Therefore, the two approaches (usability inspection and usability testing) are often used in conjunction, with usability inspection identifying potential errors to improve design and subsequent usability testing with users determining whether there

Goal	Order a patient's medication in an EHR.
Subgoal	Select system operation for ordering a patient medication.
Action 1	Click the medication order entry tab.
System response	The system displays physician order entry screen.
Action 2	Click the medication text box.
System response	The cursor appears in a text box.
Action 3	The user types in the first three letters of the medication.
System response	A list of medications with the same three letters appears.
Potential problem	The medication the user wants does not appear in the list, potentially causing the user to select a medication they did not want to order.
Action 4	The user selects a medication.

Table 16-1   Example of a Cognitive Walk-through for a Physician User Ordering a Medication

are serious user problems. Selecting the most appropriate usability evaluation method, given a particular system, will depend on the considerations of time and expense, with usability inspection methods requiring less investment of both. However, to ensure that systems meet user needs, observing or interviewing end users of those systems should never be replaced. Furthermore, the costs and efforts associated with conducting usability testing of HIT systems have been shown to be reasonable, and the approach can be done in a highly cost-effective way. For example, usability testing of HIT applications does not require expensive usability laboratories but rather can be conducted "on location" or "in situ" within the healthcare organizations where the system will be deployed. Furthermore, the costs associated with data collection have been shown to decrease by using low-cost video cameras and inexpensive computer screen–recording software such as Hypercam.[21,22]

Usability and HIT Safety

In recent years, a growing body of literature on commercially available HIT and EHR systems indicates that some system features and poorly designed user interfaces may actually introduce and cause health professionals to make new types of medical errors. These errors are often not detected until the system has been released and is being used in complex clinical settings. These errors are referred to as *technology-induced errors*.[23] Furthermore, without proper testing with end users before releasing systems, it has been shown that some HIT systems may be dangerous to use, leading to potential harm to patients. Even systems that may have been tested to ensure they pass traditional software testing during their development may be found to "facilitate" or "induce" errors when used in real healthcare settings, in real work situations, and under real-world conditions that were not fully tested during commercial development.

 HIT PRO EXAM TIP Healthcare information systems need to be extensively tested before going live to prevent technology-induced error.

Previous work has shown that HIT systems may have a number of consequences on clinical performance and cognition, which may be inadvertent and in some cases negative. For example, work by Kushniruk and colleagues has shown that certain design of screen layouts in EHRs may lead clinical users to become "screen-driven," where they are overly guided by the order of information on the computer screen, thus relying on how information is presented on the screen to drive their interviews of patients and ultimately their clinical decision making.[17] Furthermore, suboptimal design of user interfaces can lead to errors that could potentially lead to patient harm. For example, screens that are cluttered and, as a consequence, obscure important information about drug allergies could potentially contribute to a physician giving patients medication to which they are allergic. Other examples include errors resulting from the inability of the user to navigate or move through the clinical user interface in order to find critical information, especially when needed during a patient emergency, where time is critical.

Use Case 16-2: Simulation Testing the System

A hospital has decided to implement a medication administration system, which will allow physicians to enter medication orders for patients electronically.[24] Nurses may access the system to see what medications they should administer to their patients, including all the information about what medication to give the patient, the dosage, and so on. The system also allows the nurses to verify that the patient is the correct patient and is linked to the medication barcoding system that allows the nurse to scan the wristband of the patient to make sure the patient is the right one and also to scan the label of the medication to make sure the medication is correct. It was expected that the system would make giving medications in the hospital safer. However, through simulation testing before the system was released, it was found that under emergency situations the system could become a hazard itself. For example, the testing showed that during emergencies there was not enough time for the nurse to go through all the checking procedures that the system required. Furthermore, it was found that if one nurse was using the system for a patient and was called away, all other users were "locked" out from viewing that patient's data on the computer. Based on this prerelease testing, it was decided that in order to ensure system safety under all conditions, an emergency override function could be invoked by users if there were serious time constraints. In addition, the system was modified to allow more than one nurse or physician to access a patient record in an emergency.

To ensure HIT safety, a variety of new methods and approaches to more fully testing healthcare information systems are beginning to appear. For example, clinical simulations are an extension of usability testing, whereby representative users are observed using a system to carry out representative tasks, much as is done in usability testing.[23] However, this type of testing is typically conducted under highly realistic conditions that closely simulate the real working environment in which a system being developed will be deployed. Once a system has been deployed, the reporting of potential technology-induced errors is also beginning to receive attention from both healthcare IT vendors and governmental organizations concerned with healthcare IT safety. Along these lines, error-reporting systems are beginning to be developed where end users can create anonymous online reports about errors that may be related to HIT that can be collected, published, and used to refine and improve the safety of commercially available HIT.

Chapter Review

The success of HIT depends on a number of human factors and requires that the systems and technologies that we develop are both usable and useful. Human factors is a broad area of study that includes consideration of a wide range of human elements within healthcare systems. Human–computer interaction (HCI) is a subfield of human factors that deals with understanding how humans use computers so that better systems can be designed. There are a number of dimensions of HCI including the technology itself, the user of the technology, the task at hand, and the context of use of the technology. It is important to consider all of these dimensions when designing and deploying HIT. Design of user interfaces in healthcare can benefit from an understanding of the capabilities and limits of human cognition. For example, knowledge about how information is best displayed to healthcare professionals borrows from fundamental work in cognitive psychology and HCI. Indeed, to design effective user interfaces, consideration of human aspects related to the processing of information, training, and potential for introduction of error must be considered. From the technological side of things, advances in user interfaces are rapidly advancing. Some of these breakthroughs have included the development of GUIs, new input and output devices, and advances in the visualization of healthcare data. Further advances include the widespread use of mobile devices and increased use of the Web and social media, allowing for access to healthcare data from many locations and supporting collaborative work practices involving multiple users. In addition, approaches to developing more effective user interfaces to HIT are also evolving, with the advent of user-centered design methods and participatory design, both of which promote increased user involvement in all stages of HIT design, implementation, and testing.

The usability of HIT has become a critical issue in developing HIT that will work effectively and be willingly adopted by end users. Usability is defined as a measure of how easy it is to use an information system in terms of its efficiency, effectiveness, enjoyment, learnability, and safety. A number of practical methods for evaluating HIT usability were described in this chapter. They included usability testing, which involves observing users of HIT carrying out tasks using a technology. The other main approach is known as a usability inspection method (heuristic evaluation and the cognitive walk-through) involving trained analysts "stepping through" or analyzing HIT and their user interfaces in order to identify potential usability problems and issues. In the chapter, the relationship between poor usability and increased chances for medical error was discussed. Along these lines, it has been increasingly recognized that some HIT systems, if poorly designed, can pose a safety hazard. Approaches for more effectively testing the safety and effectiveness of HIT systems before widespread release were described. It is important that the HIT system that is developed and deployed in healthcare settings be shown to be not only effective and efficient but also safe.

Questions

1. Human factors can be defined as what?
   A. The study of making more effective user interfaces to computer-based systems
   B. The field that examines human elements of systems

    C. The group of methods that can be used to make systems more usable

    D. The study of technology-induced errors

2. User-centered design involves which of the following?

    A. An early focus on the user and their needs

    B. Continued testing of system design with users

    C. Iterative feedback into redesign

    D. Participation of users as members of the design team

    E. All of the above

    F. A, B, C, D

    G. A, B, C

3. Which of the following is *not* a user interface metaphor?

    A. The desktop metaphor

    B. The document metaphor

    C. The patient chart metaphor

    D. The command-line metaphor

4. What are the main methods from usability engineering?

    A. Participatory design

    B. Cognitive walk-through

    C. Heuristic inspection

    D. Usability testing

    E. B, C, D

    F. A, B, D

5. Which of the following is *not* one of Nielsen's heuristics?

    A. Allow for error prevention.

    B. Support recognition rather than recall.

    C. Use bright colors to be aesthetically pleasing.

    D. Allow for flexibility and efficiency of use.

6. Which of the following is *not* true?

    A. Usability testing can be conducted inexpensively in hospitals.

    B. Usability testing should be conducted only by human factors engineers.

    C. Lack of user input in design and testing is one of the biggest causes of system implementation failure.

    D. Nurses and physicians should be involved in systems design.

7. What can technology-induced errors arise from?

   A. Programming errors

   B. Systems design flaws

   C. Inadequate requirements gathering

   D. Poorly planned systems implementation

   E. A, B, C, D

   F. A, C

8. What are the four main components of HCI?

   A. Software, task, human factors engineer

   B. Technology, task, user, context of use

   C. Software, hardware, user

   D. User, human factors engineer, usability testing lab

Answers

1. **B.** Human factors broadly examines human elements of systems, whereas systems represent physical, cognitive and organizational artefacts that people interact with (e.g. computers).

2. **G.** User-centered design involves: (1) an early focus on users and their needs, (2) continued testing of system design with users, and (3) iterative feedback into redesign.

3. **D.** The user command-line is not a metaphor; it does not represent some other object in the world.

4. **E.** The main methods used in usability engineering are: (1) the cognitive walk-through, (2) heuristic inspection, and (3) usability testing.

5. **C.** Using bright colors is not one of Nielsen's heuristics.

6. **B.** Usability testing can be conducted by professionals with varied backgrounds and not just by human factors engineers. Usability engineering methods have become more widely known and have been simplified and used by different types of IT and health professionals.

7. **E.** Programming errors, systems design flaws, inadequate requirements gathering, and poorly planned systems implementation have all been identified as factors that cause technology-induced error in healthcare.

8. **B.** The four main components of HCI are the technology itself, the task, the user of the technology, and the context of use of the technology.

References

1. Caryon, P. (Ed.) (2012). *Handbook of human factors and ergonomics in health care and patient safety*. CRC Press.

2. Kushniruk, A., & Borycki, E. (Eds.) (2008). *Human, social and organizational aspects of health information systems*. IGI Global.

3. HealthIT.hhs.gov information related to the American Recovery and Reinvestment Act of 2009. (2012). Accessed on June 20, 2012, from http://healthit.hhs .gov/portal/server.pt/community/healthit_hhs_gov__learn_about_hitech/1233.

4. Caryon, P. (Ed.) (2012). *Handbook of human factors and ergonomics in health care and patient safety*. CRC Press.

5. Preece, J., Sharp, H., & Rogers, Y. (2007). *Interaction design: Beyond human-computer interaction, second edition*. John Wiley & Sons.

6. Shortliffe, E., & Cimino, J. (Eds.) (2006). *Biomedical informatics: Computer applications in health care and biomedicine*. Springer.

7. Norman, D., & Draper, S. W. (Eds.). (1986). *User centered system design*. LEA.

8. Patel, V. L., Kushniruk, A. W., Yang, S., & Yale, J. F. (2000). Impact of a computer-based patient record system on data collection, knowledge organization and reasoning. *Journal of the American Medical Informatics Association, 7*, 569–585.

9. Baecker, R. M. (1992). *Readings in groupware and computer-supported cooperative work: Assisting human-human collaboration*. Morgan Kaufman.

10. Patel, V., Kaufman, D. (2006). Cognitive Science and Biomedical Informatics. In E. Shortliffe and J. Cimino (Eds.). *Biomedical informatics: Computer applications in health care and biomedicine*. Springer.

11. Patel, V. L., & Kushniruk, A. W. (1998). Interface design for health care environments: The role of cognitive science. *Proceedings AMIA Symposium*, 29–37.

12. The DaVinci surgical system (2012). Accessed on June 20, 2012, from www.davincisurgery.com/davinci-surgery/davinci-surgical-system/.

13. Bardram, J.E., Mihailis, A., & Wan, D. (2007). *Pervasive computing in healthcare*. CRC Press.

14. Microsoft health common user interface (2012). Accessed on June 20, 2012, from www.mscui.net.

15. Berg, M. (1999). Patient care information systems and health care work: A sociotechnical approach. *International Journal of Medical Informatics, 55*, 87–101.

16. Nielsen, J. (1993). *Usability engineering*. Academic Press.

17. Kushniruk, A., & Patel, V. (2004). Cognitive and usability engineering methods for the evaluation of clinical information systems. *Journal of Biomedical Informatics, 37*, 56–76.

18. Nielsen, J., & Mack, R. L. (1994). *Usability inspection methods*. John Wiley & Sons.

19. Zhang, J., Johnson, T., Patel, V., Paige, D., & Kubose, T. (2003). Using usability heuristics to evaluate patient safety of medical devices. *Journal of Biomedical Informatics, 36*, 23–30.

20. Research-based web design & usability guidelines (2012). Accessed on June 20, 2012, from www.usability.gov/guidelines/index.html.

21. Kushniruk, A., & Borycki, E. (2006). Low-cost rapid usability engineering: Designing and customizing usable healthcare information systems. *Healthcare Quarterly, 9*, 98–100, 102.

22. Rubin, J., & Chisnell, D. (2008). *Handbook of usability testing: How to plan, design, and conduct effective tests*. John Wiley & Sons.

23. Borycki, E., & Kushniruk, A. W. (2005). Identifying and preventing technology-induced error using simulations: Application of usability engineering techniques. *Healthcare Quarterly, 8*, 99–105.

24. Kushniruk, A., Borycki, E., Kuwata, S., & Kannry, J. (2006). Predicting changes in workflow resulting from healthcare information systems: Ensuring the safety of healthcare. *Healthcare Quarterly, 9*, 114–118.

Build- and Implementation-Related HIT Success Factors

Michael Fossel

In this chapter, you will learn how to
- Successfully implement an electronic health record (EHR) in a hospital setting
- Identify the critical issues that are required for a clinically useful build
- Ensure that your hospital implementation can support meaningful use
- Provide optimal conversion support and postconversion optimization

The implementation of healthcare information technology is on the rise and will soon reach its peak in hospital settings. Ten years ago few hospitals were "electronic," but in another ten years few hospitals will be anything but "electronic." This wave of change is only partly because of the advent of feasible technology—technology that can meet the demands of clinical use within the hospital setting. In the last several years, the major impetus to this change has been through the government's prompting, with regulatory requirements that have been accompanied by financial incentives, which will eventually shift toward unavoidable penalties. The result has been an enormous increase in the market for, and the implementation of, electronic health records. Over the next several years, as reimbursement and incentives for healthcare shift toward a single payment for care of the patient over time, the push to fully implement EHRs will continue to increase. Until now, the emphasis has been on the implementation of three distinct EHR functions.

- Access to clinical data
- Computerized provider order entry (CPOE)
- Clinical documentation

A fourth component, clinical decision support (CDS), has also become a key part of the EHR. CDS is often viewed as a distinctly different function of an EHR because it is not as much a function of a health record but instead is a dynamic function that can access a large amount of (often real-time) clinical data and use it to guide clinical care. Moreover, this support is available synchronously, rather than in retrospect or in review of previous care decisions. While decision support is not new, medical textbooks, consultations, pathways, guidelines, clinical rules, and academic articles have served the same purpose; the ability to incorporate CDS into the EHR *at the time decisions are being made* and to have them directly correlated to the health status of the patient in question is a remarkable change.

As the global surge in EHR implementations peaks and a majority of hospitals finish their implementation phase, there has been a growing emphasis on the optimization of the EHR. In the implementation phase, all clinicians receive basic training on how to navigate through the EHR, place orders, and write notes. But soon, the focus will shift to finding the most efficient and effective uses of the EHR. The optimization phase is likely to be ongoing, unlike the episodic implementation phase, and will have a different emphasis. While implementation has been driven by the need to meet regulatory requirements, the optimization phase will have a greater emphasis on clinical usability and CDS. Although regulatory requirements will still be part of the optimization phase, the focus has changed from the simple requirements of using an EHR to the more complex and sophisticated requirements that the EHR do the following:

- Interface with other systems
- Report and extract data
- Offer clinically accurate and actionable decision support

In the optimization phase, the goal is no longer to simply install the EHR and meet a simple list of requirements but rather to ensure that the EHR interface is efficient for clinical workflow, easy to learn, and able to improve clinical care. Although this emphasis is new, these are the same key elements that are the foundation for successful EHR implementations.

 HIT PRO EXAM TIP   The best implementations are those that are already focused on optimization.

Success Factors in EHR Implementations

The key to a successful implementation is that it supports clinical care. This sounds simple but is often overlooked because there is the assumption that any EHR implemented will automatically support clinical care. Case studies of EHR implementations that are only partially accomplished or fail entirely consistently reveal the same features: implementation was driven by the information systems department's viewpoint rather than by the clinician's viewpoint.

While no successful project can ignore the realities of IT and the technical issues involved in building an EHR, neither can it ignore the realities of clinical workflow. With so much emphasis now on clinical use and reliance on EHR systems, any implementation approach that is focused primarily from an IT perspective can expect less than optimal results. The causes of failure are not a lack of knowledge of the system, drive to ensure operability, or will to support good clinical care, but a lack of understanding of how the system will be used, what operability is needed, and what good clinical care consists of. Any successful EHR development and implementation project *must* include the physicians, nurses, and other clinical personnel who will be *using* the system.

In general, clinical involvement is critical not only in the design phase but throughout the successful implementation. This is true within the governance, training, and support aspects. Involvement by clinicians in the design and build phase not only is necessary to ensure that the decisions and processes reflect clinical reality but also ensures that the rest of the clinical staff perceive the system as beneficial and "buy into" the significant change in how patient care is facilitated. The clinical staff will be more likely to adopt EHR usage if they believe that clinical judgment has guided the project.

At the deepest level, the vision of the project must itself be clinical. All hospitals have many goals, and while the goals of financial success and regulatory compliance are critical to the long-term survival of a hospital, the primary goal of delivering quality patient care must remain preeminent. Without this as the primary vision, not only does the hospital eventually lose focus, but also the patient population may decide to go elsewhere, as will the clinical staff. The ability to attract and retain quality clinical personnel and to develop patient loyalty depends upon more than just the financial success of a hospital. Clinical personnel, like patients, are attracted to hospitals that are perceived as having a strong clinical mission.

Use Case 17-1: Ensuring Clinical Perspective in Interface Design

Programmers at a major EHR vendor working to improve an interface were reluctant to obtain clinical perspectives on proposed changes. When questioned about the choice of an "improved" font and color in one panel that showed the medication order and order details, the designers (correctly) pointed out that they had access to a substantial body of human factors research and that the literature clearly agreed with their suggestion for how to draw the physician's eye to the correct data. However, the physician (even more correctly) pointed out that while the literature suggested how to draw attention to a particular item of data, it did not tell the designers which data was actually important to the physician. Human factor data can help separate useful from less useful data, but the definition of which data is useful is a clinical decision. In this particular example, the designers were attempting to highlight sections of data that were relatively trivial and that would have resulted in clinical confusion, a slower workflow, and a potential increase in the risk of medical errors.

Most successful implementations consistently maintain that the primary goal of the EHR is to improve the quality of patient care. The goal of clinical improvement must not only be stated but must accurately reflect the intent of those driving the project, it must be communicated throughout the timeline of the project by the project staff, and it must be communicated to both the clinical staff and the patient population. From a purely practical standpoint (and not merely starry-eyed idealism), clinical improvement must be the vision that drives the implementation as a whole, drives the IT staff to deliver a quality project, and drives the clinical staff to adopt the changes required of them.

The Balance Between Workflow and Risk

In designing any workable EHR, there is always a balance between mitigating risk and improving workflow. This trade-off recurs repeatedly at all levels during the implementation phase. On one hand, projects can minimize risk to such an extent that you risk impeding the ability to deliver efficient and timely care; on the other hand, you can easily deliver rapid and timely care while ignoring risks altogether. One classic example is the need for clinical documentation: physicians and nurses spend much of their time documenting their care, which slows down that care but also improves quality by providing information for further care in the future. Without documentation, care would be simpler and easier, but the risk would be increased. At the other extreme, there are already examples of medication administrations (and medication wastage) that require being witnessed by a second nurse. To better manage risk, we might go further and require that every clinical decision should require a second physician to be involved and to sign off on the action. While this might decrease the rate of errors, it would certainly impede the workflow and increase the cost of care.

Use Case 17-2: Communicating the Goal of the EHR Implementation

In a large, urban, multihospital EHR implementation project in the Midwest, the chief executive officer (CEO), chief medical officer (CMO), and chief nursing officer (CNO) consistently defined (and communicated) the primary goal of the EHR project as the improvement of patient care. Physicians were encouraged to voice their concerns and their suggestions for specific improvements, on the grounds that "if the EHR does not improve patient care, then it's not worth doing." The hospital stood behind this vision throughout the project and did so at all levels of governance. The result was that when a physician could successfully argue for a design change that would result in improved care, the change was graciously accepted. If, however, the physician simply voiced concerns about the system with minimal or no detail as to how to alleviate the concern, they were gently told that if they weren't in favor of better quality patient care, then perhaps they shouldn't be in practice. It was a difficult argument for any physician to counter without undermining their professional ethics. The result was very few unfounded complaints and an adoption rate of almost 100 percent on the day of conversion.

Realistically, most decisions regarding the EHR interface and medical policy changes during implementation involve a careful balance between risk and workflow, and neither should be ignored. A typical trade-off is the ability to bypass alerts. This concern for alert fatigue, or the "cry wolf" problem, will be addressed in the following use case. Even without the complication of human fatigue with alerts, there is a clear issue of risk versus workflow when programming alerts in an EHR. For example, an EHR may alert the physician to every possible interaction, allergy, or other ordering concern, coming down hard on the issue of risk. Forcing the physician to respond to every alert may lower the risk of medication error, but it will slow patient care and may increase risk in time-critical cases.

In general, though not without exception, the two sides of this balance are represented by physicians on one side (who emphasize the need to increase the efficiency of their workflow, decrease lost time, and expedite patient care) and risk managers, quality assurance personnel, and hospital attorneys on the other (who emphasize the need to avoid risk, increase safety, and improve the quality of patient care). While both sides are correct in their concerns, any EHR implementation that ignores either view instead of finding a way to balance both concerns is asking for trouble. Quality care requires a careful assessment of both of these issues. Quality care must be timely and safe; when there is a trade-off between these two concerns (as there usually is), then both must be assessed in light of the overall quality of care, not merely in terms of risk or workflow.

Change Control Best Practices

Many large HIT systems, such as an EHR, have a great degree of customization and configuration required for local use by a particular hospital or office practice. Multiple

Use Case 17-3: Balancing Clinical Risk with Impact on Workflow

One large, national chain of hospitals had a chief medical information officer (CMIO) who was almost exclusively concerned about risk, without regard to workflow costs. He required that physicians not only see every potentially useful CPOE alert (including lower-risk diet-to-drug interactions) but that they choose a specific rationale every time they overrode an alert. Again, with an eye toward risk (including litigation risk), he required that physicians choose from a drop-down list of 17 possible reasons for overriding each alert in order to clearly document their clinical thinking. Physicians, daunted by the number of clicks, the length of the drop-down (which required scrolling through four screens to see the full list), and the loss of time, immediately discovered that they could simply click the first choice on the drop-down, thereby saving several clicks and several seconds per alert. When the CMIO queried the data after the first six months, he discovered that 99.3 percent of all such alerts were overridden for a single reason—the one listed first on the list of options. The data was reliable but invalid, because it did not accurately reflect the actual rationale used but only the easiest option to access.

environments, also known in some systems as domains, of the same base software are maintained at each organization to facilitate a controlled change process as the customization and configuration occurs. The Development environment is the environment where analysts, programmers, and application specialists "build" the customized functionality that is right for the organization. If they make a mistake in the Development environment, patients don't get hurt. Once they are done with the build, they move the new functionality into a QA/Test environment, and test engineers and analysts run multiple tests on it. (One test analyst told me his job is to try to break things!) A User Test, also known as a Train (short for training), environment is closer still to the actual live environment, with a full set of realistic patient data that allow users to "play in the sandbox" before they experience the software in clinical or business practice. The Production/Live environment—the environment that clinicians and staff use to manage actual "live" patient data—is the final destination for the new functionality that has been carefully developed and tested. After the build is moved into Production/Live, it is carefully monitored for unintended consequences for several days to several weeks.

Project Governance

Several characteristics are found in the majority of successful EHR implementation projects. These include the inclusion of clinical decision makers, reliable timelines and deadlines, and the normal (but all-too-frequently ignored) "rules of responsibility." The overall organization generally includes ownership at the executive level, with an overall project committee immediately under this level. This project committee includes clinicians and is occasionally chaired by them as well but must include the project manager, the IT department, and vendor representation. At this level, the project represents both the clinical and the technical aspects of the project. Below the project level, committee structures usually split into the technical side (encompassing the catalog, build, domains, hardware, etc.) and the clinical side (encompassing the order sets, procedures, processes, workflow, etc.). It remains imperative that close communication between the two sides be maintained, particularly in regard to the design decisions, orderables, and the interaction between the technical system and the clinical workflows, which are mutually dependent upon one another.

While the importance of including clinical decision makers (and having a clinical vision) has been discussed, the practical nature of this becomes apparent within the clinical committees. These generally include a single overarching clinical committee, with subcommittees responsible for order set design (with IT representation), both overall and by specialty. In general, the clinical committee has two major functions and a host of minor responsibilities. The two major issues are the design and maintenance of the order sets and the analysis of both current and future workflows. Of these, the former takes the most time and resources, while the latter is actually more important to success at conversion. Conversion to an EHR system can survive (and occasionally has) the absence of order sets, but it cannot survive a total absence of workflow analysis. Physicians can place individual orders, but they *must* know how to manage their patients in the new EHR environment.

The importance of timelines and deadlines becomes very obvious when they are absent. Not only are there financial and contractual costs associated with missed timelines, but the project rapidly loses all credibility when the timelines slip repeatedly. Such loss of credibility can entirely destroy any attempt to achieve meaningful use (MU), because the clinical staff becomes unwilling to believe a timeline that has repeatedly changed. They can scarcely be expected to alter their surgical schedules, clinic appointments, staffing needs, and personal time in order to accommodate a project that has proven itself unreliable.

Project Deadlines

The issue of deadlines has equal importance, if at a smaller scale, to project governance. Here, the issue is that many of the critical parts of the project are interdependent. One typical example of this is the order catalog or complete list of all items (nursing orders, lab, medication, radiology, ancillary departments, etc.) a physician might order. In the optimal case, the catalog should be complete and accurate prior to starting order set design, since the orderables within an order set would otherwise change every time the catalog was amended. Workflow analysis is dependent upon the order sets, because they determine how physicians and nurses will organize their clinical care. Training cannot be done until the workflows are determined, because the workflows determine training, and training would otherwise have to be redone every time the workflow changed. Conversion cannot occur until after training, for obvious reasons. While there is actually a reasonable amount of flexibility in order set design as the catalog is coming into final form, every time a deadline is missed in the catalog, the order set design, the workflows, or the training, there is a very real risk of compromising the conversion date. Almost every deadline has an impact on the entire project, and very few deadlines stand independent of the entire project. However, individual workers often overlook the problem of being "just a few days late." While a project may be able to survive a few missed deadlines, this can rapidly snowball, resulting in a complete failure of the heavily interdependent nature of EHR implementations. A missed deadline is a predictor of a failed conversion.

The most obvious rules of responsibility are also the most frequently ignored. These rules are easy to state and their adherence almost always guarantees project success.

Use Case 17-4: The Importance of Avoiding Schedule Delays

A 200-bed community hospital in the Southeast was "forced" to push back their date of conversion three times. By the time the actual conversion occurred, only five of the staff physicians had agreed to attend training, and while the nurses had been required to attend training, few of them were willing to take it seriously by the third time. Several physicians had instituted a betting pool on the actual date of conversion, and almost none were willing to bet on the actual date. On the morning of conversion, only seven orders were placed using the CPOE function of the EHR, thus ignoring both pleas and threats (by the CEO) regarding the necessity of CPOE. The conversion was canceled before noon. After substantial loss of money and credibility, the hospital managed to finally achieve a conversion 18 months later (with 30 percent compliance in using CPOE).

Unfortunately the rules are enforced selectively in most organizations. The rules require that when any action has been decided upon, the committee must define the following:

- *Who* is to perform the task
- *What* the task consists of
- *When* the task is to be finished
- *Where* the results are to be brought

If, for example, the committee has decided that they should obtain a legal opinion from the hospital attorney, then they should state that: "*John* is to contact the attorney and request an opinion consisting of an *e-mail* response from the attorney, which should be sent before *Thursday* at 4 p.m. to *Mary*, the committee chair."

The absence of any one of these defined items can result in committees that not only never get anything accomplished but also have no idea why they are having problems. The clinical equivalent to this occurs during cardiac arrests, when a physician yells out an order for epinephrine, without specifying who is to give it, what dose, what route, and so on. Actions require boundaries and definition.

Orderable Nomenclature

A build is only as good as its clinical utility. While technical aspects are crucial to a successful build, clinical aspects are equally crucial. The user does not see, and has little appreciation of, the technical underpinnings of the build but is immediately and keenly aware of any clinical shortcomings when using the EHR. Clinical utility defines the build success. Within the orders catalog the same observation pertains. Clinical users will be attentive to errors and to the difficulty of use within their clinical workflow. The most obvious concerns, from the clinical perspective, are the use of synonyms and order entry formats (OEFs).

Important Definitions

- **Order Catalog**   A complete list of all items or actions that can be ordered within a medical system
- **Orderable**   Any item that can be ordered from the catalog
- **Order Entry Formats (OEFs)**   All of the order details in a given orderable
- **Synonyms**   Any of several alternative names used for the same orderable

Within the orders catalog the same observation pertains. Clinical users will be attentive to errors and to the difficulty of use within their clinical workflow. The most obvious concerns, from the clinical perspective, are the use of synonyms and order entry formats (OEFs).

Common Errors

Synonyms should have *clinical meaning*. While this seems obvious, there are three commons errors: departmental naming, generic naming, and geographically local naming. In the first type of error, which is most commonly seen with radiology examinations, the department that actually performs the test (radiology, laboratory, blood bank, respiratory department, etc.) has had an historical name for the orderable, often reflecting either their own internal billing concerns or the inherited idiosyncrasies of previous decades. A common example is the order for a chest X-ray. While the official description in the system may be "XR Chest 2 view," a common synonym is "CXR" or simply "chest X-ray," terms most physicians are used to writing on paper. To ensure uniformity in how the order catalog is built, a nomenclature must be established. Conversely, there must be attention to the needs and expectations of the ordering physician. It is, after all, the ordering physician who is placing the order: the order should have a common, well-accepted nomenclature. In cases where the performing department has one name and the accepted clinical name is different, a synonym must be created in order to avoid errors and delays.

In the second common error, the catalog is restricted to generic names for medications. Unfortunately, while this is how medications should probably be listed, it is not in line with common usage and can actually be erroneous. In the case of common medications, such as over-the-counter pain medications, patients and clinical personnel often use the commercial names of these drugs. While due attention must be given to the correct form (e.g., caplets, pills, capsules, liquids, or suppository) of the drug and to combined ingredients (e.g., acetaminophen with codeine), the careful use of synonyms can speed patient care. Moreover, in the case of some medications, not only do few physicians (and sometimes few pharmacists) know the names of the generic

Use Case 17-5: Being Aware of Different Nomenclature

A large, national hospital chain converted its catalog for CPOE but continued to use the radiology nomenclature without any attention to the ordering physician's common nomenclature. On the previous paper order form, clinicians had long ordered a "Doppler" when they wanted to have an ultrasound done of an extremity when concerned for venous clots. In the previous workflow, the unit clerk would read the physician's written order and, with knowledge of the idiosyncratic order catalog, enter an order into the computer that the radiology department understood as a Doppler exam. However, not only was "Doppler" not in the electronic catalog and available to the ordering physician via CPOE, but neither was "ultrasound," "US," "clot," "vein," "venous," or several other educated guesses. On the day of conversion, one physician spent 16 minutes simply trying to locate the name of the test (that 100 percent of the clinical staff called a "Doppler") before the radiology department informed him that it was now called an "NV" (for nonvascular). No clinical physician had ever heard of an NV before, yet they were now required to use the orderable.

ingredients, but changing pharmaceutical contracts often result in changing availability over time. One example is that of topical ophthalmic drops. Inpatient pharmacies may change suppliers to keep costs down, yet the clinicians often look for (and refer to) the name of a common commercial preparation of such drops. This can lead to both errors and delays in ordering. With due regard for copyright and safety, synonyms can speed ordering without compromising quality.

The third common error in orderable nomenclature is the use of geographically local names to the exclusion of nationally used terms. Many smaller (and some larger) hospitals have gradually come to use local idiomatic names for some laboratory tests and other orderables. Even quite common terms such as "BMP," "Chem7," "basic metabolic profile," and "chemistry profile" that are used nationally may vary in actual composition from location to location. This is all the more true of terms such as "trauma panel" or "cardiology panel," which define a general medical concern but lack an accepted definition. There is a temptation to accept purely local nomenclature on the grounds that "that's what we've always called it and everyone knows the name already." But, in reality, new physicians come not only from anywhere in the nation but from anywhere in the world. Synonyms should reflect common (global) usage rather than regional usage. In the case of the "basic metabolic panel" (regardless of the actual composition of the panel), there may be good reason to have several common synonyms. However many synonyms there are, at least one synonym must reflect accepted global usage.

A final caveat can be made to restrict synonyms that might increase risk. Several hospitals have chosen to remove both the abbreviation BMP (basic metabolic profile) and the abbreviation BNP (beta naturetic peptide) from their catalogs on the grounds that these two abbreviations are often confused, whether spoken, written, or searched in a computer and that safety considerations require the test names be used in full. This sort of concern, which may actually restrict the use of synonyms, is worth consideration, but the overall concern needs to be finding a balance between the ease of workflow (finding the orderable) and the risk of error (confusing orderables). In general, synonyms are useful to clinicians, and widely accepted synonyms are essential to a quality catalog, but care needs to be taken so as not to introduce patient safety issues with overly broad usage of synonyms.

The most common error within the orderable is either to include unnecessary OEFs or, even worse, to actually require using unnecessary OEFs. Within the individual orderable, the OEFs are necessary to define the details of the orderable, but too many OEFs can slow medical care. In every case of defining an orderable, the question must be asked: "Is this OEF *necessary*?" In many cases, the OEF is unnecessary and simply slows care without any gain in quality. In many cases, the designers of EHRs have assumed that all prior (paper) OEFs must be maintained in the electronic version. In the computer world, much of the information that had to be included in a paper order can now be found easily from anywhere in the hospital at any time. Common examples are the OEFs within radiology orders. In the paper world, these were needed on the paper order that accompanied the patient to radiology, since the entire paper chart was not available during transport. In the electronic world, however, a patient's EHR is available hospitalwide. Most hospitals have therefore removed radiology OEFs for pregnancy

Use Case 17-6: Invest Time before Conversion to Avoid Risk and Save Clinician Time

A community hospital in Iowa discovered that physicians could (if they weren't careful) easily order Mylanta 60 ml, intravenously (IV). Mylanta is an oral antacid medication not meant to be given IV but could be given IV if someone tasked to execute the order simply followed the physician's instructions and was not thinking critically about the order. While this order would (ideally) not be filled by the pharmacist nor administered by the nurse, the fact that the order was permitted by the system was felt to be a foolish and unnecessary risk and necessitated a complete review of the catalog.

Editing the options within an OEF can be time-consuming, but it will save time and energy in the long run. While the EHR implementation project might need to allocate someone for a week to edit these OEFs to avoid patient risk, if it isn't done, then the outcome is that each physician will waste a few extra seconds every time they place an order. Over the course of a year, the wasted clinical time, including all patients and medical staff, can add up to several days. This waste will take resources out of the overall hospital budget as the costs rise per nurse, per physician, and per patient. OEFs must be pared down to the essentials prior to EHR conversion. Any other action wastes money, wastes time, and increases risk.

status, oxygen use, transport type, and so on. This information, which is critical to good care and to radiology, can now be found in the EHR. Even OEFs that are clearly necessary, such as the reason for exam in the case of radiology tests, can often be reduced to a manageable drop-down or even, in the case of clinically limited order sets, defaulted into the clinical problem addressed in the same order set. For example, an order set for pneumonia should default the reason for a chest X-ray exam as "pneumonia."

An almost equally common and unnecessary design mistake with OEFs occurs when the details within an OEF are not edited for clinical applicability. In the case of medication orders, the route of administration is necessary, but not all medications can be given by all possible routes. An orderable for common IV antibiotics must have an OEF for routes of administration, and this OEF must include the choice of IV. An orderable for common oral antacids, however, should *not* include the choice of "IV" among the routes of administration. In many builds, the OEF for routes of administration is taken from a general list and is not edited for clinical accuracy. Since this list is often several dozen items in length, the lack of editing slows patient care as the physician is forced to weed through not only the two to three options that are clinically appropriate and that might reasonably be used for the patients but also the two to three dozen other options that are entirely unreasonable. This slows patient care, but also more importantly, it increases the risk of medication error. OEFs that permit the ordering by unsafe routes should not be listed.

Order Sets

Correctly used, order sets can be effective tools because they speed up care, increase safety, and reduce medical errors. The best order sets not only represent the best practices but provide the flexibility to respond to individual patient circumstances and still increase efficiency. Order sets are not "cookbook medicine," but they are recipes. Like all recipes, they can give you extremely useful guidelines and ensure a good outcome, but like any recipe, they can be adapted to produce a different outcome when necessary. While most hip-replacement patients fit nicely into a Hip-Replacement Order Set, some patients will have additional medical problems, some will have surgical complications, some will have allergies, and some will do something unexpected. A good order set reflects the best care, but it allows user modifications to respond to individual patients. An order set can never prevent poor care; the most it can do is make it harder to deliver poor care.

 HIT PRO EXAM TIP   Order sets when used properly can be effective tools in speeding up care, increasing safety, and reducing medical errors. The best order sets provide flexibility to respond to individual patient circumstances.

In any EHR implementation project, a clinical committee oversees the design, deadlines, and insertion of order sets into the domain. This committee is also responsible for ensuring the clinical and technical appropriateness of the order sets. The clinical committee also ensures that the hospital has all of the order sets it requires in response to clinical, financial, and regulatory needs and that all of the order sets comply with the institutional design parameters and nomenclature. A subcommittee, or physicians representing a clinical specialty, develops the design of the individual order sets. This subcommittee, or group of physicians, also ensures that the details of the order set are accurate and appropriate for actual patient care.

Order Set Design Rules

Several "rules of good design" should be followed by institutions in order to ensure that the order sets they create are successful.

- **Standard nomenclature**   The name of any order set should not only immediately suggest its content but also should be the first guess when searched for by a user. The overarching rule is that naming should be "intuitive and consistent." Using an intuitive name lowers the risk of errors and lost time both in choosing an order set (in which the name alone should make it clear what the order set should be used for without confusion or error) and in searching for an order set (the most likely search parameters should always result in finding the order set). A new physician, or a physician using an unfamiliar order set, should be able to guess at the likely name and find it immediately without delay and without frustration. Names should make sense.

- **Standard internal organization**   Again, the rule is simple: the internal organization of the orderables and the orderable categories should be intuitive and consistent. The value of consistency is that users will always be able to locate individual orderables, even when using an unfamiliar order set or in an unfamiliar medical setting. Historically, this is the same organizing framework that was used to place admitting orders to a hospital and, with a handful of different eponyms and slightly different arrangements, generally begins with an order to admit and then a diagnosis, vital signs, nursing orders, laboratory orders, and medication orders. In general, there is every reason to simply adopt (or adapt) the framework previously used for paper orders with a few caveats. Some hospitals feel that medication orders (since they carry the most risk) should be "higher" in the order set to avoid inadvertent placing of orders that might not be intended. Certain orders such as blood bank orders may be brought together, even though they encompass disparate types of orders (laboratory, IV, consent, nursing, medications) that would otherwise be separated. Note that some content vendors, for example Zynx, Provation, and BMJ, suppliers of commercially available content used by organizations to create order sets, offer their own proprietary order set organization. This order set organization does not need to be followed, even in hospitals with a Zynx subscription. Finally, most commercially available order sets offer the option of having subcategories, which should be used with moderation, because they can slow down care.

- **Concise and efficient design**   Almost invariably, order sets are too long. The optimal order set is one screen (more realistically, two) and requires no clicking or scrolling. Common orders are prechecked, and rarely used orderables are absent. As a quick rule of thumb, any suggestion that an order—or a comment line—be added to an order set should require thoughtful justification. Every time an order is added "to make it easier," the order set becomes longer and harder to use, so the question should be whether the added order is justified. There is almost no such thing as an order set that is too short. This same attention to efficiency and utility applies to using the fewest possible subphases (if any), the shortest possible drop-downs (if any), and the least number of unchecked orders (if any). Some hospitals have argued that, in the interests of safety, order sets should never contain any prechecked orders. While this is an understandable position, it undercuts the value of order sets and generally prevents widespread adoption. Even with safety in mind, an order set is optimal when it cannot be made any easier to use.

- **Flexible design and maintenance**   Many vendors offer the option of saving order sets once an individual user has prechecked, chosen options and even added to the standard orderables of the order set. Even hospitals that initially chose to disallow this option have generally permitted its use later. The purpose of the order set, to push an accepted standard of care, is not undercut by this usage. The user can always place orders either way; the previous option merely makes it simpler to do so. Regardless of how order sets are used, however, they must be maintained. In many cases, order sets need to respond rapidly to changes in medication (e.g., antibiotic drug resistance, newer oncology medications), new clinical data, and changing regulation. As a general rule, order sets should be reviewed at least annually as well as whenever new data warrants review.

> ## Use Case 17-7: Strive for Unambiguous Order Set Titles
>
> A Michigan hospital had an order set called Acute Pn Abd Fe. Several physicians assumed that this was for patients who had abdominal pain secondary to iron (Fe) ingestion, since iron ingestion does cause abdominal pain. Although the order set was actually intended for female (Fe) patients with abdominal pain, the corresponding order set for males was named Acute Pn Abd Male (spelling out the gender fully). Good usage would have been to (at least) spell out "female" as they had spelled out "male." A better choice would have been to have named the order set Acute Abdominal Pain, Female or another unambiguous title.

Home Folders

Home folders (also called *modal order entry windows*) are the screens that come up initially when a physician wants to place an order. In some of the initial EHRs, these screens consisted of no more than a search window, requiring that every order or order set be typed out, character by character. Most EHRs have now evolved to include the ability to search on the first few characters (making searching faster and easier), as well as allowing users to build "favorites" folders, which include their most common orders or order sets.

The most efficient way to place an order is not to search but to click. The most efficient way to use favorites folders is not to build them but to have them already built. The most effective ways to place orders, having them face-up and available by a single click when the user wants to place an order, are possible because of a general rule of clinical care: most things that were ordered yesterday will be ordered again today. This is equally true for single orders and for order sets; each specialty has its own typical orders and order sets. Physicians almost never need to find obscure orders by searching the entire catalog. Unfortunately, this design principle is rarely employed by EHR vendors but can almost always be used effectively by an individual hospital. There are two key design rules.

- Every specialty needs its own home folder.
- The folder should contain only those orders that are in daily (or weekly) use.

In the case of the first rule, a specialty is defined by similarity of workflow and limited by project resources. In some smaller hospitals, there may be only three to four specialty folders, typically including the emergency department, surgery, hospitalists, and pediatrics. In larger, academic centers, there may be as many as several dozen specialty folders, each fashioned by the few physicians (e.g., pediatric neurosurgeons) who share a common workflow.

Despite training and potential value, some physicians never create their own favorites folders, and their workflow is consequently inefficient. Having daily orders and order sets directly in front of a physician enables rapid and efficient ordering and can even be used to "steer" patient care. For example, having the "preferred" hospital antibiotic available with a single click makes it far less likely that the physician will order the more expensive antibiotic that requires searching and modification.

The optimal home folder then includes only frequently placed orders and is visually organized for rapid location and ordering. There should be few (or no) drop-downs or options. OEFs should be defaulted in whenever possible. In some cases, an order can be placed in the home folder twice, each with a different OEF. For example, in an emergency department there are two common reasons for ordering a chest X-ray, either for chest pain or for respiratory problems (dyspnea, shortness of breath, or cough). Many hospitals have therefore placed two chest X-ray orders (for the two different reasons listed here) on the emergency department home folder, enabling rapid radiology ordering. This same principle can apply to common drugs that have two commonly used doses or to IVs that have several common rates of infusion. In each case, the question remains the same: which orders (and which OEFs) are the most commonly ordered for that group of physicians?

The best examples of this approach have gone further and used color or other visual cues to decrease search time even more. They have also included orderables immediately followed by the OEF options that are in daily use, thus ensuring that any common OEF can be ordered by a single click.

Clinical Decision Support

CDS has come into its own over the past decade and, at least in principle, includes not only simple alerts but more sophisticated pop-ups, order trees, references, calculators, and rules that are meant to improve patient care by offering advice to the physician. Most of these are synchronous, in that they are dynamic and offer advice at the moment the clinical decision is being made (real time) rather than in retrospect (asynchronous). Given the complexity of medicine and the overwhelming and rapidly increasing medical literature, no physician, perhaps even within their own specialty, can realistically keep up with all of the available current evidence. To the extent that the computer can be used to improve medical care, the use of clinical decision support is laudable and can be effective.

Too often, however, clinical decision support can actually increase risk. The most common problem occurs with the use of pop-up alerts (e.g., for allergies or drug interactions) that occur so frequently that the physician no longer notices them. This "cry wolf" phenomenon is universal and can severely impede medical care. The risk is not so much that the unnecessary alert will slow down medical care and prevent the adoption of CPOE (both of which do occur) but that recurrent, unnecessary alerts will result in the physician ignoring an alert when it is actually beneficial and even necessary. Any physician who has just seen 99 alerts that had no clinical relevance and that slowed their workflow can routinely be expected to ignore the next one, even if that alert is critical to patient survival. Human beings are unable to maintain vigilance when there is a low frequency of significant information.

The key is to design and implement alerts and rules that are necessary and that will have an effect on patient care, rather than simply designing and implementing rules that may occasionally be useful and important. In using clinical decision support, wishful thinking and pious intentions will predictably decrease the quality of patient care and patient safety. Data, intelligence, sophistication, and knowledge of human nature, with careful attention to real-life clinical workflow, are required.

Any CDS intervention will fail if it is delivered to the wrong person at the wrong time. If the CDS doesn't precisely match the workflow, it becomes "white noise" and merely drowns out other information that might be useful. Successful use of CDS requires that you always answer several key questions every time you propose to present clinical advice.

- What is the *crucial piece* of information?
- Who *requires* it?
- What is the *best format* for the information?
- What is the *best point in the workflow* to present the information?

Any time you present the wrong information or give it to the wrong person, in the wrong format, or at the wrong point in time, you fail. Worse yet, you will actually undermine the value of all other attempts to support clinical decision making, even if the other attempts are done perfectly. *Poorly designed decision support is worse than no decision support.* To learn more about clinical decision support, including design principles for effective clinical decisions support, see Chapter 19.

Use Case 17-8: Avoiding Poorly Designed CDS

A single physician was observed for three hours during a busy shift in the emergency department. During this time, he experienced six pop-up alerts, warning him about drug allergies and drug interactions. In every case he bypassed these alerts; every one of these alerts was later reviewed and felt to be appropriate. At the end of the three-hour period, the physician was asked if he had noticed any alerts during the morning. He denied having seen any alerts, let alone having bypassed them. His behavior, not atypical, had become automatic, and he had ceased to even notice potentially important information. Frequent alerts, particularly if they do not result in a change in the clinical decision, result in habituation and inattention. Had there been a significant alert, this physician, like many others, would likely have ignored it. *Poorly designed clinical decision support increases patient risk.*

EHR Conversions

The majority of conversions are now done as "big-bang" conversions, rather than unit-by-unit conversions, although many hospitals still convert the emergency department first, followed by inpatient wards. The important principle is to avoid having patients with simultaneous paper and electronic charts, especially for orders in general and medications in particular. Since the emergency department is, in some sense, isolated from inpatient care, it can be converted independently as long as some care is taken during the admission process. The same, again with due care, can be said of the independent conversion of labor and delivery units or ambulatory clinics. In accordance with this point, CPOE is (within any unit and often for all inpatients) all-or-nothing. Clinical documentation, however, can be (and often is) implemented on a more gradual basis.

Regardless of other considerations, EHR conversions should occur when patient census (number of patients in the hospital) and staff stress can be minimized, if feasible. This is true with regard to the time of year (e.g., avoiding seasonal increases in admission), day of the week (weekends may mean a quieter surgery schedule), and time of day (early morning is often used).

Conversion support typically consists of personnel in a command center (handling issues and change control) and superusers on the clinical wards (handling direct support for the users). Typically, there is a specific hotline for physician support and, likewise, specific superuser support on the clinical wards for the physicians. Within the command center, organization is key. The primary point of organization is change control. Some issues, such as those that are patient critical, must be managed immediately. But, most issues require at least a short time to consider the ramifications to the system and to clinical workflow. All issues, even patient critical issues that may be documented retrospectively, require documentation. Every issue must have the following considerations:

- How critical is this issue? What is the priority?
- What resources will this issue require to be fixed?
- What else will happen to the system, or to workflow, if the change is made?

Every issue should be logged, given a priority, and dealt with by a defined chain of command, even when done on an emergent basis. On the morning of conversion, critical decisions are typically made in real time (i.e., immediately). Less critical decisions are still made quickly, and all decisions that have been handled are then reported in a staff meeting, typically every 12 hours. By the end of the conversion period (usually 1 to 2 weeks), decision making generally settles into a more leisurely pattern, and decisions begin to be made on a daily basis, with staff meetings held on a similar schedule. After the conversion period, decisions gradually resume the baseline pace and require consideration by a committee structure, which meets perhaps every several weeks or even every several months. Support for EHR users follows a pattern similar to that of decision making, and by the end of the first two weeks there will be some support in-house during the day, with limited support available by phone during the nights.

Physician Support Issues

There is generally a need for physician-specific support, with both a physician hotline and superusers specifically for physicians. In addition, most conversions attempt to increase the number of physicians, who may either have clinical duties or serve as superuser support for those who do have clinical duties. This assumes that such additional personnel are available and have flexibility in their schedules, which may well not be the case. Often the department heads, CMO, chief of staff, or other administrative physicians will provide support during the conversion period, or outside physician consultants may be hired.

Postconversion Issues

Postconversion, a number of issues must be addressed. After conversion, the hospital must assess the success of the project, modify the governance structures for long-term functions, and optimize both the system and the users.

Postconversion assessments require that the hospital determine their goals and means of measuring successful attainment of those goals before the conversion to an EHR system begins, usually in a project charter. After conversion, the hospital must then measure its success by carefully comparing the goals specified in the charter with the actual results attained and then deciding on the next steps.

Governance changes are generally of two sorts. Much of the project governance gradually ties up the work and ends, while other parts of the governance, particularly the clinical structures, adapt and become permanent parts of the hospital structure. Typically, for example, the committee that oversaw the development of order sets must now continue to review, update, and maintain such order sets on a permanent, ongoing basis.

Optimization of the system is usually clearly defined. System issues must be fixed and closed, but there are also long-term issues such as upgrades that need to be taken care of. Often ignored but crucial to long-term success is the optimization of the users and their workflow. A large number of clinical users have typically learned just enough of the system to survive conversion but will need to be reevaluated and receive additional training if they are ever to become adept and efficient at using the system. The use of favorites, macros, filters, and customizable settings is often forgotten or scarcely learned at all and will require that the trainers "circle back" and help such clinical users improve.

Finally, successful hospitals use the postconversion period to reassess clinical workflows and clinical decision support. Most clinical workflows were designed prior to conversion, in an attempt to provide optimal guidance, but these workflows are often found to be imperfect once conversion occurs. A good hospital will use its remaining clinical governance to review workflows and "touch up" any workflows that need improvement. Clinical decision support is likewise usually imperfect. The most typical problem is that there are too many alerts, and they should be pared down or redesigned. The reevaluation and redesign of clinical decision support should be ongoing and permanent.

System Patching and Updates

As stated elsewhere in this book, there are many systems, large and small, even in a medium-sized healthcare enterprise. Almost all of them require software and hardware upgrades and/or patches on an intermittent basis. Small patches are generally scheduled quarterly and large upgrades are done every 1–3 years. There are many approaches to rolling out patches and upgrades in a healthcare environment. Some principles behind these approaches deserve a mention. Since the main objective of a healthcare organization is high-quality patient care, planning for a patch or upgrade starts with analyzing the effect of the change in software functionality on clinician and staff work and workflows. Once the changes are analyzed and identified, training to optimize clinician and staff use of the newly patched or upgraded software is planned and executed. Simultaneously, HIT technical staff begin staging the patch or upgrade for installation. If possible, testing the change on non-production/non-live environments is highly recommended. Especially for large upgrades, a mini-implementation, complete with a command center and around the clock "go-live" support should be planned and carried out. Finally, a postmortem meeting and a lessons learned write up should be done, so that future patches and upgrades benefit from the experience.

Chapter Review

In this chapter, I reviewed many aspects of EHR implementation in a hospital setting. The key features of a successful implementation are clinical workflow and an attention to patient care. IT critically supports but cannot drive the project nor define its success. Governance, design considerations, the catalog and its orderables, the order sets, and clinical decision support must all aim to improve clinical use and strengthen the quality of patient care provided. Implementations should minimize user stress and patient risk and must have a clearly defined structure for handling change control. Once the EHR has been implemented, systems converted, and the system optimized, some aspects of any implementation, such as order set maintenance, optimization of workflow, and clinical decision support, become ongoing and permanent operations.

Questions

To test your comprehension of the chapter, answer the following questions and then check your answers against the list of correct answers at the end of the chapter.

1. Why is the implementation of EHRs on the rise?

    A. Hospitals need to find better ways to use their employees.

    B. It's because of the government's prompting, with regulatory requirements that have been accompanied by financial incentives.

    C. All of the above.

    D. None of the above.

2. What is the key to a successful implementation?

    A. It is done as quickly as possible.

    B. It uses a lot of a hospital's resources.

    C. It supports clinical care.

    D. It doesn't bother the hospital staff.

3. When developing orderable nomenclature for an EHR system, what are the three most common errors?

    A. Too many orderables, poor spelling, and poor layout

    B. Departmental classifications, brand name classifications, and regionwide classification

    C. Departmental naming, generic naming, and geographically local naming

    D. No order entry formats, no place to write an order, and too many choices

4. When used correctly, order sets can do which of the following?

    A. Be effective tools because they speed up care, increase safety, and reduce medical errors

    B. Help doctors and nurses diagnose patients without spending much time with them

    C. Eliminate errors in reporting infectious diseases

    D. Reduce the amount of time a patient waits in an emergency room

5. Successful use of clinical decision support requires that you always answer several key questions every time you propose to present clinical advice:

    • What is the *crucial piece* of information?

    • Who *requires* it?

    • What is the *best format* for the information?

    • What is the *best point in the workflow* to present the information?

    A. True

    B. False

6. What are two key design rules in developing home folders in an EHR?

   A. Making them visually pleasing and easy to see.

   B. Ensuring that all doctors have their own folder and can access it from anywhere.

   C. Every specialty needs its own home folder, and the folder should contain only those orders that are in daily (or weekly) use.

   D. All specialties can find their folders from home, and the folder has all orders they have ever created.

7. What is an important principle during the conversion stage?

   A. To manage the conversion piece by piece over several weeks

   B. To make the conversion during a busy time at the hospital so you can see how it will work quickly

   C. To make sure all hospital staff gets a chance to voice their concerns

   D. To avoid having patients with simultaneous paper and electronic charts, especially for orders in general and medications in particular

Answers

1. **B.** Implementation of HIT is on the rise because of the government's prompting, with regulatory requirements that have been accompanied by financial incentives.

2. **C.** The key to a successful implementation is that it supports clinical care.

3. **C.** When developing orderable nomenclature for an EHR system, the three most common errors are departmental naming, generic naming, and geographically local naming.

4. **A.** Correctly used, order sets can be effective tools as they speed up care, increase safety, and reduce medical errors.

5. **A.** Successful use of clinical decision support requires that you always answer several key questions every time you propose to present clinical advice:

   • What is the *crucial piece* of information?

   • Who *requires* it?

   • What is the *best format* for the information?

   • What is the *best point in the workflow* to present the information?

6. **C.** Two key design rules in developing home folders in an EHR are that every specialty needs its own home folder and the folder should contain only those orders that are in daily (or weekly) use.

7. **D.** An important principle during the conversion stage is to avoid having patients with simultaneous paper and electronic charts, especially for orders in general and medications in particular.

412

References

1. Frankovich, J., Longhurst, C. A., & Sutherland, S. M. (2011). Evidence-based medicine in the EMR era. *New England Journal of Medicine, 365,* 1758–1759.

2. Vishwanath, A., Singh, S. R., & Winkelstein, P. (2010). The impact of electronic medical record systems on outpatient workflows: A longitudinal evaluation of its workflow effects. *International Journal of Medical Informatics, 79,* 778–791.

3. Longhurst, C. A., Parast, L., Sandborg, C. I., Widen, E., Sullivan, J., Hahn, J. S., Dawes, C. G., & Sharek, P. J. (2010). Decrease in hospital-wide mortality rate after implementation of a commercially sold computerized physician order entry system. *Pediatrics, 126,* 14–21.

HIT Connectivity and Interoperability Opportunities and Challenges

David Liebovitz

In this chapter, you will learn how to
- Identify the purpose and uses of pertinent healthcare terminologies in the electronic health record
- Identify commonly used medical terms and devices
- Describe the role of mobile and ubiquitous computing in healthcare
- Describe data flows across HIT systems and the implication of standards
- Understand the principles of healthcare data exchange and standards, workflow design and assessment, and their relationship to patient care

Rounding in the Hospital

The inpatient environment presents numerous opportunities for the effective delivery of healthcare information. Imagine, for a moment, a large hospital with 500 beds, with 75 devoted to intensive-care patients. In such an environment, at any moment in time, some patients are improving as expected, some are stable but haven't yet turned the corner for definite improvement, and, unfortunately, some are deteriorating. Taking this scenario a bit further, if a new parameter for a patient, say blood pressure or temperature, was recorded that clearly moved the patient out of the "improving" category and into the deteriorating category, how might this data point serve as a trigger for immediate evaluation?

To address scenarios like this one, it is helpful to consider the data flows that are required. First, a data element is acquired from a patient. In a simple context, you could imagine that a temperature is entered into an electronic medical record (EMR) system after having been obtained from a patient-care technician whose job is to assist nurses in their clinical duties. For the temperature value to be interpreted by the EMR, the fields in the system need to understand that this is a numerical value (say, 100.6) and its units (for example, degrees Fahrenheit). Once data is recorded in this manner, syndrome recognition algorithms can come into play. In this context, consider that there is a syndrome entitled systemic inflammatory response syndrome (SIRS). This particular syndrome recognizes emerging severe infections as well as other severe inflammatory states. Since there are specific criteria that define SIRS, if temperature is an element, then a change in temperature could indicate that a patient has now developed SIRS, a negative prognostic indicator, and send a message to a caregiver. For the EMR to recognize newly entered temperatures, all locations within the EMR that record temperature must be available to the SIRS decision support engine, and all values should be consistent regarding their units (Fahrenheit versus Celsius) and also be explicit regarding their source (e.g., oral temperature versus ear sensors) in order for criteria to be appropriately assessed for SIRS.

In this context, it's helpful to consider that EMRs also receive data directly from medical devices. For example, in an intensive-care unit, patients may have a sphygmomanometer cuff attached that periodically and automatically inflates and records a blood pressure. This value can be directly interfaced to the EMR. In this example, to raise the complexity a bit, it often exists as a "temporary value" that can then be verified and accepted into the system by the nurse taking care of the patient. This holding pattern before acceptance is necessary since sometimes a transmitted reading may have an error if, for example, the patient moves her arm, such that automatic instantiation into the record might lead to erroneous decisions. The transmission of information from a biomedical device into an EMR is referred to as a *bedside-medical* (or biomedical) *device interface* (BMDI).

The complexity of directly transmitting information from a device into an EMR is readily evident. How does the EMR know which patient's data is coming in? How does the device identify which patient's information is being relayed? Is the same process followed for every device connected to a patient? To address these issues, communication standards would be beneficial, but they are not yet comprehensive, and proprietary approaches are common. An applicable common language approach is evolving through the Integrating the Healthcare Enterprise (IHE) initiative. Specifically, the IHE Patient Care Device (PCD) domain and framework profiles address numerous aspects of this process (www.ihe.net/pcd/).

At this point, we have taken clinical information from a monitor, and a nurse has recorded the value in the context of the EMR. What's next? At a macro-level view within the organization, if a dashboard notification process has been established and this new data element results in an algorithm generating an alert, then a page or other notification message might be transmitted to a surveillance or rapid response team (RRT), letting them know the patient may require further attention. If not, this information will be reviewed in the normal course of clinical workflow.

To understand device considerations when working in a hospital, it is essential to describe briefly the physician workflow. Depending on the setting (community or academic hospital) and the clinical service (e.g., organ transplant versus psychiatry), workflow and information needs may differ substantially. In the hospital, the general medical service provides a useful example to illustrate the concept in more depth, given its breadth of coverage of medical conditions. In addition, a slightly more complex academic workflow is used as an example. In this setting, acutely ill patients are not sick enough to be in an ICU but are cared for by a team. The team typically consists of an attending physician, a resident physician (who has completed medical school and at least one year of residency), one or more interns (in their first year of residency), and one or more medical students, either third or fourth year. In some organizations, pharmacists and nurses also round with this team. *Rounding* implies visiting the patients and reviewing their conditions and plans of care. The first thing in the morning, the interns arrive and talk to the physicians who worked the night before to find out what happened overnight. Traditionally, this also implies sitting down at a computer and extracting key content to paper so they'll be ready when their attending or supervising physician asks for updates. Device improvements to this "prerounding" process by interns are potentially available but still limited in their practical use.

Some current approaches to devices, though, are enabling them to become more useful for these medicine team members. For example, many hospitals have implemented wireless access (after a biomedical device team verifies lack of significant interference with hospital equipment and sufficient coverage throughout the facility). As a consequence, portable devices are now available. Laptops on carts, often referred to as COWS for "computers on wheels" (or WOWS for "workstations on wheels" to avoid patients misconstruing terminology), are often available. These devices interact similarly to the desktop computers except for their bulky portability. Alternatively, vendors are now starting to provide small form-factor device-specific applications to connect to the central EMR database. Typically, these applications only transiently retain data to address security and privacy concerns but, in turn, often provide limited functionality. For example, information retrieval may be enabled, while full-note writing or order entry capability might not be available. This will evolve such that portable devices, while interacting with the same database, will do so via a device size–specific interface such that touch screens, for example, would have larger buttons than applications navigated with a mouse. Vendors are adapting their applications to take advantage of such built-in or native capabilities of mobile devices. As a result, changes are also occurring in the user interface to accommodate smaller screen size and limited keyboard entry. Additionally, by having native applications optimized for running on the device, such as Android OS or Apple (iOS), other native tools within the device such as image capture, voice recognition, or typing tools can be more easily and effectively leveraged for further time savings and convenience. With the increasing demand for mobility and the competitive nature of the industry, most EMR features will ultimately become available regardless of the device. As a result, the intern will have the answer when the attending physician asks about the latest lab results, when the most recent radiology or cardiology test was performed, and what the results were. Further, when rounding, orders could be updated and note addendums added through voice recognition via an iPhone. Applications that further emphasize specific history elements to ensure safe patient handoffs among team members are starting to enter the healthcare market.

In another hospital context, when a patient requires transfer from one facility to another (acute or ambulatory), faxing is often the most common mode of communication and providing handoffs. The Healthcare Information Technology Standards Panel (HITSP) produced a spreadsheet that illustrates the range of content that may be included in clinical document architecture documents, available at http://publicaa .ansi.org/sites/apdl/hitspadmin/Matrices/HITSP_09_N_451.pdf.

A more efficient option, health information exchanges (HIEs) are now in place in many areas of the United States (Figure 18-1). One model is that of a record locator service where medical history information isn't stored at the level of the HIE, but instead links are available pointing back to the source systems to retrieve standardized documents from the source medical record. While these services show substantial promise, EMR users already struggle to assimilate content, sometimes conflicting, within a single EMR. When confronted with an array of disparate information from many systems, finding essential information needed to make a key medical decision can become more difficult. Various strategies to compile information at the HIE level are also under development.

A particularly challenging step in delivering care is at the time of discharge from an acute-care facility. When they are sent home or to a subsequent facility for additional care, patients need to understand their medications, receive education regarding next steps to maintain their health, have follow-up appointments, and understand any other information provided at discharge. The primary-care outpatient physician who follows

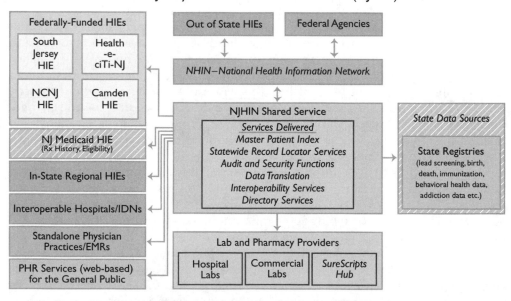

Figure 18-1   New Jersey Health Information Network HIE example. Reprinted from the State of New Jersey, State HIT Operational Plan, Figure 1.1, www.nj.gov/health/bc/documents/hitc10/hit_operational_plan_onc.pdf.

the patient also needs the same level of communication. Even with a common EMR across multiple venues, opportunities exist for gaps in communication. For complex patients with multiple health problems seen in several contexts, a variety of EMRs are often involved, greatly increasing the risk for error. One way to improve communication is a patient-maintained electronic record, personal health record, or patient portal, often provided by a commercial web site where the patient has access to and controls much of the information in the record. While patient-maintained portals have garnered some limited success, "tethered" portals attached to a given medical center's EMR have seen a steady increase in adoption. When multiple organizations are involved, an easy means for patients to "walk away" with essential content and for the next physician to receive information is critical. Two examples in this context include the My Medication List from the National Library of Medicine (Figure 18-2) and direct messaging solutions such as the Direct Project to providers recently introduced in the United States. (See the Direct Project at http://directproject.org/content.php?key=overview.) Solutions like these, and especially the latter, offer ease of use and secure communication of potentially otherwise unavailable information.

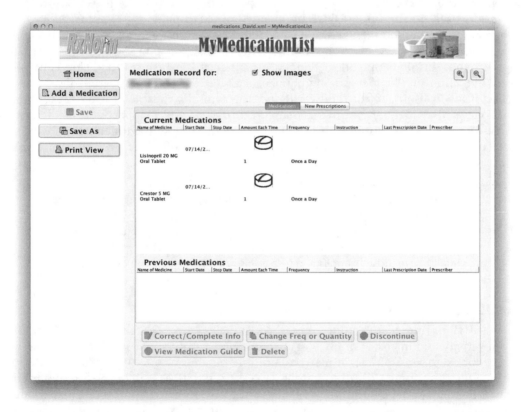

Figure 18-2   My Medication List. Reprinted from the National Library of Medicine leveraging RxNorm, http://mml.nlm.nih.gov.

Use Case 18-1: Modified Early Warning System

Rapid response teams have been established at many medical centers to intervene quickly when a patient's medical condition deteriorates. The potential benefits of an RRT include preventing cardiac arrests or avoidable transfers into critical-care units. (For more information on rapid response teams, see www.aarc.org/resources/rapid_response/.) Leveraging the electronic medical record and interfaces to medical devices (e.g., bedside monitors), these systems no longer require an individual to manually identify a critically ill patient and notify the appropriate care team. Some hospitals are now utilizing frequent reports leveraging sophisticated analysis of specific discrete data in the electronic record (Modified Early Warning System [MEWS]; see www.ncbi.nlm.nih.gov/pubmed/18693867) to identify patients at risk of deteriorating.

One additional consideration in the inpatient-care context is the use of dashboard views focused on appropriate or recommended care. Hospitals are incentivized to discharge patients as soon as medically stable and to prevent readmission for the same condition within a certain amount of time. Furthermore, hospitals strive to ensure that all care that should happen does happen (e.g., prevention against blood clots) and all care that shouldn't happen doesn't happen (e.g., receiving an incorrect medication or dose of medication). To that end, EMRs are now typically capable of real-time reports and views that identify cases of missing and/or receiving inappropriate treatment. Access to this information on a mobile device would improve the timeliness and accuracy of the interventions by those clinicians tasked to identify and correct the problems in real time.

 TIP   A key area of focus and a common source of error in most hospitals are the handoffs or sign-outs between providers (often physicians) at shift change. Effective sign-outs are critical to safe handoffs among care providers. Well-designed information views and reports, available on mobile devices, can facilitate and improve those handoffs and help minimize missing or mistaken communication.

Outpatient Practice

Using HIT in outpatient settings presents many challenges. These include aspects of connectivity and interoperability that are particularly problematic in an outpatient setting. For example, a physician may see multiple patients at one time located in three different exam rooms. Providing seamless access to an EMR as a physician cares for each patient and ensuring they are viewing and taking action on the appropriate patient are significant challenges. Anecdotally, a similar problem can occur in the emergency room where physicians care for multiple patients at any given time. Various approaches to facilitate physician access and prevent errors include the following:

- Permitting multiple logons to the system at the same time from devices located in each room (with a subsequent impact on system performance)

- Using portable devices with strong wireless connectivity carried from room to room with no change in user login required

- Linking devices and patients to specific exam rooms to avoid searching for the patient or selecting the incorrect patient off a list or schedule

- Using smart cards/biometric recognition for fast switching from one device to another (logging out on one device and logging in on another, picking up where the user left off)

The typical steps involved in an ambulatory visit by a patient include the following:

1. Calling the office to schedule an appointment at some point prior to the visit.

2. On the day of the appointment, check-in by a staff member who "arrives" the patient into the system, typically at a desktop PC.

3. "Rooming" the patient by bringing them back to an exam room where a medical assistant typically measures and records vital signs. (In some practices, the physician performs these tasks.) Increasingly some blood pressure cuffs, thermometers, and scales now interface directly with the EMR, avoiding manual data entry by the staff. Communication options with the EMR include Wi-Fi, Bluetooth, Zigbee, and other proprietary wireless protocols.

4. The physician then enters the room to perform a history and exam of the patient, document their findings, and plan and enter any orders.

5. Once the physician has finished, the nurse or medical assistant may see the patient for any remaining tasks as a result of the physician's orders.

6. Finally, the patient returns to the front desk to make any additional appointments and/or provide payment as required by insurance or other agencies.

If the specific physician is not familiar with the patient's history, the physician may appear to be distracted by the computer and not focus on the patient when trying to review what has transpired since the last visit and collect additional history. The typical physician interaction with the computer includes navigating and "clicking," as well as typing into the EMR.

Voice recognition (VR) software, where the clinician speaks into a microphone and software translates voice to text, is now more common because the technology has improved considerably in the last few years. In addition, voice files that contain the user's profile and preferences can be stored on the network and accessed from any device with a microphone, overcoming a previous limitation of a single device being voice enabled.

Now that practices have become incentivized through meaningful use federal incentives (http://healthit.hhs.gov/portal/server.pt?open=512&objID=2996&mode=2) to offer patient portals, patients can often review selected chart content and plans from their visit online. Common features of portals include access to data such as laboratory results, medication lists, and upcoming appointments as well as messaging features between the patient and provider.

Device considerations in the outpatient context include devices for the exam room, shared/open areas, and front-office staff who greet and depart the patient. Many options exist, and no "fits all" solution has been defined. For physicians, placing the device to facilitate eye-to-eye contact with the patient (conversely avoiding the physician turning her back to the patient while using the EMR) and inviting patient viewing of the EMR are considered optimal. Outside the usual venues where care is provided (typically office and hospital), mobile options are also a consideration. Frequently, a physician on-call is contacted by an answering service. A number of mobile devices and solutions exist that have replaced the trusted pager. Common and suggested characteristics include minimal caching of patient-related information on the device, end-to-end encryption, and EMR-specific passwords in addition to any device security. Currently, paging services are not often directly integrated into mobile EMR solutions, yet after connecting to the person calling, the physician can at least open the mobile EMR to review selected content now available through many vendor-sponsored apps and then electronically place orders including eprescriptions relayed via Surescripts. These mobile EMR apps tend to follow similar safeguards as described for still-distinct answering-service applications. Access to referential information is also common on desktop computers as well as mobile devices. A number of providers offer mobile solutions in this arena including ePocrates, Medscape, and UpToDate. As clinicians become more familiar with electronic records and other related information and notification via smartphones, seamless access from the answering service to the mobile EMR and to anticipatory and referential information will be possible.

Use Case 18-2: Mobile Device and Clinical Reference Tools

As a physician on call, you receive a page from a female patient with typical urinary tract infection symptoms, and after assessing her condition, you would like to begin treatment. Unfortunately, she has allergies to the three most commonly prescribed antibiotics, and the fourth option you might consider is not readily apparent. The ideal workflow would include access to all relevant patient information, a set of embedded and actionable guidelines for common conditions, the ability to prescribe electronically (referred to as eprescribing or eRx), and the ability to document clinician thoughts and actions, thereby approximating care provided in a physical setting.

 TIP In an ideal office, monitors are placed such that patients and physicians are able to share the display and physicians are able to maintain eye-to-eye contact with patients and avoid becoming focused on the keyboard with their heads down. Large (e.g., 21 inches or bigger) and mobile displays, which can be pushed to the side while physicians can face patients, constitute one option.

Future Directions

The future is bright for improvements to HIT connectivity and information interoperability. From a connectivity perspective, devices to monitor a patient's health will have options for feedback directly to the patient, such as warning of status changes in the patient's health or feedback to a care team that might contact the patient as the patient's condition changes. Additionally, diagnostic device portability will be enhanced, such as portable ultrasound devices with automatic uploading to office EMRs. It was hardly conceivable just a few years ago that physicians could electronically prescribe for their patients while both might be on vacation miles apart. This has now become routine. As communication protocols and options increase, more seamless exchange of summary and discrete data will become possible from within an EMR. Pilots to integrate state-based communication systems into EMRs are already underway. EMRs will better facilitate the patient downloading not just summary documents but their entire records ready to be uploaded and shared with services that will interpret and highlight key concerns for patients to address with their physicians. Lastly, EMR software will no longer be stand-alone islands of information but will enable integration with an extensive array of actionable reference materials, both patient-specific and population-centric. As all of these potential improvements and enhancements are realized, patients can work more closely with their providers to actively manage their health based on the latest recommendations specific to them.

Commonly Used Medical Terms

The following sections define commonly used medical terms.

Common Specialties/Body Systems/Disease Processes

Cardiology   This means relating to the heart and blood vessels.

> **Arrhythmia**   This is abnormal electrical activity in the heart producing abnormal beats (atrial fibrillation is a common example).
>
> **Congestive heart failure**   This is an abnormal pumping function of the heart leading to too much fluid (congestion) on the side of the heart before the pump or in the lungs.
>
> **Coronary artery disease**   This is an atherosclerotic plaque-based narrowing of the coronary arteries that provide essential oxygen to the heart. A heart attack (myocardial infarction) occurs if one of the three main arteries or their branches becomes suddenly blocked.

Gastroenterology   This means relating to the gastrointestinal system from the esophagus to the anus.

> **Cirrhosis**   This is progressive fibrosis (scarring) of the liver significantly impairing function.
>
> **Esophageal reflux disease**   This is an abnormal release of contents from the stomach back into the esophagus leading to inflammation and changes of the esophagus lining.

Inflammatory bowel disease   This is an inflammation within the intestinal tract with bleeding, strictures, and abnormal function with different syndromes (Crohn's disease and ulcerative colitis, for example).

Pancreatitis   This is an inflammation of the pancreas generally from pancreas enzymes often from pancreatic duct blockage from gallstones or alcohol use.

Peptic ulcer disease   This consists of abnormal changes in the lining of the stomach related to stomach acid and changes in stomach protection barriers.

Nephrology   This means relating to the kidneys and urinary tract.

Chronic kidney disease   This is the impaired blood filtering capacity of the kidneys.

Kidney failure   This is a significant loss of kidney function usually requiring ongoing treatment such as dialysis.

Nephrotic syndrome   This is a loss of filtering integrity of the kidneys leading to protein loss in the urine.

Neurological   This means relating to the brain and nervous system.

Seizures   These are abnormal synchronized electrical activities in the brain giving rise to various syndromes (groups of clinical findings).

Stroke or cerebrovascular accident   This is a loss of blood flow to an area of the brain resulting in death of brain tissue and various syndromes.

Oncology   This means related to the study and treatment of cancer.

Pulmonary   This means relating to the lungs.

Asthma   This is reversible airway constriction accompanied by inflammation.

COPD   This stands for chronic obstructive pulmonary disease; it is often associated with smoking and loss of lung tissue.

Interstitial disease   This is an inflammation and/or fibrosis of the cell network between airspaces within the lung.

Pneumonia   This is infection and inflammation within the lung.

Rheumatology   This includes disorders of the joints, soft tissues, and autoimmune diseases.

Inflammation   This is a reaction of the body to stimuli perceived as harmful, including cell migration to the area, changes in blood vessels and proteins.

Urology   This means relating to surgical issues of the kidney and urinary tract.

Cystitis   This is a bladder infection.

Nephrolithiais   This is kidney stones.

Select Medical and Clinical Roles

Advanced practice nurse or nurse practitioner   This is a nurse who has additional training and an expanded scope of responsibilities such as placing orders and who often works under the supervision of a physician. This nurse also often works as a primary-care practitioner.

Attending/admitting physician   This physician is ultimately responsible for the care of a patient during a hospital stay.

Consulting physician   This is commonly a specialty physician whose services are requested by an attending physician during an inpatient stay or by a primary-care physician in an outpatient context.

Dental Assistant (DA)—A Dental Assistant (DA) assists a dentist or other dental office staff in the care of dental patients.

Fellow   This is a physician receiving specialty training following residency.

Hospitalist   Typically this is an internal medicine or family medicine–trained physician whose practice is confined to hospitalized patients on medical-care units.

Intern   This is a physician in the first year of residency (a first-year resident). This person is often not fully licensed by the state until sometime during the year.

Medical student   These are individuals in training, usually for four years, typically following college, who are pursuing either a medical doctor (MD) degree or a doctor of osteopathy (DO) degree.

PharmD   These are pharmacists with a professional degree in pharmacy, which includes several years of education, post a bachelor's degree and significant practical experience.

Physician assistant   This is a medical professional who has a specific course of training and typically works as a provider under the supervision of a physician.

Primary-care physician   This is typically an internal or family medicine physician who cares for a diverse array of a patient's chronic problems over many years.

Providers   This generally refers to clinicians allowed to enter orders, usually physicians, nurse practitioners, and physician assistants. (Midlevel providers generally are nurse practitioners and physician assistants.)

Rapid Response   Rapid response teams are teams of physicians, nurses, and other clinicians who are called to assess and treat acutely deteriorating patients in non-ICU hospital units. The aim of a rapid response intervention is to prevent respiratory or cardiac arrest, and/or to medically stabilize a patient.

Referring physician   This is a physician requesting additional care from another provider, by sending a patient either to a hospital or to a specialty physician.

Resident   This is a physician receiving additional training in a specialty following medical school, typically three to six years.

Senior medical student   This is a medical student in the fourth (last) year of medical school.

Specialty physician   This physician has received additional training in a focused medical or surgical specialty and typically treats a narrower range of conditions. An example of a medical specialty is cardiology, and a physician in that specialty is a cardiologist.

Unit Assistant (UA) or Patient Care Technician (PCT)—A UA or PCT assists nursing, medical, and unit coordinator staff in caring for patients on their assigned hospital unit..

Select Hospital Care Units

MED/ SURG   MED/SURG is short for Medical/Surgical. A MED/SURG unit is a hospital inpatient care unit that treats a variety of acutely ill patients admitted by surgeons or medical physicians. MED/SURG patients are not as seriously ill as ICU patients.

OR   An Operating Room (OR) is the place where surgeries or operations occur in a hospital.

PACU   PACU stands for Post Anesthesia Care Unit. In some hospitals, it's called the recovery room. This is the hospital unit where patients go after surgery so that they can be monitored carefully to ensure a smooth awakening after anesthesia. They are then discharged from the PACU to another care unit in the hospital, or directly to home if they experienced a "same day surgery."

PCU   A Progressive Care Unit (PCU) is a hospital unit that treats patients whose needs are not acute enough for an ICU, but are too complex for a regular hospital care unit.

Procedural room   A procedural room, also known as a procedure room, is a room in a hospital where relatively minor medical, surgical, and radiology procedures are performed on patients by medical staff. Theses rooms are often equipped with fluoroscopy, which is a type of medical imaging that shows a continuous X-ray image on a monitor. Fluoroscopy is used to guide the physician as she performs a procedure, such as insertion of a catheter to monitor pressure from inside the heart, as well as many other types of procedures.

TCU   A Transitional Care Unit (TCU) is a special care unit in a hospital that provides intensive care nursing and medical services to patients as a transition from full ICU care to regular care.

Trauma Center   A trauma center is a hospital or a unit within a hospital that provides comprehensive emergency medical care to patients suffering traumatic injuries. Trauma centers have varying capabilities which are identified by "Level" designators. Level I is the highest level, or most capable trauma center designation, going down to Level III, which is the lowest. A few states have five designated levels, in which case Level V is the lowest.

Miscellaneous Medical Terms

Code Blue   This is a term used in a hospital or other medical setting for a patient requiring resuscitation, usually due to respiratory or cardiac arrest.

Float room   A float room, also known as an "on-call" room, is a small room in a hospital where medical, radiology, or surgical residents (or other overnight medical staff) can sleep, shower, and rest when not actively caring for patients.

Patient Acuity   The concept of patient acuity is based on the reality that patients have different levels of severity of illness. A more acutely ill patient has higher nursing and medical needs and is likely to consume more resources during an episode of care than a less acutely ill patient.

STAT   Stat is a common term used in medical settings to indicate that a thing or an action is needed immediately. Ordering modules of EHRs usually have an order priority as one of the modifiers for orders. Stat is one of those priorities, routine is another.

Major Categories of Clinical Documentation

Allergies   Allergies are typically medication related and include the specific agent and the reaction to the agent. This should be differentiated from "adverse reaction" such as nausea, which is often not a true allergy.

Chief complaint   This is the primary reason a patient is seeking care together with the duration of the complaint if appropriate. It is often solicited by a nurse or medical assistant.

Diagnosis   While there isn't necessarily consensus among providers as to the definition, this is often considered the reason(s) patients are receiving care at a given point in time.

Family history   This typically includes first-degree relatives (parents, offspring, siblings) given significant shared genetic history with the patient. Further relatives can be important in syndrome mapping.

History of present illness   This is the narrative chronology of the current medical illness. It's often documented in the patient's own words and includes parameters such as duration, severity, and alleviating factors.

Impression, assessment, and plans   Included in most physician notes (office notes, hospital progress, and admission notes), these provide an overall summary for the patient and include a list of active problems connected with the associated plans for each problem.

Medication list   This is a summary of medications including dose, frequency, and route. While not typically linked to indications for the medications, this may be required in the future.

Medication reconciliation This is the process of comparing the list of medications reported by the patient prior to the current status change (e.g., office or emergency visit or hospital stay) with the intended list of medications from that point forward.

Past medical history This involves resolved or inactive medical issues. This overlaps with the problem list, and as with diagnosis, it is frequently a source of controversy. In some EMRs, it's used to represent a comprehensive list of both active and resolved problem list items.

Past surgical history This is a list of past surgical or operative procedures.

Problem list This is a list of ongoing medically relevant issues that persist across visits. It should use the most appropriately descriptive term available within a set of terms (e.g., "mild intermittent asthma" instead of "asthma"). It's typically recorded as a codified term using either SNOMED or ICD-9 vocabulary.

Results These include both discrete data recorded via a flow sheet (laboratory) and narrative documents (radiology, cardiology, etc.) that may include additional discrete data points.

Review of systems This is a list of potential symptoms used to determine whether any are present to ensure no potential symptom is missed. It typically covers a variety of body systems and is documented as either positive (e.g., patient has chest pain) or negative (e.g., patient denies shortness of breath).

Social history This includes lifestyle issues including occupation, alcohol, drug, and tobacco usage, exercise, and diet.

Common Devices and Technology

Electroencephalogram (EEG) This test measures and records electrical activity in the brain. Electrodes are attached to the patient's head and connected by wires to a computer that records the brain's electrical activity as a series of wavy lines. An EEG can aid in the diagnosis of various neurological conditions such as seizures.

Glucose Monitor A glucose monitor is a test system used to measure the amount of sugar (glucose) in a person's blood. A patient self-administers the test with the device at home, work, or school.

Magnetic Resonance Imaging (MRI) scans These leverage magnetic fields induced in nuclei to image soft tissues more clearly than CT scans. Two- and three-dimensional and functional reconstructions are possible. No ionizing radiation is produced but contraindicated with metal implants.

Nuclear Stress Test A nuclear stress test, or thallium stress test, is a nuclear imaging examination that shows how blood flows into the heart muscle, at rest and during activity. This test requires that a patient undergo part of the exam while walking on a treadmill, or, for patients unable to exercise, to receive a medication to stress the heart.

Positron Emission Tomography (PET)   PET is a digital imaging technology, often performed in conjunction with CT scanning, that can detect subtle differences in how a patient's tissues use substances such as glucose. This test is often used in care of cancer patients.

Sphygmomanometer   This is also known as a blood pressure cuff with pressure meter. It now also includes biomedical device interfaces (BMDIs) for readings to download directly into EMRs.

Ultrasound   This is the use of sound waves to image body tissues.

Ventilator   For patients with difficulty breathing on their own and require mechanical assistance, this is a device that uses a variety of methods to improve a patient's level of oxygen in the blood stream. Positive pressure and various triggered events instill different concentrations of oxygen to patients through nasal, oral, or tracheal breathing tubes for patients who cannot breathe on their own.

X-ray and CT   This is the use of X-rays to image body tissues. Two- and three-dimensional reconstructions are possible with computed tomography (CT). X-rays contain ionizing radiation that in high enough doses harms tissue over time.

 CompTIA EXAM TIP   An outpatient or inpatient nuclear medicine department uses very small amounts of radioactive material to diagnose and treat disease. For diagnostic imaging, special cameras detect radiopharmaceuticals that are analyzed by computers to provide precise pictures of the area of the body being imaged. For treatment, radiopharmaceuticals go to the target organ or body system to provide therapeutic treatment.

Procedure-Related Terms

Cardiac catheterization   This is a procedure in which catheters are fed through the arterial system back into the heart to measure pressures and to inject dye to assess heart valves and the coronary arteries on the surface of the heart.

Cardiac stents   These are types of tubes that hold the coronary arteries open and improve oxygen supply to the heart muscle. They are introduced, if needed, during cardiac catheterizations and may require specific blood thinners for defined periods afterward to avoid clotting.

Central line   This is a catheter that is inserted in the large blood vessels near the heart and used to monitor heart-related central venous pressure and to administer medications.

Central venous pressure   This measurement provides information about the filling pressure of the heart that tends to reflect hydration status and other parameters.

Coronary artery bypass graft   This is the use of segments of arteries or veins to provide blood supply around blockages of the coronary arteries.

Interventional radiology   This is a radiology specialty in which biopsies or intravascular procedures are performed directly with imaging assistance.

Intra-arterial line   This is a catheter (thin tube) introduced into arteries to provide pressure readings, administer organ-targeted medications, or perform procedures. Arteries are high-pressure vessels carrying blood away from the heart.

Intravenous line (IV)   This is a catheter (thin tube) introduced into veins to provide medications and IV fluids. Veins are low pressure and return blood to the heart.

Pulmonary artery catheter   This is a catheter inserted via the venous system through the heart and into the arterial system supplying blood to the lungs. It is used to measure blood pressure in the lungs and to estimate filling pressure of the left side of the heart.

Evidence-Based Medicine Terms

Evidence pyramid   A stacked listing of potential sources of information for which the confidence level of conclusions increases progressively. Systematic reviews that summarize well-constructed double-blind randomized controlled trials are at the top of the pyramid. (These types of primary studies randomly allocate subjects to treatment or placebo and hide this information from patients/researchers.)

Gold-standard tests   These are definitive tests to establish a diagnosis and often require an invasive procedure such as a biopsy.

Meta-analyses   This is a study of studies. Primary studies are compared and combined, when appropriate, to increase the value of the conclusions.

Number needed to treat   This represents how many individuals must receive a treatment to avoid a specific negative outcome. For example, 60 patients without known heart disease would need to be treated with cholesterol lowering agents to prevent one heart attack in 5 years.

Positive and negative predictive values   The positive predictive value indicates how often a patient with a positive test really has the disease. The negative predictive value indicates how often a patient with a negative test result truly doesn't have the disease.

Primary and secondary literature   Primary literature refers to initial research data collection from clinical trials. Secondary literature refers to aggregated views based upon primary literature.

Sensitivity and specificity   Sensitivity refers to the percentage of patients with a disease a test can pick up. Specificity refers to the percentage of patients without the disease that the test correctly identifies as not having the disease.

Commonly Used HIT Terms

The following sections define commonly used HIT terms.

Terms Related to EHR Implementation

Barcode medication administration   This is the process of using a barcode scanner to ensure the right medication is administered at the proper time to the correct patient.

Benefits realization analysis   In an EMR deployment context, this refers to a list of predetermined potential benefits (such as decreased turnaround times for orders and fewer severe adverse medication errors) and their measurement before and following EMR deployment.

Billing systems   These are often distinct systems linking to diagnostic codes representing services performed.

Biomedical device interface   This is the connection via some type of intermediary device that facilitates communication between bedside monitors and IT systems.

Change control   Before updates or changes are introduced into an EMR, standardized testing in preproduction domains occurs to ensure all consequences of the change are anticipated.

Clinical data repository   This is the database housing clinical information about patients optimized for rapid entry and retrieval at a single patient level.

Clinical decision support   In a medical record context, this refers to a broad array of design characteristics and functions intended to support safe and effective decisions. Examples may include how results are organized or whether order entry options are made available or hidden if inappropriate. Similarly, alerts that trigger guidance or warnings such as regarding a patient allergy, drug dose, or drug interaction constitute decision support. This topic is covered in more detail in another chapter.

Clinical documentation   This generally refers to notes and forms entered by nonprovider members of the care team.

Communication and training strategies   In an EMR deployment context, this refers to ensuring users remain up-to-date regarding the system status and to providing an array of training options on system functionality. This topic is covered in more detail in another chapter.

Computerized provider order entry (CPOE)   This is the electronic entry of orders for patients by providers (physicians and midlevel providers).

Domain management   In an EMR context, this typically refers to the group of software environments hosting multiple test systems as well as the live production system used by the organization.

Encounter   This refers to a healthcare event, generally also billable, such as an outpatient or emergency room visit or an extended hospital stay.

Enterprise data warehouse   This is a database optimized for data retrievals across many patients with variables normalized (mapped to common scales) for appropriate interpretation; it often includes information from the primary EMR as well as other systems (financial, external reference, and so on).

Laboratory information systems (LIS)   This is system supporting workflow within a laboratory department capturing data output from equipment in the lab via interfaces including chemical analyzers typically then made available to the broader EMR.

Medication administration record   This is the list of medications with dose, route, date, and a time of administration.

Pharmacy information systems   This is a system supporting workflow within a pharmacy. Most commonly, this system exists as a component of an integrated enterprise medical record system. Often the intermediary, this system provides order verification and dispensing information between physician orders and nursing medication administration documentation. It usually has the same medication alerting capability as order entry component. Inventory, billing, and formulary can be additional integrated functions.

Picture archiving and communication system (PACS)   These systems provide file management for the complex array of images generated from many radiology exams and include image-viewing capability. DICOM (digital imaging and communications in medicine) is the standard used for handling, storing, and exchanging the image content.

Progress notes   This generally refers to physician notes but may include clinical documentation.

Radiology information systems (RIS)   This is a system supporting workflow within a radiology department, often including patient scheduling, result reporting, and image tracking.

Registration systems   This is the transactional system used to track and record patient demographic information and encounters in the healthcare organization.

Scheduling systems   This refers to the system of scheduling events for patients, typically including visits, diagnostic tests, and procedures.

Usability, utility, and workflow   Usability refers to how successfully (effectiveness, efficiency, and satisfaction) a given tool is used. Utility refers to the array of functionality available with a tool. Workflow refers to the sequence of steps involved in performing a particular action. These topics are covered in more detail in other chapters.

Workflow analysis   In an EMR deployment context, this refers to a careful examination of current workflow, mapping an ideal state to serve the goals of the process and then integrating the new EMR into a new workflow state as close as possible to the ideal.

Major Standardized Clinical Terminologies

CMT   This is Kaiser Permanente's open source terminology solution integrating commonly used terms across SNOMED CT, LOINC, and drug terminology.

ICD-9-CM   This is a classification system used for assigning diagnosis codes to inpatient encounters and outpatient office visits.

ICD-10   This is a classification system in use in most countries outside the United States that includes many more codes than ICD-9 as well as additional details about the specificity of a given code. Implementation in the United States has been delayed several times since it was initially proposed.

National Drug Code (NDC)   NDC is a unique three segment number that is a universal product identifier for commercially-available human drugs. Drug manufacturers are required to submit a list of all drugs manufactured, prepared, propagated, compounded, or processed to the Food and Drug Administration (FDA). These drugs are assigned National Drug Codes. Some HIT systems refer to the National Drug Codes as NDCID. In that case the ID means identifier, thus National Drug Code Identifier (NDCID).

RxNorm   This is a cross-mapping set of brand and generic medication names enabling interoperability among medications, their attributes, and pharmacy knowledge base systems.

SNOMED CT   This provides core terminology for EMR systems with 311,000 concepts organized into hierarchies.

Health Information Exchange

Continuity of care document (CCD)   This is a summary document used for information exchange.

Health information exchanges (HIEs)   These are hubs for exchanging medical information among clinical entities. Approaches include record locator services and master patient indices pointing back to source systems or stored clinical summaries and content.

Health IT Policy Committee (HITPC)   This is a federal advisory committee making recommendations on nationwide health information infrastructure including standards for exchanging patient information.

Health IT Standards Committee (HITSC)   This is a federal advisory committee making recommendations on standards, specifications, and certification criteria for the exchange and use of health information.

Privacy, confidentiality, and security   Privacy addresses the rights of patients to withhold sharing information. Confidentiality refers to ensuring identifiable information is further shared only based on consent or as required by law. Security refers to the systems and structures in place to preserve the confidentiality of patient information.

Use Case 18-3: SNOMED CT in Practice

Using a standardized terminology such as SNOMED CT to capture clinical syndromes and problems benefits both efficient workflow and decision support. For example, in an emergency room a variety of complaints are encountered, and any individual physician may miss emerging trends. By using a standardized terminology such as SNOMED CT to capture diagnoses encountered, related diagnoses may be grouped according to the terminology and provide warnings into emerging trends for infectious diseases. Similarly, by capturing problem list items with a standardized terminology and an associated hierarchy of terms, decision support can be focused on specific sets of patients without inappropriately interrupting care for other patients.

Chapter Summary

In this chapter you learned that both the inpatient and outpatient healthcare environments present numerous opportunities for the effective delivery of healthcare information. Through the development of healthcare information technology (HIT), including electronic medical records (EMRs), this delivery of healthcare information has been sped up and improved. EMRs are typically capable of real-time reports and views that identify cases of missing and/or inappropriate treatments. Access to this information helps improve the timeliness and accuracy of interventions to correct the problem. This is a real benefit of HIT.

The common workflow in an inpatient setting is improved by providing health care professionals better and quicker access to information for patients under their care. In particular, physicians benefit, because they often have limited time to see their patients. Health information exchange (HIE) is now in use in many parts of the country and helps the transfer of patients from one facility to another. Finally, once a patient is ready to be discharged from an inpatient facility, patient-level access to an EMR helps provide them with the necessary tools for managing their own care.

We also discussed using HIT in outpatient settings and the challenges that venue can present. These challenges include aspects of connectivity and interoperability that are particularly problematic in an outpatient setting. For example, a physician may see multiple patients concurrently, who are located in three different exam rooms. Providing physicians seamless access to EMRs as they care for each patient, and ensuring physicians are viewing and taking action on the appropriate patient are significant challenges.

A critical step for healthcare systems (both inpatient and outpatient) to find the devices that best suit their needs (from portable laptops to voice recognition software) is to conduct a workflow assessment and to consider the data flows that are required in their organization. These evaluations help them determine the electronic devices that will help their organization provide the highest possible level of patient care. Inpatient and outpatient facilities have different needs and many options exist. While no "fits all" solution has been defined, through careful consideration of workflow design and the necessary flow of data, there are many HIT solutions that can help improve the level of healthcare information exchange and patient care. The use of HIT is relatively new and constantly improving, and we believe that the future is bright for improvements to HIT connectivity and information interoperability.

Finally, in this chapter we provided you with a list of commonly used medical and device definitions that will be helpful as you work with HIT.

Questions

1. Which of the following are typical roles within a healthcare organization whose jobs include interacting with a patient's medical records?

   A. Attending physician

   B. Pharmacist

   C. Dietician

   D. All of the above

2. The transmission of information from a biomedical device into an EMR is referred to as what?

   A. BMDI

   B. Transfer of data operation

   C. EDI

   D. Electronic information update

3. Assuming an organization has established a dashboard notification process, a nurse takes clinical information from a monitor and records the value in the context of the EMR. What is the next step?

   A. Inform the patient of their care and what procedures will take place in order for them to be released home.

   B. A page or other notification message might be transmitted to a surveillance or rapid response team (RRT), letting them know the patient may require further attention.

   C. A message will be sent to the billing department letting them know what information was taken and how the patient should be billed.

   D. A notice will be sent to the nurse's station that the value was recorded correctly, and they can move on to the next patient under their care.

4. What is a primary benefit of having wireless access in hospitals?

   A. Patients can e-mail their families with progress reports more frequently.

   B. Nurses and doctors can keep abreast of news outside of the hospital while they are on duty.

    C. Portable devices, such as laptops or computers on wheels, can assist a medical team with their rounding responsibilities.

    D. None of the above.

5. Prior to the advent of HIT, when a patient required transfer from one facility to another (acute or ambulatory), faxing was often the most common mode of communication and handoffs. A more efficient option is now in place. What is it?

    A. E-mailing health information prior to transfer

    B. Health information exchanges (HIEs)

    C. Data exchange services (DESs)

    D. Overnight mail services

6. A key area of focus and a common source of error in most hospitals is the hand-off or sign-out between providers (often physicians) at shift change.

    A. True

    B. False

7. Through meaningful use incentives, patient portals have been developed where patients can often access which of the following?

    A. Laboratory results

    B. Medication lists

    C. Upcoming appointments

    D. All of the above

8. What is a continuity of care document (CCD)?

    A. List of a patient's current prescriptions

    B. Document that a patient keeps to track the doctors they see

    C. Summary document used for information exchange

    D. Tabular printout of a patient's laboratory results

9. What kind of analysis needs to take place before a new EMR can be integrated?

    A. Workflow analysis

    B. System requirement analysis

    C. Deployment analysis

    D. None of the above

10. Using a standardized terminology such as SNOMED CT to capture clinical syndromes and problems benefits both efficient workflow and decision support by doing which of the following?

    A. Grouping related diagnoses according to the standardized terminology and providing warnings into emerging trends for infectious diseases

   B. Focusing decision support on specific sets of patients without inappropriately interrupting care for other patients.

   C. All of the above

   D. None of the above

Answers

1. **D.** Attending physician, pharmacist, and dietician are all typical roles within a healthcare organization that use medical records in patient care.

2. **A.** The transmission of information from a biomedical device into an EMR is referred to as a bedside-medical (or biomedical) device interface (BMDI).

3. **B.** At a macro-level view within the organization, if a dashboard notification process has been established and this new data element results in an algorithm generating an alert, then a page or other notification message might be transmitted to a surveillance or rapid response team (RRT), letting them know the patient may require further attention.

4. **C.** Many hospitals have implemented wireless access that enables portable devices for medical team members. Laptops on wheels are often referred to as COWS for "computers on wheels" (or WOWS for "workstations on wheels" to avoid patients misconstruing terminology). These devices interact similarly to the desktop computers except for their bulky portability.

5. **B.** In a hospital context, when a patient requires transfer from one facility to another (acute or ambulatory), faxing is often the most common mode of communication and providing handoffs. A more efficient option, health information exchanges (HIEs) are now in place in several areas of the United States.

6. **A.** A key area of focus and a common source of error in most hospitals are the handoffs or sign-outs between providers (often physicians) at shift change. Effective sign-outs are critical to safe handoffs among care providers. Well-designed information views and reports, available on mobile devices, can facilitate and improve those handoffs and help minimize missing or mistaken communication.

7. **D.** Now that practices have become incentivized through meaningful use federal incentives to offer patient portals, patients can often review selected chart content and plans from their visit online. Common features of portals include access to data such as laboratory results, medication lists, and upcoming appointments as well as messaging features between the patient and provider.

8. **C.** A continuity of care document (CCD) is a summary document used for information exchange.

9. **A.** In an EMR deployment context, workflow analysis refers to a careful examination of current workflow, mapping an ideal state to serve the goals of the process and then integrating the new EMR into a new workflow state as close as possible to the ideal.

10. **C.** Using a standardized terminology such as SNOMED CT to capture clinical syndromes and problems benefits both efficient workflow and decision support. By using a standardized terminology such as SNOMED CT to capture diagnoses encountered, related diagnoses can be grouped according to the terminology and can provide warnings into emerging trends for infectious diseases. Similarly, by capturing problem list items with a standardized terminology and an associated hierarchy of terms, decision support can focus on specific sets of patients without inappropriately interrupting care for other patients.

Additional Study

This chapter has given you a good start to understanding HIT connectivity and interoperability opportunities and challenges. Here are a few key resources to further your learning on this important topic. These resources, especially healthit.hhs.gov, are frequently updated to reflect ongoing changes on these evolving topics.

Office of the National Coordinator for Health Information Technology (includes all supported initiatives including adoption, innovation, and health information exchange): http://healthit.hhs.gov

Unified Medical Language System: www.nlm.nih.gov/research/umls/

PCAST Report on Health Information Technology: www.whitehouse.gov/sites/default/files/microsites/ostp/pcast-health-it-report.pdf

HIPAA and HITECH Privacy and Security Related Information: www.hhs.gov/ocr/privacy/hipaa/understanding/index.html

CHAPTER 19

Fundamentals of Clinical Decision Support

Bharat R. Rao, Charles Denham

In this chapter, you will learn how to

- Identify and explain the key elements of a clinical decision support (CDS) system
- Present the increasing value and importance of clinical decision support systems for clinical and administrative use in today's healthcare environment
- Examine the pitfalls of clinical decision support and barriers to successful adoption and how to overcome these issues
- Compare decision support capabilities and customizability

Healthcare is undergoing a dramatic transformation, fueled by economic, social, regulatory, and technological drivers. Clinicians in the healthcare systems of tomorrow will be tasked to deliver more efficient and safer care at lower costs while improving patient outcomes—all within a rapidly changing environment of new diagnostic tests, specialized treatments, and evolving healthcare knowledge and regulations. Clinical decision support systems are a vital component of any institution's healthcare strategy to meet these goals.

Consider the following hypothetical scenario.

Use Case 19-1: Avoiding Adverse Drug Events

In the spring of 2012, an elderly patient is correctly diagnosed with a severe pneumonia infection caused by Gram-positive bacteria that are resistant to most antibiotics. The physician prescribes the antibiotic of choice for this condition. The physician also carefully examines the patient's electronic health record (EHR), notes that the patient is taking a medication for depression, and renews the prescription. The two drugs react adversely, leading to a condition called Serotonin Syndrome, where high levels of a chemical produced by the body (serotonin) build up in the brain and cause toxicity. Fortunately, the signs of this condition—mental changes, muscle twitching, excessive sweating, trouble with coordination, and so on—are noticed quickly, and the antibiotic medication is changed before any further damage occurs.

Physicians occasionally prescribe medications that are considered to be classified as erroneous prescriptions or medication errors. A small percentage of these events actually cause harm to the patient and are considered *adverse drug events* (ADEs). Given the vast numbers of medication ordering, this kind of error and subsequent ADEs occur more frequently than one might expect. Technically an adverse drug event is an injury resulting from the use of a drug; ADEs can be caused by medication errors (e.g., accidental overdose, providing a drug to the wrong patient) or by adverse drug reactions (e.g., allergic reaction, side effects such as excessive bleeding or vomiting). The National Priorities Partnership (NPP) convened by the National Quality Forum estimates that 50 percent of the 1.9 million ADEs that occur in hospitals each year are preventable.[1] The numbers are staggering: the NPP report notes that preventing medication errors "provides a $21 billion opportunity to save on wasteful healthcare spending as well as prevent unnecessary deaths." In its landmark report "To Err is Human," the Institute of Medicine estimated that up to 7,000 deaths in the United States each year are due to preventable medication errors.[2]

The ADE described in Use Case 19-1 could have been prevented in a number of ways.

- A pop-up alert to the physician warning of the potential interaction at the time when the antibiotic was prescribed
- Clinical rules that predicted the risk of Serotonin Syndrome for the medication given to this patient
- Clinical guidelines for the treatment of pneumonia (or indeed for the treatment of depression)

These interventions are all examples of the ways clinical decision support systems suggest alternatives to patient care to the clinician, leading to increased patient safety, reduced costs, and better patient outcomes.

Use Case 19-1 illustrates two additional important points:

- While EHRs provide the foundation for improving patient outcomes and reducing costs, CDS plays a crucial role in achieving these goals.
- CDS should be reviewed and updated on a regular basis to prevent the knowledge base from becoming obsolete.

The FDA issued a drug safety communication on this particular drug-drug interaction in 2011,[3] a few months before the hypothetical patient encounter described. Unless the knowledge base that supports the CDS is routinely updated to stay consistent with changing medical guidelines, it will quickly become obsolete.

The Scope of Clinical Decision Support

The meaningful use Final Rule defines clinical decision support as "HIT functionality that builds upon the foundation of an EHR to provide persons involved in care decisions with general and person-specific information, intelligently filtered and organized, at point of care, to enhance health and health care."[4] This reinforces the earlier point that CDSs are vital components to leverage the power of an EHR to achieve an institution's cost, patient safety, and outcome goals.

A general definition is provided by Osheroff et al.[5] wherein "Clinical Decision Support is a process for enhancing health-related decisions and actions with pertinent, organized clinical knowledge and patient information to improve health and healthcare delivery." This definition deliberately eliminates the notion of an EHR, so as to include non-EHR and even paper-based methods for delivering CDS interventions. For the purposes of this chapter, we will assume the foundation of an EHR for all CDSs.

Components of CDS

All CDS systems are based on a knowledge base, which is a database of compiled clinical information of drug interactions, guidelines, diagnoses, procedures, and other knowledge sources in a computer-interpretable form. Most modern EHR systems include a CDS knowledge base, at least for the common CDS use cases, such as drug-allergy and drug-drug interactions. Examples of commercial knowledge bases include the Drug Therapy Monitoring System (WoltersKluwer Health) and the National Drug Data File Plus (First Data Bank), these products can be incorporated as a module into EHR software.

In addition, CDSs require two essential processes:

- **Submit patient-specific information**   A way of entering or importing patient data from the EHR (or even a paper chart) into the CDS
- **Generate patient-specific recommendation**   A method to combine the patient-specific information with the knowledge base to come up with a recommendation

These processes may be performed either by the computer or manually by the clinician.

CDS Continuum

For a CDS to achieve its goals of improving patient outcomes and reducing costs, the knowledge in the knowledge base must be evidence-based. Early CDSs were expert systems that helped the clinician with diagnosing conditions or prescribing medications. Today's CDSs cover a wide spectrum of clinical scenarios, from providing nationally endorsed guidelines to allowing individual clinicians to customize order sets to include their medications of choice.

A recent Agency for Healthcare Research & Quality (AHRQ) publication on CDSs, *Enabling Health Care Decision-making Through Clinical Decision Support and Knowledge Management,*[6] defines a continuum of decision support based upon the degree of automation of two essential processes: submitting patient-specific information and generating patient-specific recommendations, illustrated in Table 19-1.

The *classical definition of CDS* is a system that takes individual characteristics of the patient into account to develop patient-specific assessments and recommendations that are presented to the clinician to aid in clinical decision making. Examples include basic alerts, automatic reminders that remind the clinician of a particular action, order sets, drug-dosage calculations, and care-summary dashboards (e.g., the quality of care delivered as measured by quality metrics). For classical CDS, the mechanisms for both submitting patient-specific information and generating patient-specific recommendations are done by the computer.

This definition does not cover a growing number of *knowledge management* systems that provide information relevant to the characteristics of a specific clinical situation but that require human interpretation of the information by the clinician to apply at the point of care for a specific patient. There are two kinds of knowledge management systems:

- **Information retrieval tools**   These are electronic tools designed to aid clinicians in the search and retrieval of context-specific knowledge from information sources based on patient-specific information from an EHR to support clinical decisions for a specific care situation. Examples include an info button in an EHR that, when selected, provides access to context-sensitive information. In these situations, patient-specific information is automatically submitted, but the clinician must review the relevant knowledge (e.g., a guideline) to determine the correct action.

- **Knowledge resources**   These are tools that consist of distilled primary literature in an electronic form that allows the clinician to select content that is germane to a specific patient to support clinical decision making. Examples of knowledge resources are solutions such as Epocrates and MD Consult, which provide clinical recommendations, up-to-date lists of drugs, and so on. For these systems, both essential processes are manual (see Table 19-1).

CDS Continuum	Mechanism for Submitting Patient's Information	Mechanism for Generating Patient-Specific Recommendation
Classical CDS	Automated (by computer)	Automated (by computer)
Information retrieval tool	Automated (by computer)	Manual (by clinician)
Knowledge resources	Manual (by clinician)	Manual (by clinician)

Table 19-1 Continuum of Clinical Decision Support

Implementing CDS Interventions

The fundamental goal of any CDS is to drive changes in care delivery that will improve care processes and outcomes by adhering to agreed-upon best practices and guidelines. The CDS does so by providing interventions into care delivery; the manner in which these *CDS interventions* are provided into the care process is critical to successfully meeting the institution's goals to improve cost, patient safety, and outcomes.

Selecting Clinical Goals for CDS Intervention

CDS interventions are goal-driven. The first step is to determine the target objective.

Use Case 19-2: Selecting CDS Clinical Goals

The CMO of General Hospital wants to select clinical goals to best target CDS efforts. The CMO looks at a meaningful use measure, specifically, "assess all patients for risk of venous thromboembolism (VTE) upon hospital admission and provide pharmacologic prophylaxis to all patients with moderate to high risk of VTE." This brings up the question, how should CDS clinical goals to target CDS interventions be selected?

Generally speaking, targets must be aligned with institutional and stakeholder priorities. Without leadership buy-in, it will be hard to get sufficient funding for effective CDS. Similarly, without buy-in from clinicians, even the best CDS interventions will be ignored. Further, targets must be reasonable—choosing targets that are too difficult to achieve will lead to failure. Osheroff et al.[5] present some general considerations for selecting specific CDS goals:

- **Select goals that optimize impact** CDS should provide clinical, financial, and operational benefits. General Hospital's CMO notes that reducing the incidence of VTE will reduce the institution's morbidity and mortality statistics (clinical), decrease the length of stay and avoid potential penalties for poor outcomes (financial), and reduce the utilization of overburdened resources (operational). Reducing VTE could also increase patient satisfaction. With the number of potential benefits, the CMO must also consider the cost of this intervention and the opportunity cost of selecting this intervention versus another.

- **Consider goals that are well suited to CDS interventions**   The VTE goal is suitable for a CDS intervention, because well-established criteria exist for determining VTE risk and selecting the VTE prophylaxis. Additionally, it requires intervening early (upon admission) in a supportive role, rather than modifying care plans that have already been created (which could lead to user frustration on the part of the clinician). Avoid goals based on subjective data, and avoid scenarios where the clinicians would view the intervention as a potential threat (substituting for their skill or overriding their decisions).

- **Measure the baseline**   Before implementing a CDS tool, it is important to establish baseline performance. The CMO measures VTE assessment compliance and follow-up and finds General Hospital to be at 60 percent, whereas adherence to another potential CDS intervention (e.g., beta-blockers at discharge to AMI patients) is at 95 percent. The opportunity for improvement is much higher for VTE prophylaxis. The ability to introduce a rule or some type of decision support by itself doesn't justify the action; a crucial factor in the selection of CDS interventions is the ability to impact the institution's performance.

- **Start simple and small, take a team approach, and build upon successes**   General Hospital's analysis identifies seven high-priority goals that could have a significant impact. Resisting the temptation to go for a "big bang," the CMO suggests a pilot for VTE prophylaxis. The CMO secures buy-in for the approach from the CEO and CIO and recruits two physicians, four nurses, one IT professional, and one pharmacist for the pilot. The interventions are designed after careful adherence to the Five Rights framework (see the section "The CDS Five Rights Framework"). The results after just six months are dramatic—for the select group of patients in the pilot, compliance to VTE assessment is now at 97 percent, VTE occurrences are greatly reduced compared to the rest of the hospital, and there are no significant adverse effects for the pilot group. The pilot also identifies gaps in the IT infrastructure of General Hospital. Subsequently, the VTE program is implemented across the entire hospital, along with two other goals, but only after instituting education and training sessions to prepare the clinicians for the changes in their workflow. Within a year, General Hospital's quality metrics in the selected clinical areas are among the highest in the region.

TIP Settling for small quick wins, especially early on, is critical to the long-term success of CDS.

The CDS Five Rights Framework

As more organizations digitize the medical record, there is growing consensus that CDS has great potential to improve healthcare quality and reduce costs. Selecting the goal is only the first step. A proper implementation of CDS is critical to achieving these goals.

 TIP Implementing an effective CDS intervention requires considering many dimensions (the "what, who, how, where, and when"), beyond the high-level clinical goal ("why intervene").

The CDS Five Rights approach proposed by Osheroff and colleagues[5] provides a framework for configuring the "what, who, how, where, and when" dimensions that are critical to create effective CDS interventions. The Five Rights framework asserts that for every proposed intervention, the CDS team must consider each of these five dimensions. Carefully optimizing all dimensions of the CDS Five Rights will ensure that CDS interventions achieve the desired goals of patient safety, clinical effectiveness, and satisfaction (for both patients and clinicians) and that they make optimal use of resources.

A brief summary of the framework follows. (For a detailed discussion of this framework, refer to the online resource by Osheroff et al.,[5] which is highly recommended for those wanting to implement CDS in their institutions. Note that the CDS Five Rights are different from the Five Rights of Medication Use and the Five Rights of Imaging.)

The Right Information (What)

After selecting a clinical goal (e.g., VTE), the first question is, "What information should we communicate to the user to support clinical decision making?" The primary intent should be to rely on well-established clinical guidelines and nationally recognized quality metrics. Furthermore, the information must be actionable—effective in guiding decisions and actions. The information must be concise, relevant to a specific patient and their situation, and well aligned with institution and user core values.

The Right Person (Who)

It is critical to consider communicating relevant information to all members of the care team, including physicians, nurses, pharmacists, patients themselves, and their caretakers. Who *not to present to* is equally important; the recipient must be in a position to make a decision or act on this information based upon their role, or it will be a waste of effort.

The Right Intervention Format (How)

There are many types of interventions; this is described in detail in the next section.

The Right Channel (Where)

This relates to how the information about the intervention will be delivered to the user. CDS for the clinicians will increasingly happen through the EHR or via mobile devices, but for CDS for the patient, their personal health record, a website, or a smart app may be more effective.

The Right Time in Workflow (When)

Information must be presented when it is most needed to make a decision or take action. Presenting information too early or too late will be ineffective; further, the context is also important (e.g., reminding the clinician about a routine immunization in an emergency situation is counterproductive).

Exploring the "How" Dimension: Types of CDS Interventions

Most modern-day EHRs either have tools to support CDS interventions built into the EHR or provide ready interfaces for integrating with a rich variety of CDS tools developed by many health information technology vendors. The lack of standards and system interoperability can make integration of third-party suppliers challenging.

There is no universally accepted methodology for classifying CDS interventions. Osheroff et al. provide a taxonomy of CDS interventions based on their typical presentation and user interaction. There are four main types of CDS interventions, further categorized into ten types, as described next.

CDS During Data-Entry Tasks

- **Smart documentation forms and flow sheets**   This category includes static and dynamic forms (which adapt or flex based on a patient's conditions) and flow sheets to help clinicians provide the correct documentation for adhering to and measuring the quality of care, ensuring proper reimbursement, providing proper information for continuity of care, and meeting legal and regulatory environments. Many prompts are intended to reduce clinical errors of omission or commission. Examples include checklists, documentation templates for a given problem, self-assessment forms, questionnaires, nursing documentation, medication administration records, referral forms, data flow sheets for preventive care, and so on. Figure 19-1 illustrates basic CDS associated with documentation. Once the clinician completes the assessment on the form, the CDS rules associated with the evaluation automatically place orders and notifications related to the evaluation.

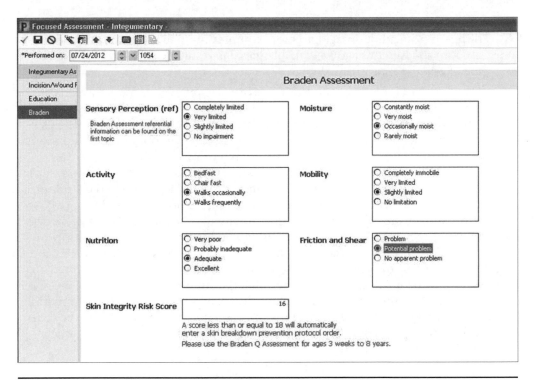

Figure 19-1 Basic CDS associated with form documentation. Reprinted with permission from Cerner Corporation. © 2012 Cerner Corporation. All rights reserved.

- **Order sets, care plans and protocols** Order sets are predefined templates of standard orders for conditions, diseases, or procedures that promote adherence to the standard of care and provide better documentation. Order sets can be static (fixed), dynamic (adjusting to patient-specific information, such as allergies and comorbidities), conditional (e.g., suggested based upon admitting diagnosis), grouped (into protocols or care plans that suggest a sequence of order sets), and cross-institutional and cross-encounter (to manage patient care across multiple encounters and even at home). Order sets are typically based on nationally developed standards and are available from many vendors (e.g., Zynx Health, Elsevier) but can also be customized at the institution level and even down to the individual clinician.

- **Medication parameter guidance** These proactive CDS interventions ensure that drug dosing, frequency, and delivery information adhere to the standard of care because drug dosing errors constitute 37 percent of all preventable medication errors.[7] Frequently implemented as dosing tools that take into account patient weight or body surface area, these interventions run the gamut from a simple check, for example, if a drug dosage is within guidelines (e.g., to avoid potentially serious adverse patient impact from incorrect decimal point or units), to optimizing dosage based upon patient age (pediatric dosage is often different from adult dosage), to more complex mechanisms that take into account the patient's age, weight, allergies, lab results (e.g., kidney function) to suggest the appropriate dosage.

- **Interruptive alerts** Considered "reactive" CDS interventions, these alerts are prompted by some new information that has just become available, typically a new drug prescription or order entered into the EHR by the clinician. The CDS recognizes a potential error, a patient safety issue, or an opportunity to prevent an ADE and raises an immediate flag and interrupts the clinician workflow. Examples include warnings about drug-allergy and drug-drug interactions, drug-dosage alerts, additional documentation to justify ordering potentially unnecessary expensive tests or procedures, and warnings to order required tests (e.g., to check kidney function) and to suggest potentially cheaper drugs (e.g., generics or recommended pharmacy formulations). Alerts of this type typically rely on third-party medication databases maintained by the external organization and customized by the organization implementing the EHR. Figure 19-2 shows an example of a medication-allergy alert that the clinician receives during the order process. Once the alert triggers, options include links to additional information regarding the alert, agreeing with the recommendation and removing the order or overriding and providing a reason based on additional information that is available to the clinician.

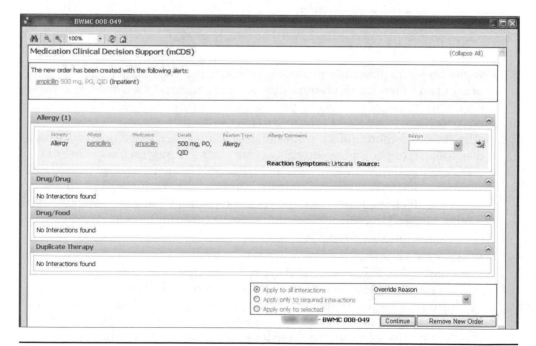

Figure 19-2 Medication-allergy alert. Reprinted with permission from Cerner Corporation. © 2012 Cerner Corporation. All rights reserved.

TIP Interruptive alerts are typically the most overused—primarily because of their simplicity. The risk is they become ineffective because of overuse, and users may ignore or override the alert without considering the information presented. Furthermore, alerts can be particularly effective if used mostly in situations where it is extremely likely that the user will accept the recommendation (i.e., to change care as suggested by the alert).

CDS During Data-Review Tasks

A common way CDS is used in clinical practice is during a clinician's review of individual or aggregate patient information. The following are examples of CDS utilization during clinical data review:

- **Relevant data summaries (single-patient)**   A concise summary of all relevant information about a specific patient can be useful for clinicians during patient care. Examples include broad dashboard views with a number of disparate elements of the EHR in one view as well as patient-specific summaries of immunization history, quality metrics, highlighted items of concern (e.g., during rounds), unusual findings and test values, and key patient parameters.

- **Multipatient views**   A concept similar to individual patient summaries presented in a concise way across a group of patients to allow prioritization of resources to the most important and urgent care situations. Examples include Emergency Department (ED) tracking systems for newly admitted patients, operating room status monitors that include postoperative summary of key issues (e.g., antibiotics, ventilator parameters, medication dosing), and inpatient summaries that alert nurses and physicians to pending events, status changes, and patients who are at risk for serious complications such as sepsis or the need for a specialized team to intervene because of a rapid deterioration in patient condition. Many of these dashboards are displayed on large monitors in a given venue with specific patient information hidden and are accessible to broad groups of clinicians.

- **Predictive and retrospective analytics**   As the amount and complexity of patient information and medical knowledge increases, analytics is playing a correspondingly larger role in patient care. There are hundreds of opportunities for analytics in the context of CDS, and an in-depth discussion of analytics is beyond the scope of this chapter. Unlike prior CDS tools that are more real-time, the practice of analytics supports the visualization of data over time, creates comparative benchmarks, detects trends, and facilitates data drill-downs that are essentially for quality improvement. Examples include retrospective quality, clinical and financial performance charts, benchmarks, surveillance tools, predictive tools to identify high-risk patients (for example, for hospital readmission or to assess cardiac risk), drill-down tools to identify adherence to standards of care (potentially at the clinician and patient level), and comprehensive reports that merge clinical, financial, quality process, and outcomes data for clinicians and administrators.

CDS During Assessment and Understanding Tasks

The amount of knowledge required for a given clinical decision often exceeds what a clinician might recall from experience. In these instances, CDS offers references and advice tailored to the issue facing the clinician. The following are examples of CDS used in assessment and diagnostic tasks:

- **Filtered reference information and knowledge resources** These tools deliver information from knowledge sources into clinician and patient workflow. Examples include info buttons with links to web-based resources for side effects for prescribed drugs, clinical evidence related to items within a patient's particular medical problems, links to immunization and screening schedules, explanations of order sets, and risk calculators.

- **Expert workup and management advisors** This category consists of more sophisticated decision support that takes into account a number of patient parameters and can suggest a course of action or treatment(s) optimized for those conditions. Examples include systems that review patient symptoms, signs, test results, and similar input and that then suggest a potential diagnosis and treatment (e.g., proprietary tools from vendors as well as third-party suppliers such as DxPlain and Iliad), as well as computer-aided image diagnosis systems that detect potential abnormalities in medical images (e.g., mammography screening) and photos (dermatology applications). Figure 19-3 is an example of a more complex CDS screen that takes into account a number of patient factors to suggest therapy to prevent venous thrombotic events, or clots in the lower extremity that can be more dangerous if dislodged and travel to the lung. Some of these tools can be quite advanced, going beyond diagnostic assistance to suggest potential therapies; for instance, the TrueGene system analyzes whole-gene sequences of the HIV virus to recommend the best therapeutic combination of medications for HIV patients. Additional CDS tools are also being developed for use by patients and the broader consumer community. These include smart apps for diet, exercise, medication management, diabetes care, and so on.

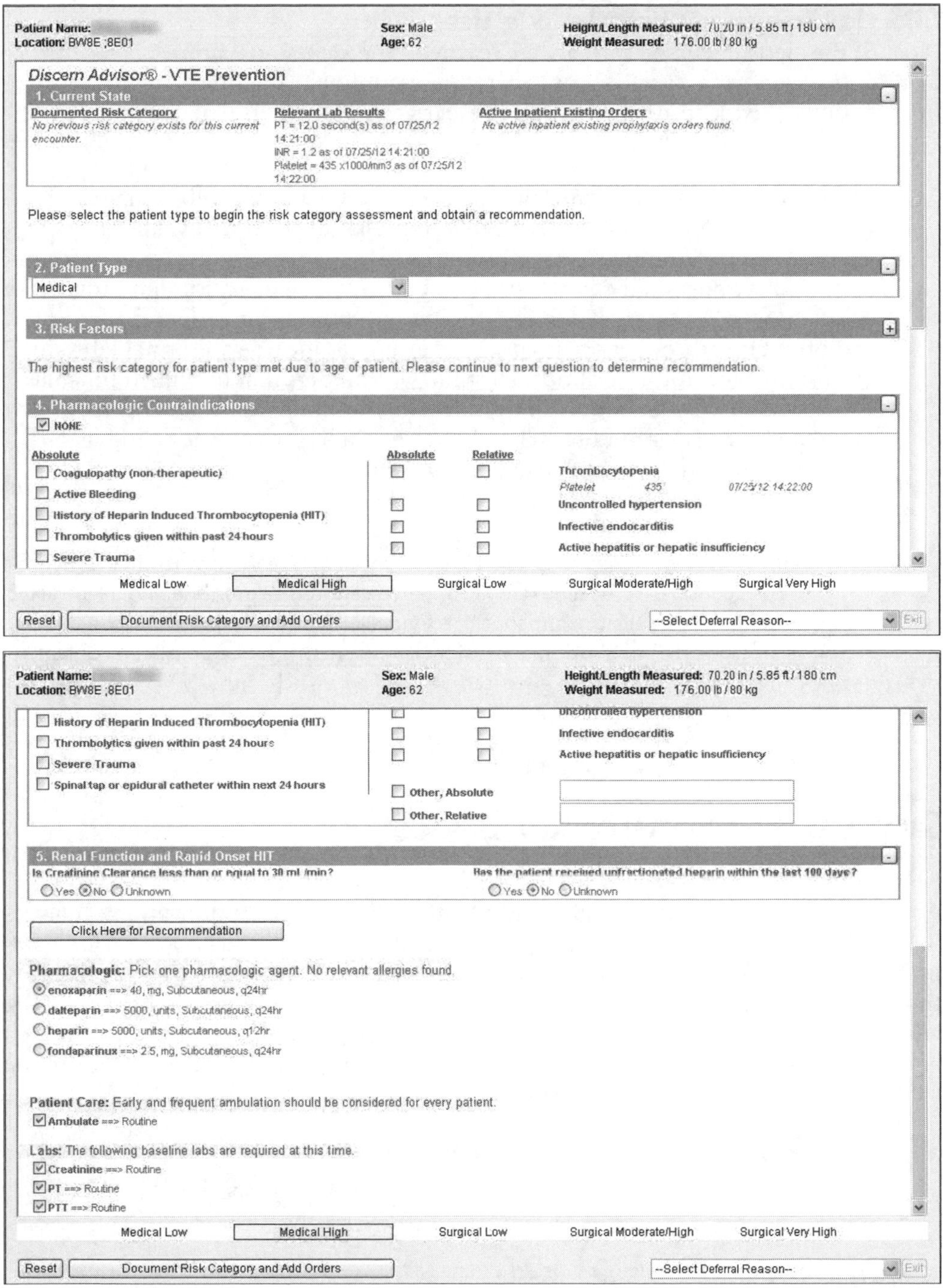

Figure 19-3   Complex CDS alert. Reprinted with permission from Cerner Corporation. © 2012 Cerner Corporation. All rights reserved.

CDS Not Triggered Directly by a User Task

Most of the alerts discussed earlier were reactive—the alerts were a direct consequence of a recent user action, such as an order or prescription. This final category of CDS interventions is asynchronous; these alerts are triggered by events that occur outside the typical clinician workflow.

- **Event-driven alerts and reminders** These interventions may be data-driven (alerts, for example, for a lab result that indicates an abnormal value) or time-triggered (reminders, for example, that a patient is overdue for an immunization). Reminders can detect the absence of events (medication not ordered for a patient where indicated) and can remind the clinician or patient that an important event has not occurred. Other examples include abnormal lab values, critical imaging findings, abnormal studies, reminders that too much time has elapsed from when a critical lab or procedure should have been performed, ventilator and urinary catheter checks, and reminders to monitor patients on therapies with a high risk of adverse drug events.

 TIP Asynchronous alerts can often be written in tandem with their synchronous counterpart. As an example, if a medication is prescribed and a lab result is abnormal, an alert might appear to the clinician synchronously. If the patient is already on a medication and a new lab result suggests a possible problem, the ordering clinician or another care giver can be notified asynchronously via message, pager, or other type of communication.

Success Factors for an Effective CDS Implementation

An Agency for Healthcare Research and Quality (AHRQ) CDS publication[6] analyzes 312 evidence-based studies on the effectiveness of CDS and builds upon earlier landmark studies.[8,9] This study reviewed multiple features of electronic CDSs to identify those that were associated with improved clinical practice through the use of a CDS. Nine attributes of CDS were identified as being highly correlated with three desired endpoints, namely, adherence to performing preventive care, adherence to performing a clinical study, and adherence to prescribing a treatment.

- Automatic provision of decision support as part of clinician workflow
- Provision of decision support at time and location of decision making
- Provision of a recommendation, not just an assessment
- Integration with charting or order entry system to support workflow integration
- Promotion of action rather than inaction

- No need for additional clinician data entry
- Justification of decision support via provision of research evidence
- Local user involvement in the development process
- Provision of decision support results to patients as well as providers

As expected, many of these items are strongly correlated with the Five Rights framework.

The Benefits of CDS

When correctly implemented, CDS has the potential to have a profound impact on patient safety and outcomes and can improve efficiencies and reduce costs. Individual studies have shown tremendous impact. However, the evidence when viewed across the entire spectrum of CDS implementations is mixed. Understanding where CDS systems have had success can help create strong buy-in and demonstrate positive results with any new CDS implementation.

The AHRQ publication on CDS,[6] which includes a meta-analysis and review of many studies, states that there is strong evidence to believe that CDSs have positively impacted select healthcare process measures and improved outcomes. There is moderate to low evidence that CDSs have had positive impact on efficiencies, economic outcomes and use, and implementation outcomes. Note that moderate to low evidence is not the same as "no evidence" nor is it the same as "evidence that CDSs do not work." These qualifications often indicate that not enough scientific studies have been conducted that examine that specific question and the body of the scientific evidence is not sufficient to support the conclusion with a strong conviction.

The evidence and body of literature around CDS are rapidly growing. The number of hospitals and ambulatory practices that have fully automated their care processes continues to grow, and as the percentage increases and CDS becomes more prevalent, additional data will be available for review. Widespread adoption of CDS and increased use of standards and knowledge sharing will only increase the number of success stories and correspondingly the evidence to support CDS.

Here are a few of the key findings in reviewing specific examples of CDS implementations to improve healthcare processes and clinical outcomes:

- There is strong evidence that CDSs, when integrated into CPOE and EHR systems, have increased adherence by providers of ordering recommended treatments, both in the inpatient and outpatient settings.

- There is also strong evidence that automatic delivery of preventive care reminders to clinicians at the point of ordering improves the ordering of preventive care practices.

- There is moderate evidence that CDSs increase adherence of providers to ordering recommended tests.

- There is moderate evidence that CDSs improve patient morbidity.

TIP The success of the second and third items depended on the system not requiring a mandatory clinician response; in other words, allowing the physician to disregard the alert appears to be correlated with increased compliance.

Tables 19-2 and 19-3 summarize these and other key findings.

As shown in Table 19-3, there is moderate evidence that CDS improves economic outcomes via lower treatment costs, lower total costs, and greater cost savings, and that it increases provider satisfaction. Studies indicate there is more than tenfold variability in reported cost savings.

Key Question	Strength of Evidence
Recommended preventive care service ordered/completed	High
Recommended clinical study ordered/completed	Moderate
Recommended treatment ordered/prescribed	High
Length of stay	Low
Morbidity	High
Mortality	Low
Health-related quality of life	Low
Adverse events	Low

Table 19-2 Positive Impact of CDS on Healthcare Process Measures and Clinical Outcomes

Category/Key Question	Strength of Evidence
Changes in workload and efficiency for the user	
Efficiency	Low
Changes in use and implementation outcomes	
Healthcare provider acceptance	Low
Healthcare provider satisfaction	Moderate
Healthcare provider use	Low
Changes in economic outcomes	
Cost	Moderate

Table 19-3 Positive Impact of CDS in Other Areas

Avoiding the Pitfalls of CDS

Although CDS has significant potential to improve care, when designed and implemented incorrectly, it has the potential to misguide clinicians and introduce error. Instead of individual clinicians making isolated mistakes in care, broadly implemented CDS systems can impact multiple users, with the potential of both positive and negative patient outcomes. Osheroff et al.[5] identify two areas of concern regarding CDS implementations.

Potential Problems with CDS

Users can quickly become disenchanted when CDS interventions do not deliver expected benefits or, even worse, are perceived as unhelpful or harmful. The following are common problems associated with CDS interventions:

- Improper integration into workflow leading to poor user adoption.
- CDS focused mainly on interruptive alerting, which leads to users ignoring alerts, overriding alerts by default, and alert fatigue—a common cause of user frustration.
- End users are not educated about workflow changes and potential benefits and their vital role in realizing these benefits.
- Trying too many interventions at once—we recommend that widespread CDS implementations be done only after testing the CDS implementation on a smaller group of stakeholders.
- Lack of maintenance of the knowledge base, resulting in obsolete interventions.
- Not linking interventions tightly to goals, leading to ineffective interventions.
- Failure to engage key stakeholders, including clinicians (physicians, nurses, pharmacists, and other care providers), IT staff, patient representatives, and hospital and ambulatory practice executives.

Avoiding Potential Problems with CDS

A successful CDS program will help determine performance-improvement and organizational decision-making priorities and, in concert with change management and communication processes, will leverage the technology infrastructure and create processes to systematically measure outcomes, examine workflows, and create interventions. Some key factors of successful CDS programs include the following:

- Well-defined decision-making and governance processes. It is vital to tightly link CDS to institutional improvement imperatives and get buy-in from executive leadership.
- A team approach that includes all relevant stakeholders. As Osheroff et al. say, CDS is done *with* recipients of CDS, not *to* them. For CDS to succeed, clinicians

must accept CDS as a decision-making aid and not as a substitute for their clinical judgment.

- Sufficient resources to measure the impact of CDS interventions (both positive and unexpected consequences).

- A strategy for keeping the knowledge base current.

- CDS implemented within the context of an institutional culture of patient safety and performance improvement. CDS is not an end in itself.

When all these factors are included, CDS implementers can create a structured, goal-based, team-oriented approach to CDS, leading to positive results for all stakeholders and improvements in quality and cost outcomes.

Patient Safety: A Critical System Property

One of the fundamental reasons for CDS implementation is to improve patient safety by eliminating errors and increasing adherence to evidence-based standards. In this section, we delve deeper into the critical area of patient safety.

It has become abundantly clear that the following issues are a new reality to healthcare:

- Patient safety must be considered a critical system property of any HIT solution.

- To generate the greatest benefits and lowest risk associated with healthcare information technology solutions, they must be considered as part of a socio-technical system, and human performance dynamics are core to optimizing safety and performance.

- Safe care, in fact great care, exists at the intersection of leadership, practices, and technologies. Engaged leaders must ensure that best and better practices are adopted while leveraging technologies such as CDS and HIT as enablers of such practices.

- Health information technology innovations such as CDS can introduce new risks that must be managed proactively and with vigilance.

- Reimbursement for healthcare is changing (as highlighted in other chapters) with new models such as value-based purchasing (VBP) that emphasize transparency of quality and cost for purchasers of healthcare. HIT and CDS will be critical aspects of those new payment structures.

Critical System Property

Overuse, underuse, and misuse of healthcare procedures, devices, and medications have been established as a major cause of healthcare harm and waste with more than 200,000 deaths and as much as 30 percent of the $2.6 trillion expended for healthcare in the United States alone. A large fraction of patients face potential harm in industrialized nations and likely even more in less developed nations. When considering any improvements to the current systems of healthcare, preventable adverse events must be included as intrinsic to any improvement approach. The 1999 Institute of Medicine (IOM) report "To Err is Human: Building a Safer Health System," and the 2002 IOM report "Crossing the Quality Chasm: A New Health System for the 21st Century" that followed it, established that the majority of harm is because of systemic problems and not human error.[2,10]

Sociotechnical System

The Institute of Medicine report "Health IT and Patient Safety: Building Safer Systems for Better Care" released in 2011 established that HIT must be considered a key element of sociotechnical systems. Cultural and work process engineering are vital elements to the success of HIT systems. The report established that safer systems begin with user-centered design principles and includes adequate testing and quality assurance assessments conducted in actual or simulated clinical environments, or both. The report declared that designers and users of healthcare IT should work together to develop, implement, optimize, and maintain healthcare IT products.[11]

Leadership, Practices, and Technologies

Safe care and great care exist at the intersection of leadership, practices, and technologies. The performance envelope of any new solution is defined by those three spheres, and this framework may be applied to consideration of changes in workflow and care. Engaged leaders assure that performance is continually optimized by adherence to best and better evidence-based practices. Technologies must be considered as an enabler of those practices. Adoption of any technology without clearly understanding best and better practices of CDS can lead to similar issues as those encountered with systems such as computerized prescriber order entry (CPOE) solutions where HIT can mitigate or accelerate errors and healthcare harm. Leaders must practice the four As of innovation adoption:

- **Awareness** Be aware of performance gaps or opportunities for improvement of patient care as measured by outcomes, processes, structure, and patient/caregiver measures.

- **Accountability** Make the proper personnel accountable for changes in behavior that will be required to safely adopt the technology or impact a change in care or performance.

- **Ability** The staff must be able to make the changes. Awareness and accountability are not enough—organizations must be able to make changes, which requires investment of hard financial resources and soft capacity resources to succeed.

- **Action**   Action is the final common pathway to ensure success. Actions, when taken in aggregate, result in successful performance improvement through the implementation of new practices or technologies.

Because safety in a human system is a team endeavor, everyone must own it, from the board of trustees to the frontline care providers to the IT team, or safety will remain an accidental attribute.[12]

Unintended Risks

There are a number of possible risks associated with CDS and its implementation. New systems introduce new workflow changes that must be understood. Overuse, misuse, and underuse of testing can introduce incidental findings that require unnecessary follow-up and additional interventions. Physicians in training may rely on CDS tools to the detriment of the clinical skills they need collecting a patient's history and performing a detailed exam. Workflow redesign with multidisciplinary teams can minimize risk by collaborating on changes.

Value-Based Purchasing

The cost of harm and inefficiencies of the healthcare system is driving transparency of quality and cost. Consumers, purchasers, and employers will utilize available information on safety, best practice, and standards reported by providers to guide their purchasing. CDS systems should facilitate doing the right thing for patients, which in the future will result in properly getting paid.[13]

U.S. Healthcare Trends Driving CDS Adoption

A number of U.S. and global market, economic, government and regulatory trends are driving the increased adoption of EHR technology and the use of CDS.

Impact of Regulatory and Economic Trends on CDS Adoption

The meaningful use Final Rule[4] requires eligible hospitals and critical access hospitals to "implement one clinical decision support rule related to a high priority hospital condition along with the ability to track compliance with that rule." Many institutions will implement this aspect of meaningful use via tools and CDS functionality provided by their EHR vendor, leading to the widespread adoption of CDS in the United States. As discussed earlier, several other dimensions need to be considered beyond just the CDS tool for a successful implementation. For more information on meaningful use, please see Chapter 11.

The current fee-for-service reimbursement model pays for procedures rather than outcomes. Many payers (both CMS and private payers) are providing incentives for hospitals to use CDS (for example, with electronic prescribing systems) and in some cases are creating penalties for the nonuse of CDS in specific high-cost disease areas.

Finally, there is increasing focus on exponential increase in the cost of healthcare. Recent projections forecast a 70 percent increase in healthcare costs over the next decade, with 2019 healthcare costs projected to total $4.5 trillion, which would consume almost 20 percent of the 2019 GDP.[15] CDS has been identified as one of the key opportunities to help reduce the projected growth.

All these trends suggest the next decade should see a huge growth in the need for CDS in U.S. institutions and continued studies regarding the effectiveness of CDS.

The Impact of Technology Trends on CDS Adoption

The stimulus provided by the Health Information Technology for Economic and Clinical Health (HITECH) Act will lead to increased adoption of EHRs and the development of standards, facilitating the deployment of CDS within and across institutions. Healthcare providers are becoming increasingly tech-savvy—80 percent of physicians use smartphones—and are using the Internet to access knowledge resources in routine care.[16] (For more information on HITECH, see Chapter 11.) The development of Internet technologies such as service-oriented architectures enables the wide dissemination of CDS interventions within and across institutions. This approach also makes it possible to develop centralized and standardized knowledge resources that are updated regularly (at a single location) and yet accessed and utilized in a uniform fashion across the country, avoiding the need for knowledge maintenance at each institution. The recent trend toward cloud-based EHRs (particularly in small outpatient settings) and patient health records also opens up intriguing possibilities for CDS.

Three other fundamental technology trends will further accelerate the need for CDS.

- Available information about a single patient increases more each year: images of greater resolution, increasing number of laboratory tests, new tumor markers, and, eventually, whole-gene sequences for patients and tumors.

- The number of available therapies and associated diagnostic tests continues to expand.

- Published knowledge (evidence-based guidelines) from clinical studies and publications that evaluate treatment outcomes and patient risks is increasing. Some estimates suggest that the amount of medical knowledge available will double every three to four years.[17]

Well-designed EHRs with sophisticated CDS tools will enable clinicians to evaluate the expanding body of knowledge, consider the latest therapies, and synthesize all this information in the context of increasingly precise patient information at the point of care.

Chapter Review

There is widespread agreement and a growing amount of evidence to suggest CDSs have the potential to significantly improve patient safety, reduce adverse events, potentially improve efficiency, reduce costs, and improve long-term health outcomes. The key to a successful CDS implementation is a goal-oriented and team-oriented approach that engages all relevant stakeholders across the enterprise. The CDS Five Rights framework provides a systematic blueprint for using CDS interventions to improve outcomes by considering the "what, who, how, where, and when" of CDS interventions. Multiple success factors drive successful implementation and adoption in the EHR, including getting clinician buy-in, carefully integrating the system into workflow, and paying careful attention to how the intervention is delivered. An over-reliance on interruptive alerting can lead to user frustration and alert fatigue, with alerts eventually being ignored. A number of CDS-associated pitfalls can be prevented by obtaining executive alignment and developing processes for governance, knowledge maintenance, and careful measurement of CDS impact. Most important is the mantra to do CDS "with" users rather than "to" users.

There are many success stories for CDS, and the number of well-constructed CDS implementations is growing rapidly. This is primarily a result of the focus at the national level to improve the quality of care and the recognition of the role of CDS to improve patient safety, leading to a number of direct and indirect incentives for CDS adoption. Patients too are becoming increasingly technology friendly and are beginning to demand CDS for their own use, pushing their clinicians to adopt CDS. Emerging technologies are making CDS easier to implement, changing the question from "if CDS?" to "when CDS?"

Questions

To test your comprehension of the chapter, answer the following questions, and then check your answers against the list of correct answers at the end of the chapter.

1. CDS is possible only with an electronic health record.
   A. True
   B. False

2. Which of these is/are essential CDS processes? (Select all that apply.)
   A. Submitting patient-specific information
   B. Gathering team consensus
   C. Generating patient-specific recommendation
   D. Gathering user-specific preferences

3. CDS is intended for many kinds of users, not just for doctors, nurses, and other care providers.

   A. True

   B. False

4. Which of these is/are *not* one of the Five Rights of CDS as defined by Osheroff and colleagues?[5] (Select all that apply.)

   A. The right information (what)

   B. The right reason (why)

   C. The right person (who)

   D. The right intervention format (how)

   E. The right channel (where)

   F. The right time in workflow (when)

5. Alerts are the most effective form of CDS intervention.

   A. True

   B. False

6. Which of these is/are potential benefits of CDS? (Select all that apply.)

   A. Improved patient safety

   B. Improved patient outcomes

   C. Improve efficiencies

   D. Increased clinician satisfaction

   E. Increased patient satisfaction

   F. Reduced care costs

   G. Reduced ADEs

Answers

1. **B. False.** Although CDS is greatly enhanced with the use of robust electronic delivery tools, it can be used even with paper-based infrastructures. The discussion in this chapter is relevant to implementing CDS in all kinds of settings; nevertheless, a well-designed IT backbone will typically result in a more structured and effective CDS implementation.

2. **A and C.** The two essential CDS processes are "submit patient-specific information" (a way of entering or importing patient data from the EHR, or even a paper chart, into the CDS) and "generate patient-specific recommendation" (a method to combine the patient-specific information with the knowledge base

to come up with a recommendation). Arriving at consensus is important in selecting a clinical goal, and gathering user preferences is helpful in designing effective CDS interventions, but these are not considered essential CDS processes.

3. **A.** True. Certainly care providers such as doctors, nurses, and pharmacists are major users of CDS. However, many other institutional personnel, such as administrators, department heads, and members of the executive team (including finance, purchasing, and IT) also make use of CDS (for example, with analytics reports). In addition, patients and their care givers can also make effective use of CDS. This trend is growing to include the general population, who can use CDS to monitor diet, monitor activity, and maintain health.

4. **B.** The right reason is not one of the five rights of CDS. The correct reason to intervene is decided before by the CDS team, when it chooses the clinical goal behind the CDS intervention. The CDS Five Rights approach proposed by Osheroff et al.[5] provides a framework to create effective CDS interventions. The Five Rights framework asserts that for every proposed intervention, the CDS team must configure each of the "what, who, how, where, and when" dimensions.

5. **B.** False. Alerts can be very effective when used correctly, but more often than not, alerts are overused, leading to alert fatigue—wherein the user tends to ignore the alert because it is used too often. There are at least ten different kinds of CDS interventions.

6. **A, B, C, D, E, F, G.** An effective CDS implementation can have a positive impact on any or all of patient safety, outcomes, and satisfaction (for both users and patients), and can improve efficiencies and reduce ADEs and costs.

References

1. Preventing medication errors: A $21 billion opportunity. Available from www .nehi.net/bendthecurve/sup/documents/Medication_Errors_%20Brief.pdf.

2. IOM (Institute of Medicine). (2000). *To err is human: Building a safer health system.* National Academy Press.

3. Serious CNS reactions possible when given to patients taking certain psychiatric medications. (2011). Available from www.fda.gov/Safety/MedWatch/ SafetyInformation/SafetyAlertsforHumanMedicalProducts/ucm265479.htm.

4. Eligible hospital and critical access hospital meaningful use core measures measure 10 of 14. (2010). Available from www.cms.gov/Regulations-and-Guidance/ Legislation/EHRIncentivePrograms/downloads/10_Clinical_Decision_Support_ Rule.pdf

5. Osheroff, J.A., Teich, J.M., Levick, D., et al. (2012). *Improving outcomes with clinical decision support: An implementer's guide, second edition.* Healthcare Management and Information Systems Society.

6. Lobach, D., Sanders, G.D., Bright, T.J., et al. (2012). *Enabling health care decision-making through clinical decision support and knowledge management.* Agency for Healthcare Research and Quality.

7. Bobb, A., Gleason, K., Husch, M., et al. (2004). The epidemiology of prescribing errors. *Archives of Internal Medicine, 164*, 785–792.

8. Kawamoto, K., Houlihan, C.A., Balas, E.A., et al. (2005). Improving clinical practice using clinical decision support systems: A systematic review of trials to identify features critical to success. *British Medical Journal, 330*, 765.

9. Bates, D.W., Kuperman, G.J., Wang, S., et al. (2003). Ten commandments for effective clinical decision support: Making the practice of evidence-based medicine a reality. *Journal of the American Medical Informatics Association 10*, 523–530.

10. IOM. (2001). *Crossing the quality chasm: A new health system for the 21st century.* National Academy Press.

11. IOM Report Brief. (Nov 2011). *Health IT and patient safety: Building safer systems for better care.* The National Academy of Sciences.

12. National Quality Forum (NQF 2010). *Safe practices for better healthcare–2010 update: A consensus report.* NQF; 2010.

13. Denham, C.R. (2009). The no outcome-no income tsunami is here: Are you a surfer, swimmer, or sinker? *Journal of Patient Safety, 5*, 42–52.

14. American Recovery and Reinvestment Act of 2009 (ARRA). (2009). United States Congress.

15. Truffer, C.J., Keehan, S., Smith, S, et al. (2010). Health spending projections through 2019: The recession's impact continues. Available from www.healthaffairs.org.

16. Physician opinions of the American Medical Association. (2011). Available from www.jacksoncoker.com/physician-career-resources/newsletters/Monthlymain/Jul/2011.aspx.

17. Stroetmann, B., & Aisenbrey, A. (2012). Medical knowledge management in healthcare industry. *World Academy of Science, Engineering and Technology, 64*, 557–562.

CHAPTER 20

Organizational Success Factors in Healthcare Informatics Implementation

Greg Forzley, Rick Lemoine, J. Michael Kramer

In this chapter, you will learn how to

- Understand HIT-based processes that span the entire continuum of healthcare service
- Understand the context and functions of different information systems relative to the type and location of care
- Develop effective clinical governance or manage existing governance across complex decisions and organizational structures
- Understand types of customizable content and executable knowledge used in health information systems
- Manage customizable content and configuration using appropriate evidence-based guidelines, clinician engagement, and organization governance
- Manage content and system enhancement changes using a standard prioritization method
- Understand success factors for managing governance, HIT content, and decision making

HIT and Continuum of Care: Understanding the Context of Organizations and HIT

HIT is implemented in a wide variety of organizations and across a number of care processes, from small single-physician practices to large health systems and integrated delivery networks (IDNs) (see Figure 20-1). Healthcare informaticists must consider all of these settings and often manage the flow of information between them. Table 20-1 presents example entities that informaticists and HIT professionals must coordinate with, and also presents sample tools and technologies they use to promote effective integration. Organizations that consider the flow of information across facilities and episodes of care will ultimately be more successful in managing the overall care of the patient and achieving lower costs. When the details of a patient's healthcare are accessible at any time from any location, there will be less redundant healthcare expense in the form of repeated tests, delays in care, and inefficient use of a provider's time.

Recently, the 2010 Patient Protection and Affordable Care Act (PPACA) created reimbursement models that pay incentives based on managing patients' health across multiple settings including ambulatory, hospital, and home healthcare, over a period of one to three years as defined by each contract. Referred to as accountable-care organizations (ACOs), each is charged with demonstrating lower costs of care for defined populations of patients across certain diseases and procedures (see Use Case 20-1). Organizations that successfully implement HIT and manage the flow of information across these complex scenarios will manage costs, deliver a higher-quality care than their competition, and thrive with the new reimbursement models. Whether you implement technology in a small practice or a large integrated delivery system, HIT leaders must govern these systems in the context of a larger organization and even across the healthcare community. Knowledge of the organizational contexts, their systems, governance, and how decisions are made is critical to successful HIT implementations. This chapter discusses success factors in implementing and governing HIT within and across healthcare organizations, the decision-making/knowledge management processes for managing the configuration and optimization of the system over time to assure high-quality care, and the methods of managing change including tracking change requests and maintaining and changing content within the systems.

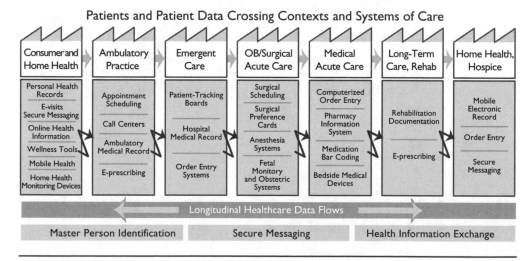

Figure 20-1 Healthcare venues and the flow of information across specific systems

Definition	Description
Accountable-care organization	A network of doctors and hospitals that share responsibility for providing care to patients across groups of physicians, hospitals, and other health organizations. The authority to create contracts for accountable-care organizations was established by the Patient Protection and Affordable Care Act in 2011.
Acute hospital care	Traditional inpatient care process where the patient is admitted and discharged for a defined episode of care.
Electronic health record (EHR)	Considered a comprehensive digital medical record that organizes all information related to a person with a focus on the health of the patient over a defined time frame. Very few organizations have this ability, intention, or breadth of care.[1]
Electronic medical record (EMR)	The record typically used for providing diagnostic or therapeutic care within a single context of care.
Episodes of care	All services associated with an optimal care for a specified medical problem, physician office visit, procedure, hospital stay, and phone call. Healthcare typically does not reimburse for the outcome of care across multiple episodes unless the patient is enrolled in an accountable-care or similar organization.[2]
Health information exchange (HIE)	The mobilization of information across organizations using a community or national health information architecture. It is a regional, state, or national network providing connections to access stored patient health information and message providers across disparate systems. For meaningful use measures, organizations must form an HIE across separate business entities and health record vendors using specific message and data standards.[3]
Home health	Wide range of healthcare services administered outside of an acute-care or skilled nursing facility.
Hospice	A form of skilled nursing care focused on the treatment of the terminally ill.
Integrated delivery system	A network of healthcare organizations under a parent corporation or other agreement. May include a healthcare management organization (HMO), provider network, provider organization, long-term care, home health, and hospice organization.
Long-term care or skilled nursing	Medical and nonmedical care provided to people with chronic illness that meets treatment requirements. Most long-term care is administered in residential and skilled nursing facilities where supportive services such as nutrition, dressing, and bathing hygiene can be managed by a nurse or skilled caregiver. Therapeutic care such as physical and occupational therapy may be administered. Documentation requirements vary significantly from typical acute-care settings.[4] Medical record requirements for physician documentation tend to address a specific goal of treatment and are often summarized on a monthly basis including physician notes. Medications are prescribed using traditional outpatient processes and do not leverage a traditional inpatient pharmacy.

Table 20-1 Principles and Definitions of Broad Organizational Context

Definition	Description
Longitudinal healthcare record	The accumulation of visits, problems, medications, and diagnostics results that span the life of the patient regardless of the organization or context of care. As patients often receive care across disparate geographies, rarely does this exist in one EMR or EHR.
Physician organization	Physician group, linkage, practices, or alliances that allow the group to manage financial integration, quality, and information across the continuum of healthcare services.
Quality measure	A definition of care process or outcome focused on a condition or disease associated with some type of scientific or research-based evidence. Typically defined by a national standards body, payer, or professional organization. Access to many measures is available at the national quality measure clearinghouse.[5]
Summary of care record	A summary care record formatted according to meaningful use standards. It must electronically incorporate, at a minimum, the following data elements: patient name; gender; race; ethnicity; preferred language; date of birth; smoking status; vital signs; medications; medication allergies; problems; procedures; laboratory tests and values/results; the referring or transitioning provider's name and contact information; hospital admission and discharge dates and locations; discharge instructions; reason(s) for hospitalization; care plan, including goals and instructions; names of providers of care during hospitalization; and names and contact information of any additional known care team members beyond the referring or transitioning provider and the receiving provider.
Transitions of care	The movement of a patient from one setting of care (hospital, ambulatory primary care practice, ambulatory specialty care practice, long-term care, home health, rehabilitation facility) to another. Currently, the meaningful use measures that use transitions of care require there to be a receiving provider of care to accept the information. Therefore, a transition home without any expectation of follow-up care related to the care given in the prior setting by another provider is not a transition of care for the purpose of stage 2 meaningful use measures because there is no provider recipient. A transition within one setting of care does not qualify as a transition of care.

Table 20-1 Principles and Definitions of Broad Organizational Context *(continued)*

Exercise 20-1: Information Flows for an Uncomplicated Surgical Procedure

In this exercise, review Use Case 20-2 and identify each transition of care. For example, a transition might be named "Physician Office to Emergency Room."

1. Make a table with the following columns: Transition Name, Stakeholders, Key Information, and Activities Prior to Transition.

   a. In the subsequent rows, identify the transition, and list the information management functions for each of the transitions.

b. Identify the stakeholders who would be interested in information in each of these transitions.

c. List the information or activities performed at each transition.

2. Advanced: After reading the section "Knowledge Management" and Table 20-2, review the case again, but this time create a table noting all the content in the case that may have been used and must be maintained and the team or person in your organization who is responsible for this work.

3. Advanced: After reading the section "Knowledge Management," list the teams in your organization that manage the changes to the executable knowledge that is used.

Use Case 20-1: Uncomplicated Case: Healthcare Across the Continuum

Mrs. Jones is a 55-year-old woman who works at a local college in a small, rural Michigan community. Mrs. Jones receives her healthcare from a local four-physician practice. She keeps her own personal health record, which includes her allergy record and blood pressure (beta-blocker) medications. She contacts her physician and schedules appointments in the practice's appointment system via a web site. Recently Mrs. Jones has been having intermittent right-sided abdominal pain made worse by fatty foods. The pain suddenly worsens, so she sees her primary physician, who refers her to the local emergency room. The emergency room doctor sees on the electronic emergency department (ED) tracking board that Mrs. Jones has arrived. Based on her severity of pain, he decides to see her next. After seeing her and reviewing information available in the EMR, he orders appropriate studies. Based on the results, the ED physician schedules a follow-up with a surgeon for a cholecystectomy (removal of the gallbladder). Mrs. Jones returns home with detailed instructions and a summary of her condition. Meanwhile, the surgeon schedules an appointment for Mrs. Jones and, anticipating a future surgery, books the case in the surgical scheduling system. During the appointment, the surgeon does an evaluation and documents a pre-operative exam in his office. Later that week, Mrs. Jones arrives in the pre-operative waiting area of the local hospital where the anesthesiologist and surgeon review the pre-operative documentation and problem list transmitted from the surgical clinic to the hospital EMR. Mrs. Jones is taken to the operating room where the anesthesiologist administers anesthetic medications and documents monitored physiological changes within the anesthesia record system. During the laparoscopic surgery, the case becomes more complicated and has to revert to an open cholecystectomy through a larger incision. Two tissue specimens are sent to pathology. Following surgery, Mrs. Jones is transferred to the postanesthesia care unit (PACU) to recover. After a few hours she is moved to the acute-care inpatient unit. The surgeon's physician assistant completes the post-operative hospital admission for Mrs. Jones and, after reviewing her home medications, uses a post-operative cholecystectomy order set to electronically order a standard set of IV fluids and pain medications for her. After she is in the hospital for a few days, the physician assistant and surgeon discuss pathology findings, use the e-prescribing system to prescribe home pain medications, enter the discharge order, and select discharge instructions. Later that day, Mrs. Jones arrives home, and a home health nurse visits to review effects of medications and teach her how to manage the abdominal wound. Finally, Mrs. Jones follows up with her regular physician when fully recovered. In this integrated system, at each change in venue and with each care provider, Mrs. Jones' information is immediately available in the EMR, thus eliminating the need for every clinician to ask and document the same information.

Health System Governance to Assure High-Quality Systems, Continuity of Care, and Communication: A Cross-Continuum Model

Governance by definition is comprised of the groups or leadership and their actions that collaboratively manage an organization. It is an organizational process that includes defining expectations, allocating resources, managing change, and measuring performance. Effective governance is essential to achieve EMR system success. A successful governance model is flexible, timely, transparent, and cognizant of the many disciplines using the EMR. The governance model provides the structure and mechanisms for managing the EMR and the organization across all phases of the HIT life cycle including planning, implementation, stabilization, optimization, and subsequent maintenance of the system (see Chapter 21 and Figure 20-1 for this life cycle). Without governance, organizations often make decisions that are poorly considered, benefit isolated stakeholders, and increase the number of reactive changes in managing the system. Poorly governed organizations respond to the crisis of the moment and do not have an overall plan to achieve the outcomes intended by implementing the EMR.

Governance must include business owners, clinical leaders, and information technology support. These people manage resources, policy, strategy, and the work plans of various teams across departments and the organization; are responsible for assuring high-quality business processes; and develop metrics to monitor and control the projects including project goals and business objectives. If the system's goals are not clearly articulated and measured, goals cannot be achieved. Governance assures that results are achieved and communicated.

In addition to responsibility for the operational framework of an EMR, a governance structure, such as the one depicted in Figure 20-2, manages complex decisions, balances

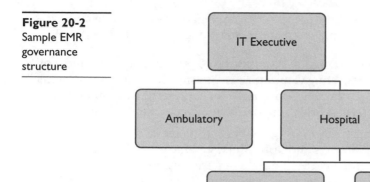

Figure 20-2
Sample EMR
governance
structure

scarce resources, and manages strategic plans for future implementations. The following are key areas of focus for governance teams and their leaders:

- **Scope and prioritization**   *Scope creep* is a frequent consequence of EMR implementation. Once users gain even a small degree of familiarity with the EMR, they begin to see alternative ways to perform their role or problems technology can help solve. This is particularly common in nondirect patient care areas such as quality monitoring, communication between disciplines, and various regulatory/compliance issues. Information technology is such that there is always an opportunity to add or change the systems. Healthcare is seemingly abundant in resources to many stakeholders, but when managing a complex system, this is not so. Prioritizing/pacing organizational change becomes an essential function.

- **Finance**   Financial issues go beyond the original purchase price and yearly operating license. Personnel issues account for a large percentage of an EMR budget. Maintenance and upgrade fees and the addition of various new modules and functionality not included with the original installation all add to the ongoing cost of keeping the EMR current and running. The addition of new modules may require hiring additional personnel, an additional yearly expense.

- **Change management**   Changes to an EMR are inevitable. Effectively managing changes in EMR function and content is an essential element of governance. The time, effort, and resources spent in establishing an ongoing change management process that is objective and responsive to user needs can provide a generous return to the organization (i.e., fewer problems to manage).

Governance structures vary widely from one organization to the next. Some are more successful than others. Depending on the size and complexity of an organization, multiple layers of governance may be required.

The following are example constituents of governing groups that guide and oversee the effective development and implementation of HIT and EHRs in healthcare.

- **Information technology executive committee**   Typically a subcommittee of the Hospital Executive Steering Committee responsible for approving projects and their budget. In general, high-cost items are considered with other major capital projects on a regular basis as part of a multiyear planning cycle.

- **Ambulatory and hospital technology operations team**   Provides operational direction for ongoing projects and leadership as issues arise within the EMR operations. Membership includes a number of organizational executives in key leadership positions such as chief operating officer (COO), chief information officer (CIO), chief medical information officer (CMIO), and chief quality officer (CQO).

- **Evidence-based medicine council (EBMC)**   Concerned primarily with content issues of the EMR as they affect physicians and medical practice. Though the committee is multidisciplinary, physicians are the predominate members. Nursing, pharmacy, and quality departments are also major contributors. This group typically focuses on clinical decision support and standardized, systemwide, evidence-based order sets.

- **EMR operations (EMROPS)**   Includes representation from all groups and levels of users across the organization. Their primary areas of interest are issues that affect process and workflow within the EMR. Nursing and pharmacy play vital roles, but the success of the committee depends on the participation of all user groups.

Success Factors and EMR Governance

A successful governance structure in any organization has a number of key characteristics as listed here:

- It is inclusive of and accountable to all relevant stakeholders.

- Governance and guiding principles are based on the organization's mission, and principles are incorporated into the work of the team.

- It strives for transparency to all constituents to assure decisions are fair and equitable to all parties involved.

- The team leaders utilize online collaboration tools such as Google documents, SharePoint, and others to facilitate optimal involvement in the discussion and dissemination of the decision-making process and knowledge coming from the organization and governance teams.

- It is responsive and highly communicative within the organization.

Use Case 20-2: Sharp Healthcare Governance Model

At Sharp Healthcare, a multihospital system in San Diego, California, there are three levels within the governance structure, listed here in descending order of position, within the organization:

- **Executive management subcommittee**   Responsible for controlling and approving project budgets

- **EMR steering committee**   Responsible for operations and has a "buck stops here" mind-set, which is important when consensus is not possible among various users

- **Operational group**   Responsible for change management and communications and is the main interface between IT professionals and users

The best way to illustrate how the various groups function and work together is through the problems/issues/projects paradigm. Individual user problems are generally handled at the operational level by the clinical informaticists and their leadership team, which is the operational group. Related user problems are sometimes grouped together and described as an issue or theme for larger investment and effort. These issues are often handled at the EMR steering level. When multiple issues are addressed or viewed as a project, that then becomes the responsibility of the executive management subcommittee. These larger projects must be managed by the executive steering teams because of frequent budgetary considerations. Organizations establish a set of criteria such as costs of change and hours to build, train, or communicate before escalating to the steering team. Once all the important factors are understood, the teams and leadership can organize and communicate the sequence and rationale for any changes proposed.

 TIP   A governance structure often has to decline or defer a request. The governance team must respond to executive, special, unplanned requests. Two principles may be valuable in saying no. First, always give an immediate answer. Second, keep the "vision" and optimism in your messaging, such as "Dr., we received your request yesterday to improve the surgical tracking board. We have determined that this is not a quick change. We are focusing on improving medication safety in the OR right now. When we are done with this work, we will consider new projects. We would welcome your input in the next round of prioritization."

Additional approaches very important to successful governance are described in the following sections.

Executive Buy-in, Participation, and Support

One of the key factors to success is an executive at the highest level or senior management in an organization. EMR operations in many large organizations now focus across venues, typically inpatient and ambulatory care. Patient care is now focused across disparate venues, and any changes to the EMR can affect clinical workflow at any given point. Health information systems are now considered more strategic enablers in the overall success of patient-care delivery of services within an organization and require engagement and support by executive leadership. Decision makers, governance, and managers must have their backing, budget, and authority to lead the organization through what may be the organization's largest change in a decades.

Integration with Existing Governance Structures

Healthcare organizations are highly structured and are often a complex collection of committees, boards, and councils. For success, tight integration of the EMR into current clinical activities necessitates cooperation with nursing councils, medical executive committees, practice management organizations, and numerous others. The challenge is to avoid conflict and repetitive decision making across these many groups.

Communication

Communication can be the most difficult and important processes in an EMR implementation and subsequent life cycle. Considering the rapid changes in healthcare and technology and the busy clinician suffering from information overload, it is necessary to communicate using multiple methods and repeated cycles for major changes. This is a particular conundrum for community-based systems with mixed employed and independent medical staff. Announcements and forms of communication should be tailored by location, individual, and type of user. In addition, the road map for EMR changes, upgrades, and future deployment should be accessible to all users. An internal or Intranet-type web site is a common way to provide access to communications.

 TIP Tools within the EMR, screen savers, and other options within the routine practice workflow can be very effective for timely and clear communication of information within an organization. Have a plan for communication of routine, unexpected, and even downtime situations. Test the plan. Consider how to communicate if systems are down or there is a network failure. Such planning is required by the Health Insurance Portability and Protection Act (HIPPA). More importantly, it will happen, so have a plan!

Multidisciplinary Membership

While EMR governance may not be democratic, it should be broadly based. Multidisciplinary means more than just physician and nursing participation. Pharmacy is a key department with considerable impact and dependence on the EMR. In addition, other ancillary departments such as physical and occupational therapy, dietary, cardiac, and other services have unique and compelling reasons for representation. Depending on the scope of EMR activities, representatives from medical records, quality, finance, and legal/compliance may need to be included. Participation by upper-level management is a prerequisite.

Infrastructure Support

The governance of an EMR requires access to various types of infrastructure support. While the administrative requirements may reside within the information systems department, other functions of the EMR may require specialized support. From time to time the change management process may benefit from a review by experts in Six Sigma or Lean technique. These techniques are discussed in Chapter 21. Communication may require assistance from individuals in the marketing or public relations departments, and Internet/web expertise is helpful.

Use Case 20-2: Designing and Configuring the System

After EMR vendor selection, the next step of implementation for an organization is typically the design and configuration of the system. Senior executives recognized that designing a single EMR with computerized provider order entry (CPOE), medication administration, and physician documentation presented challenges beyond any project previously faced by the organization. A design team was formed with 120 members including more than 20 physicians and representatives from all clinical disciplines and all levels of management. The design team had its own administrative support as well as three Six Sigma process improvement specialists known as *black belts* to facilitate discussion and decision making. The commitment of senior leadership was evident by three senior vice presidents who participated. The design team made three long-distance visits lasting five days each to the vendor's corporate office during the design process. Member physicians participated in two of those visits to help develop a feasible project scope. (It is invaluable to visit and examine the potential EMR system in use and in an actual healthcare setting if possible.) Community physicians were reimbursed for their time and travel. One advantage to the distant off-site location was the ability to focus on the project and significantly reduce the normal distractions of their day-to-day responsibilities. Once the design sessions were completed, the collective group created and installed a system that met the expectations of the organization and governance leaders.

Knowledge Management: What Kinds of Knowledge Must Be Managed and Maintained by HIT Professionals and a Systems Governance Team?

There are two major functions of an information management team that are often overlooked and difficult to sustain:

- Initial and ongoing data and functional standardization of the broad EMR
- Specific standardization and maintenance of the organization's customizable content within the EMR, often referred to as *executable knowledge*

HIT Team Sustaining Function 1: EMR Standards and Structure

As was described in Use Case 20-1, even with a relatively straightforward scenario like Mrs. Jones there is a considerable amount of data shared and incrementally new information added to her record during the numerous handoffs and transitions of care along the way. Management of the patient over the course of a defined illness or condition involves multiple clinicians and their views of data at each step of the process (nurses, physicians, pharmacists, and support staff in the office and hospital). Within an EMR, one challenge clinicians collaborating with informaticists face is ensuring relevant data is accessible easily to the clinicians in a succinct and useful format that supports efficient and effective care. The vendor often provides some of this structure, but a significant number of options within the EMR are configurable by the organization. Summary screen and flowsheet layout, menu choices, how documents are organized, alignment of similar data coming from different systems, and many more are design decisions for the team to consider.

In the case of Mrs. Jones, a number of functional tools in the EMR allowed rapid sharing of information in many ways:

- Electronic messaging tools in the physician office allowed the patient to view the physician's electronic documentation in her personal health record.
- Electronic patient-tracking board capabilities and an electronic record in the emergency room provided access to the physician office data and an opportunity for additional exam and diagnosis documentation.
- Consistent terminology and discrete pre-operative and post-operative information in the EMR-provided data that is readily accessible and meaningful to both the surgeon and the anesthesiologist.
- Home care instruction and prescriptions created in one EMR can be shared across multiple EMRs and integrated into the personal health record maintained by the patient.

As described by Michael Zack[6] more than a decade ago, information technology is the infrastructure that provides "a seamless pipeline for the flow of explicit knowledge." Information technology, when well constructed into the workflow, enables capturing knowledge; defining, storing, categorizing, indexing, and linking digital objects corresponding to knowledge units; searching for ("pulling") and subscribing to ("pushing") relevant content; and presenting content with sufficient flexibility to render it meaningful and applicable across multiple contexts of use.

Given the importance of consistent and concise information in caring for patients, the managers of the EMR must design the EMR to be a well-organized data and knowledge management system. Each function and content area must be defined and standardized. Each function must have an organizational business owner, a documented specification and justification for its construction, and a process to manage exceptions to a standard or a change to existing functionality. The process for enhancement request change management, as discussed in the next section, is also important.

The importance of an effective governance structure and HIT team cannot be overemphasized. In the absence of well-formed governance and HIT management team, an explicit implementation and optimization plan, and detailed management of data and knowledge, the EMR can be a disparate source of information with confusing and conflicting points of view. Health information experts are instrumental in the implementation and standardized use of medical terminologies. This is essential for the user experience and to manage the growing number of interfaces linking multiple systems within most organizations and across the community. As stewards of EMRs, the HIT professionals' skill set, ongoing training, and learning will become increasingly important as clinicians rely more on updated evidence-based practices within technology.

 TIP   It is essential that HIT professionals follow the emerging national standards of the Office of National Coordinator for Health IT (ONC) HIT Standards Committee. The Health IT Standards Committee, a federal advisory committee, provides recommendations on health IT standards issued to the ONC for consideration and approval. These standards are required to meet meaningful use and will drive substantial work of your teams. The ONC policy and standards committees publish the recommendations for problem lists, lab systems, medications, information transmittal, security, and many others. These recommendations substantially extend the definitions of meaningful use and EMR certification.[7]

HIT Team Sustaining Function 2: Management of Executable Knowledge

Knowledge management in the context of healthcare is the use of technology to enable people to create, capture, store, retrieve, use, and share knowledge. Two key areas typically considered part of knowledge requiring management are order sets and clinical decision support (CDS); some narrowly (and naively) think of CDS as limited to rules or alerts. CDS specifically is often considered a higher-level function of the EMR, once basic functionality has been established. CDS is covered in more detail in Chapter 19. In addition, there is also substantial non-evidence-based content that must be included in these systems to assure a reliable process of care. Many of the rules and order sets drive workflow, billing, and nonclinical performance. Therefore, we consider executable knowledge to be all of the configurable content that is installed and executed by the base EMR functions.

Evidence-based practice design and evidence-based process design are essential functions of a knowledge-based team (more about this in Chapter 21). Defined by Dr. Gordon Guyatt and others in the early 1990s, "Evidence-based medicine requires new skills of the physician (/clinician), including efficient literature-searching, and the application of formal rules of evidence in evaluating the clinical literature."[8] A HIT team must engage clinical leadership in a decision-making process that leverages both clinical experts and those skilled in evaluating the evolving scientific literature. With a structured approach, the team can avoid anecdotal and personal opinion in guiding change and systematically evaluate and document the rationale for change. Engaging clinicians in the process provides a meaningful rational for change. This work collectively becomes the science of clinical informatics, process engineering, and evidence-based practice.

Engagement of Clinicians in Knowledge Systems

One underlying goal of best practices in a healthcare setting is to reduce unnecessary variation of information, actions, and risk by clinicians through the use of evidence-based practices. Educational institutions, professional and quality organizations, expert collaborations, and health systems develop national and international best practices regularly. For these to be successfully integrated into direct patient care, local clinicians direct the design and adaptation of these evidence-based resources into local clinical processes. Given the constraints of the electronic record, advisory committees that include clinicians with the authority to develop clinically effective content management processes and structures for decision making are necessary and effective ways for gaining adoption and successful integration into the everyday workflow.

 TIP Organizations need to track change requests and include evidence for the change request using web-based database tools. In addition to tracking the evidence, teams must address challenging and sometimes competing requests using levels of evidence. Not all published literature has the same value, is relevant to day-to-day practice, or should justify change. For the advanced HIT leader, there are additional resources that describe the evidence hierarchy and should be considered for your organization.[9]

Success Factors in Knowledge Management

Leadership and governance are essential to successful knowledge sharing. Without top-level support to constantly update knowledge resources (see Table 20-2) and mid-level guidance to manage tools and resources, the activity of learning and performing according to evidence-based medicine becomes transient and unreliable. Responsibility to track and manage the body of knowledge and accountability to consistently keep content up-to-date and used by clinicians in their daily practice must be clearly defined throughout the organization and integrated into existing decision-making structures. In addition, a structure of reliable issue management and decision making must be in place. Online social media and other collaboration tools increasingly facilitate knowledge management. Celebrating this culture and measuring its success is one strategy. We have coined the term "time to evidence-based practice." We aspire that evidence practice is disseminated within 90 days of a decision to change a practice. This is ambitious considering that the knowledge of vitamin C to prevent scurvy took 264 years![10]

Executable EMR Element	Definition and Processes to Manage
Clinical education references and resources embedded in the EMR (varies, often greater than 300)	Provide links to internal and external widely available evidence-based references, organization procedures, and other clinical references at the point of care to promote clinical effectiveness. Often embed in order sets, rules, templates, and other functions. Requires ongoing maintenance of links and content.
Custom clinical decision support rules (200 to 800 custom rules)	Present decision support logic and relevant information to support an understanding of the patient's condition, typically designed as the following: • **Synchronous** Information presented in real time to clinician based on an action • **Asynchronous** Information presented later to a clinician, often via message or some other kind of notification Frequently associated with orders but also seen with documentation and other actions within the EMR. Usually prevent an action or suggest diagnostic and treatment actions or alternatives based upon key clinical findings.
Data mining and data warehouse reports (varies, greater than 200)	Create and manage reports and dashboards to support continuous improvement through reporting of results and information. Direct users to the existing organizational and vendor-provided reports.
Data sharing definitions and common language	Define standard elements of the electronic system to provided consistency across the record. Use national standard terminology to assure "codified" terminology, ease of reporting, and exchange. (See the following exam tip.)
Electronic record education and training resources (50 to 150)	Develop resources to improve user knowledge and skill in the use of electronic systems via a uniform and centralized control process. Resources may include job aids, multimedia training modules, and pocket cards. These must be updated and maintained for new users and for all users when the system is upgraded.

Table 20-2   Table of Executable Knowledge in Healthcare Informatics (Typical Quantity of These Executable Knowledge Objects in a Standard EMR Deployment in Parentheses)

Executable EMR Element	Definition and Processes to Manage
Quality and regulatory reporting data elements (400 to 1,000 discrete data elements)	Define elements of the record that are required in support of regulatory, quality, patient safety, and others and manage a process for consistent completion. These data elements have special significance and must be carefully maintained to avoid impacting key performance measures reported out of the system.
Role-based security descriptions and configurations (100 to 200 roles)	Create security roles in the system positions that define information views, restrict activity, and present tools to the user based upon their clinical and business functions. Rules and decisions around these must be continually updated and refined.
Medication rules and alert system (varies)	Specific alerts and reminders focused on reducing/eliminating medication errors such as duplication of medicine, dosing errors, drug-drug interactions, and allergies. These rules rely on hard (no further action allowed) and soft stops (user typically provides a reason but can continue). The content is usually provided by the vendor via third-party relationships (Multum and First Databank are two common sources) and are often overly conservative because of legal and other requirements requiring ongoing refinement and management.
Pharmaceutical formulary and catalog, surgical preference cards, and nonmedication orders catalogs (greater than 2,000 items)	All of the items that can be ordered in the system, i.e., a comprehensive list of labs, pharmaceuticals, nursing care interventions, and other services that a clinician can order. These are constantly changing based on drug shortages, purchasing contracts, and service evolution.
Order sets (order groups) (greater than 500 order sets or order folders)	Acute and ambulatory systems primarily have a collection of orders that are grouped to improve the ease of ordering. These may be organized and grouped together to improve a process or clinical outcome. An example might be an order set for admitting patients with heart failure or managing a transfusion.
Standardized documentation content, structure, templates, and formatting (200 to 400 templates)	Define consistent documentation templates that contain evidence-based standard elements, national quality measures, and regulatory components. Organizations will refine these as evidence and business needs change.
Standardized enhancement and change request review processes (200 to 1,000 per year)	Create a standard review process to manage new enhancements or manage changes to the electronic record.

Table 20-2 Table of Executable Knowledge in Healthcare Informatics (Typical Quantity of These Executable Knowledge Objects in a Standard EMR Deployment in Parentheses) *(continued)*

 HIT PRO EXAM TIP Codified data and discrete data are often confused. Discrete data is captured in an EMR as a single data element in the medical record. This data can be queried and included directly in a report without manipulation. Discrete data is essential for quality measure reporting and outcomes assessment. Codified data is data that is controlled and limited to a certain set of clinical responses, and these responses (i.e., clinician-defined interface terms) are mapped to a code or a numerical value. Either the numerical value or the code can be exchanged and the meaning maintained across systems. Meaningful use requires a codified terminology (e.g., RxNorm, LOINC, ICD10, or SNOMED-CT) to be mapped to the defined interface terminologies. For example, LOINC ID 18481-2 represents the lab observation for Strep Throat Antigen. A computer system could store LOINC ID 18481-2 or "Streptococcus pyogenes Antigen to represent this test or observation." Trained informaticists are familiar with the emerging national codified terminologies and existing classifications of clinical interface terminologies along with reference terminologies such as ICD10 or SNOMED-CT. As a requirement of the 2009 American Recovery and Reinvestment Act, the HIT Policy Committee and HIT Standards Committee must develop and approve meaningful use standards that require interoperability across EMRs.[11]

Use Case 20-3: Beta-Blocker Prior to Surgery Discharge Rule

The hospital quality improvement (QI) committee noted several instances where a patient on a blood pressure medication (referred to as a *beta-blocker*) at home did not receive a dose during the perioperative period (24 hours prior to surgical incision through discharge from the postanesthesia care/recovery area). Not only is this a key patient safety concern and measure, it is also a national quality measure as defined by the Surgical Care Improvement Project (SCIP). The committee is requesting that the informatics team develop a process to assure that patients consistently receive appropriate and timely medication. Options that the team will consider in designing a solution include the use of rules or alerts to remind clinicians about the need to restart the patient's beta-blocker medication, implemented as a hard-stop rule at some point in the care of the patient that requires an order to be placed. They might also consider a link to a clinical reference at some point in their workflow to help educate users about the need for the medication. Any new rule should be consistent with that workflow and provide an easy way to do the right thing. To meet the appropriate expectations by users for any new change in the electronic record, the team will involve clinicians in the design and testing of any new intervention.

As new rules (or other changes) are created and deployed, several tips will ensure success.

- Consider implementing the rule in the background, removing the final step of interrupting clinician workflow to verify it will add value and not be perceived as a nuisance.

- Make sure clinicians see it at the right time in their workflow with well-defined clinical triggers.

- Monitor how often the rule fires and how often clinicians change their action based on the rule.

- Update or remove the rule when new evidence is identified or EMR functionality occurs in order to maintain the integrity of the rule.

- Review the purpose and definitions of the rule on a periodic basis (typically every one to two years) to reaffirm the need for the rule and validate the initial reason the rule was implemented.

The change control management process consisting of a review committee composed of clinicians and informatics experts should review all key rules and reminder alerts in the system on a scheduled basis. This includes requests for new decision support rules or changes to existing rules using a formalized submission process that facilitates tracking and reporting back any decisions and rule effectiveness. The committee also has responsibility for other changes in the electronic system but must validate any change with the higher-level steering team to avoid any conflicting software changes.

System Change Management

Change in healthcare and HIT is inevitable. The subject is covered in more detail in Chapter 21. The best EMR design decisions sometimes fail to meet the rigor of daily operations. Users who were initially reticent in their adoption frequently become advocates for innovation. New and often improved functionality is common in the EMR industry. This section covers change management as it relates to technology. There are several strategies regarding change management, and the best and most successful have these recurring themes:

- **Transparency**   Ensure users at all levels who have suggested some type of change are kept apprised of the progress of their suggestion through approval, validation, testing, and deployment.

- **Tracking**   Change management suggestions are cataloged and tracked from start to finish. The clinical owner should be identified and receive updates when important milestones are reached. The tracking system should provide reporting options to evaluate the change management process.

- **Organization**   Grouping change management requests or tickets by owner, by entity, and by priority is extremely useful, especially when this information is visible to all concerned.

- **Prioritization**   Create a process for assigning the importance of suggested changes. Rather than relying strictly on when changes are submitted, a weighting system with multiple criteria determines resources and priority.

Use Case 20-4: Sharp Healthcare Enhancement Request Process

Prior to evaluating and making fundamental improvements to the change request process, the organization had more than 1,000 outstanding change requests awaiting review and approval. After significant changes to the entire management process, the organization now has approximately 30 change tickets under review at any given time with an equal number of new requests. Several factors were critical to that success:

- A clinical owner is assigned to every ticket.
- A member of the informatics team becomes the process owner until the change is completed.
- Priorities are assigned at a full meeting of the informatics team.
- A three-minute time limit for presenting changes was established.
- Six parameters are used to weigh the importance of the request: quality, safety, regulatory/compliance, productivity, finance, and scope.
  - A score of 0 to 3 is assigned to each parameter according to a rigorous and objective process.
  - The average of the first five parameters is multiplied by the score of the scope parameter to determine the importance.
  - The ticket is then assigned the resulting score and passed on to analysts and programmers within information systems with the intent that the assigned priority be maintained for the rest of the process.
  - An exception is made for "quick fixes." These are defined as a process with the equivalent work effort of changing the name of an order set within the EMR. The intent is to turn these around rapidly and, as a result, score quick wins with users who submit changes and see results quickly.

The highest value a change ticket can score is 45 by the process described, so quick-fix tickets are assigned a score of 50. This particular method borrows heavily from the experience of the informatics team at other institutions and may not be applicable in all situations. Two key success factors include informaticists with a clinical background and tight adherence to the scoring criteria.

Testing New Tools

EMR vendors routinely upgrade their solutions, and making changes or adding incrementally new modules or applications to an existing EMR presents additional challenges. It is incumbent upon user organizations to test EMR upgrades and new functionality thoroughly. Customization by the organization of the vendor's standard product often creates unique scenarios that may compromise EMR function or integrity. Testing is carried out in a nonproduction environment where the new module can be tested without the fear of impacting the clinician workflow because of system crashes and delays or compromising patient safety. Several rounds of testing may be necessary, starting with simple scenarios to confirm basic functionality and compatibility and progressing to more detailed integration testing that includes any external systems interfaced to the primary EMR.

New and/or additional EMR software should be tested in as close to a real-world environment as possible. Information system professionals can perform basic integration and compatibility testing. Clinical users bring to the testing environment a unique set of experiences and knowledge essential for thorough evaluation. Typical clinical scenarios are developed that test the system in ways users might as they provide care as well as scalability of the new application and are intended to uncover unintended consequences. A successful testing scenario is one that reveals problems and failures. These scenarios are cataloged and reused in future testing. Other organizations that have implemented the new or upgraded software are also great sources of information. While documentation provided by the vendor can provide some clue to potential consequences, there's no substitute for sharing experience within the user community. Some vendors offer web sites to facilitate this communication.

 TIP A number of organizations create units or security roles for a subgroup of clinicians referred to as *early adopters*. These roles and locations have been identified as willing participants in evaluating change and providing feedback and understand the software may not be perfect during the initial testing. Typically, several dozen users are assigned these roles and will test new functionality and provide valuable insights into the maturity of the technology and potential cost of the change. These early adopters become change leaders. They should be visible and allowed time to share their experiences with colleagues.[10]

Vendor Feedback

The investment in a modern EMR represents a substantial financial commitment by an organization and potentially the start of a long-term relationship with the vendor. A healthy relationship includes regular face-to-face meetings with executives from both sides focused on improving the system and less on assigning blame if there is a problem. Most organizations have an internal road map, reviewed at least annually, that describes over a specific period of time when upgrades are planned, external influences that impact the EMR, and a number of other factors. Working directly with the vendor to update the road map can be a valuable exercise. Customers should know the development road map of the vendor so they can make appropriate planning decisions. Vendors gain valuable insight into how clinicians actually use the system and where common workflow and other challenges occur. As healthcare moves from paper to electronic records, organizations need appropriate lead time to consider their options in terms of expanding the role of the EMR, considering their primary vendor, self, or locally developed solutions or niche vendors.

User communities are an efficient way of sharing experience. The quickest way to solving a particular problem is often a posting on a message board provided by the vendor or an independent site. One factor to consider in the selection process is the strength of the user community.

Upgrading

EMR upgrades are a fact of life. Changes occur in workflow, treatments, medications, and regulations, and all are impacted by existing functionality in the EMR. In an ideal world, upgrades would be automatic, painless, and transparent. Over time the process has improved, but there are still unanticipated issues, and for each upgrade an organization should consider the following:

- Does the upgrade require a downtime where the EMR will be unavailable and clinicians will have to use paper processes? Ideally an upgrade can be applied without bringing the system offline, or if a downtime is needed, the duration is minimal.

- If a downtime is required, can other systems be upgraded or enhanced at the same time? This allows an organization to batch upgrades and potentially minimize interruption to end users.

- How long is the estimated downtime? End users need to decide whether the downtime is long enough to warrant a switch to paper or other downtime procedures. When possible, users are provided a best-case and worst-case scenario for the length of time the system will be unavailable.

- With any change, how much training is required of end users? Some upgrades involve major changes to workflow or functionality. In these situations, users may require additional training. Any incremental training where clinicians are paid while away from their normal duties is considered an associated cost of EMR upgrades.

- Given the previous considerations, a thoughtful communication plan is developed for the upgrade process, especially when it involves downtime. A post-downtime debrief, from both information systems and end users, provides valuable information to plan for the next update.

Chapter Review

Patients and their families, national HIT standards and goals, an increasing focus on the quality and costs associated with healthcare, and competitive forces all require informaticists and clinicians to consider care provided and information flow within and outside their normal environment. HIT professionals must develop and understand the broad scope, complexity, and unique requirements of HIT in each care area. For example, regulatory and documentation requirements in rehabilitation facilities differ from those in acute care. Children's hospitals have unique considerations regarding data capture and display, medication dosing, and other factors. There are a number of organizations, such as the American Health Information Management Society, that can provide guidance and assurance to meet the multitude of information management requirements.

As healthcare regulations, quality requirements, and reimbursement models change, clinical information systems change. Implementing any new EMR functionality or module (i.e., order entry) on a given date is really just the first step of an ongoing journey. Installing information systems requires substantial investment and management of organizationwide resources. Effective leadership and management of these resources require decision-making processes that include both leaders and stakeholders organized into an effective governance structure. Guiding principles of equitable and timely prioritization, communication, transparency, and executive sponsorship are critical. HIT professionals play a significant role in assuring governance is in place and supported by executive leaders.

Finally, HIT implementation is often considered "a project," and many underestimate or don't consider the costs and efforts of ongoing knowledge management. Strategically thinking and successful organizations understand that "executable content" and the configuration of HIT systems involves thousands of decisions and ongoing updates as medical evidence and the healthcare environment evolves. Those organizations consistently implement governance teams to manage content changes such as order sets, rules, documentation templates, and process designs. HIT leaders must recognize this commitment and develop the organization structures, talent, and processes to sustain these systems into the future.

Questions

To test your comprehension of the chapter, answer the following questions and then check your answers against the list of correct answers at the end of the chapter.

1. What is the federal act that empowers the Centers for Medicare and Medicaid Services to create shared accountability for Medicare shared savings across groups of physicians, hospitals, and other healthcare providers?

   A. American Recovery and Reinvestment Act

   B. Patient Protection and Affordable Care Act

   C. Federal Employees Health Benefits Program

   D. Health Insurance and Portability and Accountability Act

   E. Medicare Prescription Drug Improvement and Modernization Act

2. The electronic medical record, electronic health record, and longitudinal health record are often used inconsistently. A hospital implements a health information system for emergency and inpatient care. What is the correct description?

   A. Electronic health record (EHR)

   B. Electronic medical record (EMR)

   C. Emergency and acute-care electronic health record (EAHR)

   D. Legal health record (LHR)

   E. A or B

3. The elements that constitute the summary of care record as defined by the meaningful use rule include all of the following except which?

   A. Discharge instructions

   B. Date of birth

   C. Vital signs

   D. Medications

   E. Final lab results

4. All of the following are requirements for an acute-care workflow and a long-term care workflow except which?

   A. Documentation in LTC and acute care includes problems, medications, and plans of care.

   B. Medications are prescribed electronically.

   C. Both workflows require physician documentation on a daily basis.

   D. Physical therapy notes are included in the medical record.

   E. Long-term care medications are provided by an outpatient pharmacy workflow and e-prescribing.

5. All of the following are considered a transition of care where a summary of care must be provided except which?

   A. Discharge of the patient to home without expectation of follow-up to another provider.

   B. Discharge of the patient to home with a follow-up to the patient's regular physician.

   C. A referral of the patient to another care provider within the same setting of care.

   D. A patient is sent to the emergency room from the primary-care office.

   E. A and C.

6. What clinical requirements(s) should you consider when designing an automated rule to "fire" in the clinical workflow?

   A. Measuring the effectiveness of the rule

   B. Defining the triggering events

   C. Maintaining the rule to match clinical evidence

   D. Creating hard stops for every rule designed

   E. A, B, and C

7. What is the least important factor when considering healthcare informatics knowledge management?

   A. Technology

   B. Process of communication to users

   C. Providers personal preferences for configuration of the technology

   D. People/culture

   E. All of the above

8. What are the elements that are part of the knowledge management scope of practice for a HIT team?

   A. Electronic record education and training

   B. Order sets

   C. Standardized enhancement and change request review processes

   D. Data mining and data warehouse reports

   E. All of the above

9. The quote "Information technology is the infrastructure that provides a seamless 'pipeline' for the flow of explicit knowledge" is attributed to which of the following?

   A. Bill Gates

   B. Edward Shortliffe

   C. Michael Zack

   D. David Blumenthal

10. All of the following are characteristics of role-based security descriptions and configurations except which?

    A. Rules can be specific to the defined position.

    B. Rules, once established, should not be flexed or adjusted for any reason.

    C. Information is presented to the user based on clinical and business functions.

    D. Each position should have limitless availability of tools to allow maximum flexibility.

    E. A and C.

    F. B and D.

Answers

1. **B.** The Patient Protection and Affordable Care Act established the Medicare Shared Savings program. The act authorizes the Centers for Medicare and Medicaid Services to establish the MSSP program and establish accountable-care organization contracts by January 2012. The MSSP creates models to manage patient populations and coordinates items and services under Medicare reimbursement. These reimbursement models require organizations to understand in detail information flows within and outside the organization across the community.

2. **B.** The electronic medical record is the best description since the medical record is serving the purposes of managing the care in one specific entity of the healthcare process. If the EMR was implemented across the continuum and was intended to manage the lifelong record for the patient, you could call it the EHR. The portion of the EHR that constitutes the summary elements across visits is considered the longitudinal health record. The portion of the medical record that is released upon patient or other legal request is the designated record set or legal health record.

3. **E.** All of the elements are included. As of October 2012, the definition of the summary of care record and a subsequent document, the transition summary, are described in the meaningful use rule and the later HIT policies and standards. Neither was defined at the time the interim meaningful use stage 2 rule was released. Final lab results are not included as a requirement of the summary of care record or transition summary. Given the large volume of and often-normal values, it is not practical to include laboratory studies in the hospital. Approximately 60 percent of patients have unresolved lab results at discharge, and of these, 15 percent can impact a clinical decision. In practice, some organizations include only preliminary or incomplete test results in the transition summary to increase awareness for subsequent care providers.

4. **C.** The statement is incorrect. AHIMA and billing standards for long-term care documentation do not require a daily progress note for care in a rehabilitation facility. Inpatient hospital care requires an admission note, daily physician progress notes, and a discharge summary to justify reimbursement for physician services and the hospital stay for most private and government payers.

5. **E.** With meaningful use stage 2, options A and C are not considered changes in settings of care that require a summary of care record. In the case where the patient is sent home without a follow-up provider, there is no provider to send the summary to. Understanding transitions of care and automating the

reporting of the completion of the summary of care record transfer will be one of the more difficult stage 2 measures.

6. **E.** Hard stops that interrupt a clinician's workflow and force them to respond should be used sparingly in the context of order entry and other clinician activities because they can impair the ability of the clinician users to perform needed tasks or enter important documentation or orders, occasionally causing a distraction that can actually have an adverse result. They should be reserved for situations that require careful consideration that result in better decision making or to meet regulatory requirements.

7. **E.** Knowledge management is a complex process that must consider governance, culture, and a large scope of specific executable content areas. Educational materials are considered in the scope of knowledge management since they often must be changed as the system is upgraded or as process improvement projects change the use of the system. An issues-tracking system will maintain the rationale and evidence for making changes to other important parts of the system such as rules, templates, and order sets.

8. **E.** While there are many more executable EMR elements, all options listed are commonly considered when implementing an EMR with the goal of using the data to improve care and support reporting.

9. **C.** Michael Zack identified the importance of information technology in supporting the flow of knowledge. He appropriately noted that it enables knowledge capture, the ability to "push" or "pull" relevant content, the ability to relate digital objects to knowledge units, and the ability to present flexible content to render it meaningful across many settings.

10. **F.** In defining role-based security access to EMR content, it is important to help the user "do the right thing." Providing appropriate tools with limits based on clinician review and input optimizes the user experience and helps avoid information overload, a frequent risk in the digital world. The assignment of rules must always be considered in the context of the clinical setting with constant monitoring, maintenance, adjustment, or refinement based on knowledge or system changes and user experience.

References

1. EMR vs. EHR: What is the difference? (2011). Available from www.healthit.gov/buzz-blog/electronic-health-and-medical-records/emr-vs-ehr-difference.

2. Hornbrook, M., Hurtado, A., & Johnson, R. (1985). Health care episodes: Definition, measurement, and use. *Medical Care Research and Review, 42,* 163–218.

3. Electronic health record incentive program stage 2. Accessed on July 2012 from www.gpo.gov/fdsys/pkg/FR-2012-03-07/pdf/2012-4443.pdf.

4. LTC health information practice and documentation guide version. Accessed on July 2012 from www.ahima.org/resources/infocenter/ltc/guidelines.aspx.

5. National quality measures clearinghouse. Accessed on July 2012 from www.qualitymeasures.ahrq.gov/tutorial/index.aspx.

6. Zack, M. Managing codified knowledge. (1999). *Sloan Management Review, 40,* 45–58.

7. HIT standards committee recommendations. Accessed on July 2012 from http://healthit.hhs.gov/portal/server.pt/community/healthit_hhs_gov__standards_recommendations/1818.

8. Guyatt, G., Cairns, J., Churchill, D., et al. (1992). Evidence-based medicine: A new approach to teaching the practice of medicine. *Journal of the American Medical Association, 268,* 2420–2425.

9. Evidence-based practice (EBP) resources. Accessed on July 2012 from www.ebmpyramid.org/samples/complicated.html.

10. Berwick, D.M. (2003). Disseminating innovations in health care. *Journal of the American Medical Association, 289,* 1969–1975.

11. HIT standards committee recommendations. Accessed on July 2012 from http://healthit.hhs.gov/portal/server.pt/community/healthit_hhs_gov__standards_recommendations/1818.

CHAPTER 21

Fundamentals of Health Workflow Process Analysis and Redesign

J. Michael Kramer, Sheila Ochylski, Jane Brokel

In this chapter, you will learn how to
- Design processes and information flows for the practice that accommodate quality improvement and reporting
- Develop a plan for a revised and optimized clinical workflow within a healthcare system that integrates meaningful use of information technology
- Develop a process map for given clinical process workflows within a complex healthcare system
- Analyze clinical workflows to design information technology that supports clinical decision making and care coordination
- Critically analyze the workflow processes in a selected clinical setting, taking into account potential gaps, areas of redundancy, delays, manual work, work volume, task time, and elapsed time
- Facilitate decision making necessary for optimizing healthcare processes
- Document clinic processes to facilitate workflow analysis and redesign
- Design and implement information technology that supports effective teamwork, fosters open communication, and enables shared decision making to achieve quality patient care
- Design and apply information technology and standardized practices that support safety and quality

Implementing health information systems across an organization brings an unprecedented magnitude of change to those organizations. This chapter reviews two major tools necessary to manage such change: process modeling and organizationwide change management. Before we discuss utilizing these tools, we will review the life cycle of change. Traditional "project management" considers project closure as a phase of a change. At this point, the project team is redeployed to other work, and the change is considered complete. In a large-scale HIT implementation project, it is necessary to sustain resources in order to manage major HIT systems in an ongoing manner after the system has been implemented. This is largely because of the rapidly evolving nature of healthcare including ever-increasing scientific evidence, regulatory updates, national healthcare quality measures, and upgrades to the system. The skills and the teams to manage ongoing change are necessary to control the ongoing work. Therefore, the concept of project closure is obsolete if organizations expect to leverage their newly implemented information systems to achieve higher levels of quality and safety.

Life Cycle of Major Information Technology Implementation and Organizational Change

To understand how health information technology can be managed, you must understand the larger context of change. As the nation implements electronic health records (EHRs) in every hospital and medical practice,[1,2] EHRs become central to each organization's operations. Therefore, the responsibility and need to sustain systems in a practice or hospital does not end with the initial implementation. Each organization will choose how to support and maintain their systems differently with varying leadership models, teams, and reporting structures. See Chapter 20 for a more detailed discussion on governance.

No matter the model of support, we have observed a very clear life cycle in implementing EHRs across our combined experience in 30 hospitals and several large ambulatory practices. The phases of large-scale HIT change can be described as planning, implementation, stabilization, optimization, and transformation. This is depicted in the first row of Figure 21-1. Planning and implementation require a great deal of diligence and traditional project management, which is clear to most organizations. The time it takes postimplementation to return to normal operations and productivity with obvious benefits of the EHR is not always appreciated. In our experience, the movement from implementation to transformation varies across organizations. The characteristics, risks, and benefits of each phase are listed and further described in Table 21-1. Despite rigorous planning and thoughtful implementation, there is still the risk of end-user workarounds.

 HIT PRO EXAM TIP   A *workaround* is a way to use the system in a fashion that it was not designed or intended. Workarounds result in unplanned and unexpected outcomes.[3] A physician might not find a lab test so instead enters an electronic order to the nurse with a typed comment to order the blood test. This results in a delay in the lab completing the test because of the extra steps required for the nurse to clarify the order for completing the test.

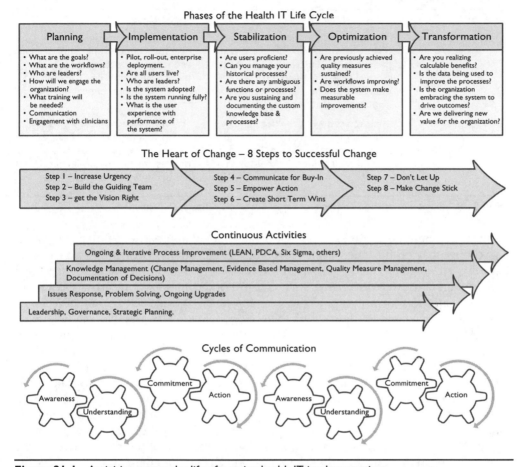

Figure 21-1 Activities across the life of a major health IT implementation

Phase	Characteristics	Risks/Benefits
Planning	Traditional project management approaches include project conception, initiation, planning, and project tracking.	Implementation requires carefully identifying and tracking project activities.
Implementation	Go-live and activation of the software. May be phased or all at once.	User support and training must be carefully planned. Monitoring usage and tracking unexpected outcomes or harms.
Stabilization	This is the period in which an organization has not yet returned to normal operations. Support resources may be less numerous. Users are finding gaps between previous workflows and new workflows.	This is a period of greatest user frustration and highest risk for workarounds and identifying recurring issues.

Table 21-1 Summary of the Life Cycle of Large-Scale HIT Change

Phase	Characteristics	Risks/Benefits
Optimization	After weeks or months, an organization returns to the new normal level of patient care. Clinicians and support personnel have identified most of the workarounds or best practices in order to continue operations.	Without careful management, users will circumvent major safety and other benefits of the system to manage day to day. This will place the system benefit at risk.
Transformation	Organizations begin to understand how to manage the system. They embrace change and leverage data in the system to inform stakeholders of their performance.	Transformation elevates an organization to a higher level. Failure to recruit or train experts on the new technology will limit this opportunity.

Table 21-1   Summary of the Life Cycle of Large-Scale HIT Change *(continued)*

Figure 21-1 introduces three additional organizational approaches to managing large-scale change that are illustrated in the second through fourth levels: organizational change management, ongoing continuous activities, and communication. Change management planning can reduce provider dissatisfaction, a prolonged stabilization phase, and a number of workarounds. Organizational change management is discussed later in this chapter. Kotter and Cohen provide a framework to develop four core activities that will help manage large change. The three long arrows, within the life cycle of change, display how organizations must develop approaches to ongoing evolution and change in the system. These activities include maintaining the system knowledge base. Chapter 20 discussed the importance of maintaining and updating the system's content (e.g., order sets, rules, and workflows) to stay current with advances in medical science, health regulation, and quality measures. Finally, with each change, organizations must maintain multiple cycles and methods of communication with all stakeholders. This is represented by the cogs in the last row of Figure 21-1.[4] Effective communication increases the awareness of the need to change, the understanding of the processes, the commitment to change, and the actions to achieve the desired changes and outcomes. These concepts are part of a theoretical model of change that is very helpful in creating a sequence of communications around major change.

 TIP   *The Heart of Change* by John Kotter and Dan Cohen[4] provides an excellent overview of change management across diverse stakeholders and an organization.

Process Management and Process Improvement

Process mapping for healthcare takes complex patient-care delivery services and organizes the collection and uses of patient information for decisions that guide patient services. This section describes a process hierarchy for workflow analysis that design HIT professionals can use to support stakeholder's planning and implementing changes. A central theme to workflow analysis and redesign of care is keeping the patient and their information centered in the approach. This section discusses five levels of process mapping, (see Table 21-2) which guide designers to consider the scope and standards of practice for key healthcare professionals, the accreditation and regulatory requirements, the Centers for Medicare and Medicaid Services (CMS) EHR meaningful use incentive program requirements, and the quality and patient safety goals.

Process Hierarchy: Levels of Mapping Process

In this section, a process hierarchy for workflow analysis and design is described to meet stakeholder needs in planning and implementing ongoing changes. The stakeholders include administrators, clinicians, department staff, and individuals who have specific tasks and functions. The first level is used by senior leaders who organize care among multiple settings for a population that will need full-service healthcare through community and referral providers. This first level is described as enterprise-to-enterprise mapping with the patient viewpoint. This viewpoint ensures there are services available and that statewide health information exchanges (HIEs) can share and move data between entities to accommodate the patient's needs for healthcare. This first level will capture the patient's broad experience of moving in and out of provider venues and processes that support the clinical practice and patient needs, financial compensation and accounting, and public obligations. Figure 21-2 illustrates what the patient may experience using healthcare services starting with the call for help and ending with a return home to self-manage their health.

While the patients perceive their care as being across visits and encounters with the healthcare system, many providers focus on care within one site such as an institution or clinic. The second level is described as venue to venue, which consists of major service lines such as emergency, surgical, or oncology services. The service line director and clinical team are stakeholders who understand care delivery. This level advances from the first level by explaining the clinical processes the patient and family are involved in. Reuse of common processes reduces variation in the healthcare professional's workflow such as medication management that applies to most venues and all service lines of care.

Level	Description
Level 1: Enterprise to Enterprise	This workflow describes referrals, full service, and community care among multiple locations for a population of patients.
Level 2: Venue to Venue	This workflow describes care for a service line in a given setting (e.g., emergency services or obstetrics).
Level 3: Roles to Patient	This workflow describes the interactions of providers with patients and with each other (role-based, patient-centered).
Level 4: Task to Task	This workflow describes the detailed steps for a procedure of care (e.g., ordering).
Level 5: Application Function	This workflow describes the use of data or information within an EHR, decision support, or exchange application.

Table 21.2 Descriptions for Levels of Mapping Process

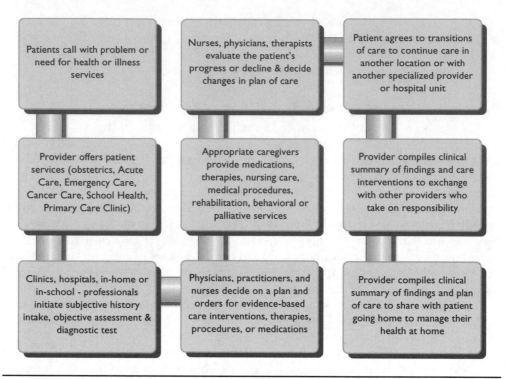

Figure 21-2 Enterprise-level processes for data, information, and knowledge use

 HIT PRO EXAM TIP For a patient undergoing surgery, typical processes include registration, admission activities, surgical preparations, shift change or handoff activities, daily care coordination, transfer and/or discharge, quality monitoring, and reporting, as well as diagnostic radiology, laboratory, and pharmaceutical services. Viewing the delivery of care as a modular activity allows reuse of defined processes within multiple venues and across multiple scenarios.

The third level is engineering role-based workflows within those clinical processes. This level will assist the healthcare professionals and leaders in emphasizing interactions with the patient while specifying multiple process requirements established by federal agencies and states who license physicians, nurses, pharmacists, therapists, and technicians. In the third level, the medication management process is viewed in more specific detail as a person-to-person workflow where three or more professional roles interact using patient data, information, and evidence-based knowledge for clinical decisions. One decision may include an order/prescription for a specific patient's diagnoses and whether to administer the medication when the patient is unstable. Later in the chapter, examples of these workflows are illustrated.

TIP Level 3 focuses on the role of clinicians with patients and within the workflow.

HIT PRO EXAM TIP   Level 3 is a patient-centered workflow, with the patient's role in the center of the swim-lane rows using a cross-functional flowchart.[5] This workflow defines the steps in each role where the communication of data, information, and knowledge within professional practices flows seamlessly to ensure proper handoffs across shifts or on a daily basis to safeguard care continuously for a patient.

Communication of information can be accomplished via electronic methods, direct conversation, or paper methods. These person-to-person handoffs identify the professional's scope of practice to care for patients, which includes their use of trended and aggregated information to evaluate patient status over time. The role-based (person-to-person) workflows use action verbs in the process steps (rectangles) to describe the activities each healthcare professional performs in a given venue (e.g., admission, clinic visit, surgery). This workflow displays questions to describe which physician or nurse decisions (diamonds) have to be made (e.g., medication management, transfer, discharge). This level of workflow is used to support the training of the healthcare professionals and support personnel.

As an example, the nurse will see the nursing process steps displayed within the workflow and can relate nursing practice steps in their use of the EHR system. Randell et al. found nurses are more likely to change their actions when they understand why the nursing process is better when using the EHR system.[6] Physicians respond similarly when they know why a given step is important. This level of workflow provides a far better illustration of the steps for each role when working with patients.

The fourth level is task to task. At this level, the detailed use of a function is described. To illustrate, how does a physician order a radiologic test that requires pretest preparations and the holding of a medication prior to and 24 hours after the test? These workflows are modular in that they are specific to a task being completed by someone. This computerized ordering step can vary from other ordering processes, and therefore a task-oriented workflow provides the orientation to the additional steps necessary. These unique tasks are limited to a few professionals or support personnel to complete, while most others don't require this level of detail.

The last and fifth level of workflow is described as functional and application flow for using patient information. These workflows are modular with less human involvement because the tracking function or decision-support logic applications are using the information based on programming. For example, the EHR's problem list may be used in several summary views, such as the continuity of care document (CCD) when extracting data for exchange with another organization or provider or within the care-planning function for nurses or ordering by physicians.

TIP   The flow of information in an EHR application, such as clinical decision support applications (covered in more detail in Chapter 5), are typically more automated than paper-based system and often require less human interaction.

Workflow for a functional application has a very limited focus such as clinical decision support or documenting allergies or supporting a specific decision. This workflow lacks the perspective of care delivery.

 HIT PRO EXAM TIP The person-to-person development of workflows displays the time-oriented interaction and steps taken for all the interdisciplinary team's processes occurring with patients.

Role-based workflows—such as those for physicians or nurses or pharmacists—identify the timely collection and documentation of patient information providing access to the data for subsequent clinical decisions. This provides a framework for how EHRs are designed to manage information for decision makers and those coordinating care with other providers or departments. The availability of patient data along with evidence-based knowledge resources (e.g., drug and disease databases, nurse procedure/intervention databases, cancer protocols) are necessary resources in the workflow to support clinical decisions and appropriate treatment steps. Person-to-person and patient-centered service-line workflows minimize the stress and better coordinate the complex activities of implementations.[7]

 HIT PRO EXAM TIP Standardizing the venues and the various workflows (role-based person-to-person, task, and functional) is useful to transfer process knowledge from one setting to the next.

Methodologies for Understanding Processes

There are several methods for understanding processes:

- Observation of current daily workflow
- Modeling workflow based on the formal scope of professional practice standards
- Simulation of the proposed workflow steps
- Quality-based deployment strategies such as Lean and Six Sigma
- Continuous workflow improvement with functional technology advances

Most organizations use business process management and modeling tools such as Microsoft Visio or others. Benefits and limitations for each method are described in the following sections. In this section, you will critically analyze the workflow processes in a selected clinical setting, taking into account potential gaps, areas of redundancy, delays, manual work, work volume, task time, and elapsed time.

Observation

Use of observation provides an opportunity to view settings and observe various patient scenarios within each setting. This method is very good for understanding the task time, manual work, delays, and multiple variations that exist within care processes for a discipline. Observation is beneficial to highlight the typical time it takes to complete a task and to identify variations in practice among professionals. While there may be a good reason for variation, a common result is unnecessary cost and inefficiency. The Lean principle of Gemba is a tool to observe workflow. "Gemba" is a Japanese word that refers to the location where value is created. The principle behind "going to Gemba" (meaning the "place where the work is being done") is commonly used by Lean experts. The foundation of this principle is to observe the actual process to get the facts and data.[8]

Modeling Workflows for Scope of Professional Practice Standards

A second method for understanding processes is modeling that is informed by the scope of healthcare professional practice. Data, information, and evidence-based knowledge are used to analyze clinical decision-making requirements.

Professional practice standards are sources to identify who, what, when, how, and where information is needed. Information technology professionals may not understand or appreciate the differences, unique responsibilities, and accountabilities for each of the healthcare disciplines that are central to patient services. The processes followed by each clinical discipline or role (such as medical assistant, nurse, or physician) are equally important to the patient's care and treatment.

 HIT PRO EXAM TIP   Spending time with clinicians (or, "Going to the Gemba,") as they provide care can help IT professionals appreciate the time and other resource constraints caregivers encounter and identify and take into account potential functionality or other gaps of the EHR or HIE.

Physicians examine, diagnose, and order medications and therapies to treat diseases and injuries or perform noninvasive or invasive procedures to improve a disease process or medical condition over time. Physicians can be specialized by the age groups they treat or in primary-care practice for all ages, while many more physicians focus on a specific body system such as cardiovascular, orthopedics, or psychiatry. (You can find more detail on care within and across venues and various medical roles and specialties roles in Chapter 1.) EHRs aggregate patient information and historical information along with drug and disease databases, laboratory, radiology and other diagnostic references, and evidence-based guidelines to support physician decisions on diagnoses, plan for care, referrals, consultations, treatment, and follow-up. Table 21-3 describes processes and decisions for different healthcare professionals. When the EHR system lacks the ability to organize and aggregate pertinent data for a specialized practice, the professional frequently finds workaround alternatives to accomplish the same function and come up with a treatment plan individualized to the patient's condition.

Roles	Activities and Decisions
Physician	• Reviews medical history (subjective); examines body systems (objective) • Orders diagnostic testing and focused assessments and care restrictions or limitations • Diagnoses disease or medical condition (e.g., diabetes, renal insufficiency) • Orders medications and treatment plan; consults other disciplines to evaluate and/or treat • Documents steps in procedures performed • Evaluates the resolution of the disease
Nurse	• Interviews and assesses human responses for functional health patterns • Diagnoses problems, risks, and needs for health enhancement • Determines what the patient and family desire for outcomes (i.e., their priorities) • Organizes and coordinates the plan of care • Schedules, educates, monitors, and documents performed interventions • Evaluates the effects for progress/decline in patient's outcomes
Pharmacist	• Reviews the patient's profile of medications, appropriate dosing, and known interactions • Verifies the medication as appropriate for indications • Consults with physician when discrepancies in drug choice, dosing, or interactions • Dispenses prescription medications • Educates and validates patient's understanding of dosing and side effects • Reviews lab tests and refills prescriptions
Therapist	• Accepts order and schedules evaluation and treatments • Evaluates current patient skills for physical, social occupation, respiratory, and speech • Shares the therapy plan and timeline for patient activities • Evaluates the patient pre- and postpatient activities • Trends the progress or lack of progress in physical or occupational abilities • Reports the progress to the provider
Technician	• Identifies and changes schedule based on order urgency • Determines appropriateness of test procedure with radiologist, consults with ordering physician • Prepares the patient by way of at home education or utilizes nursing when in facility • Conducts diagnostic test or therapeutic procedure • Evaluates patient cooperation and tolerance through test procedure • Reports critical findings to physician or nurse
Patient	• Decides to contact a healthcare professional or service • Expresses preferences and decides what patient outcomes are priorities • Learns how to recognize symptoms and manages the condition(s) • Learns when and who to contact for follow-up • Identifies who in the family is going to support them • Identifies what health resources or pharmacies to use

Table 21-3 Processes and Decisions in Scope of Healthcare Professional Practices and Patient

Nurses are the largest group of healthcare professionals in acute care and other facilities and predominant users of the EHR, providing around-the-clock coverage for patients in a number of venues. Table 21-3 highlights the major activities of the nursing process and decisions for the patient. While physicians are usually responsible for the overall management of a given disease, the nurses typically carry out the recommendations made by the physician and also address a number of patient responses including fear, agitation, confusion, nausea, acute or chronic pain, impaired skin integrity (which can lead to pressure ulcers), impaired mobility (a risk for accidental falls), and a lack of knowledge about their condition. In addition, they watch for patients who might become suicidal or aspirate (accidental entry of food or stomach contents in the airway). Nurses develop and are responsible for implementing a plan of care with evidence-based interventions to prevent problems, avoid risks and promote healthy lifestyle changes, and use evidence-based databases for nursing decisions about care that are usually different from those used by physicians. Finally, given the amount of time they spend with the patient, they tend to have a more holistic view of their care.

Patients and their families have an important role in workflows because most information from assessments and ultimately the patient's outcome is gathered from them. Table 21-3 highlights the patient's role in learning about diagnostic results and changes in treatment activities. Any workflow that doesn't include the patient is missing the most important stakeholder in patient care. Given the time they spend and their training and skills in collecting detailed assessments, nurses frequently obtain the information to evaluate the patient to detect positive and negative outcomes of a given treatment.

Pharmacists are educated in helping physicians find the best medication options for patients and are responsible for verifying the safety of medications that patients will take. Data is important to pharmacists because the age, gender, height, weight, pregnancy status, and patient's condition(s) are all relevant to medication dosing. Pharmacists and physicians rely heavily on laboratory results and vital signs and assessments from observations of signs and symptoms. Table 21-3 provides some scope of practice considerations for pharmacists.

Another broad category critical to the care of patients consists of the assorted therapies: dietitians, social workers, respiratory, physical, occupational, speech pathology, behavioral, and recreational professionals. Professionals in these groups normally focus on a specific aspect of the patient's care and, while normally autonomous, are typically involved and directed by physicians. Examples include increasing a patient's mobility and optimizing their diet and respiratory function. Table 21-3 provides some scope of practice considerations for therapists.

Technicians within laboratory, radiology, neurological testing, cardiovascular diagnostics, and other areas need information to prepare patients for a test or diagnostic exam and to ensure safe transport to perform the tests. A key responsibility of these clinicians and departments is prompt reporting of the results and timely notification to nurses and physicians when the findings are critical because these findings can dramatically alter the course of care and treatment for the patient.

Simulation

HIT technology simulation can provide a safe testing environment that allows practitioners to test new clinical processes using simulation of the technology before implementing with patients. Many simulation applications involve artificial "patients" and "providers" that can test tasks and functions to simulate care and treatment, like flight simulators used by pilots.[9] The simulation environment provides a real-life opportunity to evaluate clinical and management information systems such as EHRs, secure messaging, and exchanges with health information exchange networks in a realistic environment without the possible harm associated with real patient care. Research using simulation approaches helps inform the design and development of electronic systems.

Lean Strategy

The Lean/Six Sigma strategy has been used extensively in manufacturing and production lines to identify the most efficient production practice using less costly resources and fewer tasks and still retain the optimal value for customers. The goal when using the Lean approach is to eliminate waste or redundancies in practices while providing the best possible patient outcomes. In general, that usually means the safest care at the lowest cost with the shortest stay and no complications (i.e., eliminating unnecessary tests and complications, hospital-acquired infections, pressure sores, injuries from falls, etc.). When Lean strategies are fully leveraged, the result is optimal outcome for the patient with less work volume and minimal to no redundancy in care.

 HIT PRO EXAM TIP   When workflow is optimized, human interactions with the technology increase efficiency, decrease waste, and rely on scientific methods to decide which data are relevant rather than accepting prior methods, often based on paper or unique to an individual clinician.

The Lean approach poses critical questions to subject matter experts in a process undergoing improvement. These questions are helpful in identifying what matters most and avoiding the distraction of variation and waste. These who, what, where, how, and why questions highlight gaps, variations, unnecessary tasks, and redundancy in current practice and allow the clinical team to decide the safest and quickest ways to get to equivalent or better patient outcomes.

Business Process Management

Business process management (BPM) uses engineering activities to represent processes for the healthcare enterprise. BPM in healthcare settings often involves clinical informaticians and service-line leaders working with IT professionals and business process managers or quality managers to analyze and improve current processes. Process improvements are part of everyday activities in healthcare. IT professionals should identify and work closely with business analysts and quality staff members who are involved with improving practices for accreditation and certification.

HIT PRO EXAM TIP   Healthcare organizations and clinics should designate someone who is accountable for managing a central database of process maps/workflows. Management of workflows facilitates decision making regarding when and where workflows apply, allows for the reuse of standardization workflows across service lines, and allows for the continuous optimizing of healthcare processes (workflows). Chapter 7 covers workflow and process management in more detail.

Workflow Mapping Tools

Figure 21-3 is an example of the basic tools associated with process mapping. A structured approach can enable efficient, effective problem solving and can enhance decision making. Specific diagrams and shapes correspond to different types of activities performed to visually represent workflow.

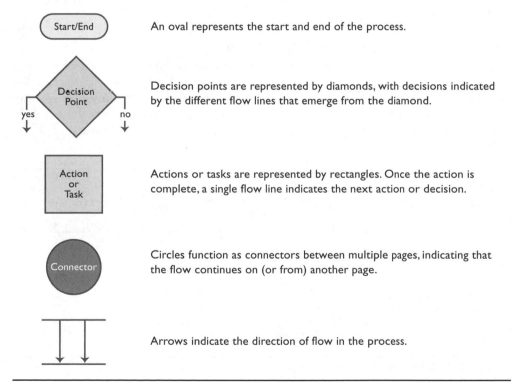

An oval represents the start and end of the process.

Decision points are represented by diamonds, with decisions indicated by the different flow lines that emerge from the diamond.

Actions or tasks are represented by rectangles. Once the action is complete, a single flow line indicates the next action or decision.

Circles function as connectors between multiple pages, indicating that the flow continues on (or from) another page.

Arrows indicate the direction of flow in the process.

Figure 21-3   Graphic representation of workflow mapping

- An oval shows where the workflow begins and where the workflow ends.
- Rectangles represent a process activity, task, or analysis necessary.
- Diamonds signify a decision-making process, usually resulting in two possible workflow directions. Most diamonds reflect a yes or no decision that has to be made; if the decision is yes, the workflow continues on the intended route, but if the answer is no, the workflow may have to go through another route to solve the problem.
- Circles represent connectors from one activity to another activity.

Workflow Diagram Example

Workflow diagrams are a graphic depiction of a course of action showing the steps in the process to accomplish a goal. Many work processes can be complex, so it is important to visually represent in detail how tasks are being completed to improve understanding and efficiency. Depending on the purpose of the map, it can be high level (abstract) or detailed. Figure 21-4 is an example of a high-level clinic visit workflow diagram.

Role-Based Swim-Lane Workflow

Figure 21-5 is an example of a role-based swim-lane workflow. Role-based swim lanes describe who is responsible for each stage, what documentation is needed, and the relationship to resources at each stage. Knowing employee roles and resource requirements allows management to easily determine weaknesses and alleviate bottlenecks. Bottlenecks represent any aspect of the workflow that impede overall cycle time of the process.

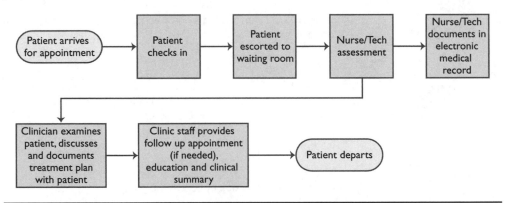

Figure 21-4 Clinic visit workflow

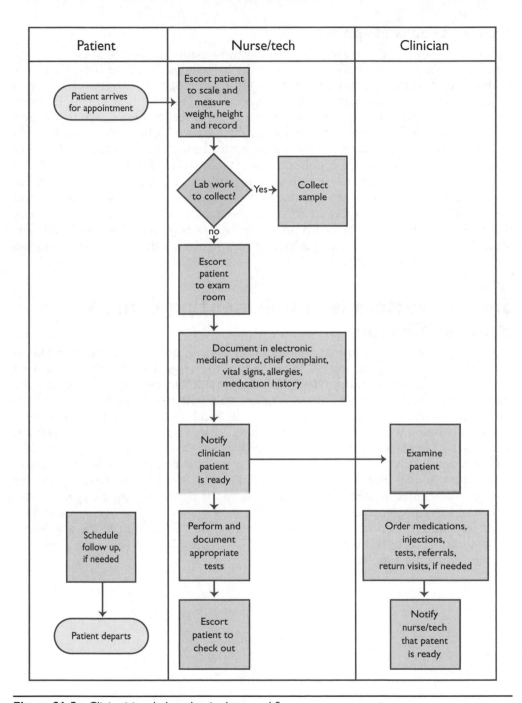

Figure 21-5 Clinic visit role-based swim-lane workflow

Value Stream Mapping

Figure 21-6 shows a value stream map. Value stream mapping is a type of process mapping or flowcharting of the value stream, which includes all of the steps (both the value-added and the non-value-added steps) in producing and delivering a service. A value stream map shows workflow from a systems perspective and can help in determining how to measure and improve the system or process of interest. Without a view of the entire stream, it is possible that individual aspects of the system will be optimized according to the needs of those parts, but the resulting total system will be suboptimal. Value stream mapping in healthcare is typically done from the perspective of the patient, where the goal is to optimize the journey through the system. Information, materials, and patient flows are captured in the value stream map. The key question to ask when determining whether an activity is value added is if the customer would be willing to pay for it. If the answer is no, the activity is nonvalue added. In healthcare, an example of a non-value-added activity is waiting time. Value stream mapping is a recognized Six Sigma methodology.[9]

Success Factors for Implementing Clinical Process Change

Designing and applying information technology using standardized practices can be an extensive, time-consuming process. When possible, leverage the vendor's standardized tools and process descriptions. When these are not suitable, incomplete, or need to be extended, you must assemble a process change team with the right skill sets, as well as subject-matter experts. A moderate-sized hospital may have 200 to 300 third-level process flows. A typical ambulatory clinic may have 50 to 75 process flows. It is useful to name each of the processes and assign a priority to map these processes explicitly. One question to ask is, Is this process well defined? If not, it may require a higher priority to determine a possible future state. Complex and ambiguous processes typically create a great deal of confusion, concern, and even risk to the patient during the implementation. The ideal implementation has *no* ambiguous processes at go-live. A knowledge manager assigned to track and manage these processes can minimize the risk. These individuals may also be experts in facilitating problem-solving events or in managing gaps in the vendor-supplied content.

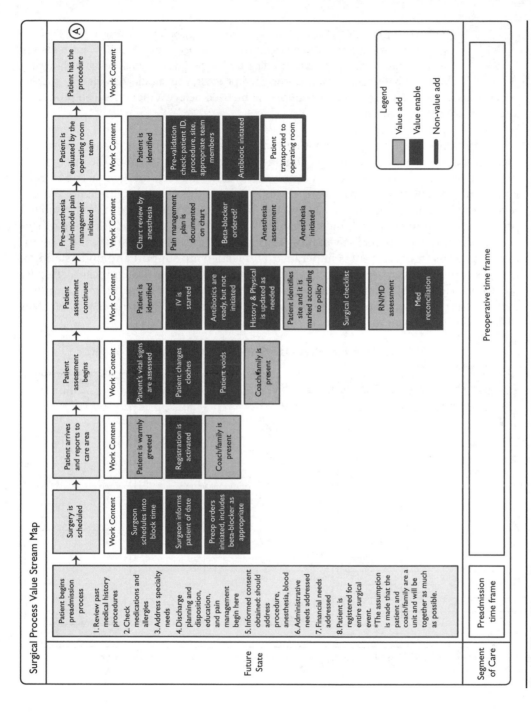

Figure 21-6 Value stream mapping

TIP   Use the SIPOC Figure 21-7 instrument (a Six Sigma tool) to simplify problem solving or to plan a large process change event. A SIPOC form identifies all aspects of a process, including the beginning, the end, and all high-level steps in between. Outside of the core process, you should also identify suppliers and customers. This high-level description can be used before a more detailed process improvement activity is used.

The implementation of the actual new steps represented in a workflow diagram is the hardest aspect of process change. Organizations often do not realize the importance of understanding processes and mistakenly rely instead on technology to resolve problems. With paper-based records, many organizations had thousands of individual order sets, many unique to specific physicians and frequently outdated. With computerized provider order entry (CPOE), most organizations appreciate the need for standardization in workflow and reducing variation among physicians. Organizationwide recognition of process improvement is imperative, and leadership support and understanding is key; simply posting a workflow diagram on a nursing unit won't significantly impact day-to-day activities. Most workflow diagrams should include a workflow improvement theory such as Lean, Six Sigma, or Total Quality Management as well as clear instructions on how to follow them.

SIPOC Diagram for Physician Specialist Procedure Consult

Revised: (date) Author: (name)

Suppliers	Inputs	Process Row	Outputs	Customers
Specialist physician		Process Trigger: Clinician needs a specialist consult for a procedure.		Ordering physician
Ward clerk		⬇		Patient
Scheduling clerk		Step 2		Primary Care Physician
Transcriptionists		⬇		Nurse
Patient		Step 3		
Nursing provider		⬇		
		Step 4		
		⬇		
		Step 5		
		⬇		
		Step 6		
		⬇		
		Done: Consulting physician communicates to ordering clinician the results of the procedure		

Figure 21-7   SIPOC chart for planning workflow mapping or problem-solving event

Exercise 21-1: Create a Simple Process Model Using the SIPOC Tool

In this exercise, review Use Case 21-1, and develop a process model and overview.

1. Describe the steps in the process including trigger and completion.

2. Identify inputs into the process.

3. Identify desired outcomes.

4. Develop a plan to engage customers and suppliers in the future state process design.

5. Advanced: After completing a process map, enhance the map by utilizing role-based swim lanes or a value stream approach.

6. Advanced: What measurement could you use to determine that the new process was being used and not the workaround?

Use Case 21-1: Physician Consult for Specialty Procedure

Mrs. Hurst is a 35-year-old woman who presented to her primary-care physician with early-onset high blood pressure. In the office she was found to have significant high blood pressure without a strong family history or other explanation. On examination, she had evidence of an abdominal bruit (an abnormal sound heard with a stethoscope over the abdomen and a sign of a narrowed renal artery). The primary-care physician treated the patient with blood pressure medications and ordered an abdominal ultrasound that identified a condition called *renal artery stenosis*. Since her blood pressure did not respond to multiple medications, the primary-care physician consults a specialist who could enlarge the renal artery using balloon angioplasty.

The doctor recently started using an EHR and is unsure how to order such a procedure. Is this an "order" like one might write for an X-ray, or is it a consult for the specialist to see the patient and then determine the appropriate course of action? Previously, the physician would communicate the intent to the nurse or office manager who would manage the details of such a workflow. Unfortunately, the physician and office manager do not know how to order the same test using the new EHR. After calling the supervisor superuser (an individual with addition training) and the EHR implementation team, everyone involved realizes that they had not developed a process to manage this type of problem. The implementation team needs to develop this process and communicate it to all involved quickly. While the team works on defining and implementing an electronic version of the paper process, the office returns to the previous method of handwriting the order and faxing it to the specialist office. In addition, the office manager calls the hospital surgical scheduling clerk who enters the request into the surgical scheduling system.

Additional Techniques

When workflow processes are viewed in isolation, they often appear quite logical and efficient enough to accomplish the end goal. When viewed more broadly across multiple disciplines, complexities arise. Frequently missed are conflicts in the priorities of different roles in an organization (e.g., tasks that nursing is accountable for versus the pharmacy).

The suggested steps for creating a process map or workflow are as follows:

1. Assemble a stakeholder planning team. The team should consist of individuals from all clinical areas and all levels with the goal of ensuring the true process is captured.

2. Determine the level of detail desired, the methodology you will employ, and the participants needed (e.g., value stream mapping, role based, SIPOC, or simple diagramming). The level of detail will depend on the problem the team is addressing and the number of handoffs between disciplines.

3. Schedule the mapping event and adequate venue, and obtain the appropriate supplies.

4. Begin the event by giving the team sufficient background on the approach you will be using. Provide an initial training in the weeks before or at the start of the event.

5. Complete the mapping event. Identify the activities in your current and future state. List them and arrange them in order.

6. Create a formal chart with standard symbols for process mapping using Microsoft Visio or Excel.

7. Create an accurate picture, and check for accuracy.

8. Identify problem areas and gaps between the current and future state.

9. Prioritize projects that will address the gaps.

Identification and Prioritization of Targets for Workflow Improvement

Information technology should be designed to support effective teamwork, foster open communication, and enable shared decision making to achieve optimal, quality patient care. Once the process is mapped, gaps between the current process and best practices will become apparent. Members of the team with the most detailed understanding of the best practices can recognize gaps and highlight them for the team. A simple approach to ranking gaps using two dimensions includes "ease of implementation" and "value to the organization." Value should be defined early in the life cycle of the program. Three common objectives for many organizations are safety, quality, and overall patient experience, with financial and provider experience as secondary benefits.

Change Management

Change management describes a structured approach to transition individuals, teams, and organizations from a current state to a desired future state. Considered an organization imperative, change management helps employees cope with and adapt to the numerous changes every industry faces. One reason change initiatives fail is because they rely on "data gathering, analysis, report writing, and presentations" instead of human, political, and symbolic elements.

Kotter defines change management as the utilization of basic structures and tools to control any organizational change effort. Change management refers to a set of basic tools or structures intended to keep the change effort under control. Ultimately, the goal is to minimize the impact on workers and avoid distractions.

Change Management Principles

Four principles for change management are as follows:

- Elicit support from people within the system (system = environment processes, culture, relationships, and behaviors, both personal and organizational).
- Understand the current state of the organization.
- Understand where you want to be, when, why, and what the measures will be.
- Communicate, involve, enable, and facilitate involvement from people, as early, openly, and completely as possible.

Kotter's Eight Steps to Successful Change

John Kotter, a leading thinker and author on organizational change management, describes an eight-stage model for understanding and managing change.[4]

Kotter's eight-stage approach to realizing significant change includes the following:

1. **Establish a sense of urgency** Inspire people to move, and make objectives real and relevant.

2. **Build the guiding coalition** Put the right people in place with the right emotional commitment and the right mix of skills.

3. **Develop a vision and strategy** Create a team to establish a simple vision and strategy and focus on emotional and creative aspects necessary to direct the change effort.

4. **Communicate the change vision for buy-in** Involve as many people as possible, communicate the essentials simply, and respond to people's needs. Declutter communications; make technology work for you rather than against you.

5. **Empower action** Remove obstacles, and enable constructive feedback and support from leaders. Reward and recognize progress and achievements, and encourage risk taking.

6. **Generate short-term wins**   Set aims that are easy to achieve. Recognize and reward people who made the wins possible. Finish current stages before starting new ones.

7. **Don't let up**   Foster and encourage determination and persistence, and encourage new projects, themes, and change agents.

8. **Make change stick**   Reinforce the value of successful change via recruitment and promotion, and develop new change leaders. Weave change into the culture.

Chapter Review

Ignoring or inadequately understanding workflows can lead to a decline in use of the EHR over time and the development of workaround steps. Workarounds can include both those within and outside an automated process. Analyzing workflows can help discover key factors to success: underuse and misuse of the EHR, workarounds clinicians find to collect or use patient information, and the need for aggregated information or reports to be available for decision making and sharing beyond the organization (often via health information exchange [HIE]). Working together, IT professionals as members of an interdisciplinary team must review existing clinical workflows when technology upgrades or the clinical evidence advances to make necessary adjustments. Creating a culture focused on process and change management and understanding workflow will help guide organizations through new technology implementations and inevitable upgrades.[9]

Questions

To test your comprehension of the chapter, answer the following questions and then check your answers against the list of correct answers at the end of the chapter.

1. Which of the following describes using health information systems in a manner not originally designed that results in unplanned and unexpected outcomes.

   A. Workflows

   B. Workarounds

   C. Tracking issues

   D. Flowcharts

2. Which of the following are life-cycle phases of large-scale health information technology changes?

   A. Workflows with workarounds and testing the technology with users

   B. Planning, implementation, quality monitoring, and improvement

    C. Planning, training, testing, and implementation

    D. Planning, implementation, stabilization, optimization, and transformation

3. Healthcare services are organized by many service lines of care such as surgical or obstetrical (i.e., maternal-child) services. Within each service, processes are organized such that they can be replicated across many services. Which of the following does not describe the healthcare general processes within venues of services healthcare?

    A. Registration, admission, daily care coordination, shift change, discharge

    B. Surgical preoperative visit, surgery, postoperative, same-day discharge

    C. Registration, dining, coding, billing, reporting

    D. Check-in, laboratory testing, radiology test, chemotherapy infusion visit, depart

    E. Emergency triage, registration, assessment, examination, education, discharge

4. The role-based workflow describes the steps in the care and information flow or evidence-based knowledge used by which of the following?

    A. Patient

    B. Physician

    C. Pharmacists

    D. Nurse and nursing assistants

    E. All of the above

5. Person-to-person cross-functional workflow describes the steps for which of the following?

    A. Electronic information collection/documentation

    B. Direct person-to-person conversation

    C. Viewing displayed reports in HIT

    D. Providing the patients a paper clinical summary

    E. All of the above

6. The role-based (person-to-person) workflow describes processes by which of the following?

    A. Using swim lanes to show the roles

    B. Describing steps in the process (rectangles) with action verbs

    C. Organizing into venues for care (e.g., admission, clinic visit, surgery)

    D. Displaying physician or nurse decisions (diamonds)

    E. All of the above

7. Which is a type of workflow with a limited ability to support a given decision that requires less human interaction and lacks the perspective of care delivery?

   A. Functional or application

   B. Role based

   C. Enterprise to enterprise

   D. Venue to venue

   E. Task to task

8. Which workflow best describes the clinical scenario of a nurse sending a secure message for follow-up to a home-care provider on research protocols involving medication administration at specific times for three days in the patient's home setting using the health information exchange network?

   A. Functional or application workflow

   B. Role-based workflow

   C. Enterprise to enterprise workflow

   D. Venue-to-venue workflow

   E. Task-to-task workflow

9. Which type of workflow describes the clinical teams as they collect and use patient information and, as a result, the decisions that coordinate care with other providers and departments?

   A. Functional or application workflow

   B. Person-to-person workflow

   C. Enterprise-to-enterprise workflow

   D. Venue-to-venue workflow

   E. Task-to-task workflow

10. Analyzing workflows can help discover which of the following?

    A. Underuse of the EHR

    B. Clinician workarounds

    C. Need to aggregate information or reports for decision making

    D. Need to extract health information for exchange

    E. All of the above

11. Identify a method that is not particularly useful in workflow analysis and redesign.

    A. Modeling workflow based on scope of professional practice standards

    B. Simulation

    C. Observing existing paper documents and replicating in electronic format

    D. Lean strategy, Six Sigma, and continuous improvement

    E. Business process management and modeling tools

12. Which is a method to articulate the tasks, time, manual work, delays, and multiple variations that exist within care processes for a discipline or with reporting process associated with many departments?

    A. Modeling workflow based on scope of professional practice standards

    B. Simulation

    C. Observation of daily activities

    D. Lean strategy, Six Sigma, and continuous improvement

    E. Business process management and modeling tools

Answers

1. **B.** A workaround is using the electronic health records, other information system, or paper-based alternatives in an unintentional way. A common example is the use of nursing communication orders in place of actual departmental orders to communicate the need for a specific test. A delay occurs while the nurse contacts the physician to determine and place the correct order with the continued risk of miscommunication. The department misreads the test and completes the test incorrectly resulting in invalid results, and the patient needs a repeat test for diagnostic accuracy.

2. **D.** In summary, with large HIT change, the stakeholders are involved from project conception with planning; activating the software, a period of time where users are unable to complete their scope of work because of gaps in workflows leading to workarounds; feeling a sense of normalcy within the clinic or hospital and optimizing practices; and embracing the change and fully using the data to determine performance to advance practice with transformation.

3. **C.** Processes within most venues have a well-defined start and endpoint and include a number of service lines during the episode of care. This option does not include any processes for care delivery, whereas the others depict general processes to consider where patient data and information are being collected from the patient and used to plan and deliver care.

4. **E.** The person-to-person role-based workflows include the patient, healthcare professionals, department staff, and support staff working collectively to identify and share the data used to make decisions in a collaborative way.

5. **E.** Role-based workflows include decisions and practice steps that may or may not make use of the technology services to ensure the critical steps of direct communication are identified in daily workflow. At some point in the future the optimization of steps not supported by technology could be supported by an application or additional information that is collected and stored.

6. **E.** All four answers describe how workflow is designed to display the steps and decisions within a process for those with a role in taking care of patients.

7. **A.** Functional workflows make use of information technology applications to assist in performing notifications automatically or to track events within the emergency center.

8. **E.** Task-to-task workflows provide additional detailed steps for less frequent activities that might occur during care delivery (e.g., a nurse identifies a patient who could receive an immunization while in the hospital). While not required per se during the hospitalization, it represents an intervention that may require coordination between the physician, nurse, and pharmacist.

9. **B.** Person-to-person or role-based workflows describe in detail the many care activities and many decisions that healthcare professionals and support staff provide. A critical step is including the patient and, frequently, family members in those decisions.

10. **E.** A workflow analysis is useful when technology is upgraded or when clinical evidence changes. In these situations it's necessary to evaluate the where, how, and when information technology supports clinical decision making and affects care coordination.

11. **C.** Existing paper-based documents are not particularly useful in designing optimal use of data, information, and knowledge for HIT systems. Providers expect significant improvements to the standardization and integration of professional processes with the EHR functions to better represent and improve patient care. This reduces the variations that lead to omissions or commissions of errors.

12. **C.** Observation of workflow will help identify some gaps, but this method alone will not help clinicians and IT professionals in discerning all potential interactions and gaps in practice workflows.

References

1. Blumenthal, D. (2009). Launching HITECH. *New England Journal of Medicine, 362*, 382–385.

2. American Recovery and Reinvestment Act of 2009 (ARRA). (2009). Accessed on June 17, 2010, from http://frwebgate.access.gpo.gov/cgi-bin/getdoc.cgi?dbname=111_cong_bills&docid=f:h1enr.pdf.

3. Halbesleben, J. R., Wakefield, D. S., & Wakefield, B. J. (2008). Work-arounds in health care settings: Literature review and research agenda. *Health Care Management Review, 33*, 2–12.

4. Kotter, J. P., & Cohen, D. S. (2002). *The heart of change: Real life stories of how people change their organizations.* Harvard Business School Press.

5. Brokel, J. M., & Harrison, M. I. (2009). Redesigning care processes using an electronic health record: A system's experience. *Joint Commission Journal of Patient Safety and Quality, 35,* 82–92.

6. Randell, R., Mitchell, N., Thompson, C., McCaughan, D., & Dowding, D. (2009). Supporting nurse decision making in primary care: Exploring use of and attitude to decision tools. *Health Informatics Journal, 15,* 5–16.

7. Brokel, J. M., Ochylski, S., & Kramer, J. M. (2011). Re-engineering workflows: Changing the life cycle of an electronic health record system. *Journal of Healthcare Engineering, 2,* 303–320.

8. Wheeler, D. J. (2004). *The Six Sigma practitioner's guide to data analysis.* SPC Press.

9. Improving patient safety through simulation research. (2012). Accessed on June 19, 2012, from www.ahrq.gov/qual/simulproj.htm.

CHAPTER 22

Reporting Requirements and Regulatory and External Factors Affecting Healthcare IT

Leland A. Babitch

In this chapter, you will learn how to
- Identify and understand external agencies and regulatory bodies that have an effect on healthcare information technology
- Determine how healthcare reform (including both legislative and payment reform) is influencing the development and use of HIT systems
- Focus efforts on key areas of risk and benefit within EMR systems as they relate to regulations and reimbursement

Healthcare reform, in the guise of payment reform and incentives, is leading to an accelerated adoption rate of electronic health records in both hospitals and physician offices.[1,2,3] Whereas physicians were previously slow to purchase systems and hospitals were reticent to invest in computerized records, the industry is seeing a significant increase in the number of new adopters each year. With those increases, the job market for trained IT professionals who understand the complexities of the healthcare system is booming.[4]

Major Governmental Agencies and Other Regulatory Bodies

Like many other industries, healthcare is highly regulated by federal, state, and other external agencies, with a primary focus on patient and caregiver safety, privacy, and compliance with health insurance rules. Each of these bodies of regulatory rules has significant impact on the way in which electronic health records are built and used. Much of the content and functionality that exists in each EHR is actually focused on compliance with these rules and reporting requirements, rather than directly related to patient care. However, the rules for safe and effective healthcare likely lead to EMRs that are more standardized in functionality, with a lower learning curve for end users; in addition, the rules eventually will lead to better interoperability between systems.

Department of Health and Human Services

Within the federal government, there is a hierarchy of agencies that have a major impact on the healthcare industry. First among them is the Department of Health and Human Services (HHS); see Figure 22-1. HHS consists of several departments that have

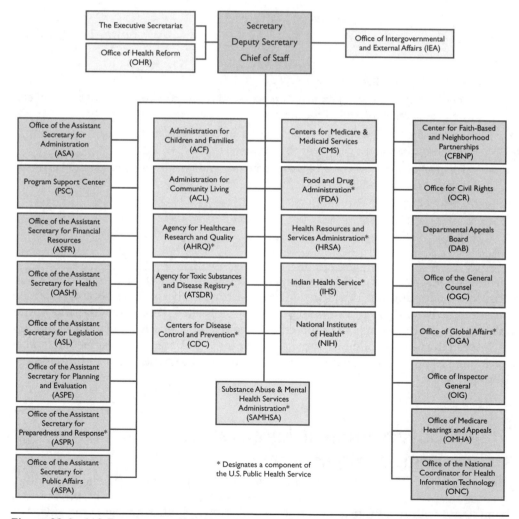

Figure 22-1 U.S. Department of Health and Human Services organization chart. Reprinted from the U.S. Department of Health and Human Services.

significant bearing on the development, implementation, and use of EHRs. They include the Agency for Healthcare Research and Quality (AHRQ), the Centers for Disease Control (CDC), the Indian Health Service, and the National Institutes of Health.

Centers for Medicare and Medicaid Services

The Centers for Medicare and Medicaid Services (CMS) are of particular significance for healthcare systems. They are responsible for overseeing both the Medicare and Medicaid programs (see Table 22-1). Combined, those two governmental payers are the largest sources of reimbursement for healthcare services in the United States and make up more than 6 percent of the gross domestic product (GDP) (see Figures 22-2 and 23-2). Overall, healthcare spending accounts for 17 percent of the GDP and is the largest industry in the United States.

Food and Drug Administration

The Food and Drug Administration (FDA) is another department within HHS. It is responsible for approving and regulating both medications and medical devices within the United States. While most electronic health records (EHRs) do not have to qualify their entire product with the FDA, certain components, especially those that involve direct patient monitoring and data transfer, are regulated by the agency. Most EHRs have prescribing components that generally follow the rules and recommendations of the FDA for safe prescribing of medications.

Medicare	Medicaid
Largest single payer in the United States, accounting for more than 6 percent of GDP spending	Expanded to include pregnant women, blind and permanently disabled individuals, and indigent and elderly patients.
Enacted in 1965	Enacted in 1965
Originally covered hospital care of the elderly population (Part A)	Originally covered impoverished children
Expanded to include physician office (Part B) care, managed care, nursing home coverage, end-stage renal disease care, and medications (Part D)	Fastest-growing portion of most state budgets
Federal oversight of the payments to ensure compliance	Overseen by each state, with significantly different rules in each locale

Table 22-1 Comparison of the Medicare and Medicaid Programs

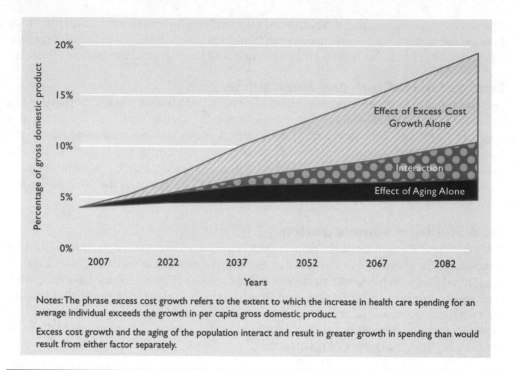

Figure 22-2 Sources of growth in projected federal spending on Medicare and Medicaid. Reprinted from the Congressional Budget Office.

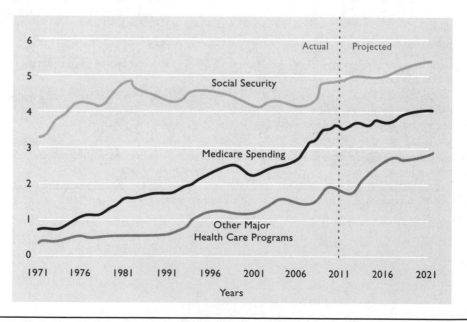

Figure 22-3 Spending for Social Security, Medicare, and other major healthcare programs (percent of GDP). Reprinted from the Congressional Budget Office.

Office of the National Coordinator for Healthcare Information Technology

A relatively new area within HHS is the Office of the National Coordinator for Healthcare Information Technology (ONC). According to its site,[5] the ONC is responsible for the following:

- Promoting development of a nationwide healthcare IT infrastructure that allows for electronic use and exchange of information

- Providing leadership in the development, recognition, and implementation of standards and the certification of healthcare IT products

- Coordinating healthcare IT policy

- Strategic planning for healthcare IT adoption and health information exchange

- Establishing governance for the Nationwide Health Information Network

In practice, the ONC is focused on certifying EHRs for meaningful use (described in the upcoming section "Meaningful Use"), promoting EMR adoption through the establishment of the regional extension centers, and creating innovation in HIT through programs like Beacon Grants. More information about ONC is available in other chapters.

Each state may also regulate medical practice, with specific rules on the scope of practice for healthcare professionals, state-specific rules for prescribing controlled substances, and medical record privacy. State laws may be more restrictive than a federal statute but can never be less so. Compliance with both federal and state regulations is a key component to the design of EHR systems and workflows.

Other Regulators

Aside from the government, healthcare organizations subscribe to many other regulatory bodies, either because of mandates linking participation in Medicare and Medicaid to compliance with those groups, because of directives from medical insurance companies, or because they seek specific accreditation and recognition for specialty areas. EHRs are a key component of documenting care that is then measured as part of these surveys, as well as a stand-alone requirement for many modern accrediting bodies.

The largest, single accrediting group for hospitals and other large health groups is the Joint Commission (JC), also known as the Joint Commission on the Accreditation of Healthcare Organizations (JCAHO, pronounced "jay-co"). With more than 19,000 member hospitals and groups, it routinely surveys sites to make sure they are in compliance with everything from fire safety to electronic signatures on notes. Preparation for and surveys by the Joint Commission can be one of the more stressful periods in any hospital system. With good planning, design, and adoption strategies, a health system may need little change to comply with their rules and requirements.

In the past, CMS required that hospitals and health systems attain and maintain Joint Commission certification. The Joint Commission remains the largest accreditor of hospitals and health systems. However, in recent years CMS has allowed other standard bodies to guarantee the quality of healthcare systems, and hospitals have started to seek certification from other agencies including the Health Facilities Accreditation Program (HFAP), International Organization for Standardization (ISO), and Det Norsk Veritas (DNV). These alternatives may be less expensive than membership in the Joint Commission or may provide a path to certification that is more consistent with the goals of the organizations that have chosen them.

Many hospitals, health systems, and other medical providers go beyond the minimum need for JC certification and seek recognition for specialty-care areas or other recognition for high-quality care. Some common designations include Trauma Center Certification (American College of Surgeons), Leapfrog Certification (the Business Roundtable), Patient-Centered Medical Home (National Committee for Quality Assurance and others), and Magnet (American Nurses Credentialing Center). All of these programs focus on quality and safety in healthcare and either require or recommend use of an EHR and use data derived from electronic systems during their award determination processes.

CMS and other insurers also mandate specific care for patients with given conditions. Core measures[6] are probably the most common goals with which hospitals and clinicians attempt to comply. They include specific guidelines for managing patients with acute myocardial infarction (heart attacks), heart failure, stroke, pneumonia, and children's asthma care. Along with those guidelines are goals for smoking cessation, substance abuse counseling, immunization, surgical care improvement (SCIP), psychiatric services, outpatient departments, perinatal care, and prevention of venous thromboembolism (blood clots). Most acute-care EHRs support compliance and reporting for some or all of these measures, though frequently the modules to support those functions are separate purchases or locally developed.

Use Case 22-1: Being Audited by the Joint Commission

Your hospital is about to undergo a planned inspection by the Joint Commission. One of the mandates of the program is that "the operative report must be written or dictated immediately after an operation or other high-risk procedure." Because of delays in transcription, your institution expects a brief postoperative note that is either handwritten or entered electronically to be placed on the chart, pending the full dictation. The JC auditors find multiple examples of missing postoperative notes and ask for a 90-day correction plan.

Your auditing of charts shows that the lowest compliance with the brief summaries is among those who are dictating notes and forgetting to handwrite a brief note. You convene a group of surgical leaders who agree to mandate the electronic documentation of the operations immediately following the procedures, which allows you to create an audit log of missing notes on a daily basis. Within 90 days, your remediation plan is successful, and JC is satisfied with the improvement.

Healthcare Reform Effect on Healthcare IT

The general belief is that increased adoption of technology will lead to what Don Berwick at the Institute for Healthcare Improvement has called the *triple aim*.[7]

- Improving the patient experience of care (including quality and satisfaction)
- Improving the health of populations
- Reducing the per-capita cost of healthcare

Unfortunately, the federal government has limited ways in which it can affect the adoption of HIT. It can regulate and mandate the use of technologies, encourage use through payments and incentives, fund research and education of IT professionals, and change the way in which it reimburses healthcare costs to encourage new patterns of care that leverage technology. At the moment, the government is trying all of those options via legislation for healthcare reform.

Overview of Healthcare Payment Models

To understand how changes in Medicare and Medicaid payments might affect healthcare delivery and HIT, it is important to understand existing models of insurance payment to hospitals and physicians. The most traditional model for payment to hospitals and physicians is known as *fee-for-service*. When reimbursed for services, patients or insurers pay for each service as the care is delivered. Originally, this sort of payment was based on the amount charged by the provider. However, over time payers and providers began to devise discount systems, bundled-care offerings, and fixed-payment mechanisms for services. Today, it is rare that any payer reimburses providers based on charges, though patients are still sometimes left to pay the full amount charged when they have no insurance coverage, have high-deductible plans, or have plans that require them to make up the difference between charges and insurance payments.

Hospital Payments

Hospitals today are typically reimbursed via one of two mechanisms. The first way is termed *per diem* (daily) charges and is akin to a fee-for-service payment, though typically charges are made at a fixed rate. The second, more common mechanism is known as the *inpatient prospective payment system* (IPPS) and is based on categorizing each stay into a diagnosis-related group (DRG).[8] DRGs are designed to cover the typical cost of care for a disease process. They guarantee a single payment for the hospital for the treatment of a problem (e.g., stroke or pneumonia). Since the payment is fixed for a given condition (though there is variability for outlier cases with complications), the hospital is accountable for care appropriate for that condition. In general, the hospital gets the same payment for a three-day length of stay as it does for a five-day stay and gets the same for a $1,000 per-day antibiotic as a $150 per-day antibiotic.

Physician Payments

Physicians, for the most part, continue to be paid on a fee-for-service basis. As independent contractors in most hospitals, they charge for each hospital day, each procedure, and each office visit they have with a patient. The dichotomy between physicians paid on a fee-for-service basis and hospitals with a comprehensive payment sometimes leaves them at odds. The physician has little or no incentive to discharge the patient quickly and no real consequences for using more expensive tests and treatments, while the hospital has every incentive to reduce the utilization of high-cost items and to look for an expedient discharge.

Payment Reform

Medicare and other payers have several ongoing experiments with providers around the country focused on changing the way healthcare is delivered by modifying the way in which they pay for services. In concept, these programs are designed to reduce high-cost healthcare utilization (hospital admissions, emergency room visits, and expensive testing) by improving access to preventative, primary-care services and better coordinating the care of patients with chronic diseases. In theory, if you can improve the amount of preventive care delivered, the result will be healthier patients who need less acute care. Additionally, if you do a better job of providing the right kind of care for your patients with key diseases (e.g., heart failure and diabetes), you can avoid more costly encounters for complications of their illnesses.

Accountable-Care Organization

The concept of the accountable-care organization (ACO)[9,10] is an attempt to align incentives for physicians, hospitals, and others in the community. The emphasis on measuring and managing a defined group of patients over a given period of time, often referred to as *covered lives*, is based on a direct relationship between Medicaid and the providers.

One model in the ACO trials includes the concept of "episodes of care" where both the hospital and the physician receive a shared, single, DRG-like payment for a hospitalization and the postdischarge period afterward. The goal is that these new bundled payment models and shared responsibility for healthcare expense will align incentives for hospitals and physicians and ultimately improve care and lower costs. Another model, termed *shared savings*, looks at the average cost of care for a population over a period of time and rewards (or penalizes) an ACO for savings or excess costs in subsequent periods.

Primary-Care Medical Home

The primary-care medical home (PCMH), also known as the medical home model, is another attempt to lower costs via improved preventative care and better oversight of patients with chronic disease.[11] Several groups including medical societies and payers can recognize physician offices as a PCMH. Recognition can bring enhanced payment for patient care to the physician practice. Healthcare information technology, according to the AHRQ website,[12] can facilitate the PCMH "by collecting, storing, and managing personal health information, as well as aggregate data that can be used to improve processes and outcomes. Healthcare IT can also support communication, clinical decision-making, and patient self-management."

Regardless of the reform mechanism, all are dependent for success on improved methods of communication between providers, real-time and longitudinal population health reporting, and tools for patient engagement. Electronic health record developers and many others in HIT are rushing to fill the need for better information systems around the concept of the ACO, PCMH, and community record. In this new model, care is no longer limited to the time during which the patient is in the office or hospital but rather becomes dependent on improved transitions of care from one venue to another and maintenance of the provider-patient relationship even when the patient is at home.

Meaningful Use

One of the provisions in the American Recovery and Reinvestment Act of 2009 is the Health Information Technology for Economic and Clinical Health (HITECH) Act.[13] HITECH has a number of provisions and specifically defines the meaningful use (MU) program.[14] MU is likely to be the biggest driver for HIT adoption over the next decade with incentives and penalties that extend as far as 2021. This broad-reaching legislation reserves $32 billion in payments to physicians and hospitals for specific use of EHRs and other systems and allows CMS and the ONC to define other programs that will further promote the adoption of electronic systems. It also assumes some $13 billion in savings so that the total price of the program will be about $19 billion.

The incentives are substantial, ranging from $44,000 to $63,750 for qualifying physicians. Eligible hospitals can receive hundreds of thousands to millions of dollars for adequate adoption of their systems. Payments are administered by CMS, and the ONC oversees the process through which EHRs become certified for meaningful use. There are several certifying groups designated by the government, and only systems that have been given their stamp of approval may be used in qualifying for incentives. Most EHR vendors have attained or are working on certification, though only as the qualifications for each stage are defined. Institutions that have chosen to use multiple vendors (best-in-breed) or to create their own EHR (homegrown) must certify their systems independently.

According to the statute, MU will be defined in at least three stages. The final rule for stage 1 has already been published,[15] and by the time this book is published, stage 2 should be clearly defined. Each stage is meant to be a progressive increase in the depth and breadth of use of HIT in hospitals and physician offices, with an increasing replacement of paper processes, improved clinical decision support, and the eventual adoption of communitywide collaborative care tools that include both caregivers and patients. The box "Meaningful Use Requirements for Stage 1" summarizes the objectives and measures hospitals and eligible providers must meet. Compliance with these metrics varies from a simple attestation or demonstration of the capability (e.g., having at least one clinical decision support rule) to the need to show a percentage of compliance, including the numerator, denominator, and any exclusions (e.g., emergency department throughput).

Meaningful Use Requirements for Stage 1

Meaningful use includes both a core set and a menu set of objectives that are specific to eligible professionals or eligible hospitals and CAHs.

- For eligible professionals, there are a total of 25 meaningful use objectives. To qualify for an incentive payment, 20 of these 25 objectives must be met.
  - There are 15 required core objectives.
  - The remaining 5 objectives may be chosen from the list of 10 menu set objectives.
- For eligible hospitals and critical access hospitals (CAHs), there are a total of 24 meaningful use objectives. To qualify for an incentive payment, 19 of these 24 objectives must be met.
  - There are 14 required core objectives.
  - The remaining 5 objectives may be chosen from the list of 10 menu set objectives.

Stage 1 Clinical Quality Measures

To demonstrate meaningful use successfully, eligible professionals, eligible hospitals, and CAHs are required also to report clinical quality measures specific to eligible professionals or eligible hospitals and CAHs.

- Eligible professionals must report on 6 total clinical quality measures: 3 required core measures (substituting alternate core measures where necessary) and 3 additional measures (selected from a set of 38 clinical quality measures).
- Eligible hospitals and CAHs must report on all 15 of their clinical quality measures.

Source: https://www.cms.gov/Regulations-and-Guidance/Legislation/EHRIncentive Programs/Meaningful_Use.html (Accessed June 29, 2012)

Stage 2, as proposed, increases the level of compliance necessary for metrics, makes the menu options in Stage 1 mandatory, and adds components focused on patient engagement and a community record. It emphasizes personal health records and health information exchange. Stage 3 will continue the trend of higher goals for metrics, while increasing the expectations for clinical decision support, electronic documentation, and sharing of health information throughout the community.

Because of MU and other programs encouraging the use of EHRs, there has been a rapid increase in the adoption of systems by hospitals and physician practices. A measure of HIT adoption frequently referred to in the healthcare informatics industry is the Electronic Medical Record Adoption Model (EMRAM) from the Health Information Management Systems Society (HIMSS). EMRAM quantifies adoption by defining several levels (1 to 7) with progressively increased use of technology. The percentage of hospitals at HIMSS stage 4 or above (the minimum most would say defines significant EMR adoption) increased from 4.4 to 30 percent in the past five years. Physician offices, as a percentage of the whole, continue to lag in terms of complex adoption (only 1.65 percent have attained HIMSS stage 4 use or above).[16] However, the number of eligible providers (EPs) that have attained stage 1 qualified meaningful use has reached 58,530, with nearly $1 billion in payments. Medicaid incentive payments (which can go to EPs in the first year for adopting, implementing, or upgrading [AIU] an EHR) total 40,700 providers, with more than $850 million in payments as of May 2012. Overall, the MU program has paid out more than $5.7 billion in its first 17 months of operation.[17]

 TIP Year 1, stage 1 meaningful use for the Medicaid program requires only that a hospital or EP adopt, implement, or upgrade a certified EHR technology. Users do not have to demonstrate actual use during the period. Year 1, stage 1 meaningful use for Medicare requires a continuous, 90-day reporting period in which hospitals and eligible providers actually attain MU criteria for all measures.

Use Case 22-2: Choosing an EHR Vendor—MU EHR Certification Considerations

Apple Valley Pediatrics is interested in adopting an EHR for their three-physician practice. They understand that there are federal incentives for meaningful use of electronic medical records but need guidance on the complexity of selecting an EHR that suits their needs and qualifies for the incentives. They research several vendors and discover that three meet their needs for pediatric patient care but that only two of the three are certified for stage 1 of MU. As they are about to eliminate the third vendor from the selection process, their office manager points out that Apple Valley has a relatively good payer mix, with only about a 4 percent rate of Medicaid patients. As pediatricians, they do not have any Medicare payments. To qualify for Medicaid reimbursement under MU, a practice needs at least 30 percent of its volume in Medicaid charges (pediatricians can get a lower payment at a 20 percent threshold). Since Apple Valley does not qualify for any MU program, they continue to pursue EHR with all three vendors, eventually choosing one that is MU certified—but because of its cost and merits in usability, not because of certification.

Electronic Prescribing

Electronic prescription generation was one of the first EMR functionalities physicians used in outpatient clinics. Since the presidency of George Bush (2004),[18] there have been federal and local incentives to promote the technology in the office,[19,20] and now it is part of the requirements for meaningful use. As of July 2011, Medicare prescribers are required to have a minimum number of e-prescriptions or face reduced Medicare payments, unless they are actively pursuing stage 1 of meaningful use.

Though growing in popularity, e-prescribing still faces some significant challenges.[21] First, controlled substances (e.g., narcotic pain relievers) are prohibited from being prescribed electronically, forcing physicians who would otherwise e-prescribe to use paper. Second, standards for e-prescribing and medication formularies are not complete, and messaging between systems can sometimes be incomplete. Also, while e-prescribing alone can allow a practice to avoid Medicare penalties, the technology itself is not an adequate qualifier for MU incentives, and as a stand-alone medical practice outside of a full EHR, it can be difficult to create workflows that successfully combine electronic prescribing with paper processes.

Regulatory Compliance and EHR Components

While most components of an EHR are not regulated by the agencies noted earlier, the work product of those systems is subject to audit by many regulators. This section focuses on physician documentation as an example of an area that is under growing scrutiny for its benefits and potential risks to healthcare providers. Of note, as of the first quarter of 2012, the percentage of hospitals that have achieved significant adoption of electronic documentation (as opposed to handwritten or transcribed) is only about 7.4 percent, according to HIMSS.[15] The low adoption rate speaks to the difficulty in getting physicians to use electronic tools for progress notes and other documents. Comparatively, 30 percent have implemented computerized provider order entry systems.

There are many benefits to the use of electronic provider documentation, both clinical and regulatory. From the perspective of patient care, an electronic note is readily available to users at multiple locations versus a paper chart, which is limited to the unit or bedside. Notes that are created electronically are also immediately available to all users, unlike dictated notes, which have to be transcribed by a typist before they are visible to other caregivers. Compliant notes must be legible, dated, timed, and signed. Notes that are created electronically generally satisfy all of those criteria.

Physician notes are a critical component for both hospital and physician reimbursement. There are guidelines for documentation put forth by CMS that describe the components necessary for billing both hospitals and professional services. The inclusion or exclusion of key sections and terms can lead to markedly different payment levels by Medicare and other insurers. Poor-quality documentation may lead to lower billing levels and/or a risk of audit and the refund of payments. Academic institutions have unique rules they have to abide by regarding documentation by residents and students and are particularly focused on appropriate and timely documentation.

In 2006, Section 302 of the Tax Relief and Health Care Act[22] established the Recovery Audit Program, which empowers recovery audit contractors (RACs) to review billings from hospitals and physicians in order to look for irregularities and automatically take back payments based on their findings. Furthermore, they have the right to review individual patient records and apply retrospective penalties to Medicare recipients, based on the type and percentage of irregularities found in documented care.

In practice, this means that poor documentation of care can lead to substantial penalties from payments already made to healthcare providers. Such irregularities include copying and pasting information from one day to the next (or from one provider to another), missing critical information, underdocumenting the complexity of care, and poorly documenting shared services between physicians and trainees or midlevel providers. Figure 22-4 gives examples of focus areas.

Reporting

Generating reports from EHRs is a key use of the systems for clinical care, compliance, and business operations. Meaningful use has dramatically increased the importance of all aspects of such reporting. Specifically, all EHRs must qualify for certification based on their ability to generate reports on the actual use of the system for critical areas such as e-prescribing, CPOE, documenting patient demographics, and reporting vital signs. Both integrated systems from a single vendor and homegrown or best-of-breed systems must demonstrate the ability to collect and report on all of the meaningful use objectives.

Other Reporting

Prior to the advent of meaningful use, hospitals developed robust reporting mechanisms for other areas focused on quality improvement with core measure criteria high on the list. While meaningful use mandates the use of electronic health records in order to meet its goals, all hospitals need to report core measure compliance, regardless of their level of electronic system adoption. Even when collected from disparate systems or paper records, the data must be aggregated and submitted via an electronic format through a certified ORYX clearinghouse,[23] which can then send the data to interested parties, including CMS and the Joint Commission.

 TIP The ORYX initiative, operational since 1999, transmits measurement data to the Joint Commission on behalf of accredited hospitals and long-term care organizations, as part of CMS certification. Certified clearinghouses can collate and transmit the data to JC from organizations.

A growing area of interest and development within EHRs and related systems is reporting on physician performance indicators. A key driver is the JC requirement for focused professional practice evaluations (FPPE) and ongoing professional practice evaluations (OPPE).[24,25] These assessments are a necessary part of the credentialing

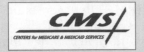

Medicare Fee for Service
National Recovery Audit Program

(July 1, 2011 – September 30, 2011)
Quarterly Newsletter

*Figures rounded to nearest tenth; Nationwide figures rounded based on actual collections. Figures provided in millions. All correction data current through September 30, 2011.

	OVERPAYMENTS COLLECTED	UNDERPAYMENTS RETURNED	TOTAL QUARTER CORRECTIONS	FY TO DATE CORRECTIONS (10/01/10-09/30/11)
Region A: DCS (Diversified Collection Services)	$43.3	$5.8	$49.1	$146.3
Region B: CGI (CGI Federal)	$60.4	$3.2	$63.6	$170.3
Region C: Connolly	$65.2	$60.7	$125.9	$260.9
Region D: HDI (HealthDataInsights)	$108.2	$6.9	$115.1	$361.8
Nationwide Totals	**$277.1**	**$76.6**	**$353.7**	**$939.4**

TOP ISSUE PER REGION
*Based on collected amounts through September 30, 2011

Region A:	**Renal and Urinary Tract Disorders:** (Medical Necessity) Medicare pays for inpatient hospital services that are medically necessary for the setting billed. Medical documentation for patients with renal and urinary tract disorders needs to be complete and support all services provided.
Region B:	**Surgical Cardiovascular Procedures:** (Medical Necessity) Medicare pays for inpatient hospital services that are medically necessary for the setting billed. Medical documentation for patients with surgical cardiovascular procedures needs to be complete and support all services provided.
Region C:	**Acute Inpatient Admission Neurological Disorders:** (Medical Necessity) Medicare pays for inpatient hospital services that are medically necessary for the setting billed. Medical documentation for patients admitted with neurological disorders needs to be complete and support all services provided.
Region D:	**Minor Surgery and other treatment billed as Inpatient :** (Medical Necessity) When beneficiaries with known diagnoses enter a hospital for a specific minor surgical procedure or other treatment that is expected to keep them in the hospital for less than 24 hours, they are considered outpatient for coverage purposes regardless of the hour they presented to the hospital, whether a bed was used, and whether they remained in the hospital after midnight.

Figure 22-4 Centers for Medicare and Medicaid Services (CMS) Medicare Fee for Service National Recovery Audit Program (July 1, 2011, to September 30, 2011) Quarterly Newsletter. Reprinted from the Centers for Medicare and Medicaid Services.

practice for physicians at every institution and require initial measurement of physician practices, with regular (more than once yearly) reevaluations of those physician metrics. Furthermore, an FPPE can be initiated for any physician whose practice standards are questioned because of an incident or concern raised by peers. While hospitals have great latitude in choosing what metrics they include in these evaluations, there is a growing trend toward using quantifiable data that can be automatically extracted from EHRs whenever possible.

Another growing area of EHR reporting is the integration of clinical data with financial systems and other operational systems for use in business applications.[26] Hospitals and health systems are building clinical data warehouses or using third-party applications to query data *in situ* in order to gain business intelligence (BI). These systems are designed to help control costs, standardize care, and improve quality through the use of advanced reporting and data mining techniques, which reveal trends in care that would otherwise be hard to identify without comprehensive and integrated data from disparate systems.

Privacy, Confidentiality, and Security

Several laws play a major role in defining the way in which EHRs operate. Arguably, the most important is the Health Insurance Portability and Accountability Act (HIPAA) of 1996,[27] which includes rules on the privacy and security of personal health information (PHI). These provisions have been in force since 2003 and 2005, respectively. They focus on the ways in which PHI can be viewed, used, and transmitted. See Figure 22-5 for the number of investigated resolutions between April 2003 and December 2011.

The Privacy Rule regulates how covered entities and business associates must handle PHI, including the following:

- Acceptable use for treatment, payment, and medical operations
- The right of the patient to access their own information and request corrections
- The need to log disclosures and report any violations of the law (intentional or inadvertent)

The act also provides for penalties for infractions, including fines and possible imprisonment, although about a third of complaints are found to have no violations and the remaining are resolved in the vast majority of cases with corrective action short of imprisonment (see Figure 22-5).

The Security Rule focuses only on electronic PHI (ePHI), whereas the Privacy Rule covers all forms. It establishes rules for developing administrative, physical, and technical safeguards for the reasonable protection of ePHI. Under the administrative umbrella, organizations must put in place and enforce policies and procedures for protecting ePHI and responding to breaches of their systems. The physical safeguards require that entities must make sure that computers and similar systems that display ePHI are secure and not visible by those who are not authorized to view the information. Technical safeguards

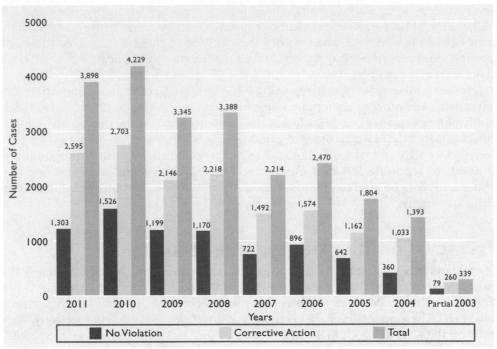

Figure 22-5 Investigated resolutions. Reprinted from the U.S. Department of Health and Human Services.

must assure that access to and transmission of ePHI is done in a compliant fashion, including risk analysis and risk management programs.

While the main goal of the HIPAA privacy and security provision may be to avoid willful and wanton misuse of PHI, there have been instances where accidental disclosures of information and even *potential* disclosures (based on inadequate system security designs) have led to significant federal penalties. While system design and good surveillance and audit practices can prevent most incidents, it is still incumbent upon every user with access to the EMR to understand the rules and regulations in this important area.

 CompTIA EXAM TIP Personal health information (sometimes called *protected* health information) includes *any* individually identifiable patient information.

The following are the definitions for *privacy*, *confidentiality*, and *security*:

- **Privacy**   Relates to the *person*. It derives from the Minimum Necessary Requirement clause of the HIPAA regulations (45 CFR 164.502(b) and 164.514(d)) and requires that covered entities take reasonable steps to limit the use or disclosure of, and requests for, protected health information to the minimum necessary to accomplish the intended purpose.

- **Confidentiality**   Relates to *data*. It refers to the practices that one takes to protect PHI such as password protection and data encryption. The information that is considered confidential may be verbal, written, electronic, or other formats.

- **Security**   Relates to practices for protecting PHI in an electronic format.

Examples of Recent Resolution Agreements

HHS Settles Case with Phoenix Cardiac Surgery for Lack of HIPAA Safeguards
Phoenix Cardiac Surgery, P.C., of Phoenix and Prescott, Arizona, has agreed to pay the U.S. Department of Health and Human Services a $100,000 settlement amount and to a corrective action plan that includes a review of recently developed policies and other actions taken to come into full compliance with the Privacy and Security Rules. OCR's investigation found that the physician practice was posting clinical and surgical appointments for their patients on an Internet-based calendar that was publicly accessible. Further, Phoenix Cardiac Surgery had implemented few policies and procedures to comply with the HIPAA Privacy and Security Rules and had limited safeguards in place to protect patients' ePHI.

HHS Settles HIPAA Case with BCBST for $1.5 Million
On March 9, 2012, Blue Cross Blue Shield of Tennessee (BCBST) agreed to pay $1.5 million to settle potential violations of the HIPAA Privacy and Security Rules. BCBST also agreed to a corrective action plan that includes reviewing, revising, and maintaining its Privacy and Security policies and procedures; conducting regular and robust trainings for all BCBST employees covering employee responsibilities under HIPAA; and performing monitor reviews to ensure BCBST compliance with the plan. The investigation followed a notice submitted by BCBST to HHS in which it was reported that 57 unencrypted computer hard drives containing PHI of more than 1 million individuals had been stolen from a leased facility in Tennessee. The enforcement action is the first resulting from a breach report required by the Health Information Technology for Economic and Clinical Health (HITECH) Act Breach Notification Rule.

Source: www.hhs.gov/ocr/privacy/hipaa/enforcement/examples/index.html (Accessed June 30, 2012)

Data Exchange and Security

There are implicit and explicit mandates to maintain the security and integrity of patient information throughout healthcare law and regulations. HIPAA regulations and MU specifically outline the need for protections built into EHR systems and regular auditing of their use. The disclosure of breaches and potential security risks is mandatory. Users are required to access the minimum amount of information that is necessary for the care and relationship with the patient.

EHR systems comply with these rules through the use of role-based access and system logging. In general, each user type (e.g., physician, nurse, lab technician) has a defined security position within the system and can access only the information that is pertinent to their relationship to the patient. Some roles restrict a user to view-only access of key parts of a medical record, while other roles may completely hide certain encounter types. For example, a radiology technician may be able to look up a patient's prior encounters but would not find visits that were for psychiatric care. Another example is the instance in which nurses may be able to view the notes created by physicians but cannot add a note themselves.

As each user accesses a patient record, EHR systems or third-party programs generally track that activity and create an audit log that is used for security reviews. Access, entries, and modifications should all be date and time-stamped for later review. Active and passive systems monitor patient access in order to determine potential threats. When a breach or a security system defect is noted, the instance must be reported and corrective action documented.

Health Information Exchange

In several areas of this chapter, I touched on the concept of a patient-centric, community-based record. Currently, there are efforts around the United States with varying levels of maturity to connect hospitals, physician offices, and others in the community via health information exchanges (HIEs). These data exchanges, generally governed by a regional health information organization (RHIO), are designed to allow providers using different electronic systems to see an aggregated view of patient data and in some cases share data across disparate systems. These efforts are complicated by the fact that the information resides in different EHRs, with different data standards, different terminologies and taxonomies, and a lack of common patient identifiers. A key function of an HIE is the integration of patient data utilizing patient-matching algorithms and normalized clinical data. The systems then deliver the combined patient record through various mechanisms including a third-party portal or via direct integration with native EHRs.

Chapter Review

Healthcare and healthcare IT are both highly regulated via a number of government and private organizations via laws, standards, and reimbursement requirements. The government and certification bodies have designed rules and regulations that are intended to protect the health and safety of patients, while at the same time encouraging the use of HIT as a way to improve care outcomes. Adoption of EHRs in hospitals and to a lesser extent physician offices is rapidly increasing. With this rapid growth, the need for expert understanding of the risks and benefits of the use of these technologies is increasing as well.

Key concepts covered in this chapter include the following:

- HIT is directly regulated in the form of protection of privacy and security of personal health information via the guarantees of the Health Information Portability and Accountability Act and meaningful use regulations.

- Components of EHRs focused on areas that are regulated cleared by the FDA under Section 510K (e.g., blood banking and patient monitoring devices) must comply with explicit federal regulations.

- Information entered in the EHR and reports from those same systems are often used to demonstrate compliance with regulation from Medicare, Medicaid, and other payers, as well as a host of other certification programs. Incentives put forth in the meaningful use program have led to a significant growth in the implementation of EHRs.

- Subsequent stages of meaningful use will increase the need for complex system design and more sophisticated reporting.

If the goals of the meaningful use initiatives are achieved, the United States will have an interoperable, patient-centric system of EHRs that can be used for care coordination across a healthcare system that rewards low-cost, highly reliable healthcare.

Questions

To test your comprehension of this chapter, answer the following questions and then check your answers against the list of correct answers at the end of the chapter.

1. What act established the Medicare and Medicaid programs?
   A. Health Insurance Portability and Accountability Act of 1996
   B. Social Security Act of 1965
   C. HITECH Act of 2009
   D. Emergency Medical Treatment and Labor Act of 1986

2. Medicare Part _____ covers care for hospitalizations.
   A. A
   B. B
   C. C
   D. D

3. Accountable-care organizations can be comprised of which of the following?

   A. Physician groups

   B. Hospitals and physician groups

   C. Entire caregiver communities

   D. All of the above

4. The triple aim does not include which of the following?

   A. Improving the patient experience of care (including quality and satisfaction)

   B. Improving the health of populations

   C. Increasing the use of electronic healthcare systems

   D. Reducing the per-capita cost of healthcare

5. Meaningful use criteria and certification for EHRs is defined by which of the following?

   A. Department of Health and Human Services

   B. Centers for Medicare and Medicaid Services

   C. The Office of the National Coordinator for Health Information Technology (ONC)

   D. The Joint Commission

6. Homegrown and best-in-breed EHRs do not need individual certification if the components are already certified for meaningful use.

   A. True

   B. False

7. Medicare and Medicaid payments for eligible providers under meaningful use are about the same.

   A. True

   B. False

8. The Recovery Audit Compliance program focuses on which of the following?

   A. Medicare under- and overpayments

   B. Cases with poor surgical outcomes

   C. Physician kickbacks from hospitals

   D. Compliance with care bundles for diseases such as pneumonia

9. What is personal health information?

   A. Any piece of information that the patient deems private

   B. Electronic information that is gathered in an EHR

   C. Information defined by each provider's Bill of Patient Rights

   D. Any information that can personally identify a patient

10. Inadvertent disclosure of protected health Information is subject to the same penalties as willful disclosures.

    A. True

    B. False

11. What are diagnosis-related groups (DRGs)?

    A. A taxonomy used for medical diagnoses in EHRs

    B. A payment mechanism that focuses on reimbursement for hospital care

    C. An analytic tool that helps determine population health

    D. A type of physician documentation

12. Core measures are defined for all of the following except which?

    A. Seizures

    B. Pneumonia

    C. Congestive heart failure

    D. Acute myocardial infarction

13. Joint Commission surveys are performed in order to do what?

    A. Gain recognition for marketing purposes

    B. Qualify for Medicare payments

    C. Get enhanced reimbursement from private insurance companies

    D. Certify electronic health record systems

14. In general, what does role-based security in EHRs help maintain the principle of?

    A. Minimum necessary requirement

    B. Meaningful use

    C. Diagnosis-related groups

    D. Accountable-care organizations

Answers

1. **B.** The Social Security Act of 1965 established Medicare and Medicaid as the first government-paid healthcare plans.

2. **A.** Part A of Medicare coverage pays for hospital care. Part B covers physician-office care, while Part D covers medication. There is no Part C.

3. **D.** Accountable-care organizations are composed of groups of providers that agree to cooperate to reduce the overall cost of care while attempting to improve quality. ACOs can include any component of the healthcare continuum.

4. **C.** While EHRs will certainly support the goals of Berwick's triple aim, they are not one of the foundational components of improving healthcare while reducing costs.

5. **C.** The ONC defines the certification criteria for electronic health records to meet meaningful use at each stage. There will be at least three stages. Certifying bodies include CCHIT and the Drummond Group.

6. **B.** False. Because homegrown systems have no prior review, they all need to be independently certified for each stage of meaningful use. Since eligible hospitals and providers that use multiple systems to satisfy MU may take an infinite number of combinations of components from each vendor, it is incumbent on the organization to get its particular combination of parts certified, even though they may all be certified on their own.

7. **B.** False. Medicaid payments are actually 45 percent higher than Medicare payments ($63,750 versus $44,000). Additionally, Medicaid payments are generally paid out over five years, while Medicare is over four years. In the first year of Medicaid MU stage 1, providers need only show evidence of adopting, implementing, or upgrading their EHR, while Medicare payments are based on 90 days of continual meaningful use.

8. **A.** RACs focus on fraud, waste, and abuse in hospitals and physician practices via automated review of Medicare and Medicaid billings and chart reviews of cases that are up to three years old. When problems are identified, penalties are applied across the board, based on the prevalence discovered in the auditing process, and can reach into the millions of dollars.

9. **D.** Personal health information is defined in the Health Insurance Portability and Accountability Act of 1996. It includes any information that can be used to identify a patient in any form (written, verbal, electronic, or other).

10. **A.** HIPAA makes no distinction between the inadvertent disclosure (or potential disclosure through poor security practices) of PHI and deliberate disclosure. While CMS may apply penalties differently, there are many examples of significant settlements against individuals and organizations where disclosure was not meant as a malicious act.

11. **B.** Diagnosis-related groups are the way in which Medicare and many other payers reimburse hospitals for patient care. They are based on the typical costs for care of a variety of disease processes and pay a single rate for the care of each disease.

12. **A.** Seizures are not part of the core measures. Core measures are defined by CMS and include treatment of acute myocardial infarction, community-acquired pneumonia, heart failure, stroke, childhood asthma, smoking cessation, substance abuse counseling, immunization, surgical care improvement (SCIP), psychiatric services, outpatient departments, perinatal care, and prevention of venous thromboembolism.

13. **B.** CMS (and most other payers and regulatory agencies) require that the Joint Commission or one of the other recognized certifying bodies certify hospitals.

14. **A.** The Minimum Necessary Requirement clause guarantees that personnel working with PHI will access the smallest subset of information necessary for their portion of care and interaction with the patient.

References

1. Accelerating progress on EHR adoption rates and achieving meaningful use. Accessed on June 2, 2012, from http://helathit.gov/buzz-blog/meaningful-use/ehr-adoptoin-rates-and-achieving-meaningful-use.

2. EHR adoption rates jump for solo practices: Meaningful use incentives and adequate preparation time to meet them have contributed to the rise. Accessed on June 2, 2012, from www.ama-assn.org/amednews/2012/03/26/bisb0326.htm.

3. Terry, N. P. (2012). Anticipating stage two: Assessing the development of meaningful use and EMR deployment. *Annals of Health Law, 21*, 103–119.

4. Needles in a haystack: Seeking knowledge with clinical informatics. (2012). Accessed on May 13, 2012, from http://pwchealth.com/cgi-local/hregister.cgi/reg/needles-in-a-haystack.pdf.

5. Office of the National Coordinator for Health Information Technology. Accessed on May 29, 2012, from http://healthit.hhs.gov/portal/server.pt/community/healthit_hhs_gov__onc/1200.

6. Accessed on April 28, 2012, from www.jointcommission.org/core_measure_sets.aspx.

7. Berwick, D., Nolan, T., & Whittington, J. (2008). The triple aim: Care, health and cost. *Health Affairs, 27*, 759–769.

8. Accessed on June 26, 2012, from https://www.cms.gov/Medicare/Medicare-Fee-for-Service-Payment/AcuteInpatientPPS/index.html?redirect=/AcuteInpatientPPS/.

9. Rittenhouse, D. R., Shortell, S. M., & Fisher, E. S. (2009). Primary care and accountable care: Two essential elements of delivery-system reform. *New England Journal of Medicine, 361*, 2301–3.

10. Accessed on June 26, 2012, from https://www.cms.gov/Medicare/Medicare-Fee-for-Service-Payment/ACO/index.html?redirect=/ACO/.

11. Grumbach, K., & Bodenheimer, T. (2002). A primary care home for Americans: Putting the house in order. *Journal of the American Medical Association, 288*, 889–893.

12. Accessed on July 1, 2012, from www.pcmh.ahrq.gov/portal/server.pt/community/pcmh__home/1483.

13. Accessed on June 13, 2012, from http://waysandmeans.house.gov/media/pdf/111/hitech.pdf.

14. Accessed on June 12, 2012, from https://www.cms.gov/Regulations-and-Guidance/Legislation/EHRIncentivePrograms/index.html?redirect=/EHRIncentivePrograms/.

15. Accessed on May 18, 2012, from www.gpo.gov/fdsys/pkg/FR-2010-07-28/pdf/2010-17207.pdf.

16. Accessed on June 29, 2012, from www.himssanalytics.org/home/index.aspx.

17. Accessed on June 28, 2012, from http://healthit.hhs.gov/portal/server.pt/document/957970/ 060612_hitpc_ehr_incentives_pdf.

18. Accessed on July 1, 2012, from http://georgewbushwhitehouse.archives.gov/infocus/technology/ economic_policy200404/chap3.html.

19. Accessed on July 1, 2012, from https://www.cms.gov/Medicare/Quality-Initiatives-Patient-Assessment-Instruments/ERxIncentive/index.html.

20. Accessed on July 1, 2012, from www.getrxconnected.com/other/NoTech/initiatives.aspx?type=notech.

21. Jariwala, K. S., Holmes, E. R., Banahan, B. F., & McCaffrey, D. J. (2012). Adoption of and experience with e-prescribing by primary care physicians. *Research in Social and Administrative Pharmacy*, [Epub ahead of print].

22. Accessed on May 11, 2012, from www.thomas.gov/cgi-bin/query/F?c109:1:./temp/~c109HX4zHm:e92447.

23. Accessed on July 16, 2012, from http://manual.jointcommission.org/releases/TJC2012A/IntroductionTJC.html#National_Quality_Measures_Cleari.

24. Edwards, M.T. (2009). Peer review: A new tool for quality improvement. *Physician Executive*, *35*, 54–9.

25. Makary, M.A., Wick, E., & Freischlag, J.A. (2011). Complying with the new alphabet soup of credentialing. *Archives of Surgery*, *146*, 642–644.

26. Glaser, J., & Stone, J. (2008.) Effective use of business intelligence. *Journal of the Healthcare Financial Management Association*, *62*, 68–72.

27. Accessed on April 27, 2012, from www.gpo.gov/fdsys/pkg/PLAW-104publ191/html/PLAW-104publ191.htm.

CHAPTER 23

Training Essentials for Implementing Healthcare IT

Cheryl A. Fisher

In this chapter, you will learn how to
- Plan, design, develop, deliver, and evaluate technology-based instruction
- Plan and implement an instructional needs assessment
- Construct a lesson plan using appropriate instructional methods
- Incorporate adult learning principles into program design
- Create a custom presentation using principles of effective multimedia presentation and Web 2.0 technologies
- Plan and conduct an effective student assessment and program evaluation

Implementing new technology into the healthcare setting can be a costly and resource-intensive undertaking. Training requirements for new technologies require an enormous amount of time, effort, commitment, and change management on the part of the organization. Training is required for those who will be involved in the initial implementation of the healthcare organization's new systems so that they will be familiar with the new capabilities and functionality now available. Because of this investment, it is imperative that best practices and sound educational design principles are applied to ensure success. Traditional face-to-face computer lab training presents many challenges and is time-consuming and resource-intensive. Because of a diverse workforce and varying schedules of healthcare providers, technology-supported design models can potentially address these limitations. This chapter will address training considerations when faced with the implementation of new technologies in healthcare settings.

Models and Principles

The first step in developing a training program is to put together a team that understands the healthcare organization's mission, the content to be delivered, the educational design considerations, and the end user's perspective. This team must then develop a training plan that is flexible, dynamic, personalized, and reflective of post-implementation training requirements in order to reinforce the concepts and to drive the successful utilization of technology adoption. Vendor-provided training sometimes falls short because of generic content delivery that does not align with the organization or is not customized enough to meet the end user requirements.

Several models should be considered when implementing training for new technologies in healthcare settings. These models guide the training developer through the appropriate steps and facilitate the incorporation of all considerations necessary for success. Instructional systems design is the analysis of learning needs followed by the systematic development of instruction to meet those needs. If such models are followed, they will facilitate the transfer of knowledge, skills, and attitudes to the learner.[1] The ADDIE model, for example, is a generic instructional design model that is used by instructional designers and training developers. The model consists of five phases: analysis, design, development, implementation, and evaluation. Table 23-1 describes what occurs in each step of the model.

One commonly accepted improvement to this model is the use of rapid prototyping. This is the idea of receiving continual or formative feedback while instructional materials are being created. This model attempts to save time and money by catching problems early while they are easy to fix.[1] In the ADDIE model, each step has an outcome incorporated in the subsequent step. Instructional design (ID) is a general term for a family of systematic methods for planning, developing, evaluating, and managing the instructional process effectively in order to promote successful learning by students.[2] Instructional systems design (ISD) is a problem-solving process that has been applied to the development of training since the 1940s. Since then, more than 100 instructional design models have emerged based on the fundamentals of the ADDIE model.

ADDIE Steps	Actions Within Each Step
Analyze	Determine needs and performance gap
Design	Write learning objectives, plan the training, and develop evaluation plan
Develop	Build the course
Implement	Teach or make training available
Evaluate	Measure effectiveness or impact

Table 23-1   ADDIE Steps and Actions

Assessing Basic Skill Level

One of the most challenging aspects of training is determining baseline skill level and the learning needs of the end users. Assessment is the process of determining these needs in order to write learning objectives directed toward these needs, and one method is through a *learning needs assessment.* A *training needs assessment* is a study done in order to design and develop appropriate instructional and informational programs and material in order to fill in the gaps.[3] However, a learning needs assessment allows you to consider both formal and informal learning needs. That is, what do they need to be trained on, and how can you best support their informal learning needs? In other words, how are the end users supported outside of the classroom?

 TIP Oftentimes the end users don't know what they need to know. Setting up general overview sessions of a new system in an auditorium prior to training and go-live can help users to start developing questions.

The next step is to determine the student's baseline knowledge and experience related to the technology to be learned. People do not learn from point zero, rather from the standpoint of their own knowledge and experience. The model seeks to motivate the student via prior experience and context to come closer to the idea of the topic. During this step, defining or describing the problem under study and sharing the objectives of the training process between trainer and participant are key.[4] Questionnaires and structured interviews are the most commonly reported methods of needs assessments. Other ways to gather information related to learning needs include observations, surveys, or group discussions. Some questions to consider when gathering information for the needs assessment include the following:

- Who is the audience, and what are their characteristics?
- What is the new behavioral outcome?
- What types of learning constraints exist?
- What are the delivery options?
- What are the online design considerations?
- What is the timeline for project completion?

Here is an example of the steps to follow when conducting a needs assessment:

1. Write objectives of what you hope to gain from the needs assessment.
2. Select an audience to sample.
   A. Consider the sample across multiple age groups, and consider those with English as a second language (ESL).
3. Collect data from participants.
4. Analyze data.

Once this information is gathered, the trainer will have a much better understanding of the baseline knowledge of the learners and any issues that seem to be prevalent among the learners.

TIP Do not assume that all users have basic computer skills and/or a working knowledge of Windows functionality. Resources or a short tutorial could be helpful to review these basic skills that many take for granted.

Design Elements

Once the learning needs are assessed, the learning objectives for the training program should be established. The general purpose for the training should be clearly defined followed by the specific learning outcomes. The learning outcomes or objectives should be measureable and criterion-based. For example, "at the end of this module (given a set of conditions), you will be able to (action verb and behavior) with (criterion with level of accuracy)." Here's a sample objective: *at the end of this module, the learner will be able to document medications with 100 percent accuracy.* When evaluating the objectives, you should look to determine completeness, practicality, feasibility, and consistency. The goal of training should be more than just knowing how and where to enter the data. The overall goal should support users to think logically and critically about how to best use the system to maximize the benefits that the system has to offer the healthcare organization and the patients. The training team and healthcare organization management have the challenge at this point of obtaining user buy-in by developing program objectives tailored to the workflow of each person's role utilizing the system. Emphasis should be placed on attitudes and benefits of the system to enhance patient outcomes.

TIP A major change such as electronic medical record (EMR) implementation often creates resistance. Firm messaging from healthcare organization leadership can help reinforce positive messaging and the fact that "the train is leaving the station, whether they like it or not."[5] Physicians can be a particularly challenging audience to engage and convince of the benefits of the EMR and organizational as well as medical leadership support is especially critical for that group of learners.

Additional design considerations should include the order of the instructional program. According to Gagne's nine events for learning, the instructor should do the following, in this order: gain the learner's attention, inform the learner of the objectives, stimulate recall of prior learning, present information, provide guidance, elicit performance, and enhance retention and transfer. Gagne's process steps for learning were developed based on an information processing model of the mental events that occur when adults are presented with various stimuli.[6] For example, to put this model into action, the instructor could tailor learning modules toward particular surgeon groups. These modules would use pre-op and post-op orders already familiar to the surgeons and provide them with the opportunity to transfer new knowledge to their already familiar work.

A major consideration for designing and developing training pertains to the delivery method of the instruction. This will depend on the organizational preference and the available resources as to whether the training will be conducted face-to-face, completely online, or using a hybrid format that includes a mix of online and face-to-face training. Training can be done by internal resources, third-party providers, or the EMR vendor, and a determination needs to be made about which groups offer the best chance for success. There are pros and cons to all approaches, and often the cost or resource impact will ultimately determine a healthcare organization's decision. The goal is to develop comprehensive training in the shortest amount of time. Often, the end users have little time and patience for training, yet it is critical that they develop the skills and competency required to safely use the new system. On average, online instruction and face-to-face instruction require similar time commitments for end users. Instructional strategies to enhance feedback and interactivity typically prolong learning time but in many cases also enhance learning outcomes.[7] Online learning has advantages such as overcoming time and distance barriers and the ability to use innovative multimedia and virtual instructional methods. It is the challenge of any instructional designer to incorporate meaningful instructional strategies that engage the learners and enhance the learning. It is also up to the organization to determine whether they have trained instructional designers on staff or whether they have the resources to outsource the required training and follow-up. Oftentimes, combinations of online and face-to-face instructional strategies are utilized in order to address the many facets of training required. Here are some examples:

- Web-based tutorials for general concepts and higher-level learning
- Instructor-led classroom training workshops facilitated by clinical subject-matter experts as well as training team members
- One-on-one short training sessions with end users for each phase of the project led by superusers, focused on clinical care and efficient interactions with the system applications
- On-request support for assistance or clarification just after go-live
- On-the-spot training via walking rounds using clinical experts to offer support
- Web-based or instructor-led training on advanced features and new enhancements after go-live and ongoing as appropriate

There are multiple ways of delivering training materials and content during educational sessions in addition to user guides, pocket reference guides, and quick-tip sheets. Posters can be developed and placed in staff workstations in order to reinforce visual displays and contact information for the user help desk. The bottom line of these multiple approaches is ultimately to develop a user-friendly rapport with the staff in order to answer questions and help problem solve. If users find they cannot get the help they need in a timely fashion, they will develop shortcuts or "workarounds" that could compromise patient safety.

The Adult Learner

When designing educational training programs for adults, success can depend on the adherence to adult learning principles that need to be embedded throughout the program. Adult learners have unique learning needs and expectations that set them apart from their younger counterparts. Adult learning has received increasing attention among educators, and a significant body of literature has established clear areas of emphasis for adult educators. These areas are typically recognized in the principles of andragogy developed by Knowles, which stresses need-to-know, immediacy of application, sharing of life experiences as a source of knowledge, independence and self-direction, and ownership of their learning as hallmarks of adult learners.[8] In other words, adult learners want to know why they should invest the time. They need to feel responsible for their learning, they bring valuable experience to the learning, they are ready to learn when the need arises, and they are task-oriented. Other noted characteristics include autonomy, self-direction, and affinity for real-life learning as key characteristics of adult learners. When developing training with adult learners in mind, the training developer must ensure that relevant training scenarios are utilized and that learning is self-paced and possibly self-directed. This can be done by creating training scenarios for different healthcare roles (i.e., physician, nurse) and by allowing for test-out options so as not to waste the time of the professional adult learner. For example, online training modules could be developed for physicians focusing specifically on order entry. Given specific concepts and opportunities for transferring knowledge, the physicians could be tested at the end of the module to demonstrate competency through applying their new knowledge. Training environments could also be made available for specific disciplines to practice their new skills. This training environment could be made accessible from every desktop with fake patient names, which will allow staff the opportunity to practice navigation within a simulated environment.

Constructing a Lesson Plan

Once the needs assessment is completed and the objectives are developed, it is time to develop a lesson plan for the targeted population. When put into simple terms, "tell, show, do, and review" is a good way to remember the steps. A sample outline for this plan could include the following:

I. Principal goal of the training

    A. Module I

        1. Learning objectives

            a. Tell: Didactic content (PowerPoint or video)

            b. Show: Demonstration of new skills to be learned (PowerPoint, video, or screen capture)

    c. Do: Learning activity to apply learned concepts (application of learned content using case scenarios)

    d. Review: Evaluation of learning (knowledge test, return demonstration)

  B. Module II (repeat previous steps)

  C. Additional resources and supporting materials

Training content should be focused on job roles and associated workflow. Vendors often provide the initial training materials and a limited amount of free training services, which should be used to train the project team and the initial set of users or superusers. These superusers will then become resources to train other staff and to problem solve, support end users, and reinforce concepts at the unit or department level. The training department should then develop customized supporting materials that are consistent with workflow and the healthcare organizations' policies and procedures.

In short, a successful training program must be tailored to an organization's environment. The materials developed should address the user roles and clinical workflow scenarios that will be familiar to the end user's daily practice. The training should focus on workflow and ultimately enhanced patient care.

 TIP The change in workflow for end users cannot be underestimated. This is often one of the primary reasons why staff will resist change and develop workarounds. To circumvent this, good relationships are critical so that staff will utilize available resources to facilitate problem solving.

Multimedia as a Method of Delivery

As multimedia becomes a more common instructional tool, researchers are finding that more than one modality (i.e., visual and auditory) is better than a single modality (visual alone) in any instructional message.[9] The implementation of multimedia can effectively enhance learning performance and retention. Incorporating multimedia tools at an appropriate time can enhance learning interests and willingness. Also, the presentation of reciprocal representations can enable students to have an in-depth understanding of a course and extend the effect of learning retention.[9]

Instructional quality of online delivery is still a common concern. Quality assurance requires a comprehensive framework of several perspectives of learners' and instructors' needs including critical analysis of teaching and learning practices with the technology platform.[10] The use of high-quality instructional and course design standards by instructors in online learning has numerous benefits as well as challenges. Moving from traditional methods of teaching to online delivery methods of instruction requires a shift in the perspectives of both the instructors and the learners.[11] When constructing instructional tutorials using presentation software, you must consider basic principles for the adult learner that will ensure the message is communicated and conveyed clearly. Here are some examples:

- Combine images with verbal text (less is more when it comes to graphics).
- Present content in logically grouped sections that allow the learner to organize for recall.
- Use a text of font size 28 to 30 (and limit yourself to one or two text styles).
- Don't use more than five lines per slide, and avoid using all capital letters.
- Use a title font size of 40 or larger.
- Minimize background colors and textures so as not to distract from the content, and be sure text color contrasts with slide background.
- Use consistent transitions.
- Unify slides and align text using bullets.
- Avoid using animation unless it is value added.

These principles are important to apply because they make the content easier to understand and avoid distraction from the information to be learned. When developing training tutorials, one of the most effective approaches includes the use of software that guides the learner through the navigational pathways. A videotaped lecture can be used for an instructional demonstration prior to allowing the participant to practice on their own. Instructional modules longer than 20 minutes tend to lose teaching effectiveness. Information overload is a real possibility, and the instructor must decide on the important points to be learned.[12]

Web 2.0 Technologies

Web 2.0 refers to the second generation of the World Wide Web. This new generation of the Web includes new features and functionality that allow for user interaction and information sharing such as blogging and social networks.[13] Despite the increasing use of Web 2.0 tools in education, there appears to be a lack of empirical evidence detailing the process educators have taken to implement them in the classroom. Providing guidance to educators on key practical issues to consider when introducing Web 2.0 into the classroom is important because it provides direction on how to overcome any unforeseen issues when undertaking this process.[14] With little guidance on how to leverage Web 2.0 in the educational context of healthcare information technology, examples and practical recommendations cited in the literature relating to Web 2.0 implementation in organizations are available.[14] Because Web 2.0 tools can be used for knowledge sharing, learning, and social interaction, these tools are now prominently used in the classroom. The tools are acknowledged in the literature to have the potential to support different educational design approaches that facilitate both self-directed and collaborative learning. Empirical research into the use of Web 2.0 tools such as wikis, blogs, and online forums is steadily increasing. The primary concerns regarding the adoption of

Web 2.0 tools are usefulness, advantages, compatibility, and technology availability. Secondary concerns are resource-facilitating conditions and peer, healthcare organization, and senior management attitudes.[15]

Training Delivery and Accommodation

For any training program to be successful, the first consideration is the audience. In other words, to whom are you speaking? It is critical to know the answers to the following:

- What do you want to communicate?
- How will the messages best be conveyed?
- When will the training be seen as most relevant?
- Where will the training take place?
- Why should the individual participate in the learning?[16]

While it might seem obvious, it is critical to keep the message clear and concise and to keep all information simple.

When formulating a training plan, consider the needs assessment findings, the diversity of your audience, and any special needs of the individuals. For example, if the didactic portion of your training has been videotaped with audio recordings and you have a participant who is hearing impaired, you will need to ensure that your training has transcripts available for this individual to read. Likewise, if you have a participant who is visually impaired, does your training meet the requirements for using screen readers or assistive devices? All training delivered online must meet the requirements of the Americans with Disabilities Act. It is required by law that all participants have equal access to educational training or that special accommodations be made if required.

Training schedules need to be flexible, and given the 24/7 nature of healthcare, it may be necessary to offer late evening or weekend training classes in order to accommodate all staff. Training content should be introduced over a period of time to avoid information overload and to progress from novice to expert concepts. This can be done using a series of modules that build on previously learned content. Readily available and easy-to-use reference material can help support the formal learned content and can reinforce learning.

 TIP   It has been the standard that the training for implementing a new EMR should occur about six weeks prior to go-live and should be delivered in no more than three-hour blocks of time. This approach will facilitate learning and retention of information. Within the three-hour blocks of time, breaks should be given, and the "tell, show, do, review" process steps should be followed.

Evaluating Learning

Effective training should focus on the user role and should be workflow-based. A common misconception of how to train is to focus on features and functions of the system. While basic knowledge about how to navigate and what icons/buttons do is important, the training ultimately should be competency-based. It is less important for users to know every button or system function than it is for users to be able to accomplish their day-to-day tasks and to ensure patient safety. While some level of basic education is needed, physicians in particular respond best when training is clinically focused on content encountered in daily practice.

Student learning and program evaluation are critical in order for the trainer to know whether they accomplished their task in delivering training. Two current working methodologies of formative assessment stress involving students in generating and using assessment information as a key assessment function. Utilizing Kirkpatrick's method of evaluation, questions to ask include the following:

- Were the students satisfied with their learning?
- Did it meet their need?
- Would they recommend it to others?
- Did their behavior (or performance) change as a result?
- Did the organization achieve its desired results from the training?

A successful training evaluation must be aligned with the organization's mission and goals, it should be a systematic process, it should be data-driven, and it should be focused on continuing improvement. The best methods for assessing student learning can be obtained from participant feedback, tests, and performance. Examples include surveys, structured interviews, and formal or informal tests. The trainers, peers, or supervisors can also make behavioral observations. The purpose for assessing student learning is primarily to determine whether knowledge gains have occurred. If the users say the training was useful and relevant, it was targeted correctly to the learning needs.

It is important to note that training does not stop at the end of the formal training sessions. Successful user adoption requires ongoing follow-up and follow-through in order to ensure that users are not creating a workaround. This happens frequently when they are unable or do not understand how to perform a task in the correct way. Walking rounds and focus groups can provide useful sources of information that require follow-up in addition to the opportunity for understanding particular areas of challenge for the users. Follow-up is also important in identifying any previous paper-based or outdated workflows that may have been missed as part of the initial review and that clinicians are still utilizing.

Program Evaluation

The overall program can be evaluated using satisfaction surveys, interviews, and knowledge outcomes.[17] The purpose is to incorporate the data and findings into the program for the purposes of improvement. Feedback can also provide useful information for necessary revisions to the overall program design and delivery, which will then become the orientation program content for new employees. Questions specific to the overall program could include the following and should be answered using a commonly accepted Likert-type rating scale:

- Please indicate your level of satisfaction with each of the following:
  - Whether the program met your expectations
  - Program content
  - Ability of presenter to communicate
  - Content and usefulness of handouts
  - Location in which program was held
  - Convenience of program day and time
  - Overall program

Utilizing a Learning Management System

Once the training program is designed and developed, one of the most efficient ways to implement the electronic content is by using a learning management system (LMS). LMS is a software application used for the administration, documentation, tracking, and reporting of training programs. A robust LMS should do the following:

- Centralize and automate administration
- Use self-service and self-guided services
- Assemble and deliver learning content rapidly
- Support portability and standards
- Personalize content and enable knowledge reuse

These platforms are particularly used to make the course materials, such as lecture slides, exercise sheets and solutions, and assignments, accessible.[18] During the past decade, LMS deployments have been utilized in most traditional educational institutions, not only to replace face-to-face instruction (e-learning) but also to combine it with computer-based instruction or hybrid learning. In addition to the delivery of learning content to students, LMSs often support interaction and cooperation with discussion, news forums, wikis, blogs, and quizzes, thus creating collaborative learning. LMSs also enable instructors to evaluate students electronically and to generate student databases where grades and progress can be charted.[18] E-learning course management systems provide educators with new tools and media to aid their teaching. For example, students can learn at their own pace at whatever time they want. These systems are not simple turnkey operations that can be implemented without some level of customization. They require an understanding of instructional design and demand a considerable amount of planning and preparation.[12] Human resources are a major consideration from the perspective of system administration and system maintenance.

Although most LMSs are commercially developed, some have an open source license, which allows for their source code to be shared. One popular set of open source software licenses include those identified by the Open Source Initiative (OSI), an organization dedicated to promoting open source software.

In recent years, e-learning has changed the traditional teaching and learning styles from teacher-centered to learner-centered. It emphasizes that the learner actively participates in the process of knowledge construction.[19] The Sharable Content Object Reference Model (SCORM) has become the standard for the tracking of records in LMSs, based on previously developed standards by the Aviation Industry CBT Committee (AICC). SCORM facilitates content acquisition from multiple providers with a single, real-time interface for recordkeeping and administration purposes. By definition, SCORM refers to a set of specifications that produce small, reusable e-learning objects when applied to course content. One advantage is these objects can be reused with other training materials.[20] For example, video clips, graphics, or learning modules might fall into this category. SCORM is a set of rules specified by the Advanced Distributed Learning (ADL) initiative that specify the order in which a learner may experience the training materials, such as using bookmarks to track progress and the opportunity to take breaks from learning without having to start over. SCORM also tracks test scores and feedback to the users. The office of the U.S. Secretary of Defense developed these standards in 1997.

Chapter Review

The task for instructional designers to train large numbers of employees on electronic medical records is a large and complex undertaking. It is increasingly apparent that innovations in information technology can deliver instruction more effectively in a wider range of contexts.[2] Anecdotal evidence suggests that projects for developing online instruction, particularly in educational settings, are often challenged by limited staff, funding constraints, and quick turnaround times. With increasingly limited resources, corporate and governmental departments responsible for designing online instruction have been reduced. Large projects requiring complex instructional design have been replaced by smaller, less complex, and less resource-intensive initiatives.[21] Having transformed traditional learning styles and sparked the interest of business communities and schools, e-learning is now regarded as an effective way to save labor and money, while enhancing learning performance.[9] Online learning using web-based computer programs for teaching can facilitate learning with instructional efficacy similar to that of traditional teaching approaches.

This chapter covered the following:

- Instructional system design and the ADDIE model as a guide for developing training
- Principles of adult learning theory and the importance of incorporating these principles into training programs
- Lesson plans and the various methodologies for developing educational content along with suggestions for evaluating student learning and program evaluation
- The use of a learning management system, open source software, and the incorporation of Web 2.0 technology to enhance learning

Ultimately, it is not the amount of time spent training or the method of delivery that is important, but the competency of the end users and their safe practices with system use that matter.

Questions

To test your comprehension of this chapter, answer the following questions and then check your answers against the list of correct answers at the end of the chapter.

1. Utilizing an instructional systems design model can facilitate the transfer of which of the following?
   A. Knowledge
   B. Attitudes
   C. Skill
   D. All of the above

2. The first step of the ADDIE model can be accomplished by which of the following?
   A. Conducting a needs assessment
   B. Asking for assistance
   C. Arranging the team
   D. Analyzing the program content

3. The best way to conduct a needs assessment is to do which of the following?
   A. Conduct a survey
   B. Conduct a focus group or structured interview
   C. Answers A and B
   D. None of the above

4. What is the final step of the ADDIE model?

    A. End the program.

    B. Evaluate the effectiveness of the program.

    C. Evaluate the return on investment.

    D. Establish a follow-up program based on learning needs.

5. When conducting a needs assessment, which of the following can be assumed?

    A. All end users have basic knowledge of computer systems.

    B. All end users have basic knowledge of Windows functionality.

    C. All end users will be receptive to change.

    D. None of the above.

6. What is the overall goal of training?

    A. To market the new system to all employees

    B. To support users to think logically and critically about how to best use the system to maximize the benefits that the system has to offer the hospital and the patients

    C. To allow all users to decide whether they want to use the system

    D. To obtain feedback on the system

7. During which step of the ADDIE model is it appropriate to write the learning objectives?

    A. Analyze

    B. Design

    C. Develop

    D. Implement

8. Learning objectives should be written based on which of the following?

    A. Criterion

    B. Accuracy

    C. A circumstance or set of circumstances

    D. All of the above

9. Characteristics of adult learners include which of the following?

    A. Are responsible for their learning, are ready to learn when the need arises, and are task-oriented

    B. Are autonomous, need direction, and do not feel responsible for their learning

    C. A and B

    D. None of the above

10. Instructional strategies to engage the learners and enhance learning include which of the following?

    A. Video and web-based tutorials

    B. Face-to-face instruction

    C. Handouts and reference material

    D. All of the above

11. When developing content using presentation software, good design principles include which of the following?

    A. An abundance of animation and a variety of background colors

    B. Consistency and uniformity of text and font sizes

    C. Excessive use of graphics and text to convey the message ("eye charts")

    D. Cartoons and humor to keep the learner's attention

12. Where can some of the best methods for assessing student learning be obtained from?

    A. Observation and attendance at training sessions

    B. Peer review

    C. Participant feedback, tests, and performance

    D. All of the above

13. What is the purpose of program evaluation?

    A. To verify the learners liked the program

    B. To make improvements and modify the training program

    C. Both A and B

    D. None of the above

14. The benefits of using a learning management system (LMS) to implement a training program include all of the following except which one?

    A. Automatic tracking of user grades and participation

    B. Incorporation of SCORM standards

    C. Administrative management

    D. Turnkey technology

15. Why is Web 2.0 technology becoming popular in education and training?

    A. Younger generations are familiar with this technology.

    B. Many frameworks exist for their use and incorporation into training.

    C. Research is beginning to show their effectiveness around collaborative learning.

    D. None of the above.

Answers

1. **D.** Use of an instructional systems design model to develop a training program can facilitate the transfer of knowledge, attitude, and skill to the learner.

2. **A.** The first step in the ADDIE model is to conduct a needs assessment and determine the gaps.

3. **C.** The best way to conduct a needs assessment is a survey or a structured focus group.

4. **B.** The final step in the ADDIE model is to evaluate the effectiveness of the program.

5. **D.** When conducting a needs assessment, it cannot be assumed that all end users have basic knowledge of computers or Windows or will embrace change.

6. **B.** The overall goal of training is to support users to think logically and critically about how to best use the system to maximize the benefits that the system has to offer clinicians, the healthcare organization, and the patients they serve.

7. **B.** The design step of the ADDIE model includes writing the objectives.

8. **D.** The learning objectives should be written based on criterion, accuracy, and a particular circumstance. For example, at the end of this module, the learner will be able to document with 100 percent accuracy.

9. **A.** Characteristics of adult learners include responsibility for their learning, are ready to learn when the need arises, and are task-oriented.

10. **D.** A challenge of any instructional designer is to incorporate meaningful instructional strategies that engage the learners and enhance the learning through the use of video and web-based tutorials, face-to-face instruction, handouts, and reference material.

11. **B.** When developing content using presentation software, good design principles include consistency and uniformity of text and font sizes.

12. **C.** Some of the best methods for assessing student learning are based on participant feedback, tests, and performance.

13. **C.** The purpose of program evaluation is to see whether the learners liked the program and to make improvements and modify the training program based on participant feedback.

14. **D.** The benefits of using a learning management system (LMS) to implement a training program include all of the options given except that it is not turnkey technology.

15. **C.** Web 2.0 technology is increasingly popular in education and training, with initial research showing effectiveness around collaborative learning.

References

1. Instructional Design home page. (2011). www.instructionaldesign.org.

2. Ozdilek, Z., & Robeck, E. (2009). Operational priorities of instructional designers analyzed within the steps of the Addie instructional design model. *Procedia: Social and Behavioral Sciences, 1*, 2046–2050.

3. Rossett, A., & Sheldon, K. (2001). *Beyond the podium: Delivering training and performance in a digital world.* Jossey-Bass/Pfeiffer.

4. Del Val, J. L., Campos, A., & Garaizar, P. (2010). LMS and Web 2.0 tools for e-learning: University of Deusto's experience taking advantage of both. IEEE Conference Presentation, Madrid.

5. Lowes R. (2004). EMR success: Training is the key. *Medical Economics, 81*.

6. Gagne, R., Briggs, L., & Wagner, W. (1985). *Principles of instructional design.* Wadsworth.

7. Cook, D. A., Levinson, A. J., & Garside, S. (2010). Time and learning efficiency in Internet-based learning: A systematic review and meta-analysis. *Advances in Health Sciences Education, 15*, 755–770.

8. Knowles, M. (1975). *Self-directed learning: A guide for learners and teachers.* Association Press.

9. Chen, Y. T., Chen, T. J., & Tsai, L. Y. (2011). Development and evaluation of multimedia reciprocal representation instructional materials. *International Journal of Physical Sciences, 6*, 1431–1439.

10. Lewis, K. O., Baker, R. C., & Britigan, D. H. (2011). Current practices and needs assessment of instructors in an online master's degree in education for healthcare professionals: A first step to the development of quality standards. *Journal of Interactive Online Learning, 10*, 49–63.

11. Dringus, L. P. (2000). Towards active online learning: A dramatic shift in perspective for learners. *Internet and Higher Education, 2*, 189–195.

12. Chan, C. H., & Robbins, L. I. (2006). E-learning systems: Promises and pitfalls. *Academic Psychiatry: The Journal of the American Association of Directors of Psychiatric Residency Training and the Association for Academic Psychiatry, 30*, 491–497.

13. TechTerms.com web 2.0. (2012). www.techterms.com/definition/web20.

14. Baxter, G. J., Connolly, T. M., Stansfield, M. H., Tsvetkova, N., & Stoimenova, B. (2011). Introducing Web 2.0 in education: A structured approach adopting a Web 2.0 implementation framework. IEEE Conference Publication, Salamanca.

15. Lau, A. S. M. (2011). Hospital-based nurses' perceptions of the adoption of Web 2.0 tools for knowledge sharing, learning, social interaction and the production of collective intelligence. *Journal of Medical Internet Research, 13*, 4.

16. Communication skills. (2011). Accessed on July 12, 2012, from http://www
.mindtools.com/CommSkll/CommunicationIntro.htm.

17. O'Niel, C., Fisher, C., & Knewbold, S. (2009). *Developing online learning environments in nursing education.* Springer Publishing.

18. Cigdemoglu, C., Arslan, H. O., & Akay, H. (2011). A phenomenological study of instructors' experiences on an open source learning management system. *Proceedings of the International Engineering Education Conference.* Nicosia/Kyrenia.

19. Chen, H. H., Chen, K. J., Chu, Y. S., Chang, W. J., & Chen, M. J. (2007). A learning management system with knowledge management capability for collaborative learning. VIC. *Proceedings of the 2007 11th International Conference on Computer Supported Cooperative.*

20. Boggs, D. (2010). *SCORM/AICC standards used in web-based learning management systems.* Syberworks.

21. Van Rooij, S. W. (2010). Project management in instructional design: ADDIE is not enough. *British Journal of Educational Technology, 41,* 852–864.

PART IV

Healthcare IT Security, Privacy, and Confidentiality

Lori Reed-Fourquet, Editor

CHAPTER 24

Building Trust

Dixie B. Baker*

In this chapter you will learn how to
- Explain the relationship between dependability and healthcare quality and safety
- Identify and explain five guidelines for building dependable systems
- Present an informal assessment of the healthcare industry with respect to these guidelines

The healthcare industry is undergoing a dramatic transformation from today's inefficient, costly, manually intensive, crisis-driven model of care delivery to a more efficient, consumer-centric, science-based model that proactively focuses on health management and quality measurement. This transformation is driven by several factors, most prominently the skyrocketing cost of healthcare delivery, the exposure of patient-safety problems, and an aging, socially networked population that recognizes the potential for using health information technology (HIT) to dramatically reduce the cost and improve the quality of care, while involving consumers as active members of their care teams.

The U.S. Health Information Technology for Economic and Clinical Health (HITECH) Act that in 2009 was enacted as part of the American Recovery and Reinvestment Act (ARRA) provided major structural changes; funding for research, technical support, and training; and financial incentives designed to significantly expedite and accelerate this transformation.[1] The HITECH Act codified the Office of National Coordinator (ONC) for HIT and assigned it responsibility for developing a nationwide infrastructure that would facilitate the use and exchange of electronic health information, including policy, standards, implementation specifications, and certification criteria. In enacting the HITECH Act, Congress recognized that the meaningful use and exchange of electronic health records (EHRs) were key to improving the quality, safety, and efficiency of the U.S. healthcare system.

* Adapted from Virginia K. Saba and Kathleen A. McCormick, *Essentials of Nursing Informatics, Fifth Edition* 265–278. © 2011 by The McGraw-Hill Companies.

At the same time, the HITECH Act recognized that as more health information was recorded and exchanged electronically to coordinate care, monitor quality, measure outcomes, and report public health threats, the risk to personal privacy and patient safety would be heightened. This recognition is reflected in the fact that four of the eight areas the HITECH Act identified as priorities for the ONC specifically addressed risks to individual privacy and information security:

1. Technologies that protect the privacy of health information and promote security in a qualified electronic health record, including for the segmentation and protection from disclosure of specific and sensitive individually identifiable health information, with the goal of minimizing the reluctance of patients to seek care (or disclose information about a condition) because of privacy concerns, in accordance with applicable law, and for the use and disclosure of limited data sets of such information

2. A nationwide HIT infrastructure that allows for the electronic use and accurate exchange of health information

3. Technologies that as a part of a qualified electronic health record allow for an accounting of disclosures made by a covered entity (as defined by the Health Insurance Portability and Accountability Act of 1996) for purposes of treatment, payment, and healthcare operations

4. Technologies that allow individually identifiable health information to be rendered unusable, unreadable, or indecipherable to unauthorized individuals when such information is transmitted in the nationwide health information network or physically transported outside the secured, physical perimeter of a healthcare provider, health plan, or healthcare clearinghouse

As noted by National Coordinator David Blumenthal, "Information is the lifeblood of modern medicine. Health information technology is destined to be its circulatory system. Without that system, neither individual physicians nor healthcare institutions can perform at their best or deliver the highest-quality care."[2] To carry Dr. Blumenthal's analogy one step further, at the heart of modern medicine lies "trust." Caregivers must trust that the technology and information they need will be available when they are needed at the point of care. They must trust that the information in an individual's EHR is accurate and complete and that it has not been accidentally or intentionally corrupted, modified, or destroyed. Consumers must trust that their caregivers will keep their most private health information confidential and will disclose and use it only to the extent necessary and in ways that are legal, ethical, and authorized consistent with the consumer's personal expectations and preferences. Above all else, both providers and consumers must trust that the technology and services they use will "do no harm."

The medical field is firmly grounded in a tradition of ethics, patient advocacy, care quality, and human safety. Medical professionals are well indoctrinated on clinical practice that respects personal privacy and protects confidential information and life-critical information services. Physicians and other medical professionals promise to uphold the Hippocratic Oath to "prescribe regimens for the good of [their] patients," to "never do harm," and to "keep secret" knowledge they acquire as they exercise their profession.[3] The American Nurses Association's (ANA's) *Code of Ethics for Nurses with Interpretive Statements* includes a commitment to "promote, advocate for, and strive to protect the health, safety, and rights of the patient,"[4] and the International Council of Nurses (ICN) *Code of Ethics for Nurses* affirms that the nurse "holds in confidence personal information" and "ensures that use of technology…[is] compatible with the safety, dignity, and rights of people."[5] Fulfilling these ethical obligations is the individual responsibility of each healthcare professional, who must trust that the information technology she relies upon will help and not harm patients and will protect their private information.

Recording, storing, and exchanging information electronically does indeed introduce new risks. As anyone who has used a desktop or mobile computer knows, it takes only a few keystrokes or screen taps to instantaneously send information to millions of people throughout the world. Try doing that with a paper record and a fax machine! We also know that nefarious "spyware," "viruses," and "Trojan horses" skulk around the Internet and insert themselves deep inside our computers' software, eager to capture our passwords, identities, and credit card numbers.

At the same time, HIT makes it possible to receive laboratory results within seconds after a biological sample has been analyzed; to continuously monitor a patient's condition remotely, without requiring him to leave his home; or to be given expert guidance and decision support specifically applicable to a patient's condition and history.

As HIT assumes a central role in the provision of care and in healthcare decision-making, the medical practitioner increasingly must trust HIT to provide timely access to accurate and complete health information and to offer personalized clinical decision support based on that information, while assuring that individual privacy is continuously protected. Legal and ethical obligations, as well as consumer expectations, drive requirements for assurance that data and applications will be available when they are needed, that private and confidential information will be protected, that data will not be modified or destroyed other than as authorized, that systems will be responsive and usable, and that systems designed to perform health-critical functions will do so safely. These are the attributes of trustworthy HIT. The Markle Foundation's Connecting for Health collaboration identified privacy and security as technology principles fundamental to trust: "All health information exchange, including in support of the delivery of care and the conduct of research and public health reporting, must be conducted in an environment of trust, based on conformance with appropriate requirements for patient privacy, security, confidentiality, integrity, audit, and informed consent."[6]

Many people think of "security" and "privacy" as synonymous. Indeed, these concepts are related—security mechanisms can help protect personal privacy by assuring that confidential personal information is accessible only by authorized individuals and entities. However, privacy is more than security, and security is more than privacy. Healthcare privacy principles were first articulated in 1973 in a U.S. Department of Health, Education, and Welfare report (entitled "Records, Computers, and the Rights of Citizens") as "fair information practice principles."[7] The Markle Foundation's Connecting for Health collaboration updated these principles to incorporate the new risks created by a networked environment in which health information routinely is electronically captured, used, and exchanged.[6] Other national and international privacy and security principles have also been developed that focus on individually identifiable information in an electronic environment (including but not limited to health). Based on these works, the ONC developed a Nationwide Privacy and Security Framework for electronic exchange of individually identifiable health information that identified eight principles intended to guide the actions of all people and entities that participate in networked, electronic exchange of individually identifiable health information.[8] These principles, described in Table 24-1, essentially articulate the "rights" of individuals to openness, transparency, fairness, and choice in the collection and use of their health information.

Principle	Description
Individual access	Individuals should be provided simple and timely means to access and obtain their individually identifiable health information in a readable form and format.
Correction	Individuals should be provided a timely means to dispute the accuracy or integrity of their individually identifiable health information and to have erroneous information corrected or the dispute documented.
Openness and transparency	Policies, procedures, and technologies that directly affect individuals and their individually identifiable health information should be open and transparent.
Individual choice	Individuals should be provided a reasonable opportunity and capability to make informed decisions about the collection, use, and disclosure of their individually identifiable health information.
Collection and use	Individually identifiable health information should be collected, used, and/or disclosed only to the extent necessary to accomplish a specified purpose(s) and never to discriminate inappropriately.
Data quality and integrity	People and entities should take reasonable steps to ensure that individually identifiable health information is complete, accurate, and up-to-date to the extent necessary for intended purposes and that it has not been altered or destroyed in an unauthorized manner.
Safeguards	Individually identifiable health information should be protected with reasonable administrative, technical, and physical safeguards to ensure its confidentiality, integrity, and availability and to prevent unauthorized or inappropriate access, use, or disclosure.
Accountability	These principles should be implemented—and adherence assured—through appropriate monitoring and other means, and methods should be in place to report and mitigate non-adherence and breaches.

Table 24-1   Eight Principles for Private and Secure Electronic Exchange of Individually Identifiable Health Information

Whereas privacy has to do with an individual's right to be left alone, security deals with protection, some of which supports that right. Security mechanisms and assurance methods are used to protect the confidentiality and authenticity of information, the integrity of data, and the availability of information and services; as well as to provide an accurate record of activities and accesses to information. While these mechanisms and methods are critical to protecting personal privacy, they are also essential in protecting patient safety and care quality—and in engendering trust in electronic systems and information. For example, if laboratory results are corrupted during transmission or historical data in an EHR is overwritten, the medical practitioner is likely to lose confidence that the HIT can be trusted to help him provide quality care. If a sensor system designed to track wandering Alzheimer's patients shuts down without alarming those depending upon it, patients' lives are put at risk!

Trustworthiness is an attribute of each system component and of integrated enterprise systems as a whole—including those components that may exist in "clouds." Trustworthiness is difficult to retrofit, as it must be designed and built into the system from the outset and conscientiously preserved as the system evolves. Discovering that an operational system cannot be trusted generally indicates that extensive—and expensive—changes to the system are needed. In this chapter, we introduce a framework for achieving and maintaining trustworthiness in HIT.

When Things Go Wrong

Although we would like to be able to assume that computers, networks, and software are as trustworthy as our toasters and refrigerators, unfortunately that is not the case. One of the more dramatic examples became the cover story for the February 2003 issue of *CIO Magazine*, which relates in detail the occurrence and recovery from "one of the worst healthcare IT crises in history"—a catastrophic failure in the network infrastructure that supported CareGroup, one of the most prestigious healthcare organizations in the United States. The source of the problem ultimately was traced to switches that directed network traffic over a highly overburdened and fragile network that was further taxed when a researcher uploaded a multigigabyte file into the picture archiving and communication system (PACS). The failure resulted in a four-hour closure of the emergency room, a complete shutdown of the network, and two days of paper-based clinical operations—a true "retro" experience for many of the physicians who had never practiced without computers. Network services were not fully recovered until six days after the onset of the disaster, and CareGroup learned a valuable lesson about network sizing and scalability.[9]

Between May 2005 and June 2006, an employee with access to electronic patient information at the Cleveland Clinic's office in Weston, Florida, downloaded the personal identification information of approximately 1,500 patients. The medical identity information stolen included patients' names, dates of birth, Social Security numbers, Medicare numbers, and home addresses. The Medicare numbers and patient identity information were ultimately used by medical services providers in Miami Dade County to fraudulently bill Medicare for approximately $8 million for medical services that had not been delivered and medical equipment that had not been supplied.[10]

Use Case 24-1: Stolen IDs Can Put Patient Safety at Risk

In 2006, a 27-year-old mother of four children in Salt Lake City received a phone call from a Utah social worker notifying her that her newborn had tested positive for methamphetamines and that the state planned to remove all of her children from her home. The young mother had not been pregnant in more than two years, but her stolen driver's license had ended up in the hands of a meth user who gave birth using the stolen identity. After a few tense days of urgent phone calls with child services, the victim was allowed to keep her children. She hired an attorney to sort out the damages to her legal and medical records. Months later, when she needed treatment for a kidney infection, she carefully avoided the hospital where her stolen identity had been used. But her caution did no good—her electronic record, with the identity thief's medical information intermingled, had circulated to hospitals throughout the community. The hospital worked with the victim to correct her charts to avoid making life-critical decisions based on erroneous information. The data corruption damage could have been far worse had the thief's baby not tested positive for methamphetamines, bringing the theft to the victim's attention.[11]

In July 2009, after noting several instances of computer viruses affecting the United Kingdom's National Health Service (NHS) hospitals, a British news broadcasting station conducted a survey of the NHS trusts throughout England to determine how many of their systems had been infected by computer viruses. Seventy-five percent replied, reporting that over 8,000 viruses had penetrated their security systems, with 12 incidents affecting clinical departments, putting patient care at risk and exposing personal information. One Scottish trust was attacked by the Conficker virus, which shut down computers for two days. Some attacks were used to steal personal information, and at a cancer center, 51 appointments and radiotherapy sessions had to be rescheduled.[12] The survey seemed to have little effect in reducing the threat—less than a year later, NHS systems were victimized by the Qakbot data-stealing worm, which infected over a thousand computers and stole massive amounts of information.[13]

Even antivirus software may not be as trustworthy as one would hope. In April 2010, computers throughout the United States began rebooting themselves when a software update caused an antivirus program to identify a normal Microsoft Windows file as a virus. The problem forced about a third of the hospitals in Rhode Island to postpone elective surgeries and stop treating nontrauma emergency-room patients.[14]

The HITECH Act introduced a federal requirement for covered entities to notify individuals whose unsecured protected health information may have been exposed due to a security breach.

 TIP Breaches affecting 500 or more individuals must be immediately reported to the secretary of the Department of Health and Human Services, who must post a list of such breaches to a public web site.

Between September 22, 2009, and April 12, 2012, a total of 435 breaches, from 47 states plus the District of Columbia and Puerto Rico, were reported on the HHS web site—affecting over 20 million individuals![15] A whopping 293 of the breaches (67 percent) were attributed to theft or loss of computer equipment, portable devices, and electronic media—the most visible and easily detected types of breaches. Thus one might surmise that this accounting may be just the tip of the iceberg of electronic breaches of health information.

The bottom line is that systems, networks, and software applications, as well as the enterprises within which they are used, are highly complex, and the only safe assumption is that "things will go wrong." Trustworthiness is an essential attribute for the systems, software, services, processes, and people used to manage individuals' health information and to help provide safe, high-quality healthcare.

HIT Trust Framework

Trustworthiness can never be achieved by implementing a few policies and procedures and some security technology. Trustworthiness requires a complete HIT trust framework that starts with an objective assessment of risk. This risk assessment must be conscientiously applied throughout the development and implementation of policies, operational procedures, and security safeguards built on a solid system architecture. This trust framework is depicted in Figure 24-1 and comprises seven layers of protection, each of which is dependent on the layers below it (indicated by the arrows in the figure), and all of which must work together to provide a trustworthy HIT environment for healthcare delivery.

Layer 1: Risk Management

Risk management is the foundation of the HIT trust framework. Objective risk assessment informs decision making and positions the organization to correct those physical, operational, and technical deficiencies that pose the highest risk to the information assets within the enterprise. Objective risk assessment also puts in place protections that will enable the organization to manage the residual risk and liability.

 TIP Patient safety, individual privacy, and information security all relate to risk, which is simply the probability that some "bad thing" will happen to adversely affect a valued asset. Risk is always considered with respect to a given context comprising relevant threats, vulnerabilities, and valued assets. Threats can be natural occurrences (e.g., earthquake, hurricane), accidents, or malicious people and software programs. Vulnerabilities are present in facilities, hardware, software, communication systems, business processes, workforces, and electronic data. Valued assets can be anything from reputation to business infrastructure to information to human lives.

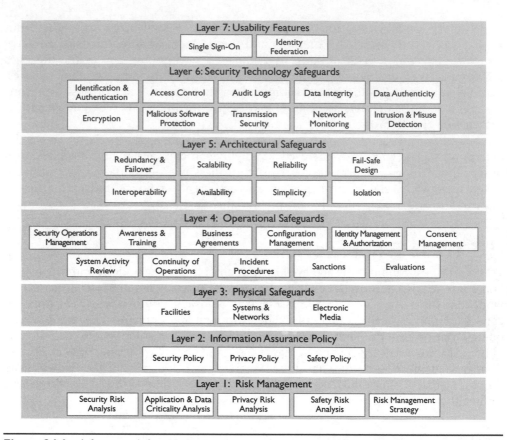

Figure 24-1 A framework for achieving and maintaining trustworthiness in health information technology comprises multiple layers of trust, beginning with objective risk assessment that serves as the foundation for information assurance policy and operational, architectural, and technological safeguards.

A security risk is the probability that a threat will exploit a vulnerability to expose confidential information, corrupt or destroy data, or interrupt or deny essential information services. If that risk could result in the unauthorized disclosure of an individual's private health information or the compromise of an individual's identity, it also represents a privacy risk. If the risk could result in the corruption of clinical data or an interruption in the availability of a safety-critical system, causing human harm or the loss of life, it is a safety risk as well.

Information security is widely viewed as the protection of information confidentiality, data integrity, and service availability. Indeed, these are the three types of technical safeguards directly addressed by the Health Insurance Portability and Accountability Act (HIPAA) Security Rule.[16] Generally, safety is most closely associated with protective measures for data integrity and the availability of life-critical information and services, while privacy is more often linked to confidentiality. However, the unauthorized exposure of private health information, or corruption of one's personal electronic health record as a result of an identity theft, can also put an individual's health, safety, lifestyle, and livelihood at risk.

Risk management is an ongoing, individualized discipline wherein each individual or each organization examines its own threats, vulnerabilities, and valued assets and decides for itself how to deal with identified risks—whether to reduce or eliminate them, counter them with protective measures, or tolerate them and prepare for the consequences. Risks to personal privacy, patient safety, care quality, financial stability, and public trust all must be considered in developing an overall strategy for managing risks both internal and external to an organization.

 TIP Resource virtualizations—from Internet transmissions to "cloud" computing—present particular challenges because the computing and networking resources used may be outside the physical and operational control of the subscriber and are likely to be shared with other subscribers.

Layer 2: Information Assurance Policy

The risk management strategy will identify what risks need to be addressed through an information assurance policy that governs operations, information technology, and individual behavior. The information assurance policy comprises rules that guide organizational decision-making, and that define behavioral expectations and sanctions for unacceptable actions. The policy defines rules for protecting individuals' private information, protecting the security of that information, and providing choice and transparency with respect to how individuals' health information is safely used and shared. It includes rules that protect human beings, including patients, employees, family members, and visitors, from physical harm that could result from data corruption or service interruption. Overall, the information assurance policy defines the rules enforced to protect the organization's valued information assets from identified risks to personal privacy, information confidentiality, data integrity, and service availability.

Some policy rules will be mandated by applicable state and federal laws and regulations. For example, the HIPAA Security Rule requires compliance with a set of administrative, physical, and technical standards, and the HIPAA Privacy Rule sets forth privacy policies to be implemented.[17] The HITECH Act's privacy and security provisions strengthened and built upon the HIPAA standards. In addition, state and local privacy and security laws will need to be translated into organizational policy rules. However, although the HIPAA regulations establish uniform minimum privacy and security standards, state health privacy laws are quite diverse. Because the HIPAA regulations apply only to "covered entities" and their "business associates" and not to everyone who may hold health information, and because the HIPAA regulations preempt only those state laws that are less stringent, the privacy protections of individuals and the security protections of health information varies depending on who is holding the information and the state in which they are located.[18]

The HIT information assurance policy provides the foundation for the development and implementation of physical, operational, architectural, and security technology safeguards. Medical practitioners can provide valuable insights, recommendations, and advocacy in the formulation of information assurance policy within the organizations where they practice, as well as within their professional organizations and with state and federal governments.

Layer 3: Physical Safeguards

Physically safeguarding health information and the information technology used to collect, store, retrieve, analyze, and exchange that information is essential to assuring that information needed at the point and time of care is available, trustworthy, and usable in providing quality healthcare. Although the electronic signals that represent health information are not themselves "physical," the facilities within which data is generated, stored, displayed, and used; the media on which data is recorded; the information system hardware used to process, access, and display the data; and the communications equipment used to transmit and route the data are. So are the people who generate, access, and use the information the data represents. Physical safeguards are essential to protecting these assets in accordance with the information assurance policy.

 TIP The HIPAA Security Rule prescribes four standards for physically safeguarding electronic health information protected under HIPAA: facility-access controls, workstation use, workstation security, and device and media controls. Physically safeguarding the lives and well-being of patients is central to the roles and responsibilities of nurses. Protecting patients requires the physical protection of the media on which their health data are recorded, as well as the devices, systems, networks, and facilities involved in data collection, use, storage, and disposal.

Healthcare organizations are increasingly choosing to rely on third parties to provide physical security for their applications and data. Third parties include EHR software-as-a-service (SaaS) subscriptions, outsourced hosting services, and cloud storage and platform offerings. The HIPAA Security Rule requires that the providers of these services sign a business associate agreement in which they agree to meet all of the HIPAA security standards. However, if a breach occurs, the covered entity remains primarily responsible for reporting and recovering from a breach. So it is essential that healthcare entities perform due diligence to assure that their business associates understand and are capable of providing the required level of physical protection and data isolation.

Layer 4: Operational Safeguards

Operational safeguards are processes, procedures, and practices that govern the creation, handling, usage, and sharing of health information in accordance with the information assurance policy. The HIT trust framework shown in Figure 24-1 includes the following operational safeguards.

Security Operations Management

HIPAA regulations require that each healthcare organization designate a "security official" and a "privacy official" to be responsible for developing and implementing security and privacy policies and procedures. The management of services relating to the protection of health information and patient privacy touches every function within a healthcare organization.

Awareness and Training

One of the most valuable actions a healthcare organization can take to maintain public trust is to inculcate a culture of safety, privacy, and security. If every person employed by, or associated with, an organization feels individually responsible for protecting the confidentiality, integrity, and availability of health information and the privacy and safety of patients, the risk for that organization will be vastly reduced! Recognition of the value of workforce training is reflected in the fact that the HIPAA Security and Privacy Rules require training in security and privacy, respectively, for all members of the workforce. Formal privacy and security training should be required to be completed at least annually, augmented by simple reminders.

Business Agreements

Business agreements help manage risk and bound liability, clarify responsibilities and expectations, and define processes for addressing disputes among parties. The HIPAA Privacy and Security Rules require that each person or organization that provides to a covered entity services involving individually identifiable health information must sign a "business associate" contract obligating the service provider to comply with HIPAA requirements, subject to the same enforcement and sanctions as covered entities. The HIPAA Privacy Rule also requires "data use agreements" defining how "limited data sets" will be used. Agreements are only as trustworthy as the entities that sign them. Organizations should exercise due diligence in deciding with whom they will enter into business agreements.

Configuration Management

Configuration management refers to processes and procedures for maintaining an accurate and consistent accounting of the physical and functional attributes of a system throughout its life cycle. From an information assurance perspective, configuration management is the process of controlling and documenting modifications to the hardware, firmware, software, and documentation involved in the protection of information assets.

Identity Management and Authorization

From a general information-assurance perspective, identity management involves the establishment and validation of the identity of each individual or entity with access to system resources; the authorization and assignment of roles, capabilities, and privileges to that identity; the control of accesses related to those entitlements, including the authentication of asserted identity; the termination of identities and authorizations; and the maintenance of the governance processes that support this life cycle. In a healthcare environment, identity management extends to assuring that patients are who they claim to be—a serious data integrity and patient safety consideration.

As noted in the previous section, medical identity theft has become a significant risk that identity-management processes and procedures must address.

Consent Management

Both federal and state laws, including the HIPAA Privacy Rule, set forth requirements for obtaining an individual's permission before collecting, retaining, or exchanging his or her personal health information. Certain types of information, such as psychiatric notes and substance abuse records, have special restrictions and authorization requirements. In addition, medical ethics require that providers obtain a patient's "informed consent" before administering treatment or retaining biological specimens. Managing these permissions and assuring that the consumer's privacy preferences are consistently adhered to across care settings is a complex process, but essential to protecting personal privacy. Today, consent management is primarily a manual process that is usually applied to an individual's complete record. However, a HITECH Act requirement calling for policy and standards for data "segmentation" that would enable an individual to specifically "segment out" specific, sensitive information for additional levels of protection will change that in the future. Current investigations and standard-development activities are exploring methods for electronically "tagging" data with metadata containing consent policies that would persist with the data as they move from provider to provider, so that these policies would be enforced consistently across time and care settings.

System Activity Review

One of the most effective means of detecting potential misuse and abuse of privileges is by regularly reviewing records of information system activity, such as audit logs, facility access reports, and security incident tracking reports. Although technology to automate system-activity review exists, few healthcare organizations use these tools; most system-activity review is conducted either manually or is semi-automated.[19] As more clinical data are generated and exchanged, the sheer volume will overpower system-activity review as a manual operation. Moreover, the HITECT Act's breach-notification requirement will require the use of forensic techniques to investigate the cause and source of breaches and to create a legal audit trail, and the need for timeliness in investigating breaches will inevitably require automated support for audit analysis. In addition, the HITECH Act's requirement to maintain an accounting of disclosures between organizations will likely use audit data as an input.

Continuity of Operations

Unexpected events, both natural and human-produced, do happen, and when they do, it is important that critical health services can continue to be provided. As healthcare organizations become increasingly dependent on electronic health information and information systems, the need to plan for unexpected events and for operational procedures that enable the organization to continue to function through emergencies becomes more urgent. The HIPAA Security Rule requires that organizations establish and implement policies and procedures for responding to an emergency. Contingency planning is part of an organization's risk-management strategy, and the first step is performed as part of a risk assessment—identifying those software applications and data that are essential for enabling operations to continue under emergency conditions and for returning to full operations. These business-critical systems are those to which architectural safeguards such as fail-safe design, redundancy and failover, and availability engineering should be applied.

Incident Procedures

Awareness and training should include a clear explanation of what an individual should do if she suspects a security incident, such as a malicious code infiltration, denial-of-service attack, or a breach of confidential information. Organizations need to plan their response to an incident report, including procedures for investigating and resolving the incident, notifying individuals whose health information may have been exposed as a result of the incident, and penalizing parties responsible for the incident. As noted above, the HITECH Act requires notification of individuals whose information may have been exposed as a result of a breach.

Not all incidents are major or require enterprise-wide response. Some PHI disclosures may be as simple as a user accidentally including PHI in a request from the help desk. Incident procedures should not require a user or helpdesk operator to make a judgment call on the seriousness of a disclosure; procedures should be clear about what an individual should do when she notices a potential disclosure.

Sanctions

The HIPAA law[20] and the HITECH Act prescribe severe civil and criminal penalties for sanctioning organizations and individuals that fail to comply with the privacy and security provisions. Organizations must implement appropriate sanctions to penalize workforce members who fail to comply with privacy and security policies and procedures.

Evaluation

Periodic, objective evaluation of the operational and technical safeguards in place helps measure the effectiveness, or "outcomes," of the security management program. A formal evaluation should be conducted at least annually and should involve independent participants who are not responsible for the program. Security evaluation should include resources and services maintained within the enterprise, as well as resources and services provided by business associates—including SaaS and cloud-services providers. Independent evaluators can be from either within or outside an organization, as long as they can be objective. In addition to the annual programmed evaluation, security technology safeguards should be evaluated whenever changes in circumstances or events occur that affect the risk profile of the organization.

Layer 5: Architectural Safeguards

A system's architecture comprises its individual hardware and software components, the relationships among them, their relationship with the environment, and the principles that govern the system's design and evolution over time. As shown in Figure 24-1, specific architectural design principles and the hardware and software components that support those principles work together to establish the technical foundation for security technology safeguards. In simpler times, the hardware and software components that comprised an enterprise's architecture were under the physical and logical control of the enterprise itself, but in an era when an enterprise may depend upon external services (e.g., a health exchange service, external back-up service) and virtualized services (e.g., SaaS, cloud storage), this may not be the case. Still, the design principles discussed below apply whether an enterprise's architecture is centralized or distributed, physical or virtual.

Redundancy and Failover

Security- and safety-critical system components and services should be engaged and integrated so that no single point of failure exists. If a given component or service fails, the system should engage a second, back-up component or service, with no breach of sensitive information, interruption of operations, or corruption of data.

Scalability

As more health information is recorded, stored, used, and exchanged electronically, systems and networks must be able to deal with that growth. The catastrophic failure at CareGroup (mentioned earlier in this chapter) resulted from the network's inability to scale to the capacity required. The latest stage in the evolution of the Internet specifically addresses the scalability issue by virtualizing computing resources into services, including software as a service (SaaS), platforms as a service (PaaS), and infrastructure as a service (IaaS)—collectively referred to as "cloud" services. Indeed, the Internet itself was created on the same principle as cloud computing—the creation of a virtual, ubiquitous, continuously expanding network through the sharing of resources (servers) owned by different entities. Whenever one sends information over the Internet, the information is broken into small packets that are then sent ("hop") from server to server from source to destination, with all of the servers in between being "public"—in the sense that they probably belong to someone other than the sender or the receiver. Cloud computing, a model for provisioning "on demand" computing services accessible over the Internet, pushes virtualization to a new level by sharing applications, storage, and computing power to offer flexible scalability beyond what would be economically possible otherwise.

Reliability

Reliability is the ability of a system or component to perform its specified functions consistently and over a specified period of time—an essential attribute of trustworthiness.

Fail-Safe Design

Safety-critical components, software, and systems should be designed so that if they fail, the failure will not cause people to be physically harmed. Note that fail-safe design may indicate that under certain circumstances, a component should be shut down or forced to cease to perform its usual functions in order to avoid harming someone. So the interrelationships among redundancy and failover, reliability, and fail-safe design are complex, yet critical to patient safety. The "break-the-glass" feature that enables an unauthorized user to gain access to patient information in an emergency situation is an example of fail-safe design. If, in an emergency, an EHR system "fails" to provide a nurse access to the clinical information he needs to deliver care, the "break-the-glass" feature will enable the system to "fail safely." Fail-safe methods are particularly important in research. where new treatment protocols and devices are being tested for safety.

Interoperability

Interoperability is the ability of systems and system components to work together. To exchange health information effectively, healthcare systems must interoperate not only at the technical level but also at the syntactic and semantic levels. The Internet and its protocols, which have been adopted for use within enterprises as well, transmit data (packets of electronic bits) over a network so that they arrive at their destination the same as when they were sent. But then, if the data are encrypted, the receiving system must decrypt the data, open electronic messages, extract content, and translate the bits into health information that its applications and users will understand. Open standards, including encryption, messaging, and transport standards, and standard vocabulary for coding and exchanging security attributes and patient permissions—e.g., HL7 Version 3 Confidentiality Code System,[21] Security Assertion Markup Language (SAML)[22]—are fundamental to implementing interoperable healthcare systems.

Availability

Required services and information must be available and usable when they are needed. Availability is measured as the proportion of time a system is in a functioning condition. A reciprocal dependency exists between security technology safeguards and high-availability design—security safeguards depend on the availability of systems, networks, and information, which in turn enable those safeguards to protect enterprise assets against threats to availability, such as denial-of-service attacks. Resource virtualization and "cloud" computing are important technologies for helping assure availability.

Simplicity

Safe, secure architectures are designed to minimize complexity. The simplest design and integration strategy will be the easiest to understand, maintain, and recover in the case of a failure or disaster.

Isolation

Isolation refers to the extent to which processes running on the same system at different trust levels, virtual machines (VMs) running on the same hardware, or applications running on the same computer or tablet are kept separate so that if one process, VM, or application misbehaves or is compromised, other processes, VMs, or applications can continue to operate safely and securely. Isolation is particularly important to preserve the integrity of the operating system itself. Within an operating system, functions critical to the security and reliability of the system execute within a protected hardware state, while untrusted applications execute within a separate state. However, this hardware architectural isolation is undermined if the system is configured so that untrusted applications are allowed to run with privilege, and then the operating system itself is put at risk. For example, if a user logs into an account with administrative privileges and then runs an infected application (or opens an infected email attachment), the entire operating system becomes infected. Within a cloud environment, the hypervisor is assigned responsibility for assuring that VMs are kept separate so that processes running on one subscriber's VM cannot interfere with those running on another VM. In general, the same security safeguards used to protect an enterprise system are equally effective in a cloud environment—but only if the hypervisor is able to maintain isolation among virtual environments. In the Apple iOS environment, apps running on an iPad or iPhone are isolated—not only are they unable to view or modify each other's data; one app does not even know whether another app is installed on the device (Apple calls this architectural feature "sandboxing").

Layer 6: Security Technology Safeguards

Security technology safeguards are software and hardware services specifically designed to perform security-related functions. All of the security services depicted in Figure 24-1 are technical safeguards required by the HIPAA Security Rule. Table 24-2 identifies a number of open standards that are used to implement these functions.

Safeguard	Standard	Description
Identification and authentication	ITU-T X.509: Information technology—open systems interconnection—the directory: public-key and attribute-certificate frameworks	Standard for public-key infrastructure (PKI), single sign-on, and privilege-management infrastructure (PMI); includes standard formats for public-key certificates, certificate revocation lists, attribute certificates, and a certification path-validation algorithm
	OASIS security assertion markup language (SAML)	XML-based protocol for exchanging authentication and authorization data ("assertions") between an identity provider and a service provider; used to enable single sign-on
	OpenID authentication	An open standard that describes how users can be authenticated in a decentralized manner
Access control	ANSI/INCITS 359-2004: Information technology—role-based access control (RBAC)	Specifies RBAC elements (users, roles, permissions, operations, objects) and features required by an RBAC system
	HL7 Version 3 confidentiality code system	HL7 V3 value set for coding confidentiality attributes
	HL7 Version 3 role-based access control (RBAC) health-care permission catalog	Permission vocabulary to support RBAC, consistent with OASIS XACML and ANSI INCITS RBAC standards
	OASIS extensible access control markup language (XACML)	XML-based language for expressing information technology security policy

Table 24-2   Many Open Standards Address Security Technology Safeguards

Safeguard	Standard	Description
Audit logging	ASTM E-2147-01: Standard specification for audit and disclosure logs for use in health information systems	Specifies how to design audit logs to record accesses within a computer system and disclosure logs to document disclosures to external users
Data integrity	FIPS PUB 180-3 secure hash standard (SHS)	Specifies five hash algorithms that can be used to generate message digests used to detect whether messages have been changed since the digests were generated
Data authenticity (nonrepudiation)	ASTM E-1762-95(2003): Standard guide for electronic authentication of healthcare information	Standard on the design, implementation, and use of electronic signatures to authenticate healthcare data
	ETSI TS 101 903: XML advanced electronic signatures (XadES)	Defines XML formats for advanced electronic signatures, based on the use of public-key cryptography supported by public-key certificates
Encryption (confidentiality)	FIPS 197, advanced encryption standard, Nov 2001	Specifies a symmetric cryptographic algorithm that can be used to protect electronic data
Transmission security	IETF transport layer security (TLS) protocol: RFC 2246, RFC 3546	Standard for establishing secured channel at layer 4 (transport) of the open systems interconnection (OSI) model; includes authentication of sender and receiver and encryption and integrity protection of the communication channel
	IETF IP security protocol (IPsec): RFCs listed at http://datatracker.ietf.org/wg/ipsec/	Standard for establishing virtual private network (VPN) at layer 3 (network) of the OSI model; includes authentication of sender and receiver and encryption and integrity protection of the communication channel
	IETF secure/multipurpose internet mail extensions (S/MIME): RFC 2633	Internet mail protocol for providing authentication, message integrity, and nonrepudiation of origin (digital signatures), and confidentiality protection (encryption)
	OASIS WS-security (WSS)	Extension to the simple object access protocol (SOAP) transport protocol used to access web services; includes encryption and digital signing of messages and exchange of security tokens, including SAML assertions

ANSI: American National Standards Institute; ASTM, ASTM International (originally American Society for Testing and Materials); ETSI: European Telecommunications Standards Institute; FIPS: National Institute of Standards and Technology (NIST) Federal Information Processing Standard; HL7: Health Level Seven; IETF: Internet Engineering Task Force; INCITS: InterNational Committee for Information Technology Standards; ITU-T: International Telecommunication Union—Telecommunication Standardization Sector; OASIS: Organization for the Advancement of Structured Information Standards

Table 24-2 Many Open Standards Address Security Technology Safeguards *(continued)*

Identification and Authentication

The identity of all entities, whether they are people or software applications, must be clearly established before they are allowed to access protected systems, applications, and data. Identity management and authorization processes are used to validate identities and to assign them system rights and privileges. Then, whenever the person or application requires access, it asserts an identity and authenticates that identity by providing some "proof" in the form of something it has (e.g., smartcard), something it knows (e.g., password, private encryption key), or something it is (e.g., fingerprint). While only people can authenticate themselves using biometrics, both people and software applications can authenticate themselves by exchanging digital certificates.

Access Control

Access-control services help assure that people, computer systems, and software applications are able to use all of (and only) the resources (e.g., computers, networks, applications, services, data files, information) they are authorized to use and only within the constraints of the authorization. Access controls protect against unauthorized use, disclosure, modification, and destruction of resources and unauthorized execution of system functions. Access-control rules are based on federal and state laws and regulations, the enterprise's information assurance policy, as well as consumer-elected preferences. These rules may be based on the user's identity, the user's role, the context of the request (e.g., location, time of day), and/or a combination of the sensitivity attributes of the data and the user's authorizations.

Audit Logging

Security auditing is the process of collecting and recording information about security-relevant events. Audit logs are generated by multiple software components within a system, including operating systems, servers, firewalls, applications, and database management systems. Many healthcare organizations rely heavily on audit log review to detect potential intrusions and misuse.

Data Integrity

Data integrity services provide assurance that electronic data have not been modified or destroyed except as authorized. Cryptographic hash functions are commonly used for this purpose. A cryptographic hash function is a mathematical algorithm that uses a block of data as input to generate a "hash value" such that any change to the data will change the hash value that represents it. Although hash functions cannot prevent modification or identify what change occurred, they can detect when the data has been changed and therefore should not be trusted.

Data Authenticity

Sometimes the need arises to assure not only that data have not been modified inappropriately but also that the data are in fact from an authentic source. This need, sometimes referred to as *nonrepudiation*, can be met through the use of digital signatures. Digital signatures use public-key (assymetric) encryption (see "Encryption" below) to encrypt a block of data using the signer's private key. To authenticate that the data block was signed by the entity claimed, one only needs to try decrypting the data using the signer's public key; if the data block decrypts successfully, its authenticity is assured.

Encryption

Encryption is simply the process of obfuscating information by running the data representing it through an algorithm (sometimes called a *cipher*) to make the information unreadable until it has been decrypted by someone possessing the proper encryption key. Symmetric encryption uses the same key to both encrypt and decrypt data, while asymmetric encryption (also known as *public-key encryption*) uses two keys that are mathematically related—one key is used for encryption and the other for decryption. One key is called a private key and is held secret; the other is called a public key and is openly published. Which key is used for encryption and which for decryption depends on the assurance objective. For example, secure e-mail encrypts the message contents using the recipient's public key (so that only the recipient can decrypt and view it) and then digitally signs the message using the sender's own private key (so that if the sender's public key will decrypt it, the recipient will be assured that the sender actually sent it).

Malicious Software Protection

Malicious software, also called *malware*, is any software program designed to infiltrate a system without the user's permission, with the intent to damage or disrupt operations or use unauthorized resources. Malicious software includes programs commonly called viruses, worms, Trojan horses, and spyware. Protecting against malicious software requires not only technical solutions to prevent, detect, and remove these intruders but also policies and procedures for reporting suspected attacks.

Transmission Security

Sensitive and safety-critical electronic data that are transmitted over open, vulnerable networks such as the Internet must be protected against unauthorized disclosure and modification. The Internet protocol was designed with no protection against the disclosure or modification of any transmissions and no assurance of the identity of any transmitters or receivers (or eavesdroppers). Internet traffic is clearly visible from every server through which it passes on its journey from source to destination. Protecting network transmissions between two entities (people, organizations, or software programs) requires that the communicating entities authenticate themselves to each other, confirm the integrity of the data exchanged (for example, by using a cryptographic hash function), and assure that data exchanged between them are encrypted.

Both the transport layer security (TLS) protocol[23] and Internet protocol security (IPsec) suite[24] support these functions, but at different layers in the open system interconnection (OSI) model.[25] TLS establishes protected channels at the OSI transport layer (layer 4), allowing software applications to exchange information securely. For example, TLS might be used to establish a secure link between a user's browser and a merchant's check-out application on the Web. IPsec establishes protected channels at the OSI network layer (layer 3), allowing Internet gateways to exchange information securely. For example, IPsec might be used to establish a virtual private network (VPN) that allows all hospitals within an integrated delivery system to openly yet securely exchange information. Because IPsec is implemented at the network layer, it is less vulnerable to malicious software applications than TLS and also less visible to users (for example, IPsec does not display an icon in a browser).

Network Monitoring

Network monitoring tools continuously monitor computer networks to detect slow or failing components, or bottlenecks in the network, that could indicate an impending or actual service outage. Network monitoring tools can detect problems caused by overloaded or crashed servers, network connections, or other devices connected to the network, and can alert system administrators when they need to take action.

Intrusion and Misuse Detection

Intrusion- and misuse-detection tools use information from network monitoring logs, system audit logs, application audit logs, and database audit logs to detect undesirable behavior. The principal difference between the two is that intrusion-detection tools attempt to detect intrusions instigated by unauthorized entities, usually from outside the enterprise, and misuse-detection tools target undesirable behavior by authorized users who are inappropriately using their rights and privileges.

Layer 7: Usability Features

The top layer of the trust framework includes services that make life easier for users. Both single sign-on and identity federation enable a user to authenticate herself once and then to access multiple applications, multiple databases, and even multiple enterprises for which she is authorized, without having to re-authenticate herself. Single sign-on often is referred to as a security service, but in fact it is a usability service that makes authentication services more palatable.

Single sign-on enables a user to navigate among authorized applications and resources within a single organization. Identity federation enables a user to navigate between services managed by different organizations. Both single sign-on and identity federation require the exchange of *security assertions*. Once the user has logged into a system, that system can pass the user's identity (along with other attributes, such as role, method of authentication, and time of login) to another entity using a security assertion. The receiving entity then enforces its own access control rules, based on the identity passed to it.

Neither single sign-on nor identity federation actually adds security protections (other than to reduce the need for users to post their passwords to their computer monitors). In fact, if the original authentication method is weak, the risk associated with that weakness will be propagated to any other entities to which the identity is passed. Therefore, whenever single sign-on or federated identity is implemented, a key consideration is the strength of the method used to authenticate the individual.

Chapter Review

Healthcare is in the midst of a dramatic and exciting transformation that will enable individual health information to be captured, used, and exchanged electronically using interoperable HIT. The potential impacts on individuals' health and on the health of entire populations are dramatic. Clinical decision support will help improve the safety and quality of healthcare. The availability of huge quantities of de-identified health information will help scientists discover the underlying genetic bases for diseases, leading to earlier and more accurate detection and diagnoses, more targeted and effective treatments, and ultimately personalized medicine.

In this chapter we have explained the critical role that trustworthiness plays in HIT adoption and in providing safe, private, high-quality care. We have introduced and described a trust framework comprising seven layers of protection essential for establishing and maintaining trust in a healthcare enterprise. Many of the safeguards included in the trust framework have been codified in HIPAA standards and implementation specifications. Building trustworthiness in HIT always begins with objective risk assessment, a continuous process that serves as the basis for developing and implementing a sound information assurance policy and physical, operational, architectural, and technological safeguards to mitigate and manage risks to patient safety, individual privacy, care quality, financial stability, and public trust.

Questions

To test your comprehension of the chapter, answer the following questions and then check your answers against the list of correct answers that follows the questions.

1. Which of the following is not one of the eight privacy principles defined by the Nationwide Privacy and Security Framework?

    A. Individual access

    B. Collection and use

    C. Accountability

    D. Trustworthiness

2. Breaches affecting 1000 or more individuals must be immediately reported to the secretary of the Department of Health and Human Services.

    A. True

    B. False

3. Which are three components of risk?

    A. Efficiency, effectiveness, and cost implications

    B. Threat, vulnerability, and valued asset

    C. Patient safety, individual privacy, and information security

    D. Reliability, scalability, and simplicity

4. Why do clouds present particular challenges in assessing risks?

   A. Clouds are likely to be shared with other subscribers.

   B. They provide too much transparency.

   C. They may be outside the physical and operational control of the subscriber.

   D. A and C

5. What components are included in an information assurance policy?

   A. Rules for protecting confidential information

   B. Rules for assigning roles and making access-control decisions

   C. Individual sanctions for violating rules for acceptable behavior

   D. All of the above

6. The HIPAA Security Rule prescribes four standards for physically safeguarding electronic health information protected under HIPAA. Which four are they?

   A. Redundancy, failover, reliability, and availability

   B. Isolation, simplicity, redundancy, and fail-safe design

   C. Interoperability, facility-access control, cloud control, and device control

   D. Facility-access control, workstation use, workstation security, and device and media controls

7. Which of the following is *not* an operational safeguard?

   A. Reliability

   B. Configuration management

   C. Sanctions

   D. Continuity of operations

8. The new push for virtualizing applications, storage, and computing power offers what dimension to your architectural safeguards?

   A. Scalability

   B. Data integrity

   C. Network audit and monitoring

   D. None of the above

9. Interoperability is the ability of systems and system components to work together.

   A. True

   B. False

10. What is a characteristic of isolation?

    A. The extent to which processes running on the same system at different trust levels, or virtual machines (VMs) running on the same hardware, or applications running on the same computer or tablet are kept separate

    B. The ability of a system or components to perform their specified functions

    C. Failure of one component will not cause people physical harm

    D. The "break-the-glass" feature that enables an unauthorized user to gain access to patient information in an emergency

11. Access controls protect against unauthorized use, disclosure, modifications, and destruction of resources and unauthorized execution of system functions.

    A. True

    B. False

12. What are two types of usability features?

    A. Data encryption and authenticity

    B. Access control and audit logs

    C. Malicious network protection and isolation

    D. Single sign-on and identity federation

Answers

1. **D.** Trustworthiness is not one of the eight privacy principles. The eight principles are individual access, correction, openness and transparency, individual choice, collection and use, data quality and integrity, safeguards, and accountability, as developed by the ONC for the purpose of guiding the actions of all people and entities that participate in networked, electronic exchange of individually identifiable health information.

2. **A.** Breaches affecting 500 or more individuals must be immediately reported to the secretary of the Department of Health and Human Services.

3. **B.** Risk is the probability that a threat will exploit a vulnerability to cause harm to a valued asset.

4. **D.** Clouds likely to be shared with other subscribers and may be outside the physical and operational control of the subscriber.

5. **D.** An information assurance policy should address all of these areas.

6. **D.** The HIPAA Security Rule prescribes four standards for physically safeguarding electronic health information protected under HIPAA: facility-access control, workstation use, workstation security, and device and media controls.

7. **A.** Reliability is an architectural safeguard, not an operational safeguard.

8. **A.** Virtualizing applications, storage, and computing power provides the capability to scale as the need and demand for these resources increases.

9. **A.** Interoperability is the ability of systems and system components to work together.

10. **A.** Isolation is the extent to which processes running on the same system at different trust levels, or virtual machines (VMs) running on the same hardware, or applications running on the same computer or tablet are kept separate.

11. **A.** Access controls protect against unauthorized use, disclosure, modification, and destruction of resources and unauthorized execution of system functions.

12. **D.** Two types of usability features are single sign-on and identify federation.

References

1. U.S. Congress. (2009). *American Recovery and Reinvestment Act of 2009 (ARRA)*. H.R. 1. February 17, 2009. Accessed on July 5, 2012, from http://frwebgate .access.gpo.gov/cgi-bin/getdoc.cgi?dbname=111_cong_bills&docid=f:h1enr.pdf.

2. Blumenthal, D. (2009). Launching HITECH. *New England Journal of Medicine*, 362, 382–385.

3. NIH. Greek medicine. Accessed on July 3, 2012, from www.nlm.nih.gov/hmd/ greek/greek_oath.html.

4. American Nurses Association. (2001). *Code of ethics for nurses with interpretive statements.* Nursesbooks.org.

5. International Council of Nurses. (2000). *The ICN code of ethics for nurses*. ISBN: 92-95005-16-3.

6. Markle Foundation: Connecting for Health. (2006). The common framework: Overview and principles. Accessed on October 2, 2012, from http://www .markle.org/health/markle-common-framework

7. Department of Health, Education, and Welfare. (July 1973). Records, computers, and the rights of citizens. Report of the Secretary's Advisory Committee on Automated Personal Data Systems. Accessed on July 5, 2012, from http://aspe .hhs.gov/DATACNCL/1973privacy/tocprefacemembers.htm.

8. ONC. (December 15, 2008). Nationwide privacy and security framework for electronic exchange of individually identifiable health information. Accessed on October 2, 2012, from http://healthit.hhs.gov/portal/server.pt/gateway/ PTARGS_0_10731_848088_0_0_18/NationwidePS_Framework-5.pdf

9. Berinato, S. (February 2003). All systems down. *CIO*, 46–53.

10. U.S. Attorney's Office, Southern District of Florida. (April 1, 2008). Press release: Miami-Dade DME and clinic owners indicted for using stolen patient

information in multi-million dollar Medicare fraud scheme. Accessed on July 5, 2012, from www.docstoc.com/docs/724092/Indictment-Remberto-Sarmiento-Perez---MIAMI-DADE-DME-AND-CLINIC-OWNERS-INDICTED-FOR-USING-STOLEN-PATIENT-INFORMATION-IN-MULTI-MILLION-DOLLAR-MEDICARE-FRAUD-SCHEME.

11. Rys, R. (March 13, 2008). The imposter in the ER: Medical identity theft can leave you with hazardous errors in health records. Msnbc.com. Accessed on July 5, 2012, from www.msnbc.msn.com/id/23392229/ns/health-health_care.

12. Cohen, B. (July 9, 2009). NHS hit by a different sort of virus. Channel 4 News. Accessed on July 5, 2012, from www.channel4.com/news/articles/science_technology/nhs+hit+by+a+different+sort+of+virus/3256957.

13. Goodin, D. (April 23, 2010). NHS computers hit by voracious, data-stealing worm. *The Register.* Accessed on July 5, 2012, from http://www.theregister.co.uk/2010/04/23/nhs_worm_infection/.

14. Tobin, D. (April 21, 2010). University hospital computers plagued by anti-virus glitch. *The Post Standard.* Accessed on July 5, 2012, from www.syracuse.com/news/index.ssf/2010/04/university_hospital_plagued_by.html.

15. HHS. (2012). Health information privacy: Breaches affecting 500 or more individuals. Accessed on July 3, 2012, from www.hhs.gov/ocr/privacy/hipaa/administrative/breachnotificationrule/postedbreaches.html.

16. HHS. (2003). Health insurance reform: Security standards, final rule. 45 CFR Parts 160, 162, and 164. *Federal Register*, February 20, 2003.

17. HHS. (2002). Health insurance reform: Standards for privacy of individually identifiable health information, final rule. 45 CFR Parts 160 and 164. *Federal Register*, December 28, 2000; amended August 14, 2002.

18. Pritts, J., Choy, A., Emmart, L., & Hustead, J. (June 1, 2002). The state of health privacy: A survey of state health privacy statutes. Second edition. Accessed on July 3, 2012, from http://ihcrp.georgetown.edu/privacy/pdfs/statereport1.pdf.

19. Healthcare Information and Management Systems Society. (2009). HIMSS Security Survey, November 3, 2009. Accessed on October 2, 2012, from http://www.himss.org/content/files/HIMSS2009SecuritySurveyReport.pdf

20. 104th Congress Health Insurance Portability and Accountability Act, public law 104-191. (1996). Accessed on October 1, 2012, from http://www.gpo.gov/fdsys/pkg/PLAW-104publ191/html/PLAW-104publ191.htm

21. HL7 Version 3 Confidentiality code system [2.16.840.1.113883.5.25]. Accessed on July 4, 2012, from http://ushik.ahrq.gov/ViewItemDetails?system=mdr&itemKey=86617000.

22. OASIS Security Assertion Mark-up Language (SAML). Accessed on July 4, 2012, from http://saml.xml.org/about-saml.

23. Internet Engineering Task Force. (August, 2008). The transport layer security (TLS) protocol. Version 1.2. RFC 5246. Accessed on July 5, 2012, from http://tools.ietf.org/html/rfc5246.

24. Internet Engineering Task Force. (November, 1998). Security architecture for the internet protocol. RFC 2401. Accessed on July 5, 2012, from www.ietf.org/rfc/rfc2401.txt.

25. International Organization for Standardization. (1996). *Information technology—Open systems interconnection—Basic reference model: The basic model.* ISO/IEC 7498-1. Second Edition, November 15, 1994. Corrected and reprinted, June 15, 1996. Accessed on July 5, 2012, from http://standards.iso.org/ittf/licence.html.

CHAPTER 25

Risk Assessment and Management

Gila Pyke

In this chapter you will learn how to
- Participate in the process of reducing the risk of any healthcare IT product or implementation
- Identify the difference between security, privacy, and other healthcare risks
- Recognize different threats and associated mitigation strategies

Risk management is the art of enabling innovation and opportunities while preparing to manage potential negative outcomes. Risk management is not about eliminating risk (that is impossible) but instead identifying it, reducing it as much as possible, informing affected parties, and preparing to respond quickly and effectively should the risk materialize.

Healthcare technology is reputed to improve patient health outcomes and reduce certain types of healthcare risk, but as with the introduction of any new system, the introduction of technology into the healthcare space introduces the potential for new risks that have to be managed. A good example of this risk-benefit balance is the introduction of healthcare information systems that provide access to health information from laboratory tests, emergency response reports, hospital discharge summaries, and patient medical histories all in one place. The benefit that this can provide to patients is obvious, but the risk that unauthorized personnel may gain access to this information is also increased as more points of access to this information are introduced. When filing cabinets contain the health files, there is only one point from which the information can be accessed. But when you have a broadly shared healthcare information system, there are many points of access.

Fortunately, once healthcare IT risks are identified and assessed, they can also be managed and additional preventative and responsive safeguards can be implemented. In the case of risks involving unauthorized access, authentication and access controls can significantly reduce such risks and enable the technology to be used more safely.

Definitions[1]

In order to better enable the reader to discuss risk management in healthcare, following are definitions of some key terms:

- **Asset** An asset is something that needs to be protected from harm or loss. In healthcare IT security terms, an asset can refer to health information itself or devices containing health information. In healthcare privacy, safety, and other risk areas, assets consist of sensitive health information, patient safety, emotional or physical well-being, etc.

- **Vulnerability** A vulnerability is a weakness that leaves the asset unnecessarily exposed to harm inherent in the design or implementation of software. In healthcare IT terms, a vulnerability can be an unnecessary connection from a system hosting live healthcare data to the Internet, a lack of virus protection, or an unnecessary open port on a firewall.

- **Threat** A threat is a possible danger that might exploit a vulnerability and cause harm to an asset. A threat can originate from natural causes (power failures, floods, earthquakes, etc., resulting in health information being unavailable), intentional misuse or attack (spying on a VIP patient's files) or error (losing or misplacing valuable health information required for a patient's treatment).

- **Safeguard** A safeguard is one of the ways that we can protect our assets against threats. A safeguard, or security control, effectively reduces or eliminates a vulnerability. For example, virus scanners (safeguard) help protect our data (assets) from exposure to viruses (vulnerability) by unauthorized individuals who want to access or destroy our data (threats or threat agents).

- **Risk**[2,3] A risk is the likelihood that a threat will exploit a vulnerability and harm an asset, resulting in an impact on the organization or the patient.[4] For example, if you are trying to protect a victim of violence/VIP's health record (asset) from being accessed by an individual with the intent to cause harm (threat), and that health record is accessible from a computer located in a public area that is often left logged in and does not require a password or any kind of credential to use (vulnerability), then there is a risk that an unauthorized individual may access poorly protected health records and use them to cause harm to the patient.

In risk management, our goal is to reduce either the likelihood of the risk or its potential harm or impact. The likelihood of the risk cited above can be reduced by making it harder for the threat to access the records (by implementing safeguards such as moving the computer into an area restricted to staff only and providing staff with training that emphasizes the need to log out when they are not using the system). The impact of the risk cited above can be reduced by removing data about the patient's whereabouts from the health record. We will explore other ways to respond to risks later in this chapter.

Exercise 25-1: Identifying, Assessing, and Mitigating Risk

Identify the asset, vulnerability, threat, risk, and impact in the following healthcare scenario. Assign a likelihood value that this scenario may occur, and identify some potential safeguards that may help lower the likelihood or reduce the severity of the impact.

Scenario

The surgical theatre in your local hospital relies on an allergy database to guide decisions on which anesthetic, medications, and other materials can be safely used on a patient during surgery. This database is also connected to the Internet for research purposes. A researcher unwittingly downloaded a virus, making the allergy database suddenly unavailable and resulting in a patient with allergies to opiates being administered morphine and suffering complications.

Risk Assessment

- **Asset**   Allergy database
- **Vulnerability**   Unnecessary Internet connection
- **Threat**   Virus
- **Risk**   Virus will be introduced to the system due to the unnecessary Internet connection and render the allergy database unavailable
- **Likelihood**   Medium or high
- **Impact**   Harm to patient health

Potential Mitigations

- Segregate database from research system, remove Internet connection (lowers likelihood)
- Install antivirus (lowers likelihood)
- Maintain paper backup of allergy data (reduces impact)

Risk Management in Healthcare IT

In healthcare IT, risk management is about assessing and reducing the risks along the spectrum of IT development—including healthcare device manufacturers, software developers, healthcare IT service providers, healthcare IT implementers, government organizations involved in healthcare, other third parties, healthcare providers, and—most importantly—patients.

Risk management in healthcare takes more lessons from the nuclear and aerospace industries than from the more traditional manufacturing or financial domains, in the sense that the ultimate impact of a risk in healthcare IT is the emotional or physical well-being of a patient. When risks can cost lives, the management of these risks becomes a priority component of healthcare IT development.

The Risk-Management Process[2]

The risk-management process is a cyclical, or spiral, process that begins with identification and assessment and returns there in order to ensure continual progress towards reducing the risks inherent in any development, implementation, or use of healthcare information technology.

At a high level, these are the steps of the risk-management process:

1. **Identification of risks**   As we move through this chapter we will discuss various methods for identifying risks that may impact the security of an application, the privacy of a patient or provider, or ultimately the safety of a patient. The first step is always to identify all possible applicable risks, regardless of how likely they are. Risks will be prioritized during the assessment step.

2. **Assessment of risks**   The risk-assessment step is the prioritization or triage step. This step takes into account the relative likelihood of a risk occurring, as well as the potential impacts of that risk, and assigns it a risk rating. A higher risk rating indicates a more serious risk that needs to be addressed first during the planning of mitigations. This prioritization is also a valuable tool for communicating with risk owners and stakeholders.

3. **Mitigation planning**   Once priority risks are identified, the next step is planning ways to mitigate them, i.e., reduce their likelihood or probability of occurrence, or reduce the potential impact if the risk does occur.

4. **Risk and mitigation tracking**   In order to ensure that mitigation plans are being implemented effectively, it is important to follow up with mitigation owners at predetermined intervals to provide support and ensure that mitigation plans will succeed.

5. **Documentation**   Once the first round of risk assessment is complete, it should be documented in a report to be used to communicate to key internal and external stakeholders so that everyone is aware of how risks are being managed.

Using one or more of the methods described below for identifying risks is recommended for the initial cycle of risk identification, such as coupling a checklist with additional follow-up interviews of key stakeholders, or leveraging a standardized questionnaire with a follow-up brainstorming session with subject-matter experts. Once the initial list of risks has been identified, the risks need to be documented in a risk register. A *risk register* is a table used to document risks throughout the risk-management lifecycle, in support of each phase. Table 25-1 is an example of a risk register.[2,5] During the first identification phase of the risk-management lifecycle, only the leftmost columns of the risk register need to be completed.

For ongoing iterations of the risk-management lifecycle, risk identification should be based off the existing risk register. Questions such as "have new risks been identified?" should be asked of key subject-matter experts and stakeholders, but conducting interviews or workshops will take less time. Often the checklists and questionnaires that are used are called "delta" or Δ assessments.

	Risk Identification			Risk Assessment				Mitigation Planning			Risk and Mitigation Tracking		
	Risk summary	Asset	Vulnerability/ threat scenario	Likelihood	Impact (note the category)	Risk rating	Modifiers (safeguards/detectability)	Mitigation	Owner	Due date	Status	Adjusted likelihood	Adjusted probability
1.													
2.													
3.													

Table 25-1   The Risk Register. (This table is available for download; see Appendix C.)

Risk Identification

The goal of the risk-identification step is to identify any and all possible risk scenarios that may adversely affect the project or solution. In order to identify risks, a project or system must be broken down into assets and scenarios so that vulnerabilities and threats can be identified.[1] Depending on the type of risk—security, privacy, data criticality, or safety—there are a few different approaches to help identify a comprehensive list of potential risks: 1) creating checklists, 2) using technology tools, 3) using questionnaires, 4) conducting interviews, and 5) holding workshops or brainstorming sessions.

Checklist Example

When building a network to host healthcare applications, a list of required security controls (such as firewalls, encryption, authentication, and audit functionality) can be used to prompt risk identification. Creating a comprehensive map of the network and then verifying the checklist against each applicable path or node can create a list of gaps or vulnerabilities. Those vulnerabilities can then be combined with a checklist of the system's assets and the potential threats to those assets to identify the security risks related to that system.

There are standardized security or safety checklists available, such as the Common Criteria Evaluation and Validation Scheme produced by the National Information Assurance Partnership (NIAP).[6] Organizations that routinely build or implement healthcare technology should leverage past risk assessments to build their own tailored risk-identification templates based on these and other standardized checklists.

Risk Assessment

Once a comprehensive list of risks has been identified, the next phase is to assess these risks and determine which risks must be prioritized for mitigation, which risks should be mitigated once the priority risks have been satisfactorily addressed, and which risks are sufficiently low that they can be accepted or removed from discussion. It is the responsibility of the healthcare provider to conduct the risk assessment.

The triage of risks enables organizations to focus their resources on implementing safeguards where they are needed most. The risk-assessment process also enables subject-matter experts to communicate about priority risks with senior stakeholders using a common language of agreed-upon concepts.

Risk assessment is composed of three sequential activities:

1. Assignment of risk likelihood and impact values
2. Prioritization of risks based on assigned values
3. Reduction of risk values based on modifiers such as existing safeguards or risk detection

Assignment of Risk Likelihood and Impact Values

In order to determine the relative priority of risks, each risk is discussed in terms of two dimensions: likelihood and impact. A risk's likelihood is the probability that this risk will materialize in the foreseeable future. Likelihood can be measured based on quantitative statistics of past occurrence if these are available (i.e., the number of distributed denial-of-service—DDOS—attacks on a network per month, where a high number infers a high likelihood of DDOS attacks occurring in the future). If statistics are not available, then a qualitative value should be assigned.

In order to ensure that all participants in the risk-management exercise are speaking the same language, an agreed-upon likelihood table should be used to assign values. Since different projects, systems, and organizations have different risks and risk tolerances, a likelihood table should be customized to that organization. Table 25-2 is an example of a likelihood table.[2,5]

	Probability	Likelihood Description
Very high	> 80%, or daily	This event may be happening on a regular basis or will likely occur soon.
High	51% to 80%, or monthly	This event is likely to occur in the near future.
Medium	21% to 50%—less than once per month but more than once per year	This event may occur in the near future.
Low	6% to 20%, or 1–2 times per year	This event is possible but highly unlikely to occur in the near future.
Very low	0% to 5%, or less than once per 5-year period	This event is not expected to occur in the near future.

Table 25-2   Example of a Likelihood Table

There are five levels of likelihood in this table. High, medium, and low are intended to be used regularly, whereas very high and very low are intended to demonstrate severe outlying events. Events such as "this happens all the time, it even happened today" would be listed as very high, and "this will probably never happen, but we wanted to document the risk anyway" would be listed as very low. An example of a very low risk could be the risk of flooding negatively impacting the availability of critical healthcare information. While the impact of such a risk is high and therefore should be considered, if the healthcare information is located in an area prone to drought that has never experienced flooding and is stored several stories above ground, then the relative likelihood of that risk would be considered very low.

TIP When the probability of occurrence is unknown due to insufficient data, a value of medium is assigned until further information is available.

Risk-Likelihood Example If the risk of unauthorized access due to insufficient role-based access control is identified but there is no information as to the motivation or likely frequency for such unauthorized access, then the likelihood is assigned a medium value. Later, when this risk is discussed with stakeholders and other safeguards are identified that might prevent the occurrence of the risk (such as restricted issuance of login credentials to the system, reducing the availability of access to unauthorized staff), then the likelihood may be lowered. (Conversely, the likelihood value may also be raised should data supporting the likelihood of occurrence be brought forward.)

The other dimension for discussing risks is the severity of the potential impact if that risk were to occur. As with likelihood, the scale for assessing level of impact should be customized to the organization assessing the risk and should be based on stakeholder and subject-matter-expert consensus. Where quantitative cost analysis is possible, impact should be measured in terms of cost. Where quantitative data is not available, a qualitative value should be assigned. Often several categories of qualitative impact are needed to be able to compare different types of risks. Table 25-3 is an example of the types of impact categories.[2,5]

In order to use a table like 25-3, where multiple categories or types of impacts are possible, the relative impact of the highest risk is the one that counts. For example, if the risk materializing may result in minor adverse attention from the media from the reputation category (which has an impact value of medium) but might also result in potential for serious injury in the safety category (which has an impact value of high), assign the risk a value of high.

TIP As with likelihood, if the potential impact of a risk cannot be estimated, a value of medium is assigned until further information is available.

	Cost (Quantitative)	Reputation	Safety	Product Functionality
Very high	Capital cost > $100M	Potential for shareholder action	Potential for multiple fatalities/serious injuries	May not be able to deliver on most critical requirements
High	Capital cost of $10M–$100M	Serious adverse attention from media and medical establishment and/or loss of clients	Potential for fatality/serious injury/severe psychiatric disability	Major shortfalls in one or more critical requirements
Medium	Capital cost of $1M–$10M	Minor adverse attention from media and medical establishment and/or existing clients	Potential for minor physical injury/emotional or mental distress	Minor shortfalls in one or more key requirements
Low	Capital cost of $100,000–$1M	Loss of reputation among public/potential clients	Potential to reduce quality of healthcare/cause anxiety	A few shortfalls in desired functionality
Very low	Capital cost < $100,000	Internal loss of reputation	Impact does not affect delivery of healthcare	System should still fully meet mandatory requirements

Table 25-3   Example of an Impact Table

Risk-Impact Example   If the same risk of unauthorized access due to insufficient role-based access control is identified but there is no information yet available as to what information may be accessible, how this unauthorized access may affect a patient's emotional or physical well-being, or whether it may affect the organization in terms of reputation or eventual financial cost, the impact category would be set to medium until more information is available about what data may be accessed without authorization and by whom. If, after further analysis, it is identified that the only information that can be accessed without login credentials is limited patient demographic information (i.e., name, age, and phone number) but no address or health information, then the impact can be reduced to very low—without home-address or health information there is likely very little cost or reputation impact for the provider or safety impact to the patient. It is important to note the impact category in the risk register or supporting documentation in order to support risk-assessment discussion with stakeholders.

Prioritization of Risks Based on Assigned Values[1,2,5]

Once each risk has been assigned a likelihood and impact value, each risk is mapped into a visual risk matrix to establish the risk's overall rating and relative priority. Figure 25-1 is an example of a risk map. In this example, the various risks are listed at the top of the map for ease of reading. They are then mapped using the likelihood and impact tables and placed in the appropriate box on the grid. The grid is divided into risk levels, with darkly shaded boxes indicating major priorities that must be addressed as soon as possible and where the majority of time and resources should be allocated. The lighter the shading in the box, the lower the prioirity

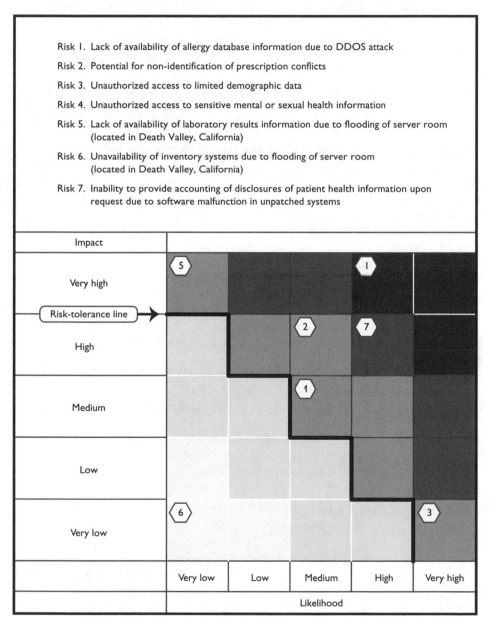

Risk 1. Lack of availability of allergy database information due to DDOS attack

Risk 2. Potential for non-identification of prescription conflicts

Risk 3. Unauthorized access to limited demographic data

Risk 4. Unauthorized access to sensitive mental or sexual health information

Risk 5. Lack of availability of laboratory results information due to flooding of server room (located in Death Valley, California)

Risk 6. Unavailability of inventory systems due to flooding of server room (located in Death Valley, California)

Risk 7. Inability to provide accounting of disclosures of patient health information upon request due to software malfunction in unpatched systems

Figure 25-1   Example of a risk map. (This figure is available for download; see Appendix C.)

The risk-tolerance line indicates the risk tolerance agreed upon by the organization performing the risk assessment.[1,2] Risks that fall below the line can be accepted. Recovery plans may still be put in place, but further efforts to reduce the likelihood or impact of the risk are not prioritized. ISO/IEC 80001 (application of risk management to IT networks incorporating medical devices) describes this phenomenon in a different way.[7] It states that the organization shall decide which of the following is most appropriate:

- The estimated risk is so low that risk reduction need not be pursued. In this case the rationale for this decision must be documented.

- The estimated risk is not acceptable. In this case risk-control measures, or in the language of this chapter, mitigations, shall be implemented.

Reduction of Risk Values Based on Existing Safeguards

Existing safeguards that reduce the potential likelihood or impact of a risk should be listed in the risk register, and the risk rating should be modified accordingly. In other words, if a healthcare information system has been designed with safeguards already in place, then the impacts or likelihoods of some risks inherent in the use of the system will be lower than upon initial assessment.

Once initial risk ratings are mapped, the next step is to identify which risks have safeguards already in place that may lower the initial risk rating. For example, for risk 1 in Figure 25-1, the likelihood of a DDOS attack on a discoverable system is high, and the impact of unavailable allergy information is very high—it can negatively impact the lives of many patients. Therefore, the initial risk rating of risk 1 is in the red (maximum-priority) category.

Upon discussion with the security team, the following safeguards are identified as already in place:

- A well-configured firewall and prevention system
- An intrusion-detection system that raises alarms if a DDOS attempt is detected

Once the safeguards have been documented in supported documentation along with their effect on the risk rating, the readjusted likelihood and impact should be updated in the risk register along with the mitigating factors.

Risk-Mitigation Planning[1,2]

There are four ways to respond to risk:

- **Accept** Weigh the cost of the risk versus the cost of mitigating it. Sometimes it is more prudent and effective to create a disaster-recovery plan or review audit logs regularly to identify an incident as quickly as possible than it is to try to mitigate the inevitable (or hard to avoid).

- **Transfer** Leverage insurance clauses, service-level agreements, and other contractual documentation to transfer the cost of recovery from a risk away from
the organization. A prime example of this is liability insurance.

- **Mitigate** Buy antivirus software, provide awareness and training, optimize
business processes, hire more people, write a profile, demand the use of encryption, or propose a controlled and well-documented activity that will reduce (not
eliminate) the risk level to the point where it is either completely tolerable or
at least tolerable enough that the focus of efforts can move to the mitigation of
other priority risks.

- **Avoid** Sometimes there is too much risk associated with something and no
effective way to mitigate the risk, so we choose to do something else and avoid
the risk altogether. This is often the least desirable or feasible action to take.

TIP For each risk in the risk register, identify which of these strategies will
be employed, the details (such as developing a recovery or log-review plan,
purchasing which kind of insurance, or implementing what kind of mitigation),
who will own these risk management activities, and when they are due. This is
necessary to enable risk tracking and reporting steps.

NOTE Formal signing of mitigation letters, or risk waivers in the case of risk
acceptance, by risk owners can be an effective way of ensuring that senior
stakeholders recognize risk-mitigation commitments.

Risk-Mitigation Tracking

Once mitigation strategies have been agreed upon, assigned, and documented, the
progress of mitigation plans must be tracked on a regular basis in order to identify
issues or obstacles and provide support to risk owners to ensure that their risks will be
mitigated. The frequency of tracking should be based on the risk rating—mitigation
plans for extremely high risks should be followed up biweekly or monthly, whereas the
progress of mitigating lower risks can be verified on a quarterly or even less frequent
basis.

Documentation and Communication

There are two audiences for risk-management documentation:

- Internal stakeholders
- External stakeholders

Communicating About Risk with Internal Stakeholders[1]

Internal stakeholders (senior management, project owners, and internal clients) must be kept informed about risks on a periodic basis as part of established reporting mechanisms, such as quarterly risk reports to the board and weekly or monthly project meetings.

The risk register should be updated prior to each reporting cycle, including any new risks that have been identified along with their mitigations, changes to mitigation plans, updates on mitigation status, and residual risk ratings for mitigation plans that have been completed. This enables stakeholders from all levels of the organization to be kept appraised of their responsibilities as risk owners and also to provide support, such as additional resources for the mitigation of risks elsewhere within the organization.

Communicating About Risk with External Stakeholders

Communicating about risk with external stakeholders is part of the closeout phase of any project and part of ongoing maintenance of any healthcare IT system. Before a healthcare IT product can be sold to a healthcare provider, before an implementer can install the hardware and software at the healthcare provider's site, and before the healthcare provider can begin using the product, risks must be managed along the entire spectrum—from software vendor to implementer to healthcare provider to patient.

In order for this to be possible, software and hardware vendors that are aware of residual risks in their products must clearly document and report these risks to the implementers who will install these products. Implementers who conduct risk assessments on the software or hardware implementation must document and communicate the residual risks to the healthcare provider, and healthcare providers must in turn include these risks in their own risk identification, assessment, mitigation, tracking, and documentation activities. Risks that may ultimately affect patients must be managed along the continuum of the development of healthcare IT, from the initial conception of a software or hardware product to the daily use of that product for providing healthcare.

Domains of Risk Analysis

There are many domains of risk that may affect a healthcare IT system. The diagram in Figure 25-2 categorizes the threats associated with mitigation strategies into the following five domains: safety, security, privacy, application criticality, and data criticality.

The risk-management cycle in each case follows the same steps. In many organizations a common risk register is used to document all categories or domains of risk, and common impact and likelihood tables are used to assess and prioritize them. The primary difference between these domains lies in the specific types of risks that are identified and minor deviations in the techniques used to identify them. In some cases subject-matter experts who have a deeper knowledge of one domain (e.g., safety) versus another (privacy) are hired to conduct risk assessments.

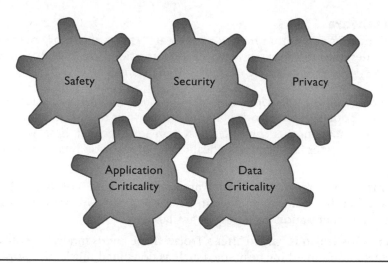

Figure 25-2 Domains of risk

Security Risk Analysis

Security risk analysis focuses on the triangle of security: confidentiality, integrity, and availability (CIA). All risks to healthcare IT assets are considered in terms of the confidentiality of the information contained in the assets, the integrity of the information contained in the assets, or the availability of the assets. Following are some examples of common security risks and their safeguards.

Threat: DOS or DDOS Attack

A denial-of-service (DOS) or distributed denial-of-service (DDOS) attack is an attempt to make a healthcare information system (asset) and the information hosted on it unavailable through flooding or overloading of the system.

Risk The hospital's decision-support software may become unavailable as a result of a DOS/DDOS attack. This is an availability risk.

Mitigations

- Implementation and configuration of firewalls, switches, and routers
- Implementation of specific preventative hardware and software
- Antivirus software
- Code reviews
- Antispyware
- Security scanning (early detection)

Threat: Malware

Malware obtains its name from malicious software. This is a category of software that is purposely designed to cause damage to an information system such as a healthcare information system. Following are examples of malware:

- **Viruses** A virus is malicious software that can copy itself and infect a computer without the user knowing. In order for a virus to spread, the infected file must be sent to another computer or system and executed there. Viruses can corrupt computer files and make healthcare information unavailable when it is most needed.

- **Worms** A worm is malicious software that makes copies of itself using a network rather than being embedded in a file like a virus. Worms can also result in healthcare information becoming unavailable.

- **Trojans** A Trojan is named after a Trojan horse and is malicious software that appears to do something desirable (such as download music files or play a video) but contains code hidden inside it that can open a backdoor and allow a malicious user to have unauthorized access to healthcare information. This is a risk to confidentiality rather than availability.

- **Rootkits and backdoors** Rootkits and backdoors are malicious software that can be installed without a user's knowledge and provide access to a computer and the information on it to an unauthorized person. Rootkits and backdoors are a threat to confidentiality of healthcare information.

- **Spyware** Spyware is malware that collects information about a computer user, such as login and password information, without their knowledge and sends it to a third party who can use it to get unauthorized access to healthcare information. Like Trojans, rootkits, and backdoors, spyware poses a risk to the confidentiality of healthcare information.

Risk The patient files stored at the doctor's office may be accessed (confidentiality risk) or modified (integrity) by unauthorized attackers, or the physician may lose access (availability) to critical health information that he or she needs to provide patient care.

Mitigations
- Educating users not to click on certain types of links or install certain types of software

- Restricting user accounts from being able to install software without the help of a technically savvy person

- Antivirus software

- Antispyware, or spyware removal, software

- Code reviews

- Regular security scans to detect rootkits and other malware as early as possible

Threat: Social Engineering

Social engineering is the act of manipulating people to provide confidential information or information that will permit an unauthorized person access to confidential information. In healthcare IT, social engineering could include posing as staff at a healthcare institution in order to gain access to a server room, impersonating an authorized user over the telephone, or various electronic means of posing as someone with a legitimate need for confidential information. A common example of social engineering is called phishing. With this technique the poser uses e-mail and a web page that appear to be legitimate to ask you to "verify your login information." In fact, you are being redirected to a false page and the sender is using the information you provide to gain unauthorized access to healthcare information.

Risk Social engineering can pose a risk to the confidentiality, availability, and integrity of healthcare information.

Mitigations

- Educating users to recognize social engineering or phishing attempts
- Effective disposal of electronic and paper media (to reduce "dumpster diving")

Threat: Spam

E-mail spam, sometimes known as junk e-mail, involves thousands of e-mail sent to as many recipients as possible with the intention of selling, advertising, or phishing for information from unsuspecting users. Spam can also involve sending bulk messages over instant messaging, mobile texting, and other forms of electronic communication media.

Risk Spam can be used to transmit viruses, phishing scams, and other threats and can also result in reduced or no availability of networks and, as a result, healthcare information. In other words, spam can pose a risk to the confidentiality, integrity, and availability of healthcare information.

Mitigations

- Educating users not to sign on to untrusted sites with their e-mail addresses, how to recognize spam messages, and not to respond to them
- E-mail filtering
- Greylisting or blacklisting services

For more information on security-specific risk analysis, see NIST SP 800-30: Risk Management Guide for Information Technology Systems.[1]

Application and Data Criticality Analysis

The purpose of application and data criticality analysis is to fulfill the HIPAA security regulation requiring healthcare organizations to have a disaster-recovery plan in place, as well as an emergency-operation plan if applications hosting critical healthcare information suddenly become unavailable. An application and data criticality analysis should identify

- Which software applications are critical to the provision of healthcare
- What data is critical to the provision of healthcare

Privacy Risk Analysis

In healthcare IT, privacy risk analysis encompasses more than the confidentiality of personal health information. It also includes

- Compliance with legislative and regulatory requirements, such as those laid out in HIPAA, and the financial or business impacts that noncompliance can have on a health organization.
- Adherence to privacy principles, such as those laid out in the OECD Privacy Principles:[9]
  - **Collection limitation** Limiting how much healthcare information is collected and where it can be collected from. Consent must be given for the collection.
  - **Data-quality principle** Information collected and used should be relevant to the purposes for which it was collected and kept up to date.
  - **Purpose-specification principle** Communicating to patients why their information is being collected, when it will be used, and under what conditions it would be disclosed.
  - **Use limitation** Limiting how and when data is disclosed and for what purposes the disclosure is being made.
  - **Security safeguards** Security safeguards should be used to protect healthcare information.
  - **Openness** Organizations should be open about their practices of using and protecting personal health information.

 TIP Informing patients about what information is collected about them supports the principle of openness.

- **Individual participation** Patients should be informed about what information is collected about them, as well as with whom it will be shared, and have the ability to correct it if they can demonstrate that it is inaccurate.

- **Accountability** Healthcare providers should be held accountable for the protection of personal health information in their custody.

NOTE Privacy-risk assessment should be conducted at the start, middle, and end of a project.

Safety Risk Assessment

While the risks identified by security, application and data criticality, and privacy risk analysis often relate to patient safety, independent safety risk assessments are necessary to ensure that all risks to a patient's safety have been considered. Safety risk assessment in healthcare IT is intended to identify any areas where technology-induced errors may introduce risks to patient safety and then follow the risk-management process to reduce them as much as possible.

NOTE Errors are introduced by poorly calibrated diagnostic imaging equipment.

Medical device and hardware manufacturers use an analysis method called "failure modes and effects analysis" (FMEA) to identify potential failures in their products.[3] Appendixes C and D of the ISO FDIS 14971[8] standard for the application of risk management to medical devices contain questions to ask when assessing device safety and conducting harm analysis. These questions can be applied to safety risk assessment in software, implementation, and healthcare-setting risk analysis as well. For example:

- What is the intended use of the device/software [in the provision of healthcare]?

- Will this device come into contact with the patient (tissues or body fluids, processing of biological materials, etc.)? What are the sterilization requirements?

- What are the accuracy requirements of the measurements?

As with all other types of risk assessment, once the risks have been identified they must be prioritized, mitigations assigned and tracked, and risks communicated with all potentially affected parties.

Chapter Review

The introduction of technology into the healthcare space reduces some risks to patients but also introduces new technology-related risks that must be managed. This chapter described the five iterative steps involved in managing risk:

1. Identifying risks
2. Assessing and prioritizing risks
3. Planning mitigations and assigning ownership for mitigation activities
4. Tracking mitigation progress and residual risk posture
5. Documenting and communicating with internal and external stakeholders

This chapter also examined the differences between security, privacy, application and data criticality, and safety risk assessment and explored the techniques used to manage risk in these specific domains.

Questions

To test your comprehension of the chapter, answer the following questions and then check your answers against the list of correct answers that follows the questions.

1. Which of these participants in healthcare IT development, implementation, and use are responsible for conducting risk assessments?
   A. Hardware and device manufacturers
   B. Software developers
   C. Healthcare providers
   D. A and B
   E. All of the above

2. Which of the following is *not* a healthcare technology asset?
   A. Ultrasound machine
   B. Rootkit
   C. Laboratory information system
   D. E-prescribing system

3. You have been put in charge of performing a risk assessment for a new software product. What should you do first?
   A. Identify information assets
   B. Identify the potential safety hazards
   C. Identify vulnerabilities
   D. Identify potential impact

4. You have completed identifying your risks. What should you do next?

    A. Assign mitigations

    B. Identify threats

    C. Prioritize the risks by impact and likelihood

    D. Report on the risks to the board

5. Which of the following mitigations does not reduce the likelihood of a risk?

    A. Antivirus

    B. Tape backups

    C. Awareness and training

    D. Access controls

6. Which of the following mitigations do not reduce the impact of a risk?

    A. Tape backups

    B. Disaster-recovery plans

    C. Firewalls and encryption

    D. Encryption

    E. A and B

    F. A, B, and C

7. What are the five steps of the risk-management process?

    A. Requirements analysis, assessment, planning, tracking, documentation

    B. Identification, assessment, planning, transmission, development

    C. Identification, assessment, planning, tracking, documentation

    D. Identification, assessment, planning, tracking, development

The following scenario should be used for Questions 8 and 9: You are conducting a risk assessment on the new clinical decision support (CDS) software that your hospital has purchased and will soon be implementing. You have identified the following risk:

- In the current design, health information will be sent to the CDS over the hospital's free wifi network and may be accessed by unauthorized individuals.

8. What is the likelihood of this risk?

    A. Medium

    B. Low

    C. Very high

    D. A and B

9. How would you mitigate this risk?

   A. Encryption

   B. Awareness and training

   C. Change the network configuration

   D. A and C

   E. B and C

10. When should you perform a privacy risk assessment?

   A. At the start of a project

   B. At the start, middle, and end of a project

   C. At the end of a project

   D. In the middle of a project

11. Why should you perform a vulnerability assessment?

   A. To identify security problems with the software

   B. To test network availability

   C. To test whether patient information will remain safe

   D. To identify whether the hospital will be able to recover from an interruption in services

12. How should you mitigate the risk of phishing?

   A. Education and awareness

   B. E-mail filtering

   C. A and B

   D. None of the above

13. What is the purpose of application and data criticality analysis?

   A. To identify which software applications and which data are the most critical

   B. To identify any risks to patient safety if applications or data are not available

   C. To identify security problems with applications

   D. To develop a disaster-recovery plan should the healthcare systems become unavailable

14. Which of the following is *not* a privacy risk?

   A. HIPAA noncompliance

   B. Informing patients about what information is collected about them

   C. Collecting health information about a patient when it is not needed

   D. Sharing health information about a patient with someone who does not provide them with healthcare

15. Which of the following is a risk to patient safety?

   A. Unavailability of an Internet connection on a nonclinical system

   B. Errors introduced by poorly calibrated diagnostic imaging equipment

   C. Hackers using the hospital e-mail servers to send spam

   D. Phishing

Answers

1. **E.** Hardware and device manufacturers, software developers, and healthcare providers are all responsible for conducting risk assessments.

2. **B.** A rootkit is malicious software that poses a healthcare technology threat, not an asset.

3. **A.** Always start with identifying what you are trying to protect, i.e., the assets.

4. **C.** After risks have been identified, they must be prioritized according to impact and likelihood.

5. **B.** Tape backups reduce the impact but not the likelihood of a risk by making sure that the information can be restored quickly.

6. **E.** Firewalls and encryption prevent risks but do not lower their impact if they do occur.

7. **C.** Identification, assessment, planning, tracking, and documentation are the five steps in the risk-management process.

8. **C.** The likelihood is very high, because anyone can access the hospital wifi at any time.

9. **D.** Encrypting the data will make it harder to access, as will changing the network so that the data is not sent over the public wifi

10. **B.** You should conduct a risk privacy assessment at the start, middle, and end of a project.

11. **A.** Vulnerability assessments identify vulnerabilities inherent in the design or implementation of software.

12. **C.** You mitigate the risk of phishing with education and awareness and e-mail filtering.

13. **D.** The purpose of application and data criticality analysis is to develop a disaster-recovery plan should the healthcare system become unavailable.

14. **B.** Informing patients about what information is collected about them supports the principle of openness and is actually a privacy practice, not a risk.

15. **B.** Errors introduced by poorly calibrated healthcare technology can have a direct impact on a patient's safety.

References

1. NIST SP 800-30: Risk management guide for information technology systems. Accessed on August 23, 2012, from http://csrc.nist.gov/publications/ nistpubs/800-30/sp800-30.pdf.

2. HL7. Cookbook for security considerations in standards. Accessed on August 23, 2012, from http://wiki.hl7.org/index.php?title-Cookbook_for_Security_ Considerations.

3. Carnegie Mellon Software Engineering Institute. Software risk evaluation method version 2. Accessed on August 23, 2012, from www.sei.cmu.edi/ reports/99tr029.pdf.

4. IEC 60812 Ed. 1.0: Analysis techniques for system reliability—Procedure for failure mode and effects analysis (FMEA) and title analysis techniques. Accessed on August 23, 2012, from http://global.ihs.com/doc document ID=60812.

5. IHE International. (October 10, 2008). IHE cookbook: Preparing the IHE pro-file security section (risk management in healthcare IT) whitepaper. Accessed on August 23, 2012, from http://wiki.ihe.net/idenx/php?title=Cookbook_for_ Security_Considerations.

6. National Information Assurance Partnership (NIAP). Common criteria evaluation and validation scheme for IT security (CCEVS). Accessed on August 23, 2012, from www.niap-ceevs.org/cc_docs/.

7. ISO/IEC 80001: Application of risk management for IT-networks incorporating medical devices. Accessed on August 23, 2012, from www.iso.org/home/store/ catalogue_tc/catalogue_detail.htm?csnumber=57934.

8. ISO 14971:2007: Application of risk management to medical devices. Accessed on August 23, 2012, from www.iso.org/iso/home/store/catalogue_ics/catalogue_ detail_ics.htm?csnumber=31550.

9. OECD (August 9, 2010). OECD Privacy Principles. Accessed on October 1, 2012, from http://oecdprivacy.org/.

CHAPTER 26

Physical Safeguards, Facility Security, Secure Systems and Networks, and Securing Electronic Media

Dennis M. Seymour

In this chapter, you will learn how to
- Understand the necessary physical safeguards for your system, including location, access, and access-control devices
- Identify and explain guidelines for building systems including office hardware, environmental controls, personal controls, and storage devices
- Understand guidelines for security and preservation of electronic media for storage devices and secure disposal of electronic media
- Assess your organization's risks related to physical security and conduct an assessment of your organization's practices for securing electronic media

Physical Safeguard Requirements

In the old days (you remember—those prior to the turn of the millennium), most of our sensitive medical records were on paper and stored in the basement of the medical center in rooms where only staff members had access. When a patient had an appointment or came into the emergency room, a staff member had to request the paper record for the clinical staff to review. The doors had locks and perhaps access codes, and the room had sprinklers and fire extinguishers—but then every other room in the medical center also had those.

In today's medical centers most of those old paper records may still be there, but they may have been scanned into the electronic records systems in use at the medical center and are rarely referenced. They might even be archived away in some off-site storage location or repository. The security of the location where the electronic data is stored has new considerations, in part based on compliance requirements and in part due to the differences between storing paper and electronic media.

Facilities' transitions from paper to electronic records are often phased and unplanned in depth. Even before the health record was electronic it is likely the office was using desktop computers for office functions such as e-mail, scheduling, and billing. Initially these functions were likely running on the local desktop and not stored centrally. At some point the organization may have moved to using servers and networking to store the data from these office operations, without considering the specific security requirements for this data. Prior to the passage of the Health Insurance Portability and Accountability Act (HIPAA) of 1996, many organizations did not consider the requirements for the security or privacy of this data. Even after HIPAA many small office environments did not have privacy or security professionals involved in their process for adding hardware, software, etc. to their office environment.

Locating Storage Devices, Network Hardware, Printers, and Other Devices

When we think about locating the devices used for our healthcare practices, we must consider certain aspects of access to the data and implement an in-depth approach to the security and privacy of the data. The systems will also need to control user access. Consider not only the storage of the data but also the display, transmission, and input/output of the data contained in the system and applications. Beginning with the desktop used to access the data, we need to consider who will have access to the keyboard and display as well as how to control who can look at the data on the computer. For example, we may have administrative staff that work in the office but should not have access to patient data. We also may have volunteers whom we permit to assist patients and visitors but again not to access the computer for patient data.

Next we must have the ability to transmit this data from the desktop to a network storage device such as a server. We must consider whether this will be a wired or wireless network connection. In either instance, we must ask whether an individual could attempt to gain access by either plugging in their own computer or accessing the wireless network with an unauthorized device. If we have a wired connection, we must consider where the cabling is run, whether overhead in a drop ceiling or within the finished walls. Either way, the wire will likely run to a data closet, which in smaller offices and facilities is often the same closet that stores administrative, cleaning, or other supplies. I have even seen routers located on a shelf in the restroom or other publicly accessible areas of the office. Access to this data can be compromised when property-security fundamentals are not applied.

Securely Handling Protected Health Information (PHI)

Your organization's processes for handling PHI should be based on implementation of best practices, and it should depend on your local assessment of the threats, vulnerabilities, and risk exposure of your location and other factors. Following are descriptions of the many pieces of the physical system you need to consider in this assessment.

PC Placement

First, you should consider whether visitors or patients can view the screens used to display patient information for scheduling, billing/insurance, or electronic medical record (EMR) data. Upon entering the physician's reception area, you often find the receptionist is behind a wall with a sliding window, with the computer placed in such a way as to prevent your view. But once you enter the office area, you may walk by half a dozen or more computers on your way to an exam room, and each computer may be clearly displaying radiology, lab, or other data with little regard to privacy of the patient data. The organization should consider the placement of each PC screen as part of its overall risk assessment strategy.

Privacy Screens

For PCs including laptops that do not permit placement to prevent "shoulder surfing," risk mitigation might include the use of privacy screens. These screens allow the user to view the screen from a direct angle, but as you change your angle of view toward the side the image becomes less and less visible. Information on the screen is not visible beyond a 45–50-degree angle.

Printer Placement

Printers should be placed in secure areas away from public access, so as to prevent data that is printed and not immediately retrieved by the user from being removed by unauthorized personnel. The same rule applies to facsimile (fax) machines. Remember that the safeguards you can implement to control electronic data on your PC or server are not effective once the data is printed.

Screensavers

Most users are familiar with screensavers; however, few actually implement them securely. The best implementation requires the user to hit CONTROL-ALT-DELETE and re-enter a password when they want to return to using their computer. This and the use of a time lockout (below) together add to a defense-in-depth strategy.

Time Lockout

Most operating systems (Windows, MAC, Android) include the ability to implement a time lockout of access to the computer. Best practices usually guide this requirement to be between 5 and 15 minutes. This time begins when the last keystroke or mouse movement occurs, so simply viewing the screen for an extended period may trigger the time lockout that starts the screensaver program.

Access to Servers, Offices, and Data Closets

Consider the security in place to simply enter your office area. Try stepping outside after the office opens, or conduct this exercise when you arrive in the morning. Exercise 26-1 toward the end of the chapter provides an expanded look at this. The Physical and Environmental (PE) Controls section of National Institutes of Standards and Technology (NIST) Special Publication (SP) 800-53 is a valuable reference for the level of security you need to consider.[1]

Data Center

The data center is the primary location where servers and other network and communications gear is maintained. The security of this location may range from limited access to extreme (such as National Security Agency, Department of Defense, or other top-secret systems). While the level of security required is based on risk, there should always be a process in place to determine which security practices will be implemented, and the specific requirements that have not been implemented based on cost or other considerations need to be documented. Exercise 26-2 toward the end of the chapter guides you through a risk assessment of your organization's data-center security.

Data Closets

The data closet is often located on each floor of a large facility and should be maintained with the same level of security as the data center. Access to the closet grants access to the network environment, meaning that anyone having access can simply plug or unplug any cable or device as they desire. At many locations data closets are often shared with engineering, electrical, or even janitorial areas, a dangerous practice. These data closets often house intermediate distribution frame (IDF) devices such as switches, hubs, routers, wireless access points, uninterruptable power supplies, and the proverbial spaghetti called cabling. In smaller clinical settings it may even contain firewalls or wireless firewall devices.

Intermediate Distribution Frame/Main Distribution Frame

An intermediate distribution frame (IDF) is a free-standing or wall-mounted rack for managing and interconnecting the telecommunications cable between end-user devices and a main distribution frame (MDF). For example, an IDF might be located on each floor (in the data closet) of a multi-floor building to route the cabling from that floor down the walls to an MDF on the first floor or basement. The MDF would contain cabling that would interconnect to the phone company or to other buildings.

Backups

System backups should be completed on a regular basis and include system-level and data-level backups. These backups may be performed at different time increments; for example, the system backups that include the operating system and all settings might be conducted on a monthly or quarterly basis, while data backups might be done weekly, daily, or, as in the case of some healthcare locations, even hourly. One surprising fact is that many organizations do not apply the same principles for physical and environmental security to the location where backups are stored. Quite often the data center has moderate to high security, while backup tapes are stored in a file cabinet in the IT section. Backup tapes should be stored with the same level of security as the data in the data center, with access to those tapes restricted to the personnel who have authorization to access the data center. Many data-loss events over the past ten years have involved backup copies of the data, not a compromise of the data center or unauthorized access to the system itself.

Access-Control Devices

Access-control devices include devices that provide both access to physical facilities and access to systems. Some devices can actually provide access to both facilities and systems, as is the case with the personal identification and verification (PIV) card and the common access card (CAC) described below.

Key Fobs

A key fob is a type of security token or small hardware device with built-in authentication mechanisms. Just as the keys held on an ordinary real-world key chain or fob control access to the owner's home or car, the mechanisms in the key fob control access to network services and information. The key fob provides *two-factor authentication*: the user has a personal identification number (PIN), which authenticates them as the device's owner; after the user correctly enters their PIN, the device displays a number that allows them to log on to the network. Because a key fob is a physical object, it is easy for the owner to know if it has been stolen. In comparison, a password can be stolen (or guessed) and used for an extended period before—if ever—the theft is detected.

Some companies now provide a service where the user's cell phone or other device can provide the same service. When the user enters their access PIN, a message is sent by the system to their cell phone with the specific number or code to enter. This code may be used only for a limited period of time and for a single login. The next time the user attempts to log in, a new code is generated and sent to their phone.

Badges

Users who are familiar with Department of Defense (DoD) systems may have seen the common access card (CAC).[2] Other users of federal agency systems may use a card called the personal identification and verification (PIV) card.[3] Many nonfederal organizations have begun implementing very similar cards. The primary purpose of these cards is to provide secure access to both facilities and systems for which the user has authorization based on their role—referred to as *role-based access* (RBA). Figure 26-1 describes the various elements of the PIV card, including displays of both the front and back of the card.[4] This PIV card (as well as the CAC) must be implemented in a specified manner in accordance with guidelines established by the Federal CIO Council.

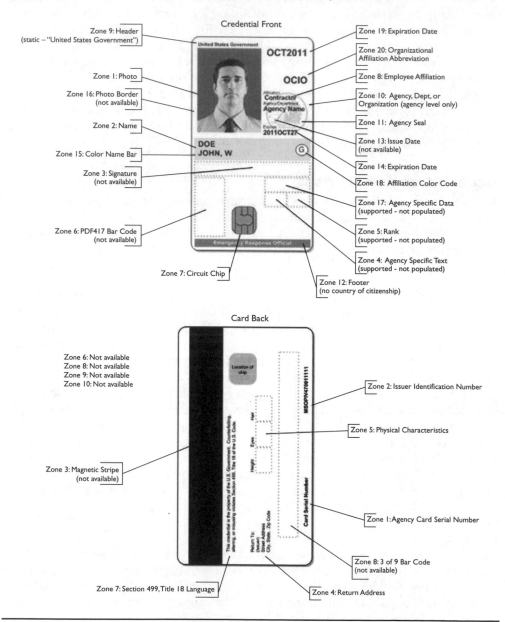

Figure 26-1 PIV card layout. Reprinted from the U.S. General Services Administration (GSA) USAccess Program, http://fedidcard.gov/credfeatures.aspx#maincontent.

Biometrics

Over the past few years the use of biometrics has increased in many areas, especially when it comes to access to facilities and IT systems. Back in the 60s, TV shows such as *The Man from U.N.C.L.E.*, *Mission Impossible*, and *Star Trek* made biometrics seem "sci-fi," but today they are very commonplace. Whether using your finger, voice, or retina, biometrics use is becoming a daily occurrence. It uses the "something you have" security principle and adds to the defense-in-depth strategy. An example of a device used to gain access to a physical location is a biometric fingerprint reader placed at the entry to the data center. This reader requires the user to place their index (or other registered) finger on the biometric reader. The screen then requests that the user add a second identification code, which might be four or more characters. The combination of something you have with a PIN (described as "something you know") provides two-factor authentication. Many devices, including tablets, laptops, and PC keyboards, now have biometric readers included in them.

Building Security Systems

Risk identification should be part of the process of working out the details of how data will be stored, and appropriate security measures to mitigate those risks should be implemented. This includes physical and environmental controls that are often in place but frequently not fully or correctly implemented. Understanding the requirements for these areas is a vital aspect of supporting the IT infrastructure.

Office Hardware

Computers and other devices should be locked to desks using appropriate cables, especially in areas where the item is accessible to the public.

Locks

Locks on safes, filing cabinets, and other storage areas must be commensurate with the risk and sensitivity of the data being stored within the area or cabinet. Consider this: at home would you store your diamond jewelry in the same drawer as your forks and knives in the kitchen? The more sensitive the information, such as backup tapes from your IT systems, the more secure the enclosure and therefore the locks must be that secure those areas.

Door Locks

Doors should be kept locked when employees are not present, and most office areas should have both a handle lock and a dead bolt lock. Keys that access doors to areas where sensitive data is stored should be controlled, and only those employees who should have access to the area should have access to the keys to that area. Consider reworking your key-control system if you have a single key storage or, even worse, you store keys in the secretary's desk drawer. Always consider who has access to the area; if the desk is left unattended and unlocked, anyone could gain access to the keys.

Environmental Controls

As you would expect from the name, these controls involve the environment in which the systems, storage, and communications reside. Again, the level of implementation of these controls must be based on the risk versus costs. While some controls must be implemented, not all must be implemented to the same level.

Heating, Ventilation, and Air Conditioning (HVAC)

The HVAC of the data center (or other area where IT equipment is stored) is vital to the health of the equipment. Place your hand beside the area of your PC or laptop where the fan is located, or simply sit with your laptop on your lap for 10 minutes. The heat generated by the central processing unit (CPU) can be over 100 degrees. Now consider that your data center may have hundreds, and in larger medical centers or universities thousands, of servers, each generating this heat. As the external temperature increases, so too does the internal temperature of the data center, so the HVAC of the data center is extremely important. Monitoring this information is also vital, including not only the temperature but also the humidity. If the humidity is too high, even a temperature in the high 70s can lead to condensation, which can cause problems with electronic circuits.

Security Lighting

The data center and data closets should have lighting even when power is lost, whether by generator power or by battery (for short-term power loss). This is both for security (so that individuals attempting to circumvent security during the power loss can be seen) and to allow IT staff to see and operate in emergency situations.

Surveillance

The ability to observe the data center may include video cameras, alarm systems, motion detectors, and other devices. Just as with other elements of physical security, the level of surveillance should be based on the risk assessment.

Fire Suppression

In an effort to prevent damage due to fires, the facility should have multiple forms of fire suppression, including handheld fire extinguishers (appropriate for the size and nature of the facility and the equipment), overhead fire suppression (which might include dry pipe, where water is always charged into the pipe; wet pipe, where water only is charged to the pipe when system is activated; or dry chemical systems, such as Halomethane, Halon 1211 or Halon 1301), and access to fire department standpipes for larger fire suppression. Staff members who routinely have access to the data center and areas adjacent to it should be trained in the use of fire suppression as well as the process for getting the system turned off.

Generator

Backup electrical power should be available, and as with other aspects of security should be based on the risk to the facility, the possibility of power disruptions, and other environmental factors. As an example, we might think a facility in an area with a history of high winds, tornados, or hurricanes would be more likely to suffer power loss than a facility in California, but a location in California might be subject to earthquakes, which could also cause the loss of power. The generator power must be implemented so that backup power is provided immediately and automatically, without requiring manual intervention.

Uninterrupted Power Supply (UPS)

The UPS provides short-term backup power to systems in the event of power loss or brownouts. In an office environment the UPS might be small and provide emergency power to a PC or other equipment so as to permit access to data in the event of power loss. In a data-closet or data-center environment, UPSs might be rack-mounted and provide power to a number of devices, again for a short period of time. In general, a UPS can provide power to devices for a period of five minutes to a few hours, dependent on the type of UPS and the amperage of the devices supported.

Other Controls

The following controls are neither physical nor environmental; however, they do tie in very closely to the implementation of those controls.

Personnel

All personnel having access to the data center should be screened. Risk and trust are an important aspect of the security and privacy of your organization's data. In addition, training your staff on their responsibility to secure the organization's data is vital, but their training should also include other areas discussed in this chapter—such as the process to use when allowing visitors into the data center or closets, the use of security devices and fire-suppression equipment, and other areas that might be part of their responsibilities.

Sensitivity Labels and Clearance

Data-storage devices should include appropriate labeling based on the type of data and data sensitivity. These labels should include instructions on who to contact should the devices be found in an unexpected place.

Securing and Preserving Electronic Media Storage Devices

Each of the storage devices discussed below needs to be considered when planning for the security and preservation of electronic media. As the organization considers the implementation of these devices, it must also consider the risks associated with each, and the strategy needed to reduce the risk of exposure due to loss or manipulation of the device and the data contained therein.

Flash Drives

Often referred to as flash memory, flash drives are small storage devices or cards that store data on flash memory. Flash memory is a nonvolatile computer storage chip that can be electrically erased and reprogrammed. It was developed from EEPROM (electrically erasable programmable read-only memory) and must be erased in fairly large blocks before it can be rewritten with new data. An important note is that just as with any storage media, these drives introduce a number of risks to the organization, including the possible undetected theft of data or the introduction of viruses or Trojans. Facilities should have policies and procedures in place for the use of these devices. The best practice is to permit only the use of flash drives which have the ability for internal encryption to prevent misuse of the data.

Personal Computers (PCs)

Personal computers, often referred to as desktop computers, frequently store at least some data locally, while most electronic health records (EHRs) and other healthcare data are stored centrally. It is important to remember that even for data intended to be stored on secure servers in the data center, authorized users have the ability to cut and paste, create screen or data "dumps," or otherwise store data on their local drive, which might not be an approved procedure. The organization should include discussion of this practice as part of privacy and security training, and should advise users that they should not circumvent processes to store data locally.

Laptops

A laptop is essentially a mobile version of the PC, making the risk of data loss significantly higher than with other devices. Generally, the laptop is intended to permit authorized user access to data while not physically at the facility. Relative to data loss, the laptop is the biggest "offender" for placing the organization at risk and the best practice is for the requirement that all laptops, even those not intended for removal from the facility, have hard disk encryption of all data.

Secure Digital (SD) Card

An SD card is a nonvolatile memory card format used in portable devices. In general the SD card requires a specific slot to access the PC or laptop; it does not use the USB slot. There are various versions of these cards, including the SD, HDSD, miniSD, and microSD. As with flash drives, using only drives with the ability to encrypt all data should be authorized for use.

External Drives

An external drive is usually larger and less mobile (although still easily transportable) than the flash or USB drive and resides outside the physical PC or laptop. External drives usually require their own power source, unlike USB or flash drives, which get their power through their connection to the computer.

Servers

A server is a computer attached to a network for the primary purpose of providing a location for shared disk access, i.e., shared storage of computer files (such as documents, sound files, photographs, movies, images, databases, etc.) that can be accessed by the workstations that are attached to the same computer network.

Network-Attached Storage (NAS)

Network-attached storage (NAS) is file-level computer data storage that is connected to a computer network and provides data access to heterogeneous clients. NAS operates as a file server and is specialized for this task by its hardware, its software, or the configuration of those elements. NAS is often made as a computer appliance—a specialized computer built from the ground up for storing and serving files—rather than simply a general-purpose computer being used for the role.

Storage Area Network (SAN)

A storage area network (SAN) is a dedicated network that provides access to consolidated, block-level data storage. The SAN generally enables storage devices, such as disk arrays, tape libraries, and optical jukeboxes, to be accessible to servers so that to the operating system, databases, and applications, these devices appear to be locally attached. A SAN typically has its own network of storage devices; these devices are generally not accessible through the local area network by other devices.

Secure Disposal of Electronic Media

Now that we have considered securing the data, the next step is to consider what we need to do when it is time to dispose of the data or the storage devices we used to store the data on. The following sections discuss how to ensure that the devices are disposed of in a manner appropriate to the type of data and the type of device.

Secure Shredding, Degaussing, and Sanitizing

Various processes and methods are in place to permit the destruction of data and media in our IT storage media, including shredding, degaussing, and sanitizing. The most important factor in deciding which is appropriate is again based on the organization's risk and mitigation policies. The overall goal is to prevent unauthorized access to sensitive information, including electronic protected health information (ePHI), PHI, and personally identifiable information (PII).

Secure Shredding

Data shredding is a data-destruction utility designed to securely erase a hard disk or digital storage device, completely removing the data and making it unrecoverable. The software utilizes an overwrite method of destroying data rather than other means of data destruction (such as degaussing or physical destruction). The downside of data shredding is that it makes the storage device unusable. Data shredding (electronic) should not be confused with the shredding of paper documents; often some confusion occurs when only the term "shredding" is used.

Degaussing

Degaussing is the process of decreasing or eliminating an unwanted magnetic field on a magnetic medium, such as a hard disk. In layman terms, degaussing converts the 0's and 1's. Due to magnetic hysteresis it is generally not possible to reduce a magnetic field completely to zero, so degaussing typically induces a very small "known" field referred to as bias. Some organizations required that degaussing occur in multiple passes—for instance, DoD practices call for at least seven degaussing passes. The advantage of degaussing is that the media is not destroyed and remains reusable for new data.

Sanitizing

Sanitizing involves the use of anonymization and other techniques to "sanitize" (often statistical) data to purge it of personally identifiable information in order to protect user privacy. Sanitizing can be used in cases where you want to remove the data and reuse the devices within the given environment.

Preventing Dissemination of PHI

The overall goal in determining which level of destruction of data to use for the organization and the specific devices must always be based on risk and the prevention of unintentional disclosure or dissemination of PHI or other sensitive data. Best practices should be followed when determining the best process to follow.

 HIT PRO EXAM TIP In preparation for the HIT Pro exam, you should complete an assessment of your organization's network and facility security. Follow the steps outlined in the exercises below to consider the areas covered by this chapter. When conducting these exercises, ensure that management is aware of your assessment and has approved the procedure. (Clearly, you would not want your efforts to be complicated by negative management reaction to a surveillance observation or a visitor who reports you, thinking you might be considering how to circumvent security.)

Exercise 26-1: Assessing Your Organization's Facility Security Risks

Office Areas

1. Walk into the office. Once inside the door where patients and visitors enter, look around and see if you can identify where PCs, laptops, printers, and other devices are visible.

2. Now act as though you are the patient being taken from the waiting room to the exam room, then from the exam room to checkout (billing, scheduling, etc.), and consider during this walk-through the same list of devices.

3. Also look for signs or other evidence of where your data closets, data center (which may not be local to your office), or other communications areas are located.

Next, you should conduct the same type of review of the areas where the data is stored or transmitted. This includes the data center, the data closet, and backups.

Data Closets

If you are authorized access to the data closets, or if an authorized individual will provide you escorted access, review the following:

1. Attempt to identify the IDF in the closet.

2. Identify the fire suppression and HVAC provided within the closet, as well as any surveillance devices.

3. Identify access-control devices, including access cards, key fobs, or biometrics if used.

4. Identify any risks you can observe, such as access issues, lock functionality, temperature or humidity, lighting, etc.

Data Center

Again, if you are authorized access to the data center, or if you can get an authorized individual to provide you escorted access, conduct a review of the following areas:

1. Prior to entering the data center, observe the signage such as warning signs, authorized-personnel-only signs, etc. Also, prior to entering determine the types of physical controls implemented, including key fobs, access cards, biometrics, two-factor authentication, etc.

2. Once you enter, determine the procedure for controlling access and visitor access to the data center, including whether the organization requires visitors to record their entry in a log book.

3. Look for fire suppression (fire extinguishers, sprinklers, etc.), security lighting, surveillance, UPSs and generators for emergency power, and HVAC.

4. Note the temperature and humidity in the data center, if displayed.

5. Note whether trash, boxes, or other items are stored in the data center. Most organizations do not permit these items in the data center to reduce fire hazards.

6. When departing, do you have to also note in the visitor log your departure time?

Exercise 26-2: Assessing Your Organization's Practices for Securing Electronic Media

Find an individual in the organization who has knowledge of how your organization disposes of electronic media, and set up a time to discuss the practices that are in place. In the interview determine whether the facility uses secure shredding, degaussing, or sanitization when disposing of electronic media. If the organization uses a combination of these methods, determine whether there is a documented procedure for the type of process to follow in different situations. For example, if a drive is defective and covered under warranty, what process does your organization follow when returning the drive to the manufacturer?

Chapter Review

This chapter addressed the physical safeguards required for your IT systems, including the location of storage devices, network hardware, and printers. Best practices regarding physical equipment were identified for the handling of PHI, including PC placement, privacy screens, printer placement, screensavers, and time lockout. Access to servers, offices, and data closets are all critical considerations. The chapter discussed how determining the level of safeguards required by your facility's data center, data closets, IDF/MDF, and backups will depend on the risks to which your facility is exposed, weighed against the costs of providing those safeguards.

Access-control devices were defined and discussed, including key fobs, badges, and biometrics. The chapter presented guidelines for building secure systems, including office hardware, environmental and other controls, and storage devices. We also discussed guidelines for securing and preserving electronic media, as well as best practices for secure disposal of electronic media, including secure shredding, degaussing, and sanitizing. The chapter concluded with a discussion of destruction of media containing PHI, and two exercises on how to conduct an informal assessment of your organization's risks related to physical security and practices for securing electronic media.

Questions

1. Which of the following is an area of environmental controls?

   A. IDF

   B. HVAC

   C. Access control

   D. Privacy screens

2. Which of the following is a storage device that is not normally internal to the PC or laptop and has its own power cord?

   A. Flash drive

   B. USB drive

    C. External drive

    D. Hard drive

3. Which of the following is a dedicated network that provides access to consolidated, block-level data storage?

    A. Servers

    B. NAS

    C. SAN

    D. SD card

4. You have chosen to delete data from a storage device. You want to ensure the data is fully destroyed, but you also want to reuse the storage media. Which of the following methods should you use?

    A. Degaussing

    B. Sanitization

    C. Shredding

    D. Either A or B

5. In our healthcare office environment, which of the following applications must be considered as possibly having sensitive data included within its storage media?

    A. E-mail

    B. Scheduling

    C. Billing

    D. All of the above

6. When determining the appropriate location of PCs, which of the following should we consider?

    A. Security of the location

    B. Ability to view the screen

    C. Whether privacy screens are available

    D. All of the above

7. When determining your organization's processes for securely handling PHI, which of the following should we consider?

    A. Personal computers

    B. Badges

    C. Key fobs

    D. All of the above

8. You can increase the ability of your PCs, laptops, and applications to prevent authorized users from gaining access by implementing which of the following?

   A. Time lockout

   B. Screensavers that are password protected

   C. Privacy screens

   D. Both A and B

   E. All of the above

9. Which of the following is a network device usually located on each floor (sometimes more than one per floor) in a larger building?

   A. MDF

   B. DMZ

   C. IDF

   D. Both A and C

10. Which of the following principles is used by a biometric device to grant physical access to systems?

   A. Something you have

   B. Something you know

   C. Both A and B

   D. Neither A or B

11. Fire suppression might be implemented in the data center by use of which of the following?

   A. Wet-pipe sprinkler system

   B. Dry-pipe sprinkler system

   C. Chemical system, such as Halon

   D. All of the above

12. Motion detectors are considered to belong to which of the following classes of environmental controls?

   A. Fire suppression

   B. Surveillance

   C. Security lighting

   D. UPS

13. Which of the following are methods for disposal of sensitive data?

   A. Secure shredding

   B. Sanitizing

    C. Degaussing

    D. All of the above

14. HVAC is a common abbreviation for which of the following:

    A. Heating, ventilation, and access control

    B. Hearing, ventilation and air filtering control

    C. Heating, ventilation and air conditioning

    D. Heart, ventricular, and aorta control

15. Which of the following is the terminology used when discussing risk associated with your IT systems?

    A. Risk management

    B. Risk assessment

    C. Risk mitigation

    D. All of the above

Answers

1. **B.** HVAC stands for heating, ventilation, and air conditioning and is one of the primary environmental controls—proper air temperature, air flow, and humidity are vital to both data centers and data closets.

2. **C.** The external drive, unlike the other storage devices listed, has its own power cord and does not get its power from the PC or laptop. The hard drive is internal to the device, and the flash drive and USB drive get their power from connection to the PC or laptop.

3. **C.** The storage area network (SAN) generally provides storage devices, such as disk arrays, tape libraries, and optical Jukeboxes, accessible to servers so that the devices appear to the operating system to be locally attached devices.

4. **D.** Because shredding makes the media unusable, it is not an option. Degaussing will remove all data but still make the storage media reusable. Sanitization removes PII but does not affect the use of the media.

5. **D.** Even though we may have policies in place that prohibit the use of e-mail for communications with the patient about specific sensitive healthcare diagnoses, etc., the fact is that users and patients could be including this in their communications. As a result, we should assume that e-mail data should be stored with the same security controls as other sensitive data systems. Clearly, patient scheduling and billing data contain personally identifiable data as well as protected health information.

6. **D.** All PCs, specifically those used to access sensitive information, should be placed in locations where only the intended viewers of the data can see it. They should also be located in a place that would make it impossible for an unauthorized person to simply pick up the device and walk out without being observed. If a device must be placed in a more public space, consider using privacy screens to allow only a limited field of view of the data being displayed.

7. **A.** Badges and key fobs are access-control devices, both for physical security and systems access, and not considered part of the process directly related to the handling of PHI.

8. **D.** Privacy screens do not prevent unauthorized users from accessing the systems or applications; they only limit the viewing area of the screen data. Both time lockout and screensavers that are password protected together (or separately) can assist in preventing unauthorized users from gaining access.

9. **C.** The intermediate distribution frame (IDF) is usually placed in the data closet, while the main distribution frame (MDF) is more centralized and located in the data center or other communications area of the facility.

10. **A.** The principle of "something you have" covers an access control device such as a key fob or badge or a part of your person such as a fingerprint, retina, etc., as opposed to" something you know," which covers passwords and personal identification numbers (PINs), etc.

11. **D.** While Halon is rarely found in use these days, it is still a viable method of fire suppression—primarily in "light-out" facilities where in general staff is not on site most of the time. Wet-pipe systems store water in the pipe at all times, while dry-pipe systems have a control valve that blocks water from the pipes over the data center until a heat or smoke detector arms the system.

12. **B.** Surveillance includes cameras, motion detectors, alarms systems, and other devices.

13. **D.** All three of these are methods for disposal of sensitive data. Secure shredding eliminates reuse of magnetic storage disks, while degaussing allows reuse but should be completed over multiple "runs." Sanitizing is more specific to the data itself; it does not affect the entire hardware.

14. **C.** HVAC is the abbreviation for heating, ventilation, and air conditioning.

15. **D.** All three are included in the process. Risk management is the larger envelope that includes the processes of identifying your risks, assessing the risks, and implementing procedures that mitigate the risks.

References

1. National Institutes of Standards and Technology (NIST). (2012). SP 800-53: Security and privacy controls for federal information systems and organizations, initial public draft. Accessed from http://csrc.nist.gov/publications/PubsSPs .html.

2. Department of Defense. Common access card requirements. Accessed from http://www.cac.mil/common-access-card/.

3. Federal Chief Information Officer Council. (2009). Personal identity verification interoperability for non-federal issuers. Accessed from www.idmanagement .gov/documents/PIV_IO_NonFed_Issuers_May2009.pdf.

4. U.S. General Services Administration USAccess Program. PIV credential features. Accessed from http://fedidcard.gov/credfeatures.aspx#maincontent.

CHAPTER 27

Healthcare Information Security: Operational Safeguards

Sean Murphy

In this chapter, you will learn how to
- Define operational safeguards
- Apply operational safeguards within a healthcare setting
- Explain the value of an information security management process that includes information security training and awareness
- Assess risk in healthcare organizations using a framework of standards-based criteria
- Identify operational safeguard fundamentals within emerging healthcare initiatives

Operational Safeguards: A Component of Information Security

Operational safeguards are correct processes, procedures, standards, and practices that govern the creation, handling, usage, and sharing of health information. They are an important piece of the "due care" and "due diligence" any healthcare organization must perform.[1,2] A distinction must be made between these and administrative, physical, and technical safeguards. While the administrative, physical, and technical safeguards are important by themselves, they must be integrated to completely protect health information and systems. To implement a process that provides layers of protection, like defense in depth, where a robust and integrated set of measures and actions are in place that focus in a variety of security areas,[3] operational safeguards must be added to any overall security program to achieve compliance.[4]

Due care and due diligence relate to processes and actions a company takes that are considered responsible, careful, cautious, and practical. Shon Harris, one of the leading experts in information security, has defined due care and due diligence as follows:[5]

> Due care: Steps taken to show that a company has taken responsibility for the activities that occur within the corporation and has taken the necessary steps to help protect the company, its resources, and employees.

> Due diligence: The process of systematically evaluating information to identify vulnerabilities, threats, and issues relating to an organization's overall risk.

Conceptually, due diligence and due care are a pathway for the flexibility a healthcare organization needs to conduct information-sharing securely, yet within the constraints of information protection.

Operational safeguards apply to information security practices that are required in all industries—banking, manufacturing, retail, etc. But this discussion will focus on the operational safeguards required for healthcare, where there are similarities but also unique challenges for providing information security.

Operational Safeguards in Healthcare Organizations

No organization can totally eliminate the risk of improper disclosure of health information. In fact, within a healthcare organization, the Heath Insurance Portability and Accountability Act (HIPAA) permits certain incidental uses and disclosures that happen as a by-product of another permissible or required use or disclosure, as long as the covered entity has applied *reasonable* safeguards.[6] An incidental use or disclosure does not invalidate an organization's operational safeguards. Operational safeguards apply to healthcare organizations because of two federal laws: the Health Insurance Portability and Accountability Act (HIPAA) of 1996 and the Health Information Technology for Economic and Clinical Health (HITECH) Act of 2009. The administrative simplification provisions of HIPAA called for the establishment of standards and requirements for transmitting certain health information to improve the efficiency and effectiveness of the healthcare system while protecting patient privacy.[7] HITECH was enacted to promote the adoption and meaningful use of healthcare information technology and addresses the privacy and security concerns associated with the electronic transmission of health information, in part through several provisions that strengthen the civil and criminal enforcement of the HIPAA rules.[8] HIPAA governs organizations that provide certain services using protected health information (PHI). Table 27-1 provides a foundational summary and definitions for some of the most important concepts and terms relevant to understanding healthcare information security.

Rule/Concept	Summary
HIPAA Privacy Rule	Implements the requirements of the Health Insurance Portability and Accountability Act (HIPAA) of 1996. Addresses the use and disclosure of individuals' health information—*protected health information* (PHI)—by organizations subject to the Privacy Rule—*covered entities*—as well as standards covering individuals' rights to understand and control how their health information is used.
HIPAA Security Rule	Establishes national standards to protect individuals' electronic personal health information that is created, received, used, or maintained by a covered entity. The Security Rule requires appropriate administrative, physical, and technical safeguards to ensure the confidentiality, integrity, and security of electronic protected health information (ePHI).
HITECH Act	Provides designated funding to modernize the healthcare system by promoting and expanding the adoption of healthcare information technology (HIT). HITECH supports the rapid adoption of HIT by hospitals and clinicians through Medicare and Medicaid incentive payments to physicians and hospitals for meaningful use of electronic health records (EHRs). It also authorizes grant programs and contracts that support HIT adoption by providing technical assistance to healthcare providers, especially in rural and underserved communities; training a HIT workforce; as well as developing standards for certification of EHR privacy and security.
Covered entity	Under the HIPAA Privacy Rule, *covered entity* refers to three specific groups— health plans, healthcare clearinghouses, and healthcare providers—that transmit health information electronically.
Business associates	A *business associate* is a person or organization (other than a member of a covered entity's workforce) that performs certain functions or activities on behalf of, or provides certain services to, a covered entity involving the use or disclosure of individually identifiable health information.
Protected health information (PHI)	All individually identifiable health information held or transmitted by a covered entity or its business associate in any form or media, whether electronic, paper, or oral, including the following: • Information concerning the individual's past, present, or future physical or mental health or condition • Information regarding the provision of healthcare to the individual • Information regarding the past, present, or future payment for the provision of healthcare to the individual • Information that identifies the individual or for which there is a reasonable basis to believe it can be used to identify the individual (e.g., name, address, birth date, Social Security number)

Table 27-1   Understanding HIPAA and HITECH: Basic Definitions[9]

What is important to the understanding of operational safeguards in healthcare is that all covered entities and business associates must put provisions in place to use PHI appropriately and not disclose any PHI inappropriately. When a covered entity or business associate does disclose PHI inappropriately, they may have committed a PHI breach. The U.S. Department of Health and Human Services (HHS) oversees the U.S. laws applicable to these breaches. Over the last several years, they have handed out numerous monetary fines (and a few jail terms) for organizations and individuals who have committed PHI breaches. Here are just a few highly publicized examples from the news headlines:

> The Alaska Department of Health and Social Services (DHSS)—the state's Medicaid agency—has agreed to pay $1.7 million to the U.S. Department of Health and Human Services (HHS) to settle possible violations of the HIPAA Security Rule, making it the second largest settlement for HIPAA violations to date.[10]

> On April 18, Emory Healthcare in Atlanta announced a data breach after the organization misplaced 10 backup disks, which contained information for more than 315,000 patients. The 10 disks held information on surgical patients treated between 1990 and 2007 at Emory University Hospital Midtown and the Emory Clinic Ambulatory Surgery Center. Of the 315,000 patient files, approximately 228,000 included Social Security numbers, with other sensitive information at risk including names, dates of surgery, diagnoses, and procedure codes.[11]

> …a former South Carolina Dept. of Health and Human Services employee, was arrested … by the South Carolina Law Enforcement Division and charged with five counts of 'medically indigent act confidentiality violations' and one count of disclosure of confidential information…[12]

As HITECH has opened the door for all 50 U.S. states to also sue for damages due to a PHI breach, the potential for an organizationally disastrous impact of just one breach is highly likely.

 TIP Per 45 CFR 164.408, if a disclosure is determined to be a breach it must be reported to the HHS immediately if it affects 500 or more individual records. At lower levels, covered entities are required to keep a log and report breaches annually.

The operational safeguards are critical to maintaining a high level of trust between the individual and the organization that uses their information. When a patient heads to their family physician for a routine check-up or visits the hospital for a more intensive procedure, they deserve to know that the information they share is kept confidential. Patients in any medical setting want to rest assured that their personal information is not going to be available to anyone other than the physicians and medical staff involved in their care. Even if patients generally trust their care providers, studies have shown they do not extend that same level of trust when the information is digitized or transferred to electronic information. In one study, 35 percent of respondents indicated they are worried that their health information will end up widely available on the Internet. Half of the respondents believe that EHRs will have a negative impact on the privacy of their health data. Only 27 percent of respondents felt computerized health records would have a somewhat positive or significantly positive effect on their privacy.

Another 24 percent said that computerized health records would have no impact on privacy at all. Interestingly, 24 percent of respondents said they don't even trust themselves with access to their own records.[13]

Beyond the impact a PHI breach can have on an organization, the impact of a healthcare provider not having access to information they need to provide diagnosis, treatment, and make any other health-related decisions can be critical. Of the traditional information security concerns—confidentiality, integrity, and availability—availability of information is uniquely and exceedingly important within healthcare.[14] The root cause of medical and diagnostic errors is often patient information that is not available when the provider needs it—at the time of patient care. Even in nonemergency situations physicians are forced to provide care, usually by asking the patient (who may or may not provide accurate information). In worse cases, a doctor may need to rely on what the family member(s) can recollect—if anything at all. Redundant tests, inefficient care, delay in treatment, and patient safety risk are all outcomes of providers lacking information—irrespective of the confidentiality or integrity concerns that are also important. Having secure information available is vital to avoiding medical errors.[15] This represents a major challenge for healthcare organizations and is illustrated in the Institute of Medicine's (IOM) report, *To Err Is Human (2000)*. The IOM also highlights the role unavailable information has in patient safety and causing medical errors.

Another aspect of information availability is system or network downtime. While these are traditionally covered by technical controls, downtime can also prevented and mitigated using numerous operational (nontechnical) safeguards. Measures like contingency planning, manual processes, and disaster recovery are ways an organization can build in extra security for information availability. And downtime is very expensive. For instance, downtime can cost a practice with six physicians nearly $35,000 per instance when the system is down for ten hours or more. If systems are down just 5 percent of the time, the data predicts the cost could top $350,000 annually. We also must factor in the cost of recovery from an unplanned event. A survey of Fortune 1000 C-suite executives showed, on average, that restoring access and availability to critical information systems (such as clinical patient record systems) would take 9 to 12 hours.[16] Clearly, periods of information unavailability are not only dangerous, as we have already examined, they are also costly—putting patients' lives at risk and healthcare organizations' reputations in jeopardy.

Now that we have seen how operational safeguards are integral to information security (particularly availability) specific to a healthcare setting, the next step is to examine common components of a robust, integrated operational safeguard program in healthcare. All of the components discussed in the following sections are required by HIPAA and HITECH.

Security Management Process

One of the first operational safeguards is an obvious security management process. This is required by HIPAA for all healthcare organizations.[17] A main provision of the security management process is that the organization must designate a "security official" and a "privacy official" to be responsible for developing and implementing security and privacy policies and procedures. This is critical, because protecting healthcare information permeates the entire organization—privacy and security of patient information is integral to every medical activity.

Identity Management and Authorization

This is an operational safeguard that applies across all industries that care about information security. Being able to establish and validate the identity of each individual or entity with access to the system; assigning roles and providing appropriate authorizations to each identity; controlling the accesses related to those authorizations, including authenticating the asserted identity; terminating the authorizations as necessary; and maintaining the governance processes that support this life cycle are best practices no matter what the business.[18] In healthcare, there are so many issues that are prevented or mitigated by implementing proper identity management and authorization processes. Obtaining unauthorized (free) care or illegally filled prescriptions via identity theft are prevalent issues—assuring that patients are who they say they are can mitigate those risks. Likewise, taking actions to enforce use of strong passwords and prohibit sharing of user credentials can prevent someone from using a doctor's credential to access the computerized order-entry system and sign orders unlawfully.

Awareness and Training Programs

The HIPAA Security and Privacy Rules require all members of the workforce to be trained in security and privacy principles. The required training should take place at least once per year. But that does not preclude real-time awareness tips and education.[19] Keeping the importance of HIPAA, safeguarding PHI, and complying with information security requirements as priorities in an organization (with dozens of competing priorities and scarce resources) is no easy task. However, a healthcare organization where safety, privacy, and security are part of the culture as opposed to a compliance requirement has a competitive advantage. And in those healthcare organizations where all employees feel individually responsible for protecting the confidentiality, integrity, and availability of health information and the privacy and safety of patients, organizational risk will be reduced and patient safety will be improved.

Risk Assessment

Risk assessment is the heart of any information security program in a healthcare organization. From a compliance perspective, HIPAA requires that an organization "conduct an accurate and thorough assessment of the potential risks and vulnerabilities to the confidentiality, integrity, and availability of electronic protected health information held by the covered entity."[20]

Even if there were no legal or regulatory mandate, any good security management process would begin and end with a risk assessment. Within a risk assessment are objective standards that are based on industry standards and accepted practices, compliant with law, and adhere to ethical principles. Within HIPAA and HITECH, a healthcare organization can defend itself against fines and penalties (and loss of public trust) by demonstrating what is called the "reasonable and prudent person" rule.[21] As mentioned before, organizations must demonstrate due diligence and due care to convince the courts that their actions were not negligent. There are numerous examples of risk assessments. In general, they are systematic, ongoing, and conducted in identifiable phases.[22] This chapter does not elaborate on risk assessments; Chapter 25 examines risk assessment in greater detail.

 CompTIA EXAM TIP HIPAA requires covered entities to protect against *reasonably anticipated threats or hazards* to the security/integrity of the e-PHI they create, receive, maintain, or transmit. They must also prevent *reasonably anticipated* impermissible uses or disclosures. A covered entity must reduce risk to *reasonable and appropriate* levels. The risk analysis process determines what is "reasonable."

 TIP See the HIMSS health IT risk assessment toolkit at www.himss.org/asp/topics_PStoolkit_RiskAssessment.asp for a variety of frameworks and other resources for conducting a risk assessment.

Software and System Development

Software and system development are important with respect to operational safeguards in that too often information security is "bolted on" at the end of development and during implementation. Operational safeguards, like risk assessments, need to be integrated into the identified phases of development—in other words, information security needs to be "built in." Managing the software and system development life cycle is akin to managing the configuration process, but it is more focused on systems or software as they are being engineered before implementation. Generally speaking, the life cycles have four development phases, listed below. However, to properly build in information security, some operational safeguards must be attended to.[23] The relative operational safeguards are listed below in italics corresponding to the appropriate development phase.

- **What** Specification of WHAT the product is to do.
  - *Initiation* *An initial threat and risk assessment will provide input for IT security requirements.*
- **How** Specification of HOW the product does it.
- **Build** Development or BUILD of the code or components that implements HOW.
  - *Design and development* *An appropriate balance of technical, managerial, operational, physical, and personnel security safeguards will help to meet the requirements determined by the threat and risk assessment.*

- **Use**   Operational deployment or USE of software or system that performs WHAT.

  - *Implementation*   *Design documentation, acceptance tests, and certification and accreditation processes are created.*

  - *Operation*   *System security is monitored and maintained while threat and risk assessments aid in the evaluation of modifications that could affect security.*

When developing software with operational safeguards built in, it is crucial to begin the process with the end in mind. A plan for disposal must also be built in to the system and software development life cycles. In accordance with archival and security standards and guidelines, the organization must plan to archive or dispose of sensitive IT assets and information once they are no longer useful.[24]

Configuration Management

Having control of how systems are developed and implemented is a crucial component of operational safeguards in healthcare organizations. Not many industries have systems as diverse as a healthcare organization. Most systems and applications within healthcare are commercial-off-the-shelf (COTS). For this reason, an operational safeguard for resources not fully developed by the healthcare organization is required. Configuration management controls provide the organization with a safe way to manage changes made to systems once they are in operation. Examples of bodies or systems that control configuration management are configuration control boards or system-change-request processes.[25]

Some of the types of systems that can be found within one healthcare organization fall into the following categories:

- Office automation IT (business and administrative functions)
- Financial systems connected to state and federal agencies as well as healthcare insurers
- EHR systems and clinical applications
- Medical devices regulated by the Food and Drug Administration (FDA) and manufactured/maintained by commercial vendors (e.g. PACS, telemetry, catherization labs).

Configuration management is an operational safeguard that creates processes for controlling how changes are made to a system and keeping records of those changes. It is good information security practices to control and document changes to the hardware, firmware, software, and documentation involved in protecting information assets. This configuration management process should be governed by the security management program an organization has in place.

Consent Management

Revisiting the importance of having operational safeguards in place to ensure public (patient) trust in the organization, having a consent management process allows a patient to know how their information will be used. It also makes it possible for patients to control the use of their information. Numerous federal and state laws cover this safeguard, and HIPAA requires a consent management process. An organization must obtain a patient's consent for collecting, retaining, or exchanging his or her personal health information. And when that information concerns behavioral health or substance abuse, additional restrictions and authorizations are needed. The consent process is extremely important as it relates to promises and obligations covered entities make to the patient. Today, these processes are primarily manual, but technologies emerging in advance of healthcare information exchanges (HIEs) and the Nationwide Health Information Network (NwHIN) are building technical methods for obtaining and maintaining consent.

System Activity Review

A comprehensive program of operational safeguards will include system activity review. This consists of trained and qualified personnel routinely reviewing records of information system activity. These can come in the form of audit logs, facility access reports, and security incident tracking reports. Being vigilant in this area can be an effective means of detecting potential misuse and abuse of privileges. The need for this activity is growing with HITECH Act's requirements for providing accounting of disclosures and notification to all patients affected by a data breach. The sheer volume of clinical and financial data will be overwhelming. Where hospitals rely on manual auditing and reporting today, they will certainly be forced to move to automatic and technical solutions for running the reports. In fact, the technology exists today; it is just underused in the healthcare industry.[26]

TIP HITECH provides that an individual has a right to receive information about disclosures made through a covered entity's electronic health record for purposes of carrying out treatment, payment, and healthcare operations.[27]

Continuity of Operations

Healthcare organizations are required to establish and implement policies and procedures for continuity of operations when unanticipated events, both natural and manmade, happen. Natural disasters, malware that causes systems to crash, and any other number of events that impede healthcare for measurable periods of time will happen. Healthcare organizations have always prepared to provide care in the face of mass-casualty emergencies or when power and water are unavailable. However, the loss of information availability or critical system access requires a different process. It is not practical to expect to go to a paper or manual process until a system or a data center is available again. Healthcare is more and more dependent on electronic health information. HIPAA requires operational safeguards that protect information continuity to be in place.[28] The plan must include a prioritization of business and clinical systems with an order of restore. When the event happens is not the time to begin deciding which systems must be restored and in what order. Those decisions must be made when all conditions are normal.

Incident Procedures

As the HITECH Act is enforced, it becomes a high priority of any healthcare organization's awareness and training program to provide employees with a clear explanation of how incidents are reported. Incidents can be a virus received in an e-mail, a medical record found in a public area, or some other breach of sensitive PHI. Not all disclosures or incidents are breaches that require notification, so healthcare organizations need to design and implement a proper response that includes a full investigation. In some cases, the organization will need to notify individuals whose health information may have been exposed. Under the HITECH Act, healthcare organizations now have the responsibility of notifying individuals when an incident is a breach that may potentially have impact.

Sanctions

The HIPAA law outlined penalties in the event of unauthorized disclosure, but the HITECH Act enacted severe civil and criminal penalties for sanctioning entities that fail to comply with the privacy and security provisions. In addition to patient notification requirements, healthcare organizations are required to penalize their employees when privacy and security policies and procedures are not followed correctly.

Evaluation

Drawing from the basic "plan, do, check, act" cycle of quality management, a healthcare organization should periodically evaluate the security management program in place.[29] This should be done at least annually and include objective measures of success. An independent review is a key component of this yearly process. That does not preclude internal review, but every effort must be made for objectivity. Another time to evaluate operational safeguards is when material changes are made within the organization that might impact the security management program. A good example of such a change would be a merger or acquisition of a new medical group practice or the opening of a new surgical service center off campus. These changes will alter the risk to which the organization can be exposed.

Business Associate Contracts

Unique to healthcare entities subject to HIPAA, business associate (BA) contracts are a source of operational safeguards. All organizations have contractual obligations and service providers that must be considered when operating a security management program. Within healthcare, HIPAA and HITECH mandate these agreements be in place and include satisfactory assurance that appropriate safeguards will be applied to protect the PHI created, received, maintained, or transmitted on behalf of the covered entity.[30]

BA agreements help manage risk and bound liability, clarify responsibilities and expectations, and define processes for addressing disputes among parties. The BA contract requires that each person or organization that provides certain functions, activities, or services to the healthcare organization involving PHI is obligated to comply with HIPAA requirements. The HITECH Act subjects the BA to the same enforcement and sanctions as the healthcare organization they support.

Healthcare-Specific Implications on Operational Safeguards

The need to implement operational safeguards applies to various industries—banking, manufacturing, energy, and healthcare, to name a handful. Across these industries, information security professionals have to be flexible enough to apply information security best practices while enabling maximum business capability at appropriate cost. Across these industries, the common constraints are the unique features of the business and how these features impact implementing security measures. Healthcare is no different. Health information security professionals need to be on top of the latest advances in information technology, including operational safeguards, all the while making accommodations for the requirements of the healthcare organization.

Medical Devices

Medical devices present a unique challenge within a healthcare environment. An increasing number of medical devices connect to the hospital network or use network resources to operate. Summarizing from the definition provided by the Food and Drug Administration (FDA), a networked medical device is a special-purpose computing system including an instrument, apparatus, or implant intended for use in the diagnosis of disease or other conditions or in the cure, mitigation, treatment, or prevention of disease, or intended to affect the structure or any function of the body.[31]

Some examples of medical devices include digital imaging machines, telemetry systems, linear accelerators, and infusion pumps. Although they are typically built upon standard IT operating systems and run well-known applications, their special-purpose nature means that the normal operational safeguards that would be appropriate in office automation IT could cause patient harm when indiscriminately applied to medical devices.[32] This fact has introduced a new term into the healthcare information security lexicon. *E-iatrogenesis* is any patient harm caused at least in part by the application of healthcare information technology (and, by extension, healthcare information security efforts). [33] This term evolves from *iatrogenesis*, which is an inadvertent adverse effect or complication resulting from medical treatment or advice from a healthcare provider.[34]

An example of e-iatrogenesis is when a prescription for a drug is not cross-referenced with the current patient medication list and the new drug causes an adverse reaction when combined with the medications the patient currently takes. Table 27-2 highlights some real-life examples of episodes of e-iatrogenesis that have occurred at various engineering stages of medical devices.[35]

Engineering Stage	Adverse Event	Contributing Factor
Requirements specification	Linear accelerator: patients died from massive overdoses of radiation.	An FDA memo regarding the corrective action plan (CAP) notes that "Unfortunately, the AECL response also seems to point out an apparent lack of documentation on software specifications and a software test plan."
Design	Pacemakers/implantable defibrillators: implant can be wirelessly tricked into inducing a fatal heart rhythm.	Security and privacy need to be part of the early design process.
Human factors	Infusion pump: patients were injured or killed by drug overdoses.	Software that did not prevent key bounce misinterpreted key presses of 20 mL as 200 mL.
Implementation	Infusion pump: underdosed patient experienced increased intracranial pressure followed by brain death.	Buffer overflow (programming error) shut down the pump.
Testing	Ambulance dispatch: lost emergency calls. An earlier system for the London Ambulance Service failed two major tests and was scuttled.	Ambulance workers later accused the computer system of losing calls and that "the number of deaths in north London became so acute that the computer system was withdrawn." The ambulance company attributed the problems to "teething troubles" with a new computer system.
Maintenance	Health information technology (HIT) devices: computer systems rendered globally unavailable.	An antivirus update misclassified a core Windows operating system component as malware and quarantined the file, causing a continuous reboot cycle for any system that accepted the software update. Numerous hospitals were affected. At Upstate University Hospital in New York, 2,500 of the 6,000 computers were affected. In Rhode Island, a third of the hospitals were forced "to postpone elective surgeries and stop treating patients without traumas in emergency rooms."

Table 27-2   Examples of Adverse Events Where Medical Device Software Played a Significant Role

Multiple-Tenant Virtual Environments

With the onset of the "cloud" computing environment, healthcare organizations looking for efficiency, cost reduction, and expert IT support are quickly entering into the virtual computing environment. Today's IT infrastructure too often suffers from single-purpose server and storage resources, which result in low utilization, gross inefficiency, and an inability to respond quickly and flexibly to changing business needs. Sharing common resources and delivering IT as a service (ITaaS) from an off-site data center promises to overcome these limitations and reduce future IT spending by as much as 47 percent.[36]

However, within the cloud data center, typical cloud providers have numerous customers. These customers have varied IT security requirements, ranging from almost none to very secure. Because healthcare is a highly regulated industry, healthcare organizations that enter into cloud computing agreements for service must ensure that their specific operational controls are in place and exercised. While subject to HIPAA and HITECH, the healthcare organization as a covered entity cannot side-step requirements to safeguard PHI because other tenants within the multiple-platform virtual environment have less rigid requirements. The lack of confidence that data and applications will be securely isolated has been a major impediment to adoption of cloud-based services in healthcare. Healthcare IT professionals must be certain that applications and data are securely isolated in a multi-tenant environment where servers, networks, and storage are all shared resources. Additionally, the contractual agreements that must be established between the covered entity and the business associate data center must also account for HIPAA and HITECH provisions for backup and recovery processes that may be more rigorous than the processes of other tenants'.

Mobile Device Management

Another buzzword in every industry is the use of mobile devices. Healthcare is no different. Many healthcare providers are enticed by the idea of allowing caregivers, administrators, and patients to use their own tablet computers, notebooks, and smartphones to access healthcare resources. However, they are concerned about the security risks—and the impact on IT operations. In fact, the pressures for mobile device use are extensive in healthcare. Statistics such as "81% of employed adults use at least one personally owned device for business use" and "Apple shipped more iPADs in 2 years than MACs in over 20 years" are eye-opening. Bring your own device (BYOD) efforts are increasing as physicians and other caregivers want to use their smartphones and tablet computers for ordering prescriptions in computerized provider order entry (CPOE).

These BYOD efforts introduce unique challenges to the operational safeguards in terms of the devices' portability, their varying configurations, and the lack of control the organization has on any third-party software already loaded on the device. Equally eye-opening statistics point to the vulnerabilities inherent in these mobile devices: "$429,000 is the typical large company loss due to mobile computing mishaps in 2011" and "1/2 of companies have experienced a data breach due to insecure devices."[37]

Operational Safeguards in Emerging Healthcare Trends

Operational safeguards impact healthcare operations in all clinical and business processes—wherever confidentiality, integrity, and availability must be assured. This is true in existing processes and legacy systems. It is also true when examining emerging healthcare trends. A few select advances and initiatives demonstrate this reality and are presented here.

Healthcare in the Cloud

As mentioned before, healthcare organizations are moving to the cloud in meaningful ways. Business associate agreements will need to become more cloud-friendly.[38] As David S. Holtzman of the Health Information Privacy Division of OCR says, "If you use a cloud service, it should be your business associate. If they refuse to sign a business associate agreement, don't use the cloud service" (during a speech at the Health Care Compliance Association's 16th Annual Compliance Institute).

It bears restating that cloud computing offers significant benefits to the healthcare sector. Healthcare providers desire quick access to computing and large storage facilities that are either not available in traditional settings or just too expensive. The need for healthcare organizations to routinely share information securely across various settings and geographies places a burden on the healthcare provider and the patient. There can be significant delay in treatment and loss of time, which translates into increased cost to the system. The benefits of cloud computing address these realities by giving healthcare organizations a way to improve healthcare services and operational efficiency—and reduce costs over the long term. The other side of the coin is that healthcare data has specific requirements under HIPAA and HITECH that cloud providers may not be prepared to follow.[39] Many cloud vendors do not appear to fully understand the importance of addressing the special considerations within healthcare.

Healthcare organizations considering cloud computing need to carefully consider the risks before taking the plunge, and then take the right steps to obtain adequate due-diligence protection. According to Rebecca Herold, CEO of The Privacy Professor, a healthcare information security professional must know the key security issues for cloud computing in healthcare:

- Cloud computing safeguards necessary to satisfy HIPAA and other privacy and security requirements, including such strategies as using "private clouds" and restricting data to servers in the United States

- The impact of the pending modifications to the HIPAA Privacy and Security Rules, in addition to the HITECH Act rules, including new standards for accounting for disclosures, on the decision about using cloud computing

- The negotiation of a HITECH-compliant business associate agreement with the cloud vendor

- How to effectively obtain assurance that cloud vendors are in compliance with HIPAA and HITECH

- Metrics to use to determine that vendors maintain compliance on an ongoing basis

- Performance issues, including availability of data and services

- Increased complexity of e-discovery if processes and/or data storage are handled using cloud computing

- Handling the transition to another cloud vendor or back to the healthcare organization without disrupting operations or conflicting claims to the data.[40]

International Privacy and Security Concerns

HIPAA security standards apply to covered entities within the United States; if your data is being hosted overseas in a cloud vendor arrangement, the same privacy and security laws may not apply. However, the international laws may even be more restrictive:

Data protection must be considered a fundamental human right....

—Testimony of Professor Stefano Rodota, Chairman, EU Data
Protection Working Party, before the Subcommittee on
Commerce, Trade and Consumer Protection of the Committee on
Energy and Commerce, 107th Cong., 1st Sess. (March 8, 2001).

The important point is for a healthcare organization to know where their data lives and how it is transferred as it is being shared and used. The physical location of data stores brings up the varying international laws governing privacy and security that come into play—they must be addressed in business associate agreements.[41]

Health Information Exchanges

As PHI becomes more digital and automated through EHRs, the movement toward health information exchanges (HIEs) is accelerating. For the most part, HIEs enable healthcare providers across the same or multiple organizations almost real-time access to clinical information, reducing the delay in information transfer in the traditional paper-based system. Built into the HIE is the ability to ensure information integrity if operational safeguards are integrated. Because of the availability of the PHI, HIEs may also provide a way for healthcare organizations to accomplish public health reporting, measure clinical quality, conduct biomedical surveillance, and perform advanced population health research.[42] But this is only true if the element of trust is present and the PHI is deemed reliable from all perspectives—those of the patient, the provider, and the HIE activity.

HIEs are subject to HIPAA rules. Patients have specific rights to how their information is used and disclosed. HIEs are required to publish their practices and inform participating patients of their individual rights. The only way to build trust is to communicate these terms and conditions clearly. The Office of the National Coordinator for Health Information Technology (ONC) has produced a "Nationwide Privacy and Security Framework for Electronic Exchange of Individually Identifiable Health Information." This framework outlines principles that, when taken together, constitute good data stewardship and form a foundation of public trust in the collection, access, use, and disclosure of PHI information by HIEs. Along with the ONC framework, the

Office for Civil Rights (OCR) published a series of fact sheets to assist HIEs in building privacy policies and explain how HIPAA applies. A summary of these two publications is found in Table 27-3.[42]

Workforce Information Security Competency

HIPAA requires that within a covered entity's environment, workforce members who need access to PHI to carry out their duties must be identified.[43] As healthcare information security processes mature over time, it is important to not only identify these individuals but ensure they are trained and competent. One model for this is the DoD's Instruction 8570.01-M, Information Assurance Workforce Improvement Program.[44] It will become increasingly important to have certification programs that aid in assessing workforce competency, because the HHS Office of Civil Rights healthcare auditing

Principle	Summary
Individual access	HIEs should provide consumers with a simple and timely means to access and obtain their individually identifiable health information in a readable form and format.
Correction	HIEs should provide patients a timely means to dispute the accuracy or integrity of their individually identifiable health information and have erroneous information corrected or a dispute documented if their requests are denied.
Openness and transparency	Policies, procedures, and technologies that directly affect individuals and/or their individually identifiable health information should be open and transparent. HIEs should provide clear notice of their policies and procedures regarding how an individual's identifiable health information is protected, used, and disclosed.
Individual choice	HIEs should provide individuals with a reasonable opportunity and capability to make informed decisions about the collection, use, and disclosure of their individually identifiable health information. HIEs should provide the opportunity and ability for an individual to make choices with respect to the electronic exchange of their individually identifiable health information.
Collection, use, and disclosure limitation	Individually identifiable health information should be collected, used, and/or disclosed only to the extent necessary to accomplish a specified purpose. Appropriate limits should be set on the type and amount of information collected, used, and disclosed, and authorized persons and entities should only collect, use, and disclose the information necessary to accomplish a specified purpose.
Safeguards	Individually identifiable health information should be protected with reasonable administrative, technical, and physical safeguards to ensure its confidentiality, integrity, and availability and to prevent unauthorized or inappropriate access, use, or disclosure.

Table 27-3 Summary of Principles from ONC's Privacy and Security Framework and OCR's Fact Sheets for HIE HIPAA Compliance

process looks at workforce security competency and assesses directly against the following criteria:

> Inquire of management as to whether staff members have the necessary knowledge, skills, and abilities to fulfill particular roles. Obtain and review formal documentation and evaluate the content in relation to the specified criteria. Obtain and review documentation demonstrating that management verified the required experience/qualifications of the staff (per management policy). If the covered entity has chosen not to fully implement this specification, the entity must have documentation on where they have chosen not to fully implement this specification and their rationale for doing so.[45]

In light of this, healthcare organizations will want to identify and qualify workforce personnel who perform information security functions focusing on the development, operation, management, and enforcement of security capabilities for the organization's systems and networks. As a condition of working information security positions, workforce competency will have to be a sustained effort, not a one-time event.

Accountable Care Organizations

An emerging healthcare organizational construct, an accountable care organization (ACO) is a legal entity recognized and authorized under applicable state law. It is composed of certified Medicare providers or suppliers. Participants come from both previously affiliated and unaffiliated healthcare organizations and work together to manage and coordinate care for a defined population of Medicare fee-for-service beneficiaries. The ACO has a shared governance that provides appropriate proportionate control over the new organization's decision-making process as priorities may conflict with individual member organizations' missions and objectives.

The motivation for participating in an ACO extends beyond a desire for improved population health. ACOs that meet specified quality performance standards are eligible to receive payments for shared savings. These shared savings come from reducing spending growth below target amounts in Medicare.[46] HIPAA allows the use and disclosure of PHI within a healthcare organization for treatment, payment, and healthcare operations by and between the hospital and its medical staff. ACOs extend the HIPAA guidelines beyond the internal healthcare organization. For this reason, ACOs will have to revisit their own internal operational safeguards with respect to HIPAA and ensure they are addressed in the framework of the ACO. An unauthorized disclosure of PHI by one member healthcare organization in the ACO could create significant risk both for the accountable care organization and its participating providers.[47]

Use Case 27-1: Expensive Data Breaches Can Occur When Operational Safeguards Are Not in Place

South Shore Hospital, based in Weymouth, Massachusetts, paid $750,000 to settle a lawsuit alleging that it failed to protect patients' electronic protected health information (ePHI).[50] The hospital is charged with losing 473 unencrypted backup computer tapes containing the names, Social Security numbers, financial account numbers, and medical diagnoses of 800,000 individuals.

It could have been more. The consent judgment credits South Shore Hospital for $275,000 the hospital spent to beef up its security measures in the aftermath of the data breach.

The data breach investigation found that in February 2010, South Shore Hospital shipped three boxes containing 473 unencrypted backup computer tapes with 800,000 individuals' personal information and PHI off-site to be erased. The hospital contracted with Archive Data Solutions of Phoenixville, Pennsylvania, to erase the backup tapes and resell them.

However, the hospital did not inform Archive Data that the backup computer tapes contained personal information and PHI; nor did South Shore Hospital determine whether Archive Data had sufficient safeguards in place to protect this sensitive information. Further complicating matters, the investigation showed that multiple companies handled the shipping of the boxes containing the tapes.

In June 2010, South Shore Hospital learned that only one of the boxes arrived at its destination in Texas. The other two boxes have not been recovered, although there have been no reports of unauthorized use of the personal information or PHI of affected individuals to date.

Experts agree that several operational safeguards should have been in place to avoid this event. The following HIPAA violations occurred:

- Internal breakdown in South Shore Hospital's policies and procedures to protect patients' ePHI

- No comprehensive security-risk analysis conducted prior to the incident

- Lack of a business associate agreement with Archive Data

- Lack of system or software life cycle management

  - Custodial responsibility does not end until disposal has been completed appropriately. Safeguarding PHI pertains to all copies of the data, whether in use at the hospital or at a business partner, and extends through the life cycle.

- Failing to properly train workforce with respect to healthcare data privacy

Meaningful Use Privacy and Security Measures

For healthcare organizations, meaningful use (MU) is a provision for financial payments of federal funds for early adopters of electronic health records under the ARRA Medicare and Medicaid EHR incentive programs. The act also establishes penalties for healthcare organizations that fail to implement EHRs and demonstrate MU against baseline criteria by a future date. To meet MU criteria, healthcare organizations must not only implement EHRs but also attest that security practices are in place to protect the confidentiality, integrity, and availability of electronic health information. Further MU is a demonstrated ability to facilitate electronic exchange of patient information, submit claims electronically, generate electronic records for patients' requests, or e-prescribe. Obviously, operational safeguards and HIPAA compliance are important considerations.

HIPAA privacy and security requirements are embedded in the ARRA Medicare and Medicaid EHR incentive programs. To meet the baseline requirements in the first stage of meaningful-use adoption, eligible providers need to "attest" that they have conducted or reviewed a security risk analysis in accordance with HIPAA requirements and correctly identified security deficiencies as part of the risk-management process.[48]

Complying with privacy and security requirements to meet MU baselines in stage 1 and subsequent stages is vital to healthcare organizations that desire to receive the ARRA stimulus funds. For many organizations, if not all, the stimulus money subsidizes a terrific cost outlay for implementing an EHR system. But failing to take privacy and security into account can be a deal-breaker. Devin McGraw, director of the Health Privacy Project at the Center for Democracy and Technology and thought leader on healthcare privacy and security issues, asserts providers and hospitals who are fined for a significant civil or a criminal HIPAA violation should be ineligible for healthcare IT incentive payments. In short, you cannot be "meaningfully using" healthcare IT if you are willfully neglecting or intentionally violating federal health privacy and security rules.[49]

Chapter Review

Healthcare organizations are in the most exciting times of change and disruptive innovation ever. The great promise of information technology (in which EHRs and information sharing play a lead role) is that it will enable providers and researchers to improve patient care dramatically and produce an equally dramatic reduction in costs over time. But underlying these improvements are the imperative components of information availability and trust. The only way to achieve information availability and trust is to have a solid information privacy and security program within a healthcare organization. At the heart of the program are operational safeguards that include a security management program, a systematic and recurring risk assessment, and workforce training and awareness.

In this chapter we have learned what operational safeguards are and how they apply within a healthcare setting. HIT professionals will need to realize and become competent in operating in the healthcare environment. We explained the value of an information security management process that includes information security training and awareness. Such a process will include a risk assessment process using a framework of standards-based criteria. Properly done, a risk assessment provides a roadmap for prioritizing improvements and maintaining compliance. Finally, we identified a few operational safeguard fundamentals with respect to their applicability within emerging healthcare initiatives. To capitalize on these, healthcare organizations must do more than acknowledge and comply with the HIPAA and HITECH requirements for privacy and security. They must use operational safeguards, one element of comprehensive administrative, physical, and technical controls, to lead their healthcare efforts over the next few tumultuous decades.

Questions

To test your comprehension of the chapter, answer the following questions and then check your answers against the list of correct answers that follows the questions.

1. What are the correct processes, procedures, standards, and practices governing the creation, handling, usage, and sharing of health information called?
   A. Technical standards
   B. Administrative safeguards
   C. Operational safeguards
   D. Physical standards

2. As operational safeguards are the robust and integrated workings of the administrative, physical, and technical standards of HIPAA Privacy and Security Rules, which term relates most to this relationship?
   A. Defense in depth
   B. Information assurance
   C. HITECH
   D. Trust framework

3. Which of these regulations is applicable to the implementation of operational safeguards in a healthcare organization?
   A. HITECH
   B. HIPAA Privacy Rule
   C. HIPAA Security Rule
   D. All of the above

4. What is a covered entity that inadvertently discloses protected health information on 500 or more individuals required to do?

 A. Report a breach to the U.S. Department of Health and Human Services

 B. Conduct an investigation to recover the data so they do not have to report it

 C. Contact the patients to see if they have had any credit report issues

 D. Ensure the records were backed up so there is another copy

5. Of the traditional information security concerns, which is uniquely and exceedingly important within healthcare?

 A. Confidentiality

 B. Integrity

 C. Availability

 D. Accountability

6. St. Mary's Hospital is interested in complying with the HIPAA requirement for a covered entity to have a security management program. Which of these actions would meet that requirement?

 A. Consult with certified HIPAA consultants on security management programs

 B. Establish a configuration control board

 C. Conduct periodic penetration tests on their network

 D. Hire a privacy official

7. As a newly certified healthcare IT professional, you recommend to the CIO at your hospital that you conduct a "Get HIP with HIPAA" poster campaign to educate hospital personnel on how to protect PHI. How do you justify your request?

 A. Marketing HIPAA counts for continuing education credits

 B. Organizational awareness and training activities are a requirement of HIPAA

 C. Posters are low-cost, high-impact communications tools

 D. HIPAA is not just an IT responsibility—others need to be "HIP to HIPAA" too

8. Which of the following statements is false?

 A. A risk assessment must be subjective because every hospital is different and only your hospital can determine what standards to assess.

 B. There are numerous standards-based risk-assessment tools.

 C. Risk assessments must be systematic and ongoing.

 D. The likelihood of an occurrence will be a subjective measure because key stakeholders must make qualitative decisions on probability.

9. What does HIPAA require of healthcare organizations?

   A. To eliminate all risks by conducting assessments and eliminating vulnerabilities independent of cost

   B. To conduct risk assessments and hire an objective third party to recommend changes

   C. To conduct risk assessments so they can have "safe harbor" protection because they have conducted due-diligence actions

   D. To protect against reasonably anticipated threats or hazards to the security/integrity of ePHI they create, receive, maintain, or transmit.

10. Your department is developing a mobile application for physicians to reconcile patients' medications taken at home with any prescribed in the office visit. At what stage of development should you initiate the required security features?

    A. At the very start and at every subsequent stage

    B. At the very start, because the security features must begin the process

    C. At any stage of development is fine—security is an independent process

    D. At the implementation stage when users can provide feedback

11. HITECH provides that an individual has a right to receive information about disclosures made through a covered entity's EHR for purposes of carrying out treatment, payment, and healthcare operations. This is the definition of

    A. Consent management

    B. Accounting of disclosures

    C. Patient bill of rights

    D. Meaningful use

12. In the exploit of an information-security vulnerability, what might medical devices cause?

    A. E-iatrogenesis

    B. Nothing—medical devices are FDA-regulated with fail-safe controls

    C. A breach notification

    D. A red-flag investigation

13. Big Bull Community Hospital signs an agreement with a "cloud" vendor to host their applications and data. The vendor will provide storage and continuity-of-operations support to include disaster recovery. As a covered entity subject to HIPAA law, Big Bull must insist on all of the following, except

    A. PHI should not be stored on shared resources with other tenant's data.

    B. Adequate bandwidth for data availability is a HIPAA requirement.

    C. Disaster recovery requirements are not lessened because other tenants compete for resources or have lesser recovery requirements.

    D. Big Bull should require the cloud vendor to sign a business associate agreement.

14. The following emerging healthcare trend enables healthcare providers across the same or multiple organizations almost real-time access to clinical information, reducing the delay in information transfer inherent in the traditional paper-based system.

    A. Health information exchange

    B. Health insurance exchange

    C. Healthcare information extranet

    D. Healthcare insurance exercise

15. Why will healthcare organizations want to identify and qualify workforce personnel who perform information security functions focusing on the development, operation, management, and enforcement of security capabilities for the organization's systems and networks?

    A. HITECH mandates basic levels of certification based on Department of Defense standards.

    B. Meaningful use cannot be achieved for EHRs without a workforce competency program. Healthcare organizations cannot receive ARRA stimulus funds today and will be exposed to fines a few years from now.

    C. The HHS Office of Civil Rights healthcare auditing process looks at workforce security competency.

    D. International privacy laws already dictate workforce competency measures, and the United States will need to catch up to be competitive globally.

Answers

1. C. This is the definition of operational safeguards.

2. A. Defense in depth is where a robust and integrated set of measures and actions focus on a variety of security areas.

3. D. All of the regulations listed are applicable to the implementation of operational safeguards.

4. A. For disclosures of 500 individuals or more, the covered entity is required to notify the U.S. Department of Health and Human Services.

5. C. Availability of PHI at the point of care is uniquely and exceedingly important within healthcare and healthcare IT security. Understanding that is what makes HIT security a distinct profession within IT security.

6. **D.** The HIPAA security management provision requires that covered entities must designate a security or privacy official.

7. **B.** Awareness and training efforts (poster campaigns are part of such activities) are required by HIPAA for covered entities.

8. **A.** A risk assessment should be based on standards that are relative to HIPAA, either through standards-setting bodies like NIST or professional organizations like HIMSS.

9. **D.** HIPAA requires covered entities to protect against reasonably anticipated threats or hazards to the security/integrity of ePHI they create, receive, maintain, or transmit.

10. **A.** Information security should be "built in," not "bolted on," to software development. At the beginning and in every stage of development, there are information security considerations that should be considered.

11. **B.** Accounting of disclosures is defined by HITECH as an individual's right to receive information about disclosures made through a covered entity's EHR for purposes of carrying out treatment, payment, and healthcare operations.

12. **A.** E-iatrogenesis is any patient harm caused at least in part by the application of healthcare information technology.

13. **B.** Adequate bandwidth is a concern, but it is not applicable to HIPAA requirements.

14. **A.** A health information exchange is described as an initiative that enables healthcare providers across the same or multiple organizations almost real-time access to clinical information, reducing the delay in information transfer inherent in the traditional paper-based system.

15. **C.** The current HHS Office of Civil Rights healthcare auditing process looks at workforce security competency. That assessment can be expected to be more rigid in the future and may include actual certification of the workforce as a credential to indicate initial and ongoing competency.

References

1. Baker, D. (2005). Dependable systems for quality care. In Saba, V. & McCormick, K. (Eds), *Essentials of nursing informatics* (4th ed., p. 239). McGraw-Hill Professional.

2. Harris, S. (2003). *CISSP all-in-one exam guide* (5th ed., p. 754). McGraw Hill/ Osborne.

3. National Security Agency. Defense in depth: A practical strategy for achieving information assurance in today's highly networked environments. Accessed in July 2012 from www.nsa.gov/ia/_files/support/defenseindepth.pdf.

4. CMS. (March 2007). 45 CFR §§ 164.314 and 164.316. Security standards: Organizational, policies and procedures and documentation requirements. HIPAA Security Series. Accessed in July 2012 from www.hhs.gov/ocr/privacy/hipaa/administrative/securityrule/pprequirements.pdf.

 5. Harris, S. (2003). *CISSP all-in-one exam guide* (5th ed.). McGraw Hill/Osborne.

 6. HHS. (December 3, 2002). OCR HIPAA Privacy: Incidental uses and disclosures. 45 CFR § 164.502(a)(1)(iii). Accessed in July 2012 from www.hhs.gov/ocr/privacy/hipaa/understanding/coveredentities/incidentalu&d.pdf.

 7. Public Law 104-191, 104th Congress. *Health Insurance Portability and Accountability Act of 1996.* Accessed from www.hhs.gov/ocr/privacy/hipaa/administrative/statute/index.html.

 8. HITECH Act Enforcement Interim Final Rule. Accessed from www.hhs.gov/ocr/privacy/hipaa/administrative/enforcementrule/hitechenforcementifr.html.

 9. HHS. (May 2003). Summary of the HIPAA Privacy Rule. Accessed from www.hhs.gov/ocr/privacy/hipaa/understanding/summary/index.html.

10. McCann, E. (June 27, 2012). Data breach leads to $1.7M fine for Alaska DHSS. *Healthcare Finance News.* Accessed from www.healthcarefinancenews.com/news/data-breach-leads-17m-fine-alaska-dhss.

11. McNickle, M. (June 5, 2012). 10 of the largest data breaches in 2012…so far. *Healthcare IT News.* Accessed from www.healthcareitnews.com/news/10-largest-data-breaches-2012-so-far.

12. Dolan, P. L. (May 3, 2012). Recent health data breaches highlight risk of inside jobs. *American Medical News.* Accessed from www.ama-assn.org/amednews/2012/04/30/bise0503.htm.

13. Caraher, K. & LaVanway, A. H. (March 8, 2011). Elevated heart rates: EHR and IT security report. Accessed from http://newsroom.cdw.com/features/feature-03-08-11.html.

14. Brockman, C. (July 6, 2012). The delicate balance of information availability and information security in healthcare [infographic]: Have you diagnosed your healthcare security program? Accessed in July 2012 from http://networkingexchangeblog.att.com/enterprise-business/the-delicate-balance-of-information-availability-and-information-security-in-healthcare-infographic.

15. Grogan, J. (May 2006). EHRs and information availability: Are you at risk? *Health Management Technology.* Nelson Publishing. Accessed from www.providersedge.com/ehdocs/ehr_articles/EHRs_and_Information_Availability-Are_You_At_Risk.pdf.

16. Gast, R. (January 13, 2012). The power of information availability: Safeguarding healthcare data. *Computer Technology Review.* Accessed from www.wwpi.com/index.php?option=com_content&view=article&id=14119:the-power-of-information-availability-safeguarding-healthcare-data&catid=331:ctr-exclusives&Itemid=2701750.

17. Borkin, S. (2003). The HIPAA final security standards and ISO/IEC 17799 (p. 6). *SANS Institute InfoSec Reading Room*. Accessed from www.sans.org/reading_room/whitepapers/standards/hipaa-final-security-standards-iso-iec-17799_1193.

18. Mackey, R. E. (April 2006). Identity management: Tackling the 400-pound gorilla (p. 45). *The ISSA Journal*. Accessed from www.systemexperts.com/assets/tutors/ISSAApril2006.pdf.

19. McLeod, L. & Nicastro, D. (April 2012). Briefings on HIPAA: Hospital undergoes one of first OCR trial audits (p. 1). *HCPro*. Accessed from http://www.hcpro.com/HIM-277556-162/Hospital-undergoes-one-of-first-OCR-trial-audits.html.

20. HHS. (July 14, 2010). Guidance on risk analysis requirements under the HIPAA Security Rule (p. 20). Accessed from www.hhs.gov/ocr/privacy/hipaa/administrative/securityrule/rafinalguidancepdf.pdf.

21. HIMSS. (Feb 2012). Introduction to the HIMSS risk assessment toolkit and security risk assessment basics (p. 2). Accessed from www.himss.org/content/files/riskAssess/RA01_RA_Toolkit_Intro.pdf.

22. NIST Special Publication 800-66 Revision 1. (October 2008). An introductory resource guide for implementing the Health Insurance Portability and Accountability Act (HIPAA) Security Rule, Appendix E: Risk Assessment Guidelines (p. E1). Accessed from http://csrc.nist.gov/publications/nistpubs/800-66-Rev1/SP-800-66-Revision1.pdf.

23. Donaldson, S. E. & Siegel, S. G. (2001). *Successful software development* (pp. 42–43). Prentice Hall.

24. Treasury Board of Canada Secretariat. (2004). Operational security standard: Management of information technology security (MITS). Accessed from www.tbs-sct.gc.ca/pol/doc-eng.aspx?id=12328&section=text.

25. Mullins, M. (June 27, 2005). Establish a configuration control board in your organization. *Tech Republic*. Accessed from www.techrepublic.com/article/establish-a-configuration-control-board-in-your-organization/5754377.

26. McGraw, D. & Hinkley, G. (February 2010). ARRA accounting of disclosures requirements: Aligning goals with emerging regulations. *eHealth Initiative*. Accessed from www.cdt.org/files/pdfs/AccountingforDisclosures.pdf.

27. HHS. 45 CFR Parts 160 and 164. (May 3, 2010). HIPAA Privacy Rule accounting of disclosures under the Health Information Technology for Economic and Clinical Health Act; request for information. *Federal Register, 75*. Accessed from www.gpo.gov/fdsys/pkg/FR-2010-05-03/pdf/2010-10054.pdf.

28. NIST Special Publication 800-53 (revision 3). (August 2009). Recommended security controls for federal information systems and organizations (p. F48). Accessed from http://csrc.nist.gov/publications/nistpubs/800-53-Rev3/sp800-53-rev3-final.pdf.

29. Oleske, D. M. (2001). *Epidemiology and the delivery of health care services: Methods and applications* (3rd ed., p. 264). Springer.

30. Bidgoli, H. (2006). *Handbook of information security, Vol. 2: Information warfare; social, legal, and international issues; and security foundations* (p. 136). John Wiley and Sons, Inc.

31. FDA. (2010). Is the product a medical device? Accessed from www.fda.gov/medicaldevices/deviceregulationandguidance/overview/classifyyourdevice/ucm051512.htm.

32. Bolte, S. (April 12, 2005). Cybersecurity for medical devices: Three threads intertwined. PowerPoint presentation to MedSun audio conference *Cybersecurity of Medical Devices*.

33. Weiner, J.P., Kfuri, T., Chan, K., & Fowles, J.B. (2007). "e-Iatrogenesis": The most critical unintended consequence of CPOE and other HIT. *Journal of the American Medical Informatics Association, 14,* 387–388.

34. Hildreth, E. A. (1965). The significance of iatrogenesis. *JAMA, 193,* 386–387.

35. Fu, K. (April 11, 2011). Trustworthy medical device software. IOM workshop on public health effectiveness of the FDA 510(k) clearance process. Accessed from https://spqr.cs.umass.edu/papers/fu-trustworthy-medical-device-software-IOM11.pdf.

36. Whitepaper (2009). NetApp, Cisco, and VMware deliver end-to-end secure multi-tenancy. Accessed from www.techrepublic.com/whitepapers/netapp-cisco-and-vmware-deliver-end-to-end-secure-multi-tenancy/1680559.

37. Hoglund, D. (2012). Healthcare wireless and device connectivity. The BYOD Healthcare Challenge—2012. Accessed from http://davidhoglund.typepad.com/integra_systems_inc_david/2012/05/the-byod-healthcare-challenge-2012.html.

38. CIO Council. (August 2010). Privacy recommendations for the use of cloud computing by federal departments and agencies. Issued by Privacy Committee and Web 2.0/Cloud Computing Subcommittee. Accessed from https://cio.gov/resources/document-library.

39. Speake, G. & Winkler, V. (2011). *Securing the cloud: Cloud computer security techniques and tactics* (p. 80). Elsevier.

40. Herold, R. Cloud computing in healthcare: Key security issues. Webinar. Accessed on May 12, 2012, from www.bankinfosecurity.com/webinars/cloud-computing-in-healthcare-key-security-issues-w-200.

41. Winkler, V. (2011). Cloud computing: Legal and regulatory issues. *TechNet Magazine.* Elsevier. Accessed from http://technet.microsoft.com/en-us/magazine/hh994647.aspx.

42. HIMSS. (2009). Accessed from www.himss.org/content/files/2009DefiningHIE.pdf.

43. CMS. (March 2007). Security standards: Administrative safeguards, *HIPAA Security Series* (p. 8). Accessed from www.hhs.gov/ocr/privacy/hipaa/administrative/securityrule/adminsafeguards.pdf.

44. DoD's Instruction 8570.01-M. (2012). Information Assurance Workforce Improvement Program, December 19, 2005 Incorporating Change 3, January 24, 2012. Accessed from www.dtic.mil/whs/directives/corres/pdf/857001m.pdf.

45. HHS. Office of Civil Rights audit criteria. Accessed from http://ocrnotifications.hhs.gov/hipaa.html.

46. CMS. (2012). Shared savings program. Accessed from www.cms.gov/sharedsavingsprogram/30_Statutes_Regulations_Guidance.asp.

47. Ziel, S. (September 27, 2010). Accountable care organizations and electronic medical record integration. Accessed from http://blog.kdlegal.com/blog/health-information-privacy.

48. ONC. (2012). Guide to privacy and security of health information v1.2. Accessed from www.healthit.gov/sites/default/files/pdf/privacy/privacy-and-security-guide.pdf.

49. McGraw, D. (February 18, 2010). A good day for health privacy. Accessed from www.cdt.org/category/blogtags/health-privacy-project.

50. Lewis, N. (May 29, 2012). Data breach costs Massachusetts hospital $750K. *Information Week: Healthcare.* Accessed from www.informationweek.com/healthcare/security-privacy/data-breach-costs-massachusetts-hospital/240001142.

CHAPTER 28

Unique Operational Safeguards in an Electronic Health Record and a Healthcare Information Exchange

John Moehrke*

In this chapter, you will learn how to

- Explain the relationship between identity, access control, authorization, authentication, and role assignment
- Identify and explain access control to data from the perspective of patient, user, and resource, as well as in the context of information use
- Identify and explain how to apply security concepts to a healthcare information exchange (HIE)

This chapter describes how to control access to healthcare information. This includes the typical rules of any business that provides specific types of data to specific types of people while forbidding access to those who don't have a need for access. Access control is an important part of any system that holds information. Even systems that simply provide a cafeteria menu use general rules to restrict those who can change the menu.

Overall, healthcare is not that different from other industries' information systems, and for many types of access to healthcare information, the same security controls found in common IT security identity and access management (IAM) can be used. But there are aspects of healthcare, related to treatment, that require some adjustments to typical access control.

---

* Portions of this chapter are adapted with permission from John Moehrke, Healthcare Security/Privacy, http://healthcaresecprivacy.blogspot.com/. © John Moehrke.

659

- **Patient safety**   Safety is not unique to healthcare, but in healthcare systems safety can have life-altering (even life-ending) consequences; this creates a complexity that is not as predictable as safety is in other industries.

- **Patient privacy**   Again, privacy is not a concern unique to healthcare, but in the context of healthcare and sensitive health topics, privacy is a more complex issue. For example, once healthcare information is released to unauthorized parties, it can't be taken back. In addition, although healthcare organizations would benefit from analyzing past data to make their operations better for future patients, this is not easy while also protecting the privacy rights of patients. Governments also want to mine the data to improve population health, but privacy concerns can arise.

- **Healthcare information exchange**   HIEs are groups of cooperating (and sometimes competing) organizations that must share information because of a common patient they are diagnosing or treating. HIEs are usually defined by geographic boundaries and are described later in this chapter.

User Identity

User identity is fundamental to controlling access, both for security and for privacy. The user's identity, known to the software, controls that user's access to an electronic health record (EHR).[1-9] It is this identity that is related to the certain data elements that the user is authorized to access. In addition, it is this identity that is recorded in security audit logs[10] for tracking what was done and by whom. The user identity is not specific to health professionals, though, because patients can also be users when they interact with their personal health records (PHRs). The user identity is also critical to system administration and maintenance. The user identity is leveraged by privacy to enable or disable access and provide appropriate accounting.

This chapter covers the specific aspects of user identity that are important to access control. This chapter does not cover everything related to user identities, such as those aspects needed by human resources and management.

Provisioning

User provisioning is the process of creating a user account, including performing the administrative steps that prove the individual represented by the user account is the correct individual. In a typical organization, provisioning is a shared responsibility among the human resources department, the managers of the department where the individual reports, and the information technology department (where the account is actually created). Larger organizations require more formal checks and balances when provisioning a user account. In addition, the process gets more complex when contractors or other short-term user accounts are needed. The provisioning step creates a user account, from which access to protected resources is provided.

In a special case of provisioning, a patient gets a user account, but there needs to be an additional step to create a binding between it and the patient identity associated with the record.

Ideally, there is only one user account per person in an organization; however, this ideal is usually never achieved. Where all systems are using the same user account per person, the user provisioning step can be simple. It is, however, common that there is some software that manages isolated user accounts, such as for laboratory, radiology, or other departmental systems. Creating all the necessary accounts is part of the user provisioning process.

Identify Proofing

Policies should be in place that document the methods used to prove that the human is who they say they are before they are allowed access to the user account, given that the user account is going to enable the individual to access sensitive healthcare information. The policies might require that a background check is done on the individual, government-issued identification is inspected, or some form of challenge and response using a previously known identifier is performed. Whatever method is used, this sets up the level of assurance that this user identity provides.

A good standard for this *identity proofing* is NIST Special Publications 800-63.[3] This document defines four levels of assurance that align well with other standards. The NIST specification is an easy-to-understand specification and is freely available, and there are many other good resources.[7,8] The following is a summary of the levels of assurance of identity proofing (these levels are different from the levels of assurance of authentication, discussed in the section "The Multiple Factors of Authentication"):

- **Level 1**   No identity proofing is required. This is typical of free Internet services such as Facebook, Twitter, Gmail, Hotmail, and so on.
- **Level 2**   This requires the user to present government-issued identifying materials that include full name, picture, address, or nationality.
- **Level 3**   This requires that the identifying information presented be proven as authentic. This is typically done through verification with the authority that issued the credentials.
- **Level 4**   This requires in-person registration and presentation of two independent identifying materials that are verified as authentic.

A digital certificate[9,10] is a specific type of user identity that is standards based and thus can be leveraged by many systems. Digital certificates are issued by a certificate authority. The certificate authority sets up the administrative capability for multiple organizations, individuals, or systems to "trust" the same certificate authority, and thus the certificate authority becomes known as a *trusted third party*. A specific example of a user provisioning policy that shows the aspects that should be included in user provisioning is a certificate policy (CP). This is a written policy that defines the methods used for digital certificate issuance and management. An X.509 certificate policy is defined in the IETF RFC-3647.[9] This certificate policy helps describe why the certificate authority should be "trusted." Note that digital certificates do not automatically mean a high level of assurance, because there are certificate authorities that will issue a digital certificate identity at level 1. Digital certificates are often issued to computer systems, services, or organizations.[11]

Another common identity system is OpenID.[12] This identity tends to be at level 1 but could be issued at a higher level of assurance. The technology is more readily available to consumers through Facebook, Google, and so on. An emerging open standard is OAuth 2.0,[13] which is a significant advancement over OAuth 1.0.[14]

Role Assignment

Roles are the mechanism used to give user accounts access permissions. Thus, during the provisioning process, it is important to define what roles the user will need to perform their job. The initial set of roles assigned is typically simply a "starter set," that is, a minimal set of roles assigned to everyone when they first start. User accounts are assigned more roles as they take on more responsibility.

It is also important to have procedures to remove unnecessary roles as a user takes on different responsibilities. A mechanism that is used to remove unnecessary roles will keep to a minimum the number of individuals who have access to resources. Having a minimal number of individuals with access permissions to resources is a best practice but should also be weighed carefully with the need to provide care. For example, when healthcare professionals takes on administrative roles, they might not need the ability to see healthcare information, but if they later need to be called upon to treat patients, then it might be best to leave access enabled.

Deprovisioning

More important than provisioning an account is to *deprovision* it when it is no longer needed. This might be when an individual retires, moves to another facility, or is dismissed. The deprovisioning should be done as soon as possible, and the date and the reason for deprovisioning should be carefully recorded.

The deprovisioning of an account in healthcare is often done through simply disabling access rather than removing the account. This is to allow the user account information to remain intact for a period of time. For example, this user account information might be needed by the medical records department to preserve the provenance of medical information, to prove signatures well into the future, or for other reasons.

User accounts that are not deprovisioned will likely stick around forever in a system, and any account that is not properly maintained presents a security vulnerability. To prevent this, an identity management system may have reports and alerts that indicate when user accounts are aging without activity. Inactivity might also be detected through the failure to change passwords on a regular basis. Regardless, there needs to be some mechanism in place to detect user accounts that are not being used so that they can be deprovisioned.

User Account Support

Not directly related to security but important to maintaining it is the user account support functions. These often include changing directory information to represent name changes or changes to a user's office location or home location.

Internal Directory vs. External Directory

A user account is often contained within a user directory, either private to the organization (internal) or public (external). Internal[15] user directories are often richly filled with contact information including many phone numbers, e-mail addresses, physical addresses, and calendars. The internal directory commonly maintains the user role assignments. In this way, an internal directory is an important asset to the operation of the organization.

External[16] directories contain information that needs to be publicly known. A specific example of this is a healthcare provider directory.[17] This kind of a directory contains information that patients and other health providers might use to discover the healthcare providers. For example, a patient might be looking for a specialist in a type of treatment they need. These external directories would contain minimal contact information, such as only the contact information of a registration or scheduling desk. An external directory would not include security roles or private contact information. An example of an external directory is one that supports the Direct Project need for certificate discovery, where the directory will contain the e-mail address and the digital certificate to use to secure the e-mail.

Authentication

Authentication in this context consists of the electronic mechanisms used to prove that someone or something is who they say they are. (This is independent of the identity proofing step that proves that an identity is being issued correctly.) There are two types of authentication: authentication used prior to issuing an identity and authentication for the use of that identity.

Essentially, the process of user authentication proves that a human is the one associated with a user identity (or user account). This might be the process used in a user interface to authenticate the "human" behind the keyboard. This also includes the process that is used to move that user authentication to other software that relies on it. An extreme example of this is the authentication that is used to authorize access to health information from another organization across an HIE.[18]

Authentication can also be used to prove that a computer system (EHR) is the system identified.[18] This can be extended to anything that can be identified, including a specific service (e.g., laboratory order manager) or whole organizations (e.g., virtual private network). Authenticating a computer system or service is often done using transport-level security[19] and digital certificate[9-11] identities.

The Multiple Factors of Authentication

Humans are hard to authenticate. When authenticating humans, security systems deal with one or more factors about that human to prove that they are indeed who they claim to be. The methods of authenticating humans have been built up over the millennium. Computers simply move these concepts to electronic technology. There are three factors[3] that we use to authenticate humans.

- Something the user knows (e.g., secret passphrase, password, personal knowledge, etc.)

- Something the user has (e.g., identity card, smartcard, security token, phone, etc.)

- Something the user is (e.g., how they look, how they behave, fingerprint, DNA, etc.)

Everyone is accustomed to using passwords to log in to computer systems. These are "secrets" that only the individual logging in knows. Even the computer should not know the actual password; rather, it knows the result of an algorithm that starts with the password (e.g., salted-cryptographic-hash). Using passwords, though, is vulnerable to "guessing," something that computers can do fast and relentlessly. This creates a need for users to create harder-to-guess passwords or change them often; however, the problem with this is that when the daily process of authenticating a user becomes hard to do, humans will get creative to thwart the system. One common example of this creativity is writing the password on a sticky note and putting it on the computer monitor for anyone to see.

Using just one of these factors is usually not enough, but using more than one tends to make the authentication step difficult. High-security environments or workflows might want to use at least two different factors. A good example of this is in the prescription of narcotic drugs. Whatever method used to authenticate the user sets up another level of assurance; this is the confidence level that the user has been authenticated with for this session. Some systems, such as the Security Assertion Markup Language (SAML),[20] will indicate the method of authentication used rather than identify the level of assurance (discussed in the section "Authentication vs. Claims About Authentication (Federated Identity)" later in this chapter).

Within an organization, the level of assurance is simply a business decision or policy. This becomes far more important when the organization must trust requests coming from another organization and, therefore, the level of assurance that those identities have. If they are not good enough, then the system should not return the resource requested. Oftentimes, much discussion and hand-wringing happens when trying to predict what level of assurance is needed to prevent unnecessary rejected requests.

Secondary Authentication

Sometimes a single authentication is not enough. For example, when requesting medical procedures, you might want to be sure that the human controlling the computer is indeed still the one authenticated. Thus, the system may need to reprompt the user for authentication credentials (e.g., password). This reprompting is part of a workflow and usually required by legal, medical, or safety rules and policies. It is done to prevent someone else from using a system that has not yet automatically logged the original user out.

Another case where a reprompt may happen is to confirm an electronic signature, or digital signature. This reprompting is required for signature events to make sure that the signature is indeed being done by the claimed identity.

Automatic Logoff

User identity, authentication, and access controls are all intended to enable proper access to information and functions while also forbidding inappropriate access. Automatic logoff functionality recognizes that the user may step away from the computer without logging off. This could lead to someone else walking up to the computer and seeing what was displayed and using the computer as if they were the original individual. To prevent this, software tries to detect when the user might not be present and take steps to protect the system. This is referred to as *automatic logoff* and is typically implemented by noting that the user interface (keyboard and mouse) has been inactive for a defined set of time. The exact time is usually different given the kind of access and the location of the access.

The term "automatic logoff" implies that the session is terminated and the user is logged out. This isn't always done, but the spirit of the criteria is to stop access to the information on the screen and to prevent more actions under this user account, until the original user can prove that they are there again. The actual methods used can be quite complex.

Authentication vs. Claims About Authentication (Federated Identity)

So far, the concept of authentication has been about the computer system confirming that the human using the computer is the one identified by the user identity. There is another process that is also called *authentication*; this is when one computer system is using the services of a second computer system on behalf of the user. The services of the second computer system will be relying on the information that it is given and thus is called a *relying party*.[1,2,3,4,6,12,20,21] Note that this concept extends well beyond just two parties.

For this process, a trusted third party creates a claim, which is a statement of the user identity, authentication method, roles being used, workflow purpose leading up to the request, and possibly other things. These claims are trusted because they are made by an entity that the relying party trusts and can confirm that the relying party truly did issue the claim. A claim that is not coming from an entity that the relying party trusts should be rejected. Thus, the requesting system does need to know what trusted third parties to use for specific relying parties.

The SAML[20] protocol defines a way to convey an identity and authentication claim (i.e., SAML assertion) to a relying party. Many enterprise-class authentication systems (e.g., Microsoft Active Directory) include the ability to create SAML assertions (e.g., information cards). The trusted third party is the organization, and thus there is only one trusted third party at each organization that needs to be trusted. This creates a federated identity, which is perhaps all the identity claims that your organization issues. This is similar to the OpenID[12] and OAuth[13,14] open standards.

Accountability

Patient care is paramount in the healthcare environment. The most effective approach to patient care involves open and cooperative access to the patient information for the diagnosis, treatment, payment, and healthcare operations. Teams of people work together to diagnose and treat a patient. Some of the team members are indirect and quite possibly remote. For example, it is common for a physician or other healthcare providers to enlist the opinion of specialists. This approach assumes and relies heavily on a well-defined and vetted user group that has been schooled in the proper ways to handle confidential information.

In a perfect world, each person who needs access to data is immediately granted access, and any inappropriate use of data is immediately blocked. The problem with this is that given the open nature of healthcare, the boundaries between justifiable need and inappropriate are elusive. Even with proper authentication and authorization controls, there is a potential for abuse. There are two philosophies to maintaining accountability: access controls and audit controls. Both methods rely on accurate authentication of the individual user. These two different philosophies are implemented in different mixtures, but it is important to understand them.

Access Control

With this method, each user account is restricted to the patient records and product functionality that the user is authorized to access. With this type of restriction, audit trails are not that important. Accountability is maintained by the technology that keeps the individuals from doing the wrong thing.

Advantages

This method prevents any misuse of patient data. An important aspect of personal data privacy is that once data has been wrongly exposed, it is very difficult to recover.

Weakness

This method does not work well in emergency situations where qualified but not previously known individuals may need to operate the equipment. This method may interfere with diagnosis and treatment in that it restricts with whom a physician can confer. As a patient transfers from one physician to another, access control needs to be updated. This puts a large burden on the information technology (IT) staff.

Audit Control

With this method, the individuals are not restricted in any way. Audit trails[18] capture all uses of patient identifiable data. In this method, the audit trail is very comprehensive. The accountability comes from training users on the proper use of the patient data and the knowledge that an audit trail will catch any misuse.

Advantages

This method will ensure that professional individuals are allowed the freedom to do the right thing when diagnosing and treating patients. Physicians and other healthcare providers are allowed to get second opinions for diagnostic and treatment purposes. In an emergency, new operators need only to have an account created; no complex access controls need to be created.

Weakness

The weakness of this method is that there is a huge number of audit trails that need to be managed, mined, and acted upon. This method relies on people not to abuse the personal data and to maintain ethical conduct. If there is no clear consequence to misuse, then this method will not work.

Balanced Access Control and Audit Control

A mixture of both access and audit control best achieves the balance of effectiveness versus safety versus security versus privacy. Using both access and audit controls follows the general concept of "failing into a safe state" in the healthcare treatment domain. What is safe in the banking industry is to forbid access; what is safe in the healthcare treatment domain is more of a balance. It's important to understand that it is a decision based on a good balance, not simply a declaration that access controls are hard or get in the way. This is not an easy balance, and HIT systems need to be flexible and dynamic; in other words, they need to be flexible to support expanding legitimate needs, and they need to be dynamic to adjust as issues become known.

- **Effectiveness**   Measure of success to provide healthcare
- **Safety**   Measure of physical harm to patient and caregivers
- **Security**   Measure of failure to achieve confidentiality, integrity, and availability of needed system/information
- **Privacy**   Measure of achieving patient privacy desires

This balance is not the same balance when the access of patient data is for reasons other than treatment. These other accesses are less time-critical and thus are best left in a mostly access control environment, which will require solid audit logging. The difference is that a delay in these workflows does not affect safety.

Regardless of the balance used for accountability, the security audit log must always be complete. The security audit logs are important to both security and privacy, but they are not the "accounting of disclosures" or even an "access report." These are reports that will leverage the security audit log but will also need to be informed by disclosures that are done outside of the EHR.[22]

Roles and Permissions

This section covers the basics of access control through roles and permissions. The classic security model that is used for many large-scale organizations is role-based access control (RBAC).[23-27] What this means is that users are grouped into roles with others who have similar access control needs. A user tends to have a set of roles that they are assigned to, not just one role. These roles have permissions assigned to them that specify to the access control engine what the users assigned to this role can do. Thus, the role is simply a grouping mechanism for multiple users and multiple permissions.

What Are Permissions?

Permissions are the building block of security access control. They are an indication of the authorization of specific actions on a class of objects. The actions are a small number of specific actions often referred to as CRUDE: create, read, update, delete, and execute.

Not all objects can be executed, and typically objects that can be executed cannot be created, read, updated, or deleted. Some examples of objects that can be executed are programs, functionality within a program, and workflows. For example, in an EHR, not all users are allowed to prescribe drugs; this would require that the individual have the execute permission on the functionality to prescribe drugs.

The class of objects tends to be the usual focus of RBAC. A class of objects is a rather open definition. It is possible to define every type of attribute as a class of objects so that the user would have permissions at the most granular level. The reality is that these classes of objects are only as small as they need to be. That is, if there is no practical reason to identify two objects, then you can identify them together as an object. The class of objects does need to be reasonable to administer or efficient to operate. Another axiom is that the class of objects will have overlap but should not have overlap without good reason. These unnecessary overlaps would just cause administrative overhead without adding any value.

Use Case 28-1: Looking at Database Permissions

To see the power of permissions, look at a database: Those in billing need access to the billing data, whereas those in diagnosis and treatment should not see this information. Those in billing need to read clinical information in order to satisfy insurance requests, but they should not be allowed to create clinical information. Those in food service need access to the dietary needs including knowledge of allergies, sensitivities, and food-related preferences.

This is a very high-level view of a simple RBAC system. Clearly, the data needs to be diced up smaller than this, and the operations such as update and delete need to be handled with care.

 CompTIA EXAM TIP Within an EHR, there are common user roles, also known as groups, such as Nurse, Physician, Physician Assistant, or Healthcare Unit Coordinator. HIT system administrators are able to set EHR permissions by specific functions that specific groups perform. For example, an attending physician may be permitted to read, write, and modify any clinical documentation on any patient under his care or whom he has been asked to consult on. A medical student may be permitted to read and write clinical documentation but not modify that "charting." Following an implementation of Computerized Physician Order Entry (CPOE), a Healthcare Unit Coordinator may no longer be able to write orders via the computer, but she would be privileged through the EHR to read any order on any patient on her unit.

Systems As Well As User Roles

Note that roles are not just for human users. Systems, services, and other organizations can be assigned roles and permissions. For example, a prescription management system would recognize a specific EHR by the system authentication and based on that system identity find that the system is authorized to create new prescriptions or update prescriptions that it had created. This remote EHR would not be allowed to do any other permission. One graphic way to show which roles have access to which objects is a truth table.

Truth Tables

A *truth table* is simply a table that shows the roles in an organization and the class of object, with the actions allowed (such as create, read, update, delete, and execute). Table 28-1 shows an example truth table.

This example shows how different roles (rows in the table) are given different action rights (cell content) to the various classes of objects (columns in the table).

Roles	Class of Objects					
	Billing Information	Demographics Information	General Clinical Information	Sensitive Clinical Information	Research Information	Dietary Information
Registration desks	CRU	CRU				CRU
Dietary staff			R			CRU
General care provider		R	CR			CRU
Direct care provider	R	RU	CRU	CRU		CRU
Emergency care provider		R	CRU			CRU
Researcher					CRUD	
Patient or legal representative	CRU	CRU	RU	RU		CRU

Table 28-1   Example Truth Table

Multilevel Data Confidentiality

Simple RBAC is not sufficient in healthcare simply because the information has so many rules applied to it that there is no simple classification scheme that can be applied. There is a set of classes of data that requires more than the typical (normal) access control protections. These classes of data are called out in regulations such as USA 42-CFR-Part 2,[28] which defines special handling for things such as drug-abuse and alcohol-abuse information when it is captured as part of a federally funded program. Individual states interpret these federal regulations in different ways. These are complex regulations that give us complex rules.

Some of these especially sensitive health topics are easier to handle than others. For example, it is rather easy to know whether your own organization includes federal funding of a drug-abuse program, but you still would need to differentiate that information gathered in general healthcare provision versus that which was discovered during a federally funded drug-abuse program. Where the sensitive health topics get more difficult for access control technology is when they are based on medical conditions such as HIV or sickle cell disease. These medical conditions are not always clear in every piece of health information, and humans are very good inference engines that can take multiple pieces of what seems to be normal health information and deduce that the patient is HIV positive, for example. This is where access control rules need to engage the same technology that clinical decision support systems (CDS) utilize.

Data Tagging with Sensitivity Codes

Some methods that can be used inside an EHR are to tag the data with sensitivity codes. The problem is that this tagging is being done using the current knowledge and current information in the patient chart. As you learn more about the sensitive topics, you learn what might expose the sensitive topic. As more information is gathered on the patient, you may be able to correlate that new information with historically not-sensitive information and expose sensitive topics. For these reasons, the tagging of health information, even inside a closed system like an EHR, is not a robust solution. Within a closed system, it may be the best solution. What is critical is the decision that is made upon disclosure, which must be made based on the best knowledge and information at the time.

Coding of Restricted Data

Sensitive health topics are usually identified with a confidentiality coding of "restricted." This identification does not indicate why the information is sensitive; for that, you would need to look at the policy that was used to declare that the information was restricted. The advantage of using a blunt code like "restricted" is that it doesn't expose the private condition, yet does tell the access control engine that there are special rules to be enforced.

Medical Records Regulations

Healthcare information is also ruled by regulations that are concerned not only with privacy but also with the quality and accuracy of the provision of healthcare. These regulations are not much different from any records management regulations, but their timeframes are greatly increased because they deal with a time frame of a human life span. In many cases, these regulations that mandate that records be maintained conflict with a patient's desire to have some healthcare episodes forgotten. Sometimes this can be handled through access control rules that will blind the information from the majority of potential uses. This is where the confidentiality coding of "very restricted" should be used.

Other Sources of Access Control Rules

There are other sources of rules that might need to be applied to healthcare information such as the following:

- **Medical ethics**   Medical ethics standards show the need to have a conversation with a patient before exposing them to the results of some life-altering results. These are often implemented as temporal restrictions on the direct exposure to the patient, such as through a PHR or patient portal, until the general provider has had this discussion.

- **Court order**   Sometimes the courts will require the exposure of information to the courts or the blocking of exposure of information to anyone other than the courts. A special case is to protect a victim of domestic abuse. These cases are usually handled through nonautomated means.

Data Treated at the Highest Level of Confidentiality

Healthcare information, when communicated, needs to be protected at the highest level of confidentiality of any part of the information being communicated. This means that if a package of data is being sent to another party and most of the information is normal health information but one diagnosis is of a sensitive nature, then the whole package must be considered sensitive. If the receiving system cannot handle sensitive information, then this package cannot be sent as is. It might be possible to revise the sensitive information, but this cannot be done if it will change the authenticity of the original authored content.

As data are handled, including internal movement of data as well as data movement externally, care must be taken not to lose privacy controls. This means that healthcare information does need to contain sufficient metadata to indicate where the information came from, including specific identifiers that may be associated with access control rules. Note that although it may seem logical to have the metadata record the access control rules to be applied to the data, this is not a good solution for the long term. Policies change over time; information does not. Thus, it is important to maintain the access control rules in the policy database and have the rules point at the data the rules control. This allows for the policy to change while maintaining strict integrity on the healthcare information.

Purpose of Use

One type of context is the purpose of use, which is a specific parameter of a request for information or a request to have something done. It indicates why the request is being made and how the requester intends to use the information. A common purpose of use is for a patient's "treatment." That is, the user is asking for this information so that they can make clinical decisions related to treating the patient. If all requests were for diagnosis or treatment, then one would not need to indicate this value on each request. However, some requests for information might be for billing purposes, research purposes, population health purposes, or quality reporting. There is an emerging vocabulary around purpose of use, coming from the HL7 standard organization. Like all vocabulary, there is a meaning behind each item that both the requestor and the relying party should understand.

Patient Privacy

The biggest deviation from simple RBAC is that the information in an EHR is about a human subject and that human subject has rights and expectations about how the information is to be used. In many cases, these rights and expectations are well aligned, and there is little impact on the RBAC rules. In other cases, the deviations can be more difficult. Privacy rights are different around the globe. In some locations, they are very strict and powerful. Generally, the privacy rights fall into seven domains:

- The purpose for the data collection should be known, limited, and stated.
- The policies and practices for handling the data should be open and transparent.
- There is a limit on the collection of information to the minimally needed information.
- The data collected should be as accurate as possible.
- The individual (patient) should have the right to see the data that has been collected and correct it if it is found inaccurate.
- The uses of the data should be recorded and accessible to the individual.
- The data should be controlled against any inappropriate use or access.

This list is often extended to requiring that the individual (patient) be fully informed before positively giving authorization for the use. This is the step that is often referred to as *consent* or *privacy consent* to differentiate it from "consent to diagnose and/or treat" or other cases where the patient positively authorizes something that is not privacy-related.

Privacy Consent Related to Purpose of Use and Access Control

Consent is not a simple binary rule. Consent can be a set of complex rules. Consent is always a binding agreement between the individual and the controller of data about that individual. The data controller can be an individual healthcare practice but may also be a federation of multiple organizations (e.g., consent at the HIE level). The binding agreement puts responsibilities upon the data controller, and thus consent rules are made up of rules that the data controller can enforce. This binding agreement needs to be captured in a way that meets the legal rules of evidence but also be able to be processed by access control enforcement, for example IHE-BPPC.[29]

This is distinct from privacy preferences, which are statements by the individual (patient) on how they want their data to be handled. This could be a very permissive set of rules or could be very restrictive. These rules could be rather unreasonable rules. Privacy preferences can be used by a data controller when formulating the binding privacy consent rules.

Where the privacy consent is aligned perfectly with organizational rules that RBAC enforces, there is no impact on the access control rules. This is the best case from a data controller perspective, because it requires no additional rules to be adhered to. In the United States, the Health Insurance Portability and Accountability Act (HIPAA) does not require a covered entity (the formal name for most data controllers in healthcare in the United States) to take on additional privacy consent rules but does give the patient the right to request their privacy preferences.

> ## Use Case 28-2: Looking at Metadata
> Some metadata explains where the data came from, some metadata explains who authored the data, and some metadata describes the type of data. The desired rule could identify a time frame that should be hidden, a type of data that should be hidden, data authored by a specific facility, or specific object (report) that can be recognized by the unique identity value. The specific way that the privacy rules would be written would be based on the specific rule desired and the available metadata to act upon it. Note that privacy rules can leverage metadata that is not typically seen as specific to privacy.

The privacy consent is often implemented in a more generic way, as privacy rules or a privacy policy. In this case, privacy rules are special handling rules that are specific to that identified individual (patient). In this way, the privacy rules can incorporate rules like "do not redisclose without getting new privacy consent from the individual."

Finally, privacy consent is often the same thing as a privacy authorization, such as when the patient authorizes a researcher to use the data for a research project. In terms of HIPAA, this is an *authorization*, but it is technically not any different from a special purpose of use in the rules of a privacy consent. That is, the patient consent specifically authorizes some individuals or roles to have specific purpose of use access to their data or a subset of their data.

Privacy consent rules can be very specific rules. A common desire is to hide specific treatment episodes because of their socially stigmatizing nature. This can be included in the privacy consent rules in many ways. This is where privacy consent rules leverage metadata or the information attributes that describe the data.

Hint
When there is a need to directly bind a specific policy and a specific piece of data, the policy rules are written to identify the data to be controlled, rather than marking the data with the policy rules around how it can be used. This is an important policy pointer axiom that the policy rule should point at the data. Specifically, the data should not include policy rules. This is because policy rules tend to change over time, whereas data is a specific record at a point in time. In this way, the data stays constant over time, whereas the policy rules governing that data can change as the patient, regulation, or circumstances adjust as desired.

Summary of Basic Access Control

Access control consists of policies and access control information. The access control information falls into some general categories: patient, user, resource, and context.

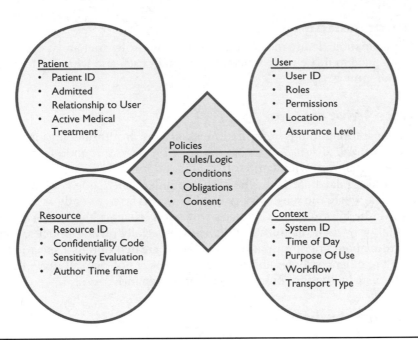

Figure 28-1 Policies vs. information used by policies

Policies are where all the logic resides (Figure 28-1). The access control information is simply available information that a policy may have included as part of the logic. For example, a consent policy may indicate that any data created during a specific time period in the past be kept very restricted to just the patient and the author of that data. It is the policy that is calling for the inspection of the access control information to determine what the access control rule will allow or deny. Thus, it is the policies that ultimately choose what information is needed. Policies are multiple levels deep, and thus higher-level policies will refer to the decisions made by lower-level policies; therefore, the highest-level policies are rationalizing between the decisions of the underlying policies.

Patient Information

The patient information includes different pieces of information about the patient, most importantly, the patient identifier, their admission status, and where they are. The patient information may contain relationships to specific user identities such as "this user identification (ID) is the patient," "this user ID is the patient's general practitioner," or "this user ID is the legal guardian of the patient." The patient information does not contain the consent rules. Consent rules are policies and thus exist in the policy space. Consent policies may be managed differently, but they are logically policies, not information.

User Information

The user information clearly includes the user ID, the roles that are assigned, the permissions assigned to those roles, where the user ID exists, and what the level of assurance of the identity is.

Resource Information

The resource information is information about the healthcare information being requested, often called *metadata*. Most information has some unique identifier that may be an externally known identifier like a laboratory order number or an internally known item like a database table entry. The confidentiality code is an assessment of the privacy risk, where the sensitivity evaluation would be a currently assessed value of how sensitive the information is. Policies will often reference the author of an object by individual or by their organization. Policies, especially privacy policies, sometimes will have rules about any information gathered or created during a specific period of time. There are other attributes about the resource that policies call upon that are not included here, including the complete chain of provenance.

Context Information

The context information is about this specific request here and now. It would include the system that is involved, the current time of day, the purpose of use for the request, an indicator of the workflow, and the security being used for transport. There are other attributes that policy may call upon that are considered context.

Policies: Where the Logic Resides

The important part to note is that policies are where the rules are. There may be multiple levels of rules, and there may be multiple locations where rules are managed. Policies will call upon information about the patient, user, resource, and context of the request. This makes up the space of access control information. For a more detailed discussion, see the access control white paper[24] or other resources.[26,27,30]

Healthcare Information Exchange

Up to this point, I have discussed access control abstractly, mostly as a discussion about what happens inside an EHR. The implementation of access control within an EHR is an essential task in healthcare because it involves a patient. I will now cover how to extend access control to an HIE.[31] An HIE is simply an extension of the healthcare information across organizational boundaries usually within a region, community, or beyond. The patient or employee may have healthcare coverage in many geographic areas.

An important aspect of HIEs is that they are often made up of healthcare provider organizations that are otherwise competing for "customers" (patients) and "employees" (providers). This is not always the case, but it is so often the case that it affects the architecture decisions. When the different parties are not competing, they will more likely just use the same EHR system in a proprietary way. Thus, this section will focus on how to satisfy access control needs when the parties are distinct and likely competing. However, the fact that they are competing does not mean they do not get benefits from the HIE. Better care for patients is in the best interest of all parties.

Push vs. Pull in an HIE

There are two general methods of exchanging healthcare information.[31] One is where information is pushed from the organization that has the information to the organization that needs it, and the other is where the one that needs the information requests the information. The first case is often simply called *push*, and the second case is called *pull*.

Push Access Control in an HIE

In the case of a push, the access control decision is mostly made completely within the source organization. That is, the source organization has some workflow that determines that information needs to be sent somewhere. An access control decision is made based on all current policies, including some general knowledge about the recipient. Once the information is sent, it is mostly in the total control of the recipient and no longer in the control of the sender. There are exceptions to this. Utilizing callback technology such as digital rights management is an exception. These exceptions are not unique to push because pull can leverage them too; however, the exceptions must be agreed to by both the sender and the recipient.

Pull Access Control in an HIE

The rest of this chapter will mostly focus on the pull model of an HIE. The pull model offers the most complexity, and it benefits the most through the use of consistent access control models. The consistency is achieved through the use of the fundamentals that were already discussed using commonly available interoperability standards. These are considered commonly available because they are unique to healthcare. Healthcare does, however, constrain these interoperability standards with specific vocabulary and behaviors.

Enforcement of Access Controls in an HIE

The enforcement of access control in an HIE is a group effort. All the parties involved in the HIE will get involved in some way with the access control enforcement. There are good resources[17,24,32,33] that discuss access control in an HIE. There are models that indicate that the access control enforcement is the sender's responsibility, others that indicate it is the receiver's responsibility, and others that indicate that the HIE itself will enforce access control. When looked at closely, all of these are actually group efforts. Ultimately, the sender, the infrastructure, and the receiver each has a role in protecting the health information. These roles are further defined in the rule of HIE access control.

The First Rule of HIE Access Control

The first rule of HIE access control is this: If the one holding the health information is not satisfied with the access control information, then the healthcare information is simply not sent. This basic rule needs to be said because many people get wrapped up in all the discussion about enabling access and forget that ultimately a deny decision is the starting point. Even if the requester has provided all the types of information that could be asked of them, the policy rules can still determine that the access control decision is "no." Ultimately, if there is no good reason to allow the information to be sent, then it clearly should not be sent. This blunt logic is not the logic that caregivers want to hear, but it is reality because sometimes their request is simply not allowed.

It is a policy decision on how this "no" is returned. The most secure way is to simply indicate no healthcare information exists, which includes denying that the patient even exists. There are others that want to enable smoother workflows through providing a hint that there is healthcare information available but the organization is not authorized to send it. The most secure method is total denial, because it doesn't expose any information, confirmed nor denied. However, there are different layers of security in an HIE. For example, if one can tell that the requesting system is a trusted system and that there are business rules in place that give assurances that the exposure is small and will be properly handled, permission might be given. Thus, a policy could determine based on the access control information what kind of a response is given.

The Second Rule of HIE Access Control

The second rule of HIE access control is this: Once the healthcare information has been transmitted, it is in the control of the recipient. This again is a rather basic rule, but it is important to the decision. If the sender is not confident that the recipient will properly handle the information, then the sender simply should not send the data (see the first rule). Thus, the sender needs to include access control rules that provide them with comfort that the recipient should be given a copy of the healthcare information. This is typically why the access control information includes the user and the context. The context speaks to the capabilities of the receiving system and how the healthcare information will be managed.

The user-based access control information speaks about the user, but it must be recognized that this is typically just the initial user who will be exposed to the information. You must recognize that for any purpose of use that includes treatment, the healthcare information disclosed will become part of the medical record at the recipient. Thus, a request for a purpose of use of "Treatment" is a request on behalf of the requesting medical record, not simply the user identified.

This rule is not as blunt as it appears; there are policies that can be communicated along with the healthcare information that would control the access at the recipient, but even in these cases, the sender must know that the recipient is going to enforce a policy before sending the healthcare information. There are standards-based methods to assure this.

Use Case 28-3: Negotiating the Policies

A policy negotiation can take place before the healthcare information is actually transferred. The policies that go along with the healthcare information are often referred to as *obligations* or *refrain policies*. The use of obligation or refrain is under the control of policies.

Everything else is in the hands of the policies. These policies should incorporate federal regulations, state regulations, regional regulations, medical ethics, professional standards of practice, organizational rules, HIE rules of engagement, and the patient consent/authorizations. An HIE is really just an extension of the access control environment. The difference is that the policy space includes the whole of the HIE, including sending and receiving systems and users (recipients).

A specific example of this is a requirement of 42 CFR Part 2, in which the data being communicated was gathered originally within a federally funded drug-abuse program. In this case, there is an obligation to not re-disclose the data without getting explicit privacy consent from the patient.

HIE Access Control Information

In an HIE, the access control information must come from the different parties in the HIE. This can be a challenge when communicating across organizational boundaries and with a competing organization. The interoperability standards used have been developed specifically with this in mind. The easiest way to describe this is through the example shown in Figure 28-2.

1. The user is authenticated, typically as part of their long-term session in the EHR.

2. At some point, the system queries the HIE and includes information about the user and context along with the query parameters requesting healthcare information, including the patient ID and type of data requested.

3. An access control service intercepts the transaction and inspects the system credentials that are used at the transport level, the user and context captured in the assertion, and the query parameters.

4. The access control service executes all relevant policies including consent policies; if the policies determine that there is reason to deny access or no reason to allow access, then the access control service responds with no results found.

5. If the information is going forward, the query is forwarded to the resource that processes it normally.

6. The receiver returns the normal results.

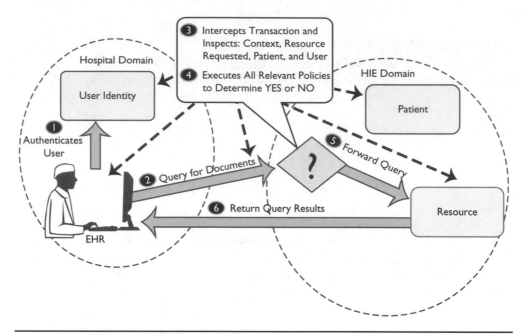

Figure 28-2 Simple HIE access control example

The user identity and authentication steps are totally within the control of the organization where the user is using the EHR. It is typical of an HIE that each organization within the HIE is responsible for the user identities from that organization. In theory, there could be a single user identity domain across the HIE, but this turns out to be too difficult to manage. Much of the concern is related to the fact that an HIE is often made up of competing organizations. Another important factor is that many of the users will have different identities within multiple organizations; these identities are different because they have different roles and responsibilities, and most importantly they are identities under the different organizations' operational environments, including medical records.

There is usually a unified patient identity domain, not just one. Unified means that there is some administrative set of rules and procedures used to create a cross-reference between the patient identifiers within each of the organizations, oftentimes with an HIE master identifier. Getting this cross-reference correct is important to access control, and specifically privacy, but is also very important for patient care and safety. There are many creative ways to do this cross-reference.

This simplified view presumes that the access control decision can be made by inspecting the query parameters and the resource access control information (metadata). Oftentimes, there needs to be more access control decisions on the return path (step 6) as well as within the EHR after the information is received. This simplified view also puts the access control decision within the HIE domain. It could be done in the hospital domain or in other types of resources. The only time that healthcare information will be returned is if the access control decision will allow it.

This simplified view shows a query and response, also known as a pull transaction. The same access control decisions can be made prior to a push transaction. The sender of the push transaction simply must predict who the user and their system capabilities are going to be. The sender clearly knows who the patient and resources are.

Metadata

In the context of access control, this chapter describes resource access control information, which is a specialization of more general-purpose metadata.[34] Metadata is associated with data to provide for specific data-handling purposes. These domains of data-handling purposes fall into some general categories. Each metadata element typically has more than one of these purposes, although there are some metadata elements that cover only one purpose. It is important to understand these domains and the purposes of metadata specific to an HIE.

- **Patient identity**   This consists of characteristics that describe the subject of the data. This includes patient ID, patient name, and other patient identity–describing elements.

- **Provenance**   This includes characteristics that describe where the data comes from. These items are highly influenced by medical records regulations. This includes human author, identification of the system that authored the data, the organization that authored the data, processor documents, successor documents, and the pathway that the data took.

- **Security and privacy**   These are characteristics that are used by privacy and security rules to appropriately control the data. These values enable conformance to privacy and security regulations. These characteristics would be those referenced in privacy or security rules. These characteristics would also be used to protect against security risks to confidentiality, integrity, and availability.

- **Descriptive**   This consists of characteristics used to describe the clinical value, so they are expressly healthcare-specific. These values are critical for query models and to enable workflows in all exchange models. This group must be kept to a minimum so that it does not simply duplicate the data and so it keeps risk to a minimum. Thus, the values tend to be from a small set of codes. Because this group is close to the clinical values, the group tends to have few mandatory items, allowing policy to not populate by choice. For healthcare data, this is typically very closely associated with the clinical workflows but also must recognize other uses of healthcare data.

- **Exchange**   This consists of characteristics that enable the transfer of the data for both push-type transfers and pull-type transfers. These characteristics are used for the low-level automated processing of the data. These values are not the workflow routing but rather the administrative overhead necessary to make the transfer. This includes the document unique ID, location, size, types of data, and document format.

- **Object life cycle**   This consists of characteristics that describe the current life-cycle state of the data, including relationships to other data. This includes classic life-cycle states of created, published, replaced, transformed, and deprecated.

All proper metadata elements are indeed describing the data and are not a replacement for the data. Care should be taken to limit the metadata to the minimum metadata elements necessary to achieve the goal. Therefore, each metadata element must be considered relative to the risk of exposing it as metadata. A metadata element is defined to assure that when the element is needed, it is consistently assigned and processed. Not all metadata elements are required; indeed, some metadata elements would be used only during specific uses. For example, the metadata definition inside a controlled environment such as an EHR will be different from the metadata that is exposed in a transaction between systems or the metadata that describes a static persistent object.

User Identity in an HIE

User identity in an HIE is more complex than patient identity or resource information. Here is a case where managing users and their roles and permissions centrally to the HIE is simply not adequate to access control. Thus, there is a need to use federated identity. An HIE consists of multiple organizations (e.g., St. Mary Hospital and St. Luke Clinic) that are accessing each other through some HIE. Each organization needs a trust bond with the HIE. This an organizational trust typically built through some operational certification and legal agreements. This is characterized in Figure 28-3.

For the purpose of use of "Treatment," the user identity is not as important in an HIE. This is not because user identity is not necessary but, rather, because most of the uses of an HIE are system to system or organization to organization. In this mode, the two systems (or organizations) need to trust that the other system has done the appropriate preconditions and will do the appropriate postconditions. This is a policy: Do not let a system connect that you do not trust has the appropriate governance. In other words, you want to be sure the client machine has done the appropriate user authentication and authorization and is otherwise a secure system. The communication is highly authenticated on both the client and the server and is fully encrypted. The result returned to the client will be properly handled, the information will be exposed only to authorized individuals, and audit logs will be captured of all accesses from that point forward. If you add a user identity to this transaction, it is mostly for a little bit better audit log on the service side.

The other side of this is that even if a user identity were provided, it would be about the user who is currently connecting. The returned healthcare information will be stored in the requesting EHR, and others on the EHR will gain access. So, although the initial connection could be access-controlled, the other future accesses within the EHR must be trusted to do the right thing.

If you look at an EHR today, it has user authentication and access controls that have been built up over time to meet the requirements of being an EHR. The user authentication likely is highly flexible to support some rather complex workflows. One of the complex workflows is the ambulatory exam room, where an administrative person

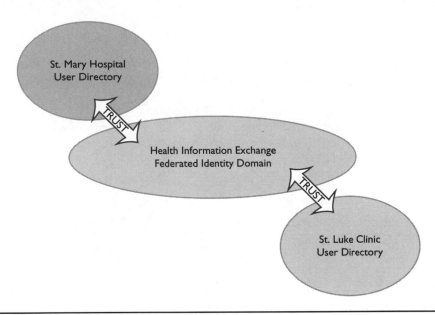

Figure 28-3 Characterization of user identify between two hospitals

walks the patient to an exam room and sets up the exam room's terminal with the right patient and then "locks the screen." Next, the nurse comes in to take the chief complaints and vital signs. The nurse logs in, enters the data, and logs out. Next, the doctor comes in for the exam, again logs in to view and enter data, and logs out. Each of these people is authenticating, but the workflow on the desktop is all about the patient. These authentication methods and authorization methods are sufficient to protect the healthcare information that is maintained in that EHR. It is possible that an organization has gone to an enterprise-class authentication system like Microsoft Active Directory or more generically Kerberos or LDAP, but this is not required.

Let's look at interacting with an HIE or other organization that requires a SAML assertion,[2] as shown in Figure 28-4 for identity management. The SAML assertion is issued by an identity provider that supports SAML. This identity provider is configured to understand specific services (relying parties) of the SAML assertions (known in SAML terms as an *audience*). The configuration will include mapping tables. Mapping tables indicate that when creating the SAML assertion for use within a specific HIE, some list of attributes need to be added to the assertion. One likely attribute is the user's role using a vocabulary known in the HIE versus the local EHR names of roles. Thus, a physician or other healthcare provider is known by a local EHR, but if the HIE wants the role to come from a different value set where the role within the HIE would be "caregiver," then it is up to the identity provider to do this mapping. This is a common thing for identity providers to do, because role vocabulary is not stable within any organization (not just healthcare) nor is it likely to be stable in the HIE. What is important to recognize is that the SAML assertion is issued by an identity provider that does this mapping. The user directory does not need to have the HIE roles.

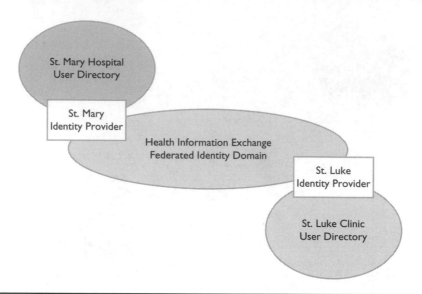

Figure 28-4 A representation of SAML

When this SAML assertion is received by the service provider, it is validated. The validation process checks that it was issued by an identity provider that is on the trusted identity provider list. This allows the service provider to support many different identity providers, likely one for each clinic and hospital connecting to the HIE. Given that all of those identity providers have normalized their roles to the HIE role vocabulary, it is clear what permissions the user should have in the context of this transaction in the HIE.

The identity provider functionality is available for most enterprise-class user-authentication systems. The WS-Trust protocol is commonly the one used to get SAML assertions issued.Federated identity decouples the task of identity management and the process of human authentication from claims of proof of authenticity within the HIE that are used for access control decisions and audit logging. The user management within any organization can be specific to that organization. Organizations are free to use proprietary means of user authentication, HTML-Forms, Kerberos, LDAP, OpenID, OAuth, or any other method. Through the conversion of these identities and authentication systems into an HIE agreed-upon federated identity, the HIE has a trusted identity system.

A few interoperability standards (such as X.509 digital certificates and SOAP) are used to support federated identity. They each have their strengths and weaknesses. The choice is often based on the technology used for the transport. Note that technologies such as SAML can bridge these environments through a trusted identity broker using WS-Trust, the interoperability standard. In this way, a user can use OpenID with their mobile device and talk to the web servers that the mobile device interfaces with. These web servers can bridge to SOAP transactions that need SAML assertions and secure e-mails that need an X.509 digital certificate.

Access Control Languages

There is much standards work on access control languages and ways to communicate policy. The most often sited is Extensible Access Control Markup Language (XACML).[34] XACML is both a policy encoding and an infrastructure for deploying access control decisions and enforcement. XACML can be used with any identity management system, although it is usually associated with SAML. There is no specific tie between SAML and XACML, although they do leverage much of the same infrastructure.

As a policy encoding language, XACML is powerful, made up of logic fundamentals that can be combined into any rules possible. The rules, however, need to invoke domain-specific vocabulary, such as for roles, permissions, object types, confidentiality codes, sensitivity evaluations, patient identities, and so on. There are also vocabularies for fractions of policies such as *purpose of use*, *obligations*, *refrain*, and *broadly applicable consent*. These vocabularies are the ones that healthcare-standards organizations are working to develop, with some of them well understood for HIE use. These vocabularies are needed regardless of whether XACML is used as the policy encoding language.

As an access control decision and enforcement system, XACML is a highly modular system; however, implementations are highly customized to fit into transactions and workflows.

CompTIA EXAM TIP   Remote Desktop Control applications allow the HIT technician to display the screen of another computer on his own computer screen via an Internet or local area network (LAN) connection. These programs allow the technician to use his mouse and keyboard to remotely control the other computer. Contemporary operating systems or their desktop interoperability add-ons like Microsoft Lync have this remote control capability built in. It allows the technician to work on a distant computer as if he were sitting in front of it.

CompTIA EXAM TIP   Before PCs and iPads were prevalent, "dumb" terminals in hospitals were more or less directly cabled to mainframe computers. Terminal emulation software allows a PC to appear to look and act like an older type of computer terminal. With terminal emulation, a user can access programs originally written to communicate with the older "dumb" terminal. Terminal emulation allows access to legacy programs via a mainframe operating system. These legacy systems (some dating back to the 1970's) are getting rare, but are still present in healthcare enterprises today.

CompTIA EXAM TIP   Layer 2 Tunneling Protocol (L2TP) is a protocol used by virtual private networks (VPNs) that supports multiple protocols and unregistered and privately administered IP addresses over the Internet. This allows the existing access infrastructure of the Internet to be used to enable a VPN.

Chapter Review

This chapter introduced the basics of access control and showed how to apply the controls to an EHR and a healthcare information exchange. The basics of access control rely on user identity provisioning and deprovisioning providing a specified level of assurance to each user identity. Human users will authenticate to computer systems using various types of authentication technology: combinations of something they have, something they know, and something they are. The access control decisions are based on the user identity but also information about the patient, the resources, and the context of the access to healthcare information. Policies are the rules that define what can and cannot be done and call upon the access control information to make the decisions. Patient privacy and consents are a subset of policies specific to that patient and their preferences. When extending access control across a healthcare information exchange, the various access control information comes together in a cooperative access control. The access control decision in an HIE delivers data only when the access control policies authorize the information to flow.

Questions

To test your comprehension of the chapter, answer the following questions and then check your answers against the list of correct answers that follows the questions.

1. Which control is responsible for confirming that the human is who they say they are?

    A. Authorization

    B. Audit

    C. Authentication

    D. Anonymization

2. In what way is accountability different in healthcare from other industries?

    A. There is no difference in accountability in healthcare from other industries.

    B. There is more balance in controlling access and monitoring access in healthcare.

    C. There is more balance in the banking industry on identify management.

    D. There is more balance in other industries on controlling access.

3. What is the level of assurance of identity proofing that requires the presentation of a government-issued identity but does not require verification of that government-issued identity?

    A. Level 1

    B. Level 2

C. Level 3

D. Level 4

4. Identity the factors that a computer uses to authenticate a human user.

   A. Something you are, have, and know

   B. Something with an image of you on it

   C. Something that you know, like a secret

   D. None of the above

5. What does SAML do?

   A. Provisions user accounts

   B. Makes access control decisions

   C. Defines an identity claim

   D. Provides an audit logging system

6. What of the following is *not* a component of RBAC?

   A. Identity, permission, roles

   B. Consent only

   C. Permission and consent

   D. Roles and consent

7. What are the operations on a class of objects that make up a permission?

   A. Identity, authentication, authorization, and consent

   B. Authentication, authorization, and identify

   C. Consent, identity, and authorization

   D. Create, read, update, delete, and execute (aka CRUDE)

8. What is the policy pointer axiom?

   A. Data should not include the policy rules; the policy rules should point at the data they apply to.

   B. Data should always be pointed to in policies.

   C. Policy rules should never point to data.

   D. None of the above.

9. What is federated identity?

   A. It includes the concepts of authentication, authorization, and identify.

   B. It provides a mechanism for communicating claims of identity and authentication to a relying party in a way that can be understood and trusted.

   C. Identity can never be federated.

   D. None of the above.

10. What standard can be used to harmonize different identity and authentication systems?

    A. WS-Trust

    B. WAP

    C. Wi-Fi

    D. WEP

Answers

1. **C.** Authentication is the control responsible for confirming that humans are who they say they are.

2. **B.** Accountability in healthcare is very much like other industries. The exceptions relate to the fact that accountability in healthcare is more of a balance between controlling access and monitoring access.

3. **B.** Level 2 requires presenting government-issued identification that includes your full name, picture, and address or nationality; it does not require that the identity be proven as authentic.

4. **A.** Identify factors are something you are (biometric), have (hardware token), or know (password).

5. **C.** SAML defines a way to convey an identity and authentication claim from one party to a relying party.

6. **A.** RBAC is a binding between an identity, role, and permission. Thus, it does not include consent.

7. **D.** The fundamental actions that make up a permission are create, read, update, delete, and execute (aka CRUDE).

8. **A.** Data should not include the policy rules; the policy rules should point at the data to which they apply.

9. **B.** Federated identity keeps local the identity management task by providing a mechanism for communicating claims of identity and authentication to a relying party in a way that can be understood and trusted.

10. **A.** WS-Trust is the standard used to harmonize different identity and authentication systems.

References

1. The national strategy for trusted identities in cyberspace. (2010). Accessed in June 2010 from www.nist.gov/nstic/.

2. Identity, credential, and access management. (2008). Accessed from www.idmanagement.gov/pages.cfm/page/ICAM.

3. Electronic authentication guide, revision 1, NIST SP800-63. (2011). Accessed from http://csrc.nist.gov/publications/PubsSPs.html.

4. Identity assurance framework: Assurance levels, draft 04. (2009). Accessed from http://kantarainitiative.org/confluence/download/attachments/38371432/Kantara+IAF-1200-Levels+of+Assurance.pdf.

5. Enterprise user authentication (EUA) profile. (2012). Accessed from www.ihe.net/Technical_Framework/index.cfm#IT.

6. Cross-enterprise user assertion (XUA) profile. (2012). Accessed from www.ihe.net/Technical_Framework/index.cfm#IT.

7. Standard guide for user authentication and authorization: ASTM E1985-98. (2005). Accessed from www.astm.org/Standards/E1985.htm.

8. Standard guide for electronic authentication of health care information: ASTM E1762-95. (2009). Accessed from www.astm.org/Standards/E1762.htm.

9. Internet X.509 public key infrastructure certificate policy and certification practices framework: RFC 3647. (2008). Accessed from http://tools.ietf.org/html/rfc3647.

10. Health informatics: public key infrastructure: part 1: Overview of digital certificate services: ISO 17090-1:2008. (2008). Accessed from http://standards.iso.org/ittf/licence.html.

11. Management of machine authentication certificates. (2007). Accessed from www.medicalimaging.org/wp-content/uploads/2011/02/CertificateManagement-2007-05-Published.pdf.

12. OpenID authentication 2.0: Final. Accessed on July 22, 2012, from http://openid.net/specs/openid-authentication-2_0.html.

13. The OAuth 2.0 authorization framework, draft in progress. Accessed from http://tools.ietf.org/html/draft-ietf-oauth-v2

14. The OAuth 1.0 protocol: RFC 5849. (2010). Accessed from www.ietf.org/rfc/rfc5849.txt.

15. Personnel white pages (PWP) profile. (2012). Accessed from www.ihe.net/Technical_Framework/index.cfm#IT.

16. Health informatics: Directory services for security, communications and identification of professionals and patients. (2005). Accessed from http://standards.iso.org/ittf/licence.html.

17. Healthcare provider directory (HPD) profile supplement. (2011). Accessed from www.ihe.net/Technical_Framework/index.cfm#IT.

18. Audit trail and node authentication (ATNA) profile. (2012). Accessed from www.ihe.net/Technical_Framework/index.cfm#IT.

19. The transport layer security (TLS) protocol: version 1.2: RFC 5246. (2008). Accessed on June 22, 2010, from http://tools.ietf.org/html/rfc5246.

20. SAML v2.0. Accessed from http://saml.xml.org/saml-specifications.

21. XSPA profile of SAML v2.0 for healthcare version 1.0. Accessed from https://wiki.oasis-open.org/security/XSPASAML2Profile.

22. Healthcare security/privacy blog. (2009). Accessed from http://HealthcareSecPrivacy.blogspot.com.

23. Information technology: Role-based access control. (2004). Accessed from www.incits.org/.

24. Access control white paper. (2012). Accessed from www.ihe.net/Technical_Framework/index.cfm#IT.

25. Health informatics: electronic health record communication: part 4: security. (2009). Accessed from http://standards.iso.org/ittf/licence.html.

26. Standard guide for information access privileges to health information. (2009). Accessed from www.astm.org/Standards/E1986.htm.

27. Standard guide for privilege management infrastructure. (2007). Accessed from www.astm.org/Standards/E2595.htm.

28. Confidentiality of alcohol and drug abuse patient records, USA 42-CFR-Part 2. Accessed from http://ecfr.gpoaccess.gov/cgi/t/text/text-idx?c=ecfr&rgn=div5&view=text&node=42:1.0.1.1.2&idno=42.

29. Basic patient privacy consents (BPPC). (2012). Accessed from www.ihe.net/Technical_Framework/index.cfm#IT.

30. Health informatics: Privilege management and access control. (2005). Accessed from http://standards.iso.org/ittf/licence.html.

31. Health information exchange: Enabling document sharing using IHE profiles. (2012). Accessed from www.ihe.net/Technical_Framework/index.cfm#IT.

32. Template for XDS affinity domain deployment planning. (2008). Accessed from www.ihe.net/Technical_Framework/index.cfm#IT.

33. Security architecture design process for health information exchanges (HIEs). NIST IR7497. (2010). Accessed from http://csrc.nist.gov/publications/PubsNISTIRs.html.

34. Healthcare security/privacy blog: John Moehrke's "Healthcare Metadata." (2012). Accessed from http://HealthcareSecPrivacy.blogspot.com.

Architectural Safeguards

Lisa A. Gallagher

In this chapter, you will learn how to
- Understand the importance of architectural safeguards for designing, building, purchasing, and implementing safe and secure IT systems and medical devices
- Know the relationship between reliability, availability, and safety as they impact healthcare IT systems
- Understand basic design considerations for high-reliability healthcare IT systems

The introduction of certain technology platforms, such as electronic health records (EHRs), has highlighted concerns about the privacy, security, and availability of patient records. But there are also many other types of IT systems and components that are used in the healthcare workflow today. For example, these are several common categories of medical devices that are used in healthcare organizations today:

- **Monitoring** Typically used to measure and track physiological aspects of patient health (for example, a heart monitor)
- **Resuscitative** Used to restore normal brain or heart function (for example, a defibrillator)
- **Surgical** Used to aid surgical procedures (for example, medical lasers)
- **Imaging** Used to obtain a medical image for diagnostic purposes (for example, an X-ray machine)

Each category listed above contains examples of medical devices that are not only implemented in technology but have evolved to contain software operating systems, to connect to and share data through information networks, and even to operate remotely through wireless technical or cellular networks. Increased use of mobile medical devices is expected to be a trend as the healthcare industry looks for new, cost-saving, and safe ways to expand and improve healthcare services (for example, to reach underserved or remote populations).

When designing or building an IT system, all aspects of the system's architecture—its individual hardware and software components—must be considered. An IT system design-and-build process demands that various architectural considerations related to the components' features, functions, and desired performance (in terms of measurable attributes or parameters of the system performance) are set out as requirements, based on the needs of the users and the operational environment. The goal and the desired outcome is to design, build, purchase, and implement safe and secure IT systems and components for use in healthcare.

Reliability

One important performance trait of an IT system is its reliability. *Reliability* is the capability of the software product to maintain a specified level of performance when used under specified conditions.[1] Table 29-1 shows several ways to specify and measure the reliability of an IT system.

 NOTE System reliability, by definition, includes all parts of the system—hardware, software, supporting infrastructure (including critical external interfaces), operators, and procedures.

For the software components of a system, a common reliability metric is the number of software faults, usually expressed as faults per thousand lines of code. This measure, along with software execution time, is key to most software reliability models and estimates.

Relationship between Reliability and Security

Software errors, defects, and logic flaws can be a cause of commonly exploited software vulnerabilities. For example, programming errors in the software of an IT system can introduce security vulnerabilities (weaknesses in the system that allow exploitation) in the following areas:

- Authentication of users (for example, improperly authenticating a potential user)

- Authorization of access rights and privileges (for example, allowing unauthorized access)

- Data confidentiality (for example, allowing unauthorized access)

- Data integrity (for example, allowing unauthorized modification or deletion of data)

- Data availability (for example, preventing data from being accessed when needed)

System Usage	Reliability Measure
System is operated frequently or continuously as a resource or workflow aid, such as most vehicles, machinery, and electronic equipment	Mean time to failure (MTTF) or failure rate
Specific mission is defined for system	Probability or percentage (without dimension)
Single mission (for example, rocket launch or airbag deployment)	Probability of one-time success
For repairable systems	Mean time to repair (MTTR)

Table 29-1   System Reliability Measures

Other problems or defects that affect security are hardware defects; inadequate site access, monitoring policies, and procedures; and lack of employee performance and monitoring policies and procedures. These are examples of "system" vulnerabilities that are not directly related to the software.

Reliability Implications for Healthcare Systems

For all IT systems, design and performance considerations are critical to meeting system mission goals and foundational to technical security considerations. The goal is to design the software and other system elements to have as few defects and failures as possible. For healthcare, the consequences of IT system failures can be severe, including:

- Risk to patient outcomes, health, and lives
- Data security breaches
- Public health implications
- Research implications
- Cost implications
- Reputational impact
- Legal/regulatory compliance implications

Reliability goals should be considered and identified for all care scenarios and processes. For hospitals, this may mean that these goals might be defined by system, department, or workflow. For a physician office, it is likely to include the workflow and integration of the IT system.

For each system or process, failure (and how it can be detected or measured) should be defined and then reliability goals associated with the desired improvement or outcome. For example, in the emergency room, one measure of failure is the percentage of patients receiving the wrong diagnosis, treatment, or medication. A reliability analysis can be conducted at the system or component level. All analyses should include the software, hardware, physical, and employee components as discussed above.

Understanding the relationship between reliability and healthcare is critical as IT systems are increasingly integrated into the clinical workflow.

Availability

System *availability* is the property of the system being accessible and usable upon demand by an authorized entity.[2] Simply put, availability is the proportion of time a system is functioning.

The availability of a system is typically measured as a factor of its reliability—as reliability increases, so does availability. No system can guarantee 100-percent reliability; therefore, no system can assure 100-percent availability.

Availability as a Component of Data Security

There are three main components, or goals, of data security (together, these are commonly called "CIA"):

- Confidentiality
- Integrity
- Availability

Information or data security is concerned with the confidentiality, integrity, and availability of data regardless of the form it may take—electronic, print, or other forms.

With respect to electronic health data, data availability is a critical issue. For any health IT system to serve its purpose, the information (for example, patient data and ancillary data—decision support data, references, alerts, etc.) must be available when it is needed. This means that the computing systems used to store and process the information, the security controls used to protect it, and the communication channels used to access it must be functioning correctly. The goal of high-availability systems is to remain available at all times, preventing service disruptions due to power outages, hardware failures, and system upgrades. Ensuring availability also involves preventing denial-of-service attacks (attacks meant to disrupt system and/or data access by users).

Maintainability

Maintainability for IT systems can be defined as the capability of the software product to be modified. Modifications may include corrections, improvements, or adaptation of the software to changes in environment, requirements, and/or functional specifications.[3] Maintainability affects both reliability and availability of IT systems and components.

Scalability

Scalability is the ability of a system, network, or process to handle a growing amount of work in a capable manner or the ability of a system, network, or process to be enlarged to accommodate that growth.[4] When an organization is considering its design or purchase requirements for health IT systems, it should also consider its ability to easily and quickly enhance the system by adding new functionality and/or storage capacity. A system that can easily "scale" to meet new requirements enables an organization to invest in technology based on current needs without having to replace the system when requirements change.

The term *cloud* or *cloud computing* is defined as a model for enabling convenient, on-demand network access to a shared pool of configurable computing resources (e.g., networks, servers, storage, applications, and services) that can be rapidly provisioned and released with minimal management effort or service-provider interaction.[5] Healthcare organizations are beginning to take advantage of the ability to "outsource to the cloud" (contract for IT services or system usage) in order to address the scalability issue. This allows the organizations to facilitate rapid provisioning of additional computing, application, and storage resources and avoid some capital expenditures.

Scalability can also be thought of as a measure of how well a system or application can grow to meet increasing performance demands. In thinking this way, one can see that scalability is a factor for both availability and reliability.

Safety

Safety in medicine is often used to mean patient safety. The Institute of Medicine (IOM) has defined *patient safety* as "the prevention of harm to patients."[6] An event during an episode of care that causes harm to a patient is called an *adverse event*. Patient safety overlaps in many ways with privacy, security, and technology concerns, which we will discuss later in this chapter.

With respect to system and software design, safety means that a life-critical system behaves as needed even when some components fail. Systems that are to be used in healthcare should be designed so that if failure occurs, it will not cause a patient to be physically harmed.

Considerations for Healthcare IT Systems

Ideally, in the early design of a system, the design is analyzed to determine what faults can possibly occur. That analysis is then used to identify the safety requirements.

 TIP The most common method used to identify possible faults is the failure mode and effects analysis (FMEA).[7]

The FMEA (see IEC 60812) provides for an evaluation of potential failure modes for processes and their likely effect on outcomes and/or product performance. Once failure modes are established, risk reduction can be used to eliminate, contain, reduce, or control the potential failures. The effects of the failure mode are described and assigned a probability based on the predicted failure rate and failure mode ratio of the system or components. Failure modes with identical or similar effects can be combined and summarized in a failure-mode effects summary. When combined with criticality analysis, FMEA is known as failure mode, effects, and criticality analysis (FMECA).

In general terms, once a failure mode is identified, it can usually be mitigated by adding extra or redundant equipment to the system. Ongoing maintenance actions are also important safety-related actions. With regard to maintenance activities, considerations must be taken to reduce operational risk by ensuring acceptable levels of operational readiness and availability.

The overall patient-safety concerns of a healthcare organization can be met only by defining system safety requirements early on in the design and/or acquisition process of a health IT system and performing a FMEA and/or FMECA analysis to identify and mitigate faults.

Safety analysis is focused on safety-critical systems or components. Reliability analysis has a broader scope than safety analysis, because noncritical failures must also be considered. Higher failure rates may be considered acceptable for noncritical systems.

Considerations for Medical Devices

Medical devices are considered safety-critical devices. They are regulated as such by the U.S. Food and Drug Administration (FDA).

 TIP The FDA reviews applications from medical-device manufacturers and approves them to sell medical devices on the open market. It also reviews any substantial changes to the medical-device system, software, or other components.

The FDA also monitors reports of adverse events and other problems with medical devices and alerts health professionals and the public when needed to ensure proper use of devices and the health and safety of patients. The FDA posts lists of recent medical-device recalls and other FDA safety communications on its safety web site, www .fda.gov/safety.

The FDA has also recently begun to oversee the deployment and use of mobile medical devices and mobile medical applications. A mobile medical device is a device that exchanges data with other devices or computers over a wireless network. Mobile applications are software programs that run on smartphones and other mobile communications devices and in most cases communicate over a cellular network. Development of mobile medical applications is opening new and innovative ways for technology to improve health and healthcare.

Consumers use mobile medical applications to manage their own health and wellness. Healthcare professionals are using these applications to improve and facilitate patient care. These applications include a wide range of functions, from allowing individuals to monitor and input their blood levels for diabetes maintenance to allowing doctors to view a patient's X-rays on their mobile communications device. The FDA encourages further development of mobile medical applications that improve healthcare and provide consumers and healthcare professionals with valuable health information very quickly.

The FDA has a public health responsibility to oversee the safety and effectiveness of a small subset of mobile medical applications that present a potential risk to patients if they do not work as intended. In order to balance patient safety with innovation, the FDA has published guidance for manufacturers and developers of mobile medical applications, including clear and predictable outlines of FDA expectations during the approval process. The draft guidance, released on July 19, 2011, defined a small subset of mobile medical applications that may impact the performance or functionality of currently regulated medical devices and therefore will require FDA oversight.[8]

Considerations for Design of High-Reliability Healthcare Systems

In the design of safety-critical systems, one of the first tasks is to adequately specify the reliability and maintainability requirements as defined by the stakeholders in terms of their overall availability needs. There are several design techniques that are important to employ when designing or evaluating an IT system or component.

Fail-Safe Design

A fail-safe system is designed to return to a safe condition in the event of a failure or malfunction. A fail-safe or fail-secure *medical* system or device is one that, in the event of failure, responds in a way that is predictable and will cause no harm to other devices or danger to patients or personnel.

A system is fail-safe not because failure is impossible or improbable but because the system's design prevents or remediates unsafe consequences of the system's failure—that is, if a system fails, it remains safe, or at least no less safe than when it is operating correctly.[9]

It is important to note also that a fail-safe design may indicate that, under certain circumstances, a component should be shut down (forced to violate its functional specification) in order to avoid harming someone.

A fail-secure component of a system secures that system (or at least the portion to which the component is dedicated) in the event of a failure either of that component or elsewhere in the system.

Fail-safe designs are particularly critical for medical devices that are connected to patients and would be part of the safety testing by the FDA.

Fault Tolerance

Fault tolerance (sometimes called graceful degradation) is the capability of the software product to maintain a specified level of performance in cases of software faults or of infringement of its specified interface.[10]

For an individual system, fault tolerance can be achieved by anticipating conditions outside normal operating parameters and building the system to deal with them—in general, aiming for self-stabilization so that the system converges towards a safe state. However, if the consequences of a system failure are catastrophic, or the cost of making it sufficiently reliable is very high, a better solution may be to use some form of duplication or redundancy (discussed next). Fault tolerance is particularly sought after in high-availability or life-critical systems.

Redundancy and Failover

One of the most important design techniques is redundancy. *Redundancy* refers to the ability to continue operations in the event of component failures through managed component repetition. In the case of information technology, it can be applied to infrastructure components such as hardware, power supply, software, and information itself. Component repetition for the purpose of providing redundancy is geared toward the avoidance of single points of failure.[11] Designing with redundant or duplicate components or resources requires creating alternate operational paths, such as backups or duplicate systems or components, that will be used if particular parts of the system fail.

Failover refers to the process of automatically switching to a different, redundant system upon failure or abnormal termination of the currently active system. Failover can be applied to a cluster of servers, to network or storage components, or to any other set of redundant devices that must provide high availability because downtime would be expensive or inconvenient. It may be implemented in hardware, software, or in a combination of hardware and software.[12]

Failover and switchover are essentially the same operations, except that failover is automatic and usually operates without warning, while the term *switchover* means that the process requires human intervention. Failover capability is designed into systems requiring continuous availability and a high degree of reliability. Failover in the context of information technology refers to the process of changing the status of a standby system to become the primary system in the case of a failure in the original primary system. Failover is commonly used in database systems as part of a high-availability and disaster-recovery (HADR) design. Failover provides a high level of fault tolerance and high availability that is transparent to the end user.[12]

Simplicity

The simpler the system or component design, the more easily or predictably the system can fail and/or recover. Simplicity in design can be seen as the opposite of complexity. For example, complex software means more lines of code, more interfaces, etc. The greater the number of code lines and/or interfaces, the greater the possibility of unforeseen errors and unsafe consequences. Complex design also results in more security concerns, because coding errors, bugs, and other factors can create greater vulnerability to security threats.

In order for a system or component to meet reliability and availability requirements and avoid security vulnerabilities, a "design-for-simplicity" approach should be used. Designs should purposefully be designed for simplicity at the component, interface, and system level and the design-review process should include consideration of simplicity.

Chapter Review

This chapter described the importance of using architectural safeguards in designing, building, purchasing, and implementing safe and secure IT systems and medical devices. When designing or building an IT system, all aspects of the system's architecture—its individual hardware and software components—must be considered. The IT system design-and-build process mandates that various architectural considerations related to the components' features, functions, and desired performance are defined in the requirements. The overall goal is to design, build, purchase, and implement safe and secure IT systems and components for use in healthcare. The reader should understand the relationships between reliability, availability, scalability, and safety. In addition, the chapter discussed the basic design considerations of a reliable system, including fail-safe design, fault tolerance, redundancy and failover, and simplicity.

Questions

1. How is a product's reliability defined?

   A. Its capability to maintain a specified level of performance when used under specified conditions

   B. The measure of the product's safety, efficiency, and effectiveness

   C. Its ease of use

   D. Assurance that the product is without fault

2. A fail-safe system is designed to do no harm.

   A. True

   B. False

3. What does FMEA stand for?

   A. Federal management event archives

   B. Failure management event archive

   C. Failure mode event analysis

   D. None of the above

4. Which agency of the government oversees the safety of devices?

   A. CMS

   B. NIH

   C. ONC

   D. FDA

5. What should systems be designed to do if they fail?

   A. Roll over to a different system

   B. Do no harm to the patient

   C. Contain backups

   D. Contain an audit of failures

6. How is a system's maintainability defined?

   A. It can be modified.

   B. It is fail-safe.

   C. It is redundant.

   D. It is rolled over.

7. How is scalability defined?

   A. A system that allows integration of multiple patient records

   B. A system capable of growth

   C. A system that is geographically diverse

   D. A system that provides multiple layers

Answers

1. **A.** A product's reliability is defined as its capability to maintain a specified level of performance when used under specified conditions.

2. **A.** A fail-safe system is one that is designed to do no harm.

3. **C.** FMEA is the acronym used for failure mode event analysis.

4. **D.** The Food and Drug Administration (FDA) is the government agency that oversees device safety.

5. **B.** If a system fails, it should be designed to do no harm to the patient.

6. **A.** Maintainability is defined as a system's ability to be modified.

7. **B.** Scalability means a system is capable of growth.

References

1. ISO. Standard 9126-1. Software engineering—Product quality: Part 1, Quality model. Accessed from www.iso.org.

2. ISO. Standard 7498-2:1989. Information processing systems—Open systems—Basic reference model: Part 2, Security architecture. Accessed from www.iso.org.

3. ISO. Standard 9126-1. Software engineering—Product quality: Part 1, Quality model. Accessed from www.iso.org.

4. Bondi, A. B. (2000). Characteristics of scalability and their impact on performance. *Proceedings of the 2nd International Workshop on Software and Performance* (pp. 195–201). ISBN 1-58113-195-X.

5. A NIST definition of cloud computing (NIST Special Publication (SP) 800-145). Accessed from http://csrc.nist.gov/publications/drafts/800-145/Draft-SP-800-145_cloud-definition.pdf.

6. Mitchell, P. H. (2008). *Defining patient safety and quality care.* (2008). Accessed from www.ncbi.nlm.nih.gov/books/NBK2681.

7. International Electrotechnical Commision. (2006). IEC 60812. Analysis techniques for system reliability—Procedure for failure mode and effects analysis (FMEA).

8. FDA. (July 21, 2011). Draft guidance for industry and Food and Drug Administration staff—Mobile medical applications. Accessed from www.fda.gov/MedicalDevices/DeviceRegulationandGuidance/GuidanceDocuments/ucm263280.htm.

9. Krutz, R. L. & Fry, A. J. (2009). *The CSSLP prep guide: Mastering the certified security software lifecycle professional.* John Wiley and Sons.

10. ISO. Standard 9126-1. Software engineering—Product quality: Part 1, Quality model. Accessed from www.iso.org.

11. Schmidt, K. (2006). *High availability and disaster recovery: Concepts, design, implementation.* Springer.

12. Chen, W., Otsuki, M., Descovich, P., Arumuggharaj, S., Kubo, T., & Bi, J. Y. (2009). *High availability and disaster recovery options for DB2 on Linux, Unix, and Windows.* IBM Redbooks. Accessed from ibm.com/redbooks.

CHAPTER 30

Healthcare Cybersecurity Technology

Braulio J. Cabral

In this chapter, you will learn how to

- Present a business case for healthcare cybersecurity
- Measure return on investment (ROI) in healthcare cybersecurity
- Understand the balance between usability and security
- Identify network and systems protection standards and technologies
- Define usability safeguards including encryption

One of the most discussed aspects of information technology in recent years is healthcare cybersecurity. It is not unusual to see news stories about compromised networks, stolen devices containing sensitive information, and cybersecurity threats to national infrastructure and security. The source of threats has shifted from bored college kids looking for peer recognition to nations involved in cyberwar initiatives. Leaders are aware of the need for rules, regulations, and laws to mitigate such threats. Governments around the world are implementing strategies to improve their cyberdefenses, such as the American Recovery and Reinvestment Act (ARRA) of 2009, which created the federal breach law; US-CERT's Control Security Program (CSSP); the Federal Risk and Authorization Management Program (FedRAMP) on cloud computing security assessment; Australia's adoption of a national approach to secure the electronic exchange of health information;[1] and the United Kingdom's Office of Cyber Security and Information Assurance (OCASIA) initiatives for cybersecurity. These are just a few examples of many other government-sponsored initiatives around the globe.[2,3] The call for awareness about the reality of threats to security and privacy in cyberspace goes out to all private industries and public agencies.

It should be clear in the minds of business leaders that security should not be an afterthought. It is the job of security professionals to educate the masses about the importance of healthcare cybersecurity and to present healthcare cybersecurity as an enabler of innovation. The cybersecurity battle waged in other industries becomes more complex in healthcare, given its particular challenges of confidentiality, privacy, and information integrity. In healthcare, the lives of patients can be at risk—as in the case of demonstrated attacks to medical devices such as insulin pumps and pacemakers vulnerable to "passive eavesdropping."[4] Life-critical alarm communication management (ACM), waveform communication management (WCM), and concerns related to privacy and identity theft in electronic health record (EHR) systems and wireless medical devices have become ubiquitous around the world.[5]

The complexity increases even more as the need arises to balance security with the availability of healthcare information to caregivers, insurance companies, and government institutions providing healthcare benefits. Situational availability of the information also complicates the scenario, adding variables such as the role played by the person using the information; the timing (emergency situations versus nonemergency)";[6] and the level of sensitivity of the information. Related to cybersecurity, these factors influence the outcomes of medical situations that might result in long and expensive legal proceedings and the loss of reputation, and in many cases lives.

Figure 30-1 shows an example of the number of actors interacting in the exchange of healthcare information.[7] The larger the network and number of actors exchanging healthcare-related records, the bigger the risk. This concept is often expressed as the

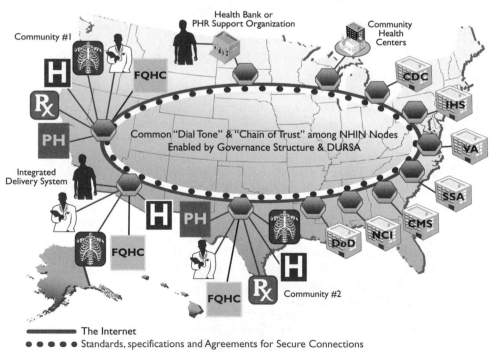

Figure 30-1 The network approach. Reprinted from the Nationwide Health Information Network Exchange Architecture Overview.[7]

CIA triad. The CIA triad includes *confidentiality* (preventing information leakage to unauthorized people), *integrity* (the prevention of information corruption or unauthorized modification of the information), and *availability* (making information available to authorized users following the established security policies of the organization).[8]

The Business Case for Healthcare Cybersecurity

The protection of sensitive information covered by the HIPAA Security Rule—such as protected health information (PHI)[9] and personally identifiable information (PII) as described in NIST Special Publication 800-112,[10] Australia's Privacy Act of 1988,[11] and the European Union member states' directive 2002/58/EC on E-Privacy[12]—and the protection of digital devices used in healthcare are obviously important. Countries around the world are engaged in developing healthcare cybersecurity regulations because they are concerned about protecting the lives of their citizens, saving billions of dollars, and protecting the reputation of their public and private healthcare organizations.

If safeguarding sensitive information is so important, the case for investing in cybersecurity in healthcare stands by itself, and the funds needed to implement the necessary safeguards should be available. However, this is far from reality. Across all industries, investments in the protection of sensitive information are less than needed, security professionals are overloaded with regulatory and technological challenges, and the demands are to do more with less. To security professionals dealing with cybersecurity threats on a daily basis, the answer is obvious: the business should invest more in healthcare cybersecurity and give security professionals the tools and resources needed to protect the organization's assets. To business leaders, it is all about the likelihood of a threat adversely impacting the information system through the exploitation of a given vulnerability (known as *risk*); the impact of the risk on the organization in cost, reputation, lives, and so on; and the level of tolerance the organization is willing to sustain for a particular risk.

Getting organizations to see healthcare cybersecurity as truly important begins not with a view of healthcare cybersecurity technology but with the human aspect of the cybersecurity program. You need to understand the role of cybersecurity professionals in the organization, but this role must be understood first by the cybersecurity professionals themselves. There is more than information security technology knowledge involved in the role of the compliance officer, cybersecurity coordinator, information systems security officer (ISSO), cybersecurity analyst, security architect, cybersecurity engineer, security and compliance auditor, or chief cybersecurity officer (CISO). There is a business related aspect to these roles, in other words, the cybersecurity professional should be someone who understands the business, increases business capabilities through technology, and contributes toward the business goals. When hiring a cybersecurity professional for any functional position within the security program, the business should be interested in an individual with the ability to respond to a business challenge with an answer such as "Let's see how we can enable the business to overcome this challenge in a secure manner" instead of a typical answer such as "We cannot do that; it is a security violation" or "It is a security risk," without providing any information about the likelihood of the risk materializing or the business impact of such a risk. Wagner[13] puts it this way:

> It's difficult to predict where the field of cybersecurity is headed, but there's a strong possibility that there will be an increasing convergence of the techie side of IT security and the more business-minded side. Companies, in other words, need cybersecurity professionals who also understand how to do business, serve customers, and design business models that work....

In other words, there needs to be that delicate balance between security and usability.

When advocating for cybersecurity, it needs to be presented as the enabler for innovation. The department or program that is developed and implements solutions to allow the business to have a leading-edge advantage over their competitors should protect the business attributes of confidentiality, privacy, integrity, and availability. The business case for cybersecurity investment is no longer purely based on the avoidance of potential risks but as a resource worth investing in. It also enables cybersecurity professionals to balance the business needs for security and the cybersecurity budget. Further, the return on investment (ROI) helps present cybersecurity as an enabler instead of being classified as an overhead to the business plan. Real-world case scenarios where cybersecurity provides a leading edge or advantage to the business should be quantified and used as a measure of ROI.

The Role of the Cybersecurity Professional in Healthcare

Up to this point, you should have a good idea of the challenges confronted by security professionals as you enter the healthcare industry or into a cybersecurity career in any other industry. Worries include daily increasing threats, limited resources, shrinking budget, and a business team that is not easily convinced about the threats you are describing. In fact, the business team might ask questions such as "What is the

Use Case 30-1: Implementing a Secure Software Development Policy

A real-world example of the contribution of the cybersecurity program to the business bottom line would be the implementation of a secure software development policy as part of the cybersecurity program. According to the policy, code developed must be scanned for security vulnerabilities in an iterative and incremental fashion during the software development life cycle instead of at the end of the development cycle. In most organizations, security comes as an afterthought or a compliance requirement, and the cost incurred because of late vulnerabilities findings is rarely calculated as part of the product's development cost. This simple proactive action can contribute to a better time to market, as well as savings in security vulnerability fixes.

likelihood of this happening to us?" and "Why should we invest in something on the assumption that it may happen?" and "How many instances of someone exploiting this threat have we had in the past year?" Of course, the ubiquitous nature of healthcare information technology today—manifesting itself in all shapes and forms including mobile devices (laptops, tables, smartphones, and so on), fax machines connected to network, security cameras, Voice over IP (VoIP), all on the same network—make the job of the security technician challenging.

Before security professionals can get the necessary funds to support a security program, they must present a compelling business case that not only talks about new threats but also presents the case in an organized manner. This layered approach to healthcare cybersecurity needs to be aligned with the business goals of the organization. It is not only about the need to place a perimeter firewall and to hire more resources to deal with the number of security-related tickets at the help desk; it's also about how these resources will impact the bottom line. Cybersecurity professionals need to determine how the healthcare cybersecurity initiative in the organization will enable the business to achieve its business goals. Healthcare cybersecurity must make the transition from its historical notion of being an overhead to the business, sometimes referred to as the *business prevention department*, to be a business-enabling asset to the organization with a demonstrable return on investment.

The Return on Cybersecurity Investment

Measuring ROI on cybersecurity investment has always been a challenge. Unfortunately, it is not a matter of straight numbers like it is with other investment types. The lack of a consistent matrix to measure security investments makes it even more difficult. Measuring, for example, the ROI on cybersecurity awareness training versus the investment in security appliances such as firewalls and web content filtering devices, and so on, are completely different things, and the resulting ROI may not be as clear as expected. One way to look at the ROI on security is from a risk reduction perspective, by measuring expected improvement against the cost associated with the improvement. To implement such an approach to ROI, the cybersecurity management system must quantify or put a value on the loss resulting from the lack of improvement. Some of these losses might include the following:

- Loss of productivity
- Loss of revenue during outages
- Loss of data and the impact of the data lost
- Cost of repair
- Cost of compromise of data due to unauthorized modification or destruction[14]

Other costs to account for are more difficult to quantify but should also be considered, such as the loss in business because of a privacy breach, legal costs, or the cost of remediation or damage control to the image of the organization.

There is no one particular way to measure ROI on cybersecurity investment, and the expected results may or may not convince the leaders of your organization of the need for investment, but you will be better prepared and will have a better chance to justify the investment through the presentation of a business case that includes an understanding of the investment and how it affects the business's bottom line.

Suggested Methods to Calculate ROI on Cybersecurity

The cybersecurity management system includes using the auditing artifacts for measuring the performance of implemented controls. The Control Objectives for Information and Related Technology (COBIT) is a set of best-practice frameworks for information security. COBIT proposes ISACA IT Audit and Assurance Guideline or G41 Calculating Return on Security Investment (ROI). The approach is "to determine the enterprise security requirements and the most appropriate measure of ROI, and establish processes to collect information to measure ROI." These are some of the questions addressed by this guideline:

- How does the business become secure?
- How much security is enough?
- How does the business know when its security level is high enough?
- How should security investment be accounted for?
- What is the right monetary and time investment to put into security?

These questions are used to compare the cost of security, the cost of a potential security breach, the cost of business continuity and disaster recovery, and the benefits of reducing the possibility of an agent exploiting a vulnerability that impacts confidentiality, integrity, availability, or privacy. It is also necessary to know how much the lack of security is costing the business, the impact of the lack of security on productivity, and what the cost-effective solutions are.[15] One way to calculate ROI is shown here:

$$ROI = (Expected\ returns - Cost\ of\ investment)\ /\ Cost\ of\ investment$$

Sonnereich[16] provides a detailed practical implementation of metrics to calculate ROI that can help you learn more about ROI and incorporate it into a cybersecurity management system. Intel Corporation proposes a similar approach based on the evaluation of cyberattacks over time, measuring the reduction of incidents as the result of implementing new security programs, putting a value on the impact of avoided incidents, and applying the results to other business areas for future value estimation. This is a process that could be automated and presented regularly to the organization's leaders in the form of a dashboard.

The Sherwood Applied Business Security Architecture (SABSA) proposes a similar approach to measuring ROI. Within the SABSA framework, ROI could be measured from a performance matrix perspective where the business drivers for security are analyzed in several ways:

- Private, personal, and business information is stored, processed, and communicated.
- The business attributes to measure are selected (in this case, privacy).
- The business attribute is defined (e.g., privacy must be protected in accordance with an authoritative definition of what constitutes privacy, such as HIPAA).
- The metric type is defined (e.g., number of reported incidents, including successful and unsuccessful attempts).
- The measurement approach to be implemented is defined.
- The performance target is defined.
- The metrics are collected and evaluated.

Another approach to measuring ROI is the use of maturity models such as Carnegie Mellon's Capability Maturity Model (CMM).[17] A newer approach to security capability measurement is the Systems Security Engineering Capability Maturity Model (SSE CMM).[18] Similar to CMM but specific to security engineering, SSE-CMM addresses three principal areas (see Figure 30-2):

- **The risk process (risk information)** Identifies and prioritizes risks associated with the development of product, systems, or services
- **The security engineering process** Develops and implements solutions to address (mitigate, transfer, or eliminate) the risks
- **The assurance process (assurance argument)** Ensures that the solution or controls established by the security engineering process are sufficient to address the risk

The assurance process can be used to gather performance measurements for evaluating the program against predetermined goals for security.

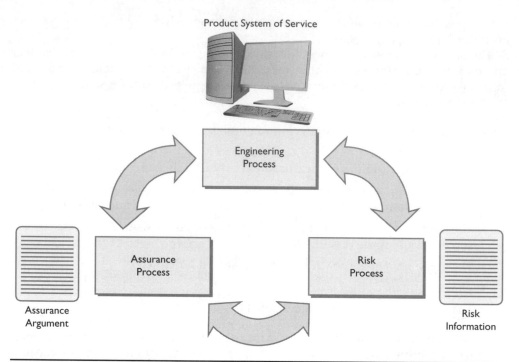

Figure 30-2 The security engineering process has three main areas.[18] Reprinted from the Systems Security Engineering Capability Maturity Model (SSE-CMM) Project. Copyright © 1995 by Carnegie Mellon University. This work is a collaborative effort of Hughes Space and Communications, Hughes Telecommunications and Space, Lockheed Martin, Software Engineering Institute, Software Productivity Consortium, and Texas Instruments Incorporated.

Balancing Usability vs. Cybersecurity

Security and usability are two concepts that often contradict each other. A particular application or information system may lose its ease of use due to implementation of security safeguards; this is commonly the case when it comes to access control, authentication, and authorization, at least from an end-user perspective. Balancing the conflicting requirements of usability and security can be a real challenge.

Usability

Usability is defined by ISO as "the effectiveness, efficiency, satisfaction with which the intended users can achieve their tasks in the intended context of product use."[19] As defined in other chapters, poor usability results in risks to patient safety, quality of data, and errors in data, such as requesting the wrong patient medications or tests or entering information in the wrong patient record.

Recent work on usability has been done by NIST, by the Agency for Healthcare Research and Quality (AHRQ), and by new grant programs at the Office of the National Coordinator (ONC) in the Department of Health and Human Services (HHS). Universal agreement on usability in the ONC HIT environment is characterized by good user-centric design (UCD) in the development of software and products.

Cybersecurity

Cybersecurity is the collection of standards, policies, processes, procedures, and technology used to protect a computer or computer system on the Internet (cyberspace) from threats to confidentiality, integrity, availability, privacy, and any other attributes considered important to the organization or individuals.

A battle between security and usability is commonly found between the software engineers who design and code the applications and the end users, whose input is usually ignored or simply not required at all. The software design/architecture often ends up with a high barrier to entry that makes the user experience intolerable and at times renders the system virtually unusable. There are hundreds of cases in which a system is implemented from an engineering perspective, without taking the end users into consideration just to end up soon abandoned by those who were supposed to benefit from it. In this section, I'm not referring to those instances in which the lack of usability is because of poor coding or a lack of the needed functionality; I'm referring specifically to the cases in which the security architect and software engineer ignore the end users, and therefore the implemented security becomes an impediment to a productive use of the healthcare information system. According to Howard et al., there are several reasons why this happens:[20]

- Designers are out of tune with how quickly users get annoyed.

- Security is almost never the user's priority; in other words, the need for security is recognized by users but can be quickly abandoned if it becomes an overhead or impediment to what they are doing; this can be considered "giving up security for the sake of functionality."

- Security designers often fail to make things obvious and easy, leaving users frustrated and looking for ways to circumvent security.

One common example is the implementation of password policies; Howard et al. describes this scenario as follows:[20]

> Let's say that, for the sake of better security, you put strict requirements on a password, such as minimum of eight characters with at least one non-alphanumeric character, and that the password is not obviously based on a dictionary word. Some users are going to have to try 20 passwords before they get one the system accepts. Then, they will either forget it, or write it down under the keyboard.

This is only one example of the many annoyances users go through that lead to the violation of security policies or to users abandoning the use of the system altogether for other solutions less constraining but not necessarily more secure.

Cybersecurity Standards and Technologies for Networks and Systems Protection

A systemic approach to cybersecurity management must begin with a clear understanding of the "big picture" (i.e., understanding the assets to be protected, the stakeholders, the impact to the organization given the realization of a threat). The only way of having such an understanding is by using standards and the necessary technology to implement the standards.

Standards

The International Organization for Standardization (ISO) defines standards as "documents established by consensus and approved by a recognized body that provides for common and repeated use, rules, guidelines or characteristics for activities or their results, aimed at the achievement of the optimum degree of order in a given context."[21] From a healthcare cybersecurity perspective or context, these rules and guidelines are intended to facilitate the protection of the confidentiality, availability, and integrity of the information as well as addressing the challenges related to the privacy in cyberspace.

Information technology and cybersecurity are not well-regulated fields; there are many technical certifications, but there are no official regulating bodies like you can find in other fields such as civil engineering, law, medicine, and so on. Standards become extremely useful, especially when security is implemented in a field such as healthcare.

In the United States, the Healthcare Insurance Portability and Accountability Act (HIPAA) provides comprehensive guidance and a legally binding framework. This was described in Chapter 13. However, HIPAA lacks the overall approach and the necessary guidance to marry cybersecurity to business goals, not to mention it is ambiguous on matters of data encryption, security strategic implementations, and other aspects of cybersecurity.

The number of organizations contributing to the development and implementation of cybersecurity standards and cybersecurity profiles continues to grow as the need to better organize and standardize cybersecurity is recognized.

NIST Special Publications 800 Standards for Cybersecurity

Organizations such as the National Institute of Standards and Technology (NIST) have developed an entire family of guidelines on cybersecurity (the NIST 800 family) covering standards including access control, audit and accountability, awareness and training, certification and accreditation, and security assessments to planning, risk assessment, and system and information integrity.[22] Many in the private sector may think of NIST standards and guidelines as concerned with government systems; however, more and more security professionals are realizing that these guidelines are applicable not only to federal systems but to any information systems and can be tailored to fit the needs of any organization.

 TIP Using standards in cybersecurity makes it easier for organizations to address security and the cybersecurity cornerstones previously mentioned in this chapter: confidentiality, integrity, and availability (CIA). Adopting an already developed standard avoids reinventing the wheel and has the advantage of using something that has already been adopted by others and proven to work.

ISO 27000 Security Standards Family

Similar to the NIST 800 special publication family, the ISO 27000 family provides the foundation for implementing and managing effective cybersecurity programs. ISO 27001 specifies Information Security Management Systems, while ISO 27002, formerly known as ISO 17799, covers security control mechanisms. The ISO 27000 family was developed by the International Standards Organization (ISO), in conjunction with the International Electrotechnical Commission (IEC), through a series of working groups including WG1 through WG3. Other standards in this family include ISO 27003, 27004, 27005, and 27006. (You can find more comprehensive detail on the road map for this standard in Arnason et al.)[23] Another international organization involved in the development of cybersecurity standards is the Information Systems Security Association (ISSA), which provides cybersecurity professional networking, educational materials, and cybersecurity certifications, among other benefits, to enhance and expand the field of cybersecurity management. Table 30-1 lists the organizations that contribute to the advancement of information management and cybersecurity, auditing, and assurance that, as a security professional in the healthcare space, you should familiarize yourself with.

Table 30-1 is not an exhaustive list of resources but will take you to the existing resources related to the current efforts to standardize cybersecurity across all industries. Similarly, organizations in the healthcare industry are collaborating to make available standards, guidance, and operating procedures directly related to protecting information and privacy in the healthcare industry. Table 30-2 lists healthcare-related resources for cybersecurity and privacy.

Organization Name	URL	Main Area of Focus
National Institute of Standards and Technology (NIST)	http://csrc.nist.gov/publications/PubsFL.html	Information systems security and security technologies guidelines
Information Systems Security Association (ISSA)	www.issa.org/	Advancing cybersecurity professionals, managing technology risks, and protecting critical information and infrastructure
Information Systems Audit and Control Association (ISACA)	www.isaca.org	ISACA describes itself as an organization for the "adoption and use of globally accepted, industry-leading knowledge and practices for information systems"[35]
International Federation for Information Processing (IFIP)	www.ifip.org/homeintro.html http://ifiptc.org/?tc=tc11	Computer and information processing including TC-11 Security and Privacy Protection in Information Processing Systems
The SABSA Institute	www.sabsa.org	Cybersecurity architecture, SABSA model certification and training
Association from Computing Machinery (ACM)	www.acm.org	Standards on cybersecurity and privacy
ISO 27000 series	www.iso.org	A set of standards dedicated to providing guidance on matters of information security

Table 30-1 Cybersecurity Standards Organizations

Organization Name	URL	Main Area of Focus
Healthcare Information and Management Systems Society	www.himss.org	Healthcare information management, security, privacy
HHS Office of the National Coordinator (ONC) for Health Information Technology	http://healthit.hhs.gov/portal/server.pt/community/healthit_hhs_gov___cybersecurity/3696 Standards and certification criteria: http://healthit.hhs.gov/portal/server.pt?open=512&objID=1195&parentname=CommunityPage&parentid=97&mode=2&in_hi_userid=11673&cached=true	Guidance and best practices
Certification Commission for Healthcare Information Technology (CCHIT)	www.cchit.org/ Security criteria: https://www.cchit.org/c/document_library/get_file?uuid=c8010f2d-8dd7-4239-9cfe-8e69ee8e75a6&groupId=18	Tests and certification for ONC on electronic health records systems
HHS Agency for Healthcare Research and Quality (AHRQ)	Health information privacy and security collaboration: http://healthit.ahrq.gov/portal/server.pt?open=512&objID=654&&PageID=13062&mode=2&in_hi_userid=3882&cached=true	Best practices and challenges in healthcare privacy and security

Table 30-2 Healthcare-Related Resources for Cybersecurity

Cybersecurity Technologies

The implementation of cybersecurity standards is comprised of two main elements: the use of technology such as encryption, content filtering, and packet analysis and the implementation of policies to safeguard the use of applications and systems. This section describes some common encryption types and the form of communication they protect, including communication via e-mail, chats, and fax.

Encryption Protocols

Encryption protocols, also known as cryptographic protocols, are used to secure data transport through the use of encryption algorithms, cryptographic keys, symmetric and asymmetric encryption, data integrity methods, and message authentication and nonrepudiation technology. The following are examples of such encryption or cryptographic protocols and their uses.

Secure Sockets Layer (SSL)

Secure Sockets Layer is an encryption protocol (also known as a cryptographic protocol) used to secure communication in cyberspace (the Internet).

TIP SSL encryption is used to protect electronic communication including communication through web browsers, e-mails, chats, fax over Internet, and Internet telephony or VoIP.

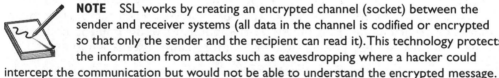

NOTE SSL works by creating an encrypted channel (socket) between the sender and receiver systems (all data in the channel is codified or encrypted so that only the sender and the recipient can read it). This technology protects the information from attacks such as eavesdropping where a hacker could intercept the communication but would not be able to understand the encrypted message.

Transport Layer Security (TLS)

TLS is considered a successor (or improvement) to SSL. It operates at the transport layer (referring to the seven layers of the Internet OSI model), which are the (1) physical layer, (2) data-link layer, (3) network layer, (4) transport layer, (5) session layer, (6) presentation layer, and (7) application layer. Through the use of this protocol, two systems or applications can authenticate each other and determine what type of encryption algorithm (set of rules for how to encrypt the data) to use. Some of the encryption algorithms used by TLS include DES and 3DES (discussed in the section "Encryption Algorithms" in this chapter). TLS is used in communication technologies such as Internet browser protocols including Hypertext Transfer Protocol (HTTP).

TIP HTTP is known as HTTPS when using TLS to protect communication over the Internet from "eavesdropping" attacks.

Pretty Good Privacy (PGP)

PGP is not an encryption protocol but instead an encryption application used to provide data encryption, data integrity validation, and communication authentication. PGP uses encryption and authentication technologies such as symmetric-key encryption and public-key encryption (also known as private/public key combination or private key infrastructure [PKI]). It also uses digital signatures through the creation of a hash or message digest using RSA or DSA signature algorithms.[24] (Learn more about message digest in the section "Encryption Algorithms.")

Hypertext Transfer Protocol Secure (HTTPS)

HTTPS is the secure implementation of the Hypertext Transfer Protocol widely used for communication across the Internet. The security of HTTP is accomplished through the use of the SSL/TLS security protocols to add the security capabilities to HTTP.

Secure File Transfer Protocol (SFTP)

Similar to HTTP, Secure File Transfer Protocol (SFTP) secures the unsecure File Transfer Protocol (FTP) through the use of the Secure Shell (SSH) protocol. It is slower than the native unsecure FTP because of the overhead added by the encryption of the data. Data encryption through SFTP supports encryption algorithms including DES, RC4, AES, and 3DES, among other industry standards, and it implements the use of key pairs or the Private Key Infrastructure (PKI) technology.

FTP Secure (FTPS)

In the case of FTP Secure or FTP-SSL, the native File Transfer Protocol is secure through the use of the Transport Layer Security and SSL protocols. FTPS can operate in two modes: the explicit mode, using the AUTH TLS command, or the implicit mode where the data transfer uses TCP port 989 and the control channel uses TCP port 990.

 TIP FTP uses TCP port 21 as the control channel and TCP port 20 as the data channel. SFTP uses port 22, the same as SSH. SSH is SFTP's underlying security protocol. FTPS in implicit mode uses TCP port 990 as the control channel and TCP port 989 as the data channel.

Encryption Algorithms

There are many types of encryption algorithms. They are limited by the length of the key supported and the number of bits required. Some of the outdated as well as faster encryption algorithms are discussed in the following sections.

Data Encryption Standard (DES)

DES developed in 1970 is an encryption algorithm. The algorithm works by shifting bits of data and by substituting bits. It uses a key (rule or cipher) to determine how the shifting and substitution will occur. At the end of this process, the data is encrypted or codified in such a manner that only someone with the key is able to unencrypt the data.

TIP By today's standards of security, DES is not considered a much secured encryption algorithm because of the limitation on the length of its key, which is limited to 56 bits. The larger the key in a particular encryption algorithm, the more difficult it would be to guess the key by brute force.

Triple DES (3DES)

Triple DES solves the limitation of the key length in DES by combining three DES keys for a total 168 bits key. 3DES is more secure than DES, but it is also three times slower, requiring three times the CPU power required by DES.

Advanced Encryption Standard (AES)

AES is considered a substitute for 3DES. Its performance is faster in both software and hardware implementations. Because of its efficiency, speed, and flexibility, AES is used in small devices such as smartphones, smartcards, and security token devices. AES supports key sizes including 128, 192, and 256 bits.

Other encryption algorithms are used to encrypt the data in such a way as to make a condensed or compressed representation of the original data through a process known as *hashing*.

 TIP Encryption algorithms including SHA-1, SHA-2, MD5, and HMAC are commonly used to protect the integrity of the data by acting as a message digest or fingerprint.

Secure Hash Algorithm (SHA-1)

Secure Hash Algorithm is used to generate a condensed representation of a message, also called a *message digest*. Given a message input of 256 bits or less, the SHA-1 algorithm outputs a message digest of 160 bits. The security of this algorithm relies on the belief that it is computationally not feasible to generate a message that corresponds to a given message digest or to find two different messages that will produce the same message digest. Given the proliferation and inexpensive availability of supercomputing power, this belief is no longer valid, and what used to be considered not feasible or too expensive can be accomplished at a very low price and in a short time today. SHA-1 is used for digital signature applications, SSL certificates, and electronic e-mails.

Secure Hash Algorithm 2 (SHA-2)

Secure Hash Algorithm 2 is considered an improvement over SHA-1. It consists of cryptographic (encryption) functions supporting digests of 256 or 512 bits. SHA-2 is used in security protocols such as TLS, SSL, PGP, SSH, S/MIME, and IPsec, among others. SHA-1 and SHA-2 are security algorithms used by federal agencies and recommended by NIST. Because of the security weakness of SHA-1, it is being substituted for SHA-2 in all government agencies, and NIST recommends its substitution in private-sector industries as well.

Message-Digest Algorithm 5 (MD5)

MD5 is also used mostly for data integrity check purposes. MD5 uses a hash function that produces a 128-bit hash value. Because of its susceptibility to collision (the ability of finding two inputs that produce the same hash), MD5 is not appropriate for use with security protocols such as SSL.

Hash Message Authentication Code (HMAC)

HMAC is a mechanism used by communication technologies to authenticate a message sent from a sender to a receiver system. HMAC combines a cryptographic hash function such as SHA-1 or MD5 and a secret key and can be used to verify both the integrity and authenticity of the message. HMAC works in the following way: the underlying hash function used (e.g., SHA-1 or SHA-2) generates a message digest (a fingerprint of the original message that cannot be altered); when the message (text) is sent, the hash is sent along with the message. The recipient can then use the hash function and input the message (text) and compare the output (digest) to the one sent along with the message. If both are the same, it is an indication that the message integrity is intact (it was not tampered with). In theory, you cannot generate the same digest from two different message inputs. The secret key is used to verify the authenticity of the sender, because this key is known only to the sender and the receiver. The strength of HMAC relies on the strength of its underlying hash function (MD5, SHA1, and SHA256).

Wi-Fi Encryption Technologies

Wi-Fi is a communication technology that allows the exchange of data through radio waves (wireless) through a computer network. Wi-Fi is based on the Institute of Electrical and Electronics Engineers (IEEE) standard 802.11.[25] Wi-Fi is used by a multitude of devices, including personal computers, tablets, smartphones, printers, fax, audio players, television sets, and medical devices, among many others. Wi-Fi communications are secure (encrypted) using several encryption protocols.

Wired Equivalent Privacy (WEP)

WEP is a security algorithm for wireless networks; the algorithm is part of the IEEE 802.11 standard. The two main functions of this protocol are to protect the WLAN network from unauthenticated users accessing the network and to protect the confidentiality of the data by encrypting the data. The data is encrypted by using a 40-bit key concatenated to a 24-bit initialization vector used in an RC4 cipher function to generate a 64- or 128-bit key. This protocol implements two forms of authentication: Open System and Shared Key authentication.

In Open System mode, no authentication is performed, but the encryption key can be used to encrypt the communication. In Shared Key mode, the client device must authenticate to the access point. Several weaknesses render this protocol not very secure, including that the size of the initialization vector is only 24 bits and is sent in clear text, and shared keys are always prompted to compromise the network because people may not secure the key properly (similar to a password written in a sticky note). Keys generated by WEP include the following: WEP-40/64-bit WEP generates a 10-digit key,

WEP-104/128-bit WEP generates a 26-digit key, and 256-bit WEP generates a 58-digit key. Many devices such as routers and gateways allow the users to enter a paraphrase and derive the key from the paraphrase. The issue with this approach is that the same paraphrase generates the same key, so if the paraphrase is weak, it is susceptible to dictionary and brute-force attacks.

Wi-Fi Protected Access (WPA)

Wi-Fi Protected Access (WPA) was developed as a quick temporary solution (or work-around) to the issues found in WEP and in expectation of the improved protocol WPA-2. Like WEP, it works in a preshared key that can be generated by the use of a passphrase and can be between 8 to 63 characters. The WPA encryption method uses a key known as a pairwise master key (PMK) generated using the preshared key and the service set identifier (SSID).

TIP The advantage of WPA over WEP is that the PMK is used to generate a temporary key or a pairwise transient key (TPK) created at the time of connection and frequently changed.

Wi-Fi Protected Access 2 (WPA2)

WPA2 supports all the functionalities of WPA (strong cryptography support based on RC4 cipher, WPA-Enterprise, and WPA-Personal). In addition, it adds strong encryption and authentication for infrastructure and ad hoc networks, reduced overhead in roaming between access points, and key derivation during authentication exchange. WPA2 supports the Counter Mode with Cipher Block Chaining Message Authentication Code Protocol (CCMP) encryption, which is based on AES.

TIP AES is the encryption algorithm used on small devices such as smartphones and smartcards because of its efficiency in speed and flexibility.

Software Vulnerabilities and Usability Safeguards

The most ubiquitous asset requiring protection is the software component of cyberspace. It is important to understand how businesses use applications and systems to exchange, store, and process information and how businesses derive strategies to preemptively deal with application-related vulnerabilities and vulnerabilities created by the users of those applications.

Historically, dealing with software vulnerabilities has been an "afterthought" for security professionals. Seldom are security professionals involved or aware of what is going on in the software engineering department, and issues related to software vulnerabilities are addressed after the software is deployed through patches or left to technology devices to protect the enterprise from threats to vulnerable applications. The price paid for this approach is high. It is more expensive to patch or fix code after it is deployed, it creates disruption to productivity, and in the case of "zero-day"[26] attacks, it is impossible to proactively prevent the attacks.

Preventing Software Vulnerabilities

To mitigate software vulnerabilities, it is necessary to introduce security at the early stages of the software development life cycle (SDLC). This may sound strange to the security professional who is used to dealing with software vulnerabilities "after the fact" through penetration testing, application vulnerability scanning, and other tools, but changing the order in which these tools are utilized so as to allow the security professional to participate in the software development life cycle goes a long way. The cybersecurity program can use strategies such as secured software development workshops, vulnerability scanning at different stages of the SDLC, and software engineering security awareness training. Also, adopting a software development life cycle that incorporates cybersecurity elements and developing security policies to be followed by the software development teams are both strategies that promote the production of more secure applications and systems and prevent software vulnerabilities.

Usability Safeguards

It does not matter how much is invested in cybersecurity, unless the users of cyberspace are aware of existing threats and make a conscious effort to follow established usability safeguards. The following are some of the most common usability safeguards implemented to protect the systems from the exploitation of vulnerabilities introduced by the users of applications and systems.

User Provisioning

Also called *identity management*, user provisioning is the process by which the system administrator or, in many organizations, the security administrator provisions the user of a system with the necessary credentials to allow users to access the system and perform their duties with the proper level of authentication and authorization.

 TIP The process of user provisioning includes verifying the identity of the user physically, through the verification of one or more forms of identification (driver's license, password, employee ID, etc.).

User Deprovisioning

As important as provisioning the user with the necessary credentials to access and operate on a system is the need for deprovisioning a user when access to the system is no longer required. This is an important aspect of safeguarding the system from internal threats. In many organizations, the network is left open to unauthorized access from users who are no longer part of the organization or do not require a particular level of access. This is because of a poor policy on user provisioning/deprovisioning and lack of user management. This issue is more accentuated in large organizations with hundreds or thousands of users.

Password Policies

Another important aspect of usability safeguards is the implementation of password policies. Usernames and passwords are the most common form of authentication. Poor password policies or the nonexistence of a password policy exposes the organization to high-impact threats that could be easily avoided if effective password policies are implemented. A password policy should include but not be limited to the following:

- **Password length and complexity** The password should comply with a predetermined length (e.g., 8 to 16 characters) including a combination of uppercase and lowercase letters, numbers, and special characters.

- **Password expiration** The policy must force users to change their password regularly (e.g., 60 to 90 days or more often).

- **Failed attempts account block** Applications and systems must implement the blockage of users after a predetermined number of failed attempts to log into the system.

- **Successful/failed attempts log** The system must maintain a log of both successful and failed attempts to the system.

- **Timeout policy** Systems must implement session timeout, forcing the user to reauthenticate after a period of idle time.

- **Password sharing policy** It must be made clear that sharing a user's password is not allowed and must give the consequences for ignoring this policy.

Security Awareness Training Curriculum

The organization must implement a security awareness and training curriculum. It does not matter how well-written security policies may be. Security policies will not do any good if no one knows of their existence. Security policies and security procedures must be socialized within the organization through the implementation of cybersecurity-related activities such as a designated day for cybersecurity awareness, mandatory annual cybersecurity awareness training and refreshers, and the use of promotional materials such as pamphlets, booklets, and so on.

Ethical, Personal, and Legal Responsibility for Cybersecurity

Cybersecurity is everyone's responsibility; it is important to make users aware of their ethical, personal, and legal responsibilities regarding their roles as users and their commitment to cybersecurity. Cybersecurity policies and standards are statements that must describe the minimum requirements, ethics, personal responsibilities, and legal responsibilities, along with the consequences for noncompliance. They should not be geared toward intimidating the users but must be clear enough to convey the fact that cybersecurity is in the best interest of the organization and of the individual.

Protecting Against Social Engineering

Awareness is the best weapon against social engineering. To protect against social engineering hackers, users must be aware of the different attack vectors used by social engineering hackers, including the following:

- **Online threats** This includes hyperlinks in e-mails (phishing) that appear to be from within a department in the organization such as human resources, cybersecurity, and so on.

- **Through the telephone** Social engineering hackers are master impersonators, and they will use their skills to try to convince the user to provide sensitive information such as passwords, confidential information, trade secrets, or any information they deem of value.

- **Through waste management and the inappropriate disposal of sensitive information** Users should be careful with how they dispose of sensitive information. Use a paper shredder for a company's or customer's related material, and limit the use of sticky notes.

- **Through sensitive conversations in open spaces and personal approaches** In many cases, we do not realize who is around us and how interested they may be in our conversations. Be aware of your surroundings and the type of conversation you have in public with colleagues, friends, and relatives in relation to your organization.

- **Knowing the organization's policies** It is important to know how your organization operates and what policies are in place; for example, knowing that it is company policy that the cybersecurity department does not request usernames and passwords over the phone or via e-mail gives you the advantage of knowing that anyone approaching you with such a request must have malicious motives.[27]

Chapter Review

This chapter provided an overview of the worldwide concerns about security in cyberspace and in particular the nationwide issues with cybersecurity in healthcare, including threats to infrastructure and the shifting of threat vectors from college kids to nation-sponsored initiatives to support the exploitation of vulnerabilities in cyberspace. The chapter covered the need for legislation and rules and the initiatives of the United States and other nations to protect themselves from threats to confidentiality, integrity, availability, and privacy in cyberspace.

Some of the latest initiatives for improving security in cyberspace discussed in this chapter included federal breach laws created under the American Recovery and Reinvestment Act of 2009, US-CERT's Control Security Program, and the Federal Risk and Authorization Management Program initiative to certify and accredit cloud computing service providers following the Federal Information Security Management Act (FISMA) risk management and security controls.

The complexity of healthcare systems and the need to protect confidentiality, integrity, and availability (CIA) are important aspects of cybersecurity and were discussed throughout the chapter. The case for investing in healthcare cybersecurity was based first on the existing threats to confidentiality, integrity, and availability and the need for compliance with regulations such as HIPAA and rules on protected health information (PHI) and personally identifiable information (PII). Historically, cybersecurity has been seen as an afterthought, or a "necessary evil," imposed by a team through the use of intimidation strategies and the imposition of constraints to the business. This team is often referred to as the *business prevention department.*

The chapter covered the relationship between cybersecurity risks, the need to present a business case, and the need to show ROI. This chapter also presented the need to balance usability versus cybersecurity and technologies used to protect the confidentiality, integrity, and availability of data. This chapter defined privacy including encryption protocols such as Secure Sockets Layer, Transport Layer Security, Hypertext Transfer Protocol Secure, and other tools and applications used for data encryption and authentication such as Pretty Good Privacy.

Overall, this chapter presented the balance between the cybersecurity professional's perspective and the business's through a synergy in which cybersecurity is viewed as an enabler to help the healthcare industry accomplish its mission. It was my intention to help leaders view cybersecurity as the set of capabilities that allows the business to maintain a competitive edge through the use of innovating technologies, with the confidence that the integrity, availability, and confidentiality of critical information is protected.

Questions

To test your comprehension of the chapter, answer the following questions and then check your answers against the list of correct answers that follows the questions.

1. Which one of the following is *not* one of the seven layers of the OSI model?

   A. Physical layer

   B. Session layer

   C. Protocol layer

   D. Transport layer

2. Which of the following is *not* an encryption protocol?

   A. SSL

   B. TLS

   C. DES

   D. WEP

3. Which of the following encryption algorithms is used on small devices such as smartphones and smartcards because of its efficiency in speed and flexibility?

   A. EAS

   B. AES

   C. SEA

   D. CSA

4. Which of the following can be used to protect communication over the Internet from "eavesdropping" attacks?

   A. HTTP

   B. HTTM

   C. HTTPS

   D. SHTTP

5. Secure Hash Algorithm is used to do what?

   A. Generate an encrypted username

   B. Generate an extended message, also called a message digest

   C. Generate a compressed representation of a message, also called a message digest

   D. Generate a copy of a message in clear text

6. Select all security protocols and encryption applications where SHA-2 can be implemented. (Choose all that apply.)

   A. SSL

   B. SSH

   C. SME

   D. S/MIME

   E. TLS

   F. All of the above

7. Which encryption algorithm is *not* appropriate for use with security protocols such as SSL/TLS because of its susceptibility to collision?

   A. SHA-2

   B. AES

   C. 3DES

   D. MD5

8. In which way do SHA-1, SHA-2, MD5, and HMAC provide data integrity protection?

   A. By encrypting the communication channel

    B. By acting as a message digest or fingerprint

    C. By obfuscating the message through a character shifting process

    D. All of the above

9. Given an input message of 256 bits or less, which security algorithm generates a message digest of 160 bits?

    A. RSA

    B. SHA-2

    C. DES3

    D. SHA-1

    E. None of the above

10. The process through which an encryption algorithm creates a condensed message or fingerprint of the original message is known as what?

    A. Hiding process

    B. Obfuscation process

    C. Hacking process

    D. Hashing process

11. Which of the following is *not* a Wi-Fi security algorithm?

    A. WEP

    B. AES

    C. WPA

    D. SSID

12. You want to use a mechanism that combines both the integrity and authenticity validation of a message; which of the following can be used?

    A. MD5

    B. HMAC

    C. HAMC

    D. SHA

13. When using WEP, which mode forces the device to authenticate itself with the access point?

    A. Authentication mode

    B. Open System mode

    C. Shared Key mode

    D. Strict validation mode

    E. None of the above

14. As the person in charge of cybersecurity in your organization, you need to develop a password policy for the organization; which of the following should be included in the password policy? (Choose all that apply.)

    A. Password length and complexity

    B. Password expiration

    C. Blocking accounts on a predetermined number of failed attempts

    D. All of the above

15. Which of the following applies to protecting against social engineering? (Choose all that apply.)

    A. Know the organization's policies on matters of password and username request.

    B. Be cautious about e-mails requesting sensitive information.

    C. Be aware of your surroundings when discussion topics of sensitive nature to the organization.

    D. All of the above.

16. Which of the following is *not* part of the user provisioning process?

    A. Verifying the identity of the user

    B. Providing credentials for authentication

    C. Providing the necessary authorization levels

    D. Removing a username from an access control list

17. Which strategies can the organization implement to prevent software vulnerabilities? (Choose all that apply.)

    A. Introduce security at the early stages of the SDLC

    B. Offer secure software development workshops

    C. Software vulnerability scanning at different stages of the SDLC

    D. All of the above

18. Why is DES *not* secured enough by today's encryption standards?

    A. Because it is two slow

    B. Because its key length is limited to 64 bits

    C. Because its key length is limited to 32 bits

    D. Because its key length is too short, limited to 56 bits

19. Which of the following technologies use the Secure Socket Layer/Transport Layer Security protocol?

    A. Chat

    B. Browsers

    C. E-mail

    D. Voice over IP (VoIP)

    E. All of the above

20. According to ISO, what is a standard?

    A. A document shared across the organization to share sensitive information

    B. A document developed and distributed by the chief security officer

    C. A document provided by a recognized organization to provide common and repeated rules and guidelines

    D. None of the above

21. Cybersecurity protects computers or computer systems from threats to which of the following?

    A. Integrity

    B. Privacy

    C. Confidentiality

    D. Availability

    E. All of the above

22. Why is it important to be aware of the potential ROI of cybersecurity investment?

    A. To help build a business case for cybersecurity investment

    B. To be able to balance the business needs for security and cybersecurity budget

    C. To present cybersecurity as an enabler instead of an overhead to the business

    D. All of the above

23. In Open System mode, what occurs with the WEP Wi-Fi security protocol?

    A. Authentication but not encryption is performed.

    B. Encryption but not authentication is performed.

    C. No authentication is performed, and encryption is optional.

    D. All of the above.

Answers

  1. **C.** The protocol layer is not one of the seven layers of the OSI model, which include the following: (1) physical layer, (2) data-link layer, (3) network layer, (4) transport layer, (5) session layer, (6) presentation layer, and (7) application layer.

2. **C.** DES is an encryption algorithm. The algorithm works by shifting bits of data and by substituting bits. It uses a key (rule or cipher) to determine how the shifting and substitution will occur.

3. **B.** Advanced Encryption Standard (AES) is used in small devices such as smartphones, smartcards, and security token devices because of its efficiency, speed, and flexibility. AES supports key sizes including 128, 192, and 256 bits.

4. **C.** Hypertext Transfer Protocol Secure (HTTPS) uses SSL/TLS to secure the communication channel through encryption; therefore, it is suitable to prevent eavesdropping attacks.

5. **C.** Secure Hash Algorithm is used to generate a condensed representation of a message, also called a message digest. Given a message input of 256 bits or less, the SHA-1 algorithm outputs a message digest of 160 bits.

6. **A, B, D, E.** SHA-2 is used in security protocols such as TLS, SSL, PGP, SSH, S/MIME, and IPsec, among others.

7. **D.** Because of its susceptibility to collision (the ability of finding two inputs that produce the same hash), MD5 is not appropriate for use with security protocols such as SSL.

8. **B.** SHA-1, SHA-2, MD5, and HMAC are commonly used to protect the integrity of the data by acting as a message digest or fingerprint.

9. **D.** Given a message input of 256 bits or less, the SHA-1 algorithm outputs a message digest of 160 bits.

10. **D.** The process of encrypting the data in such a way as to make a condensed or compressed representation of the original data is known as *hashing*.

11. **D.** The service set identifier (SSID) is not a Wi-Fi security protocol; it is the name given to identify a wireless local area network. When setting up a wireless device, you have the option of broadcasting the SSID so other devices can see it. Every device trying to connect to the wireless network must know the SSID of the network.

12. **B.** HMAC combines a cryptographic hash function such as SHA-1 or MD5 and a secret key and can be used to verify both the integrity and the authenticity of the message.

13. **C.** In Shared Key mode, the client device must authenticate to the access point.

14. **D.** When developing a password policy for your organization, you must consider items such as password length and complexity, password expiration, and blockage of account on a predetermined number of failed login attempts.

15. **D.** Knowing the organization's policies on matters of password and usernames requests, being cautious about e-mails requesting sensitive information, and being aware of your surroundings when discussing topics of a sensitive nature to the organization are all important considerations that help prevent social engineering attacks.

16. **D.** Removing a username from an access control list is part of the deprovisioning process.

17. **D.** Introducing security at the early stages of the SDLC, offering secure software development workshops, and software vulnerability scanning at different stages of the SDLC are all tactics geared toward the prevention of software vulnerabilities.

18. **D.** DES is not considered a secured encryption algorithm because of the limitation on the length of its key, which is limited to 56 bits. The larger the key in a particular encryption algorithm, the more difficult it would be to guess the key by brute force.

19. **E.** Chat, browsers, e-mail, and Voice over IP (VoIP) all use SSL/TSL to secure communication.

20. **C.** According to the International Standards Organization (ISO), a standard is a document provided by a recognized organization to provide common and repeated rules and guidelines.

21. **E.** Among other attributes, cybersecurity protection includes protecting the user's privacy and confidentiality, integrity, and availability of the information.

22. **D.** Being aware of the importance of ROI on cybersecurity investment helps build a business case for the cybersecurity budget, helps balance the business needs for security and cybersecurity budgets, and helps present cybersecurity as an enabler instead of an overhead to the business.

23. **C.** When using the WEP Wi-Fi security protocol in Open System mode, no authentication is performed, and encryption is optional.

References

1 Federal risk and authorization management program (FedRAMP). (2012). Accessed from www.gsa.gov/portal/category/102371.

2. Challenges in improving information security practice in Australian general practice. (2009). Accessed from http://ro.ecu.edu.au/ism/1/.

3. Office of Cyber Security and Information Assurance. Accessed on October 15, 2012, from www.cabinetoffice.gov.uk/content/office-cyber-security-and-information-assurance-ocsia.

4. Jamming signals to stop hackers from lethal pacemaker attacks. (2011). Accessed on June 30, 2012, from http://blogs.computerworld.com/18842/jamming_signals_to_stop_hackers_from_lethal_pacemaker_attacks.

5. Sloane, E.B. (2010). Medical device security effects of HIPAA, ARRA- and FDA-related security issues: Living in a high tech-HITECH world. NIST-OCR HIPAA Conference, May 11–12, 2010, Washington, DC.

6. Break the glass. (2009). Accessed on July 1, 2012, from www.himss.org/content/files/090909BreakTheGlass.pdf.

7. Nationwide health information network exchange architecture overview. (2010). Accessed on July 8, 2012, from www.healthit.hhs.gov/portal/server.pt/gateway/PTARGS_0_11113_911643_0_0_18/NHIN_Architecture_Overview_Draft_20100421.pdf.

8. Information security and privacy in healthcare: Current state of research. (2008). Accessed on June 30, 2012, from www.ists.dartmouth.edu/library/416.pdf.

9. Health information privacy. (2012). Accessed on July 1, 2012, from www.hhs.gov/ocr/privacy/hipaa/understanding/srsummary.html.

10. Guide to protecting the confidentiality of personally identifiable information (PII). (2010). Accessed on July 1, 2012, from http://csrc.nist.gov/publications/nistpubs/800-122/sp800-122.pdf.

11. Privacy Act 1988. Accessed on July 1, 2012, from www.austlii.edu.au/au/legis/cth/consol_act/pa1988108/.

12. Directive 2002/58/EC: Data protection in the electronic communications sector. (2002). Accessed on July 15, 2012, from http://europa.eu/legislation_summaries/information_society/legislative_framework/l24120_en.htm.

13. Breaking into the security job market. (2010). Accessed on July 1, 2012, from www.ecommercetimes.com/story/Breaking-Into-the-Security-Job-Market-69185.html.

14. The ROI of security. (2006). Accessed on July 8, 2012, from www.sei.cmu.edu/library/abstracts/news-at-sei/securitymatters200605.cfm.

15. IT audit and assurance guideline: G41 return on security investment (ROSI). (2010). Accessed from www.isaca.org/Knowledge-Center/Standards/Pages/IS-Auditing-Guideline-G41-Return-on-Security-Investment-ROSI-1.aspx.

16. Return on security investment (ROSI): A practical quantitative model. SageSecure, LLC. (2006). Accessed on October 15, 2012, from http://sonnenreich.com/wes/return_on_security_investment.pdf.

17. Systems engineering capability maturity model, version 1.1, A. (1995). Accessed from www.sei.cmu.edu/library/abstracts/reports/95mm003.cfm.

18. Systems security engineering capability maturity model. (2003). Accessed on July 8, 2012, from www.sse-cmm.org/model/model.asp.

19. Introduction to ISO 27001. (2005). Accessed from www.27000.org/iso-27001.htm.

20. Howard, M., LeBlanc D., & Viega, J. (2005). *19 deadly sins of software security: Programming flaws and how to fix them.* McGraw-Hill/Osborne.

21. Introduction to ISO 27002. (2012). Accessed from www.27000.org/iso-27002.htm.

22. Special publications (800 series). (2012). Accessed on July 8, 2012, from http://csrc.nist.gov/publications/PubsSPs.html.

23. Arnason, S. T. & Willett, K. D. (2008). *Introduction to International Standards Organization security standards.* Auerbach Publications.

24. Lucas, M. W. (2006). *PGP and GPG: Email for the practical paranoid.* No Starch Press.

25. 802.11 wireless local area networks standard. (2012). Accessed from http://grouper.ieee.org/groups/802/11/.

26. Carpenter, T. (2009). *CompTIA Convergence+ certification study guide (exam CTO-101).* McGraw-Hill/Osborne.

27. Hadnagy, C. (2011). *Social engineering: The art of human hacking.* Wiley Publishing.

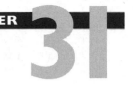

Certification of HIT Products and Systems

Karen M. Bell

In this chapter, you will learn how to
- Understand why different certification programs developed in HIT
- Identify key certification programs and processes
- Describe multiple ways of assessing HIT

Information Technology in the Clinical Setting: A 70-Year Odyssey

In order to meet our collective goal of a healthier nation, we need information technologies that will make it easier for clinicians to do their work, improve the interaction between clinicians and patients as well as among all providers, and allow for the secure reuse of data for purposes that benefit our society at large. Some of these purposes include public health surveillance, research, emergency preparedness, and improvements in the quality of care delivered. This chapter provides a historical journey of the development of healthcare information technology (HIT) products and services, describes how these products and services are evaluated, and examines the critical role and features of the certification process in assuring that HIT products are functional, secure, and reliable.

Earliest Efforts

The development of the Hollerith Tabulating Machine, a data-processing system used to tabulate 1890 census data from punch cards, was the first application of computerized technology to medicine for epidemiological purposes.[1] It was not, however, until World War II fostered the development of the first digital computers in the 1940s that the implications of applying computer technology to clinical medicine were first considered.

Dr. Larry Weed of the University of Vermont was an early pioneer in the field in the 1960s, with two major contributions: (1) a standardized way of organizing information in an outpatient medical record based on the now-familiar subjective, objective, assessment, and plan (SOAP) approach and (2) work on computer programs that could record and track this information.[2] While the mainframe systems used for these early electronic medical records were expensive, time consuming, and difficult to maintain, in the 1970s a number of model health maintenance organizations (HMOs) that provided health insurance coverage as well as care became early adopters of the technology, providing a number of insights for the next stages of clinical computing.

Among the most important of these was the recognition that biomedical applications at the time needed specialized programming languages, leading to the development in the early 70s of the Massachusetts General Hospital Utility Multi-Programming System (MUMPS).[3] MUMPS quickly became widespread and is still in use today by large clinical systems, such as the Veterans Health Information System and Technology Architecture (VistA), and many electronic health record (EHR) system vendors and developers because of its ability to scale and process very large amounts of data.

HIT Becomes Personal

It was not until the 1980s, however, with the advent of the personal computer, that the revolutionary fuse of computer use in medicine was truly lit. The base of users was widely broadened and included individuals as well as hospitals, giving birth to a new software industry. The 1990s then saw an explosion of electronic-prescribing systems, EHR systems, practice-management systems, and care-management systems—each with its own siloed existence. In spite of major advances in the field of medicine, the healthcare industry as a whole entered the twenty-first century with a hodgepodge of HIT products and systems that could not communicate with each other—and very low adoption rates for any of them.

Federal Support for HIT

With respect to HIT as an industry and as an integral part of healthcare, the first decade of the twenty-first century can best be characterized by the engagement of the federal government as a coordinating and policy-making entity. It is important to note that the government can enact policy in multiple ways. Clearly, the most effective and significant approach is through regulation, though this is a long, drawn-out process requiring publication of proposed and then final rules. Other policy-making levers include reimbursement or payment strategies, conditions of doing business with the federal government, contractual clauses, and strong, focused leadership.

 TIP A good example of the use of contractual clauses as a policy lever is the contracts that the Office of Personal Management (OPM) has in place with all of the health insurers who provide coverage for the national Federal Employees Plan, which require that they support HIT in the delivery system.

After much preliminary planning and work, the Office of the National Coordinator for HIT (ONC) was established in 2004 by Executive Order 13335 within the

Department of Health and Human Services (HHS). Led by Dr. David Brailer, the first national coordinator, its first order of business was to lay out a strategic framework that organized and set the stage for identifying and addressing the many challenges to achieving then-president George W. Bush's goal of a nationwide interoperable HIT infrastructure to improve the quality and efficiency of healthcare within 10 years.[4] In focusing on the need for HIT to support the health of the nation as well as the needs of individual consumers and patients to live healthier lives, the framework provided comprehensive long-term strategies as well as short-term solutions with a ten-year goal of widespread adoption and use of HIT in multiple settings for multiple purposes.[5]

Among the seminal pieces of work that resulted from that early framework and ONC's coordination role was the 2006 report published by the Robert Wood Johnson Foundation, "Health Information Technology in the United States: The Information Base for Progress,"[6] which established a clear definition of an EHR system for the purposes of measuring adoption. The report also outlined the barriers to adoption, particularly in the ambulatory setting. The study validated that, in addition to cost, concerns about privacy, difficulty with culture change throughout the clinical setting, and lack of interoperability among multiple EHR systems, physicians in general were reticent to purchase software and technology that they could not easily understand or evaluate themselves. This last issue was addressed in the strategic framework by ONC's plan to support the formation of a certification body that would assure clinicians that the EHR systems that it certified would meet certain standards and criteria necessary to support patient care.

Three organizations—the Health Informatics Management Systems Society (HIMSS), the American Health Information Management Association (AHIMA), and the National Alliance for Health Information Technology (NAHIT)—came together in 2005 to outline a program meeting ONC's objectives (as laid out in the strategic framework) and support the initial formation of the Certification Commission for Health Information Technology (CCHIT). CCHIT subsequently received a three-year federal contract to develop certification programs for ambulatory EHRs, inpatient EHRs, and health information exchange (HIE) organizations with the understanding that CCHIT would become a financially independent entity after this timeframe. The commission's decision-making processes were conducted independently of its founding members from the outset, and by early 2007 CCHIT was a fully independent, nonprofit organization.

While the federal contract was modified in recognition that certifying the embryonic organizations focused on health information exchange was premature at that time, CCHIT met its goals of financial and organizational independence and continued to focus on its not-for-profit mission of fostering HIT adoption through additional EHR-certification programs that are focused on consumer protection—of both the providers purchasing HIT and their patients.

 TIP Robust interoperability is still challenged by the concerns of financial sustainability, privacy and security, governance, and limited interoperability standards faced by multiple fledgling organizations developing HIE infrastructures.

These early efforts in certification clearly put the graph of EHR adoption in the out-patient arena on a consistently upward slope, as shown in Figure 31-1. However, the costs in terms of software, hardware, and lost productivity as well as the lack of interoperability among systems have remained significant barriers, particularly for physicians in small-sized practices.[7] The need for culture change was also a major barrier to more widespread adoption, given the requirements that individual job descriptions change, new skill sets be developed, and the environment structurally modified to accommodate the use of electronic equipment and information.

 TIP It can take six to twelve months for a new system to integrate into a practice and allow the practice to return to baseline levels of productivity.

These last barriers are being addressed in the current decade, as a result of the American Recovery and Reinvestment Act of 2009 (ARRA)—otherwise known as the "stimulus package." Within this legislation are two sections known as the Health Information Technology for Economic and Clinical Health (HITECH) provision, which directed the Centers for Medicare and Medicaid Services (CMS) to disperse billions of incentive dollars for the "meaningful use" of certified EHR systems and codified ONC as an office

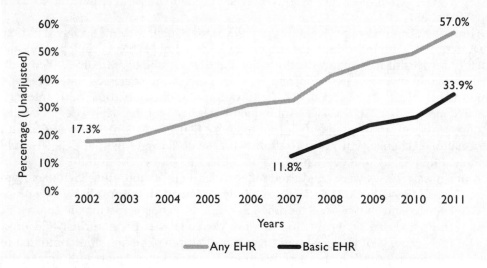

*Basic EHR defined as patient problem, medication, and allergy lists, history, and demographics; physician clinical notes; e-prescribing; and ability to view lab and imaging results electronically.

Data derived from the 2011 National Ambulatory Health Survey conducted by the Centers for Disease Control (CDC) Physician count in thousands

Figure 31-1   Physician Adoption of EHR Systems over a Ten-Year Period

within HHS that would continue to oversee and coordinate efforts to build a national HIT infrastructure. The legislation authorized ONC to disperse monies through grants, contracts, and cooperative agreements to establish programs that would support clinicians who wanted to transition from paper to meaningful use of EHRs, enrich the workforce in the realm of HIT, create statewide mechanisms for health information exchange, and study the best ways to address a number of other problems and concerns that impeded progress to the goal of widespread adoption of an interoperable HIT system.

 TIP Federal grants allow significant independent latitude to the recipient in reaching a final deliverable; cooperative agreements allow the federal government to oversee and direct the work as it progresses; and contracts have highly specified deliverables and timelines that the contractor must meet.

ONC was also authorized to regulate standards for interoperability and certification criteria for EHR systems that would support CMS's incentive program for specified licensed clinicians and hospitals who meet specified objectives and measures of meaningful use of these systems. In so doing, ONC was directed to develop a certification program to meet the objectives of the meaningful-use program. All of these efforts were to be guided by two multi-stakeholder federal advisory bodies, the Health Information Technology Policy Committee and the Health Information Technology Standards Committee, which meet regularly to develop recommendations for both ONC and CMS.

 TIP Both advisory committees meet monthly and are informed by the work done by a number of multi-stakeholder workgroups that meet with greater frequency and focus on specific issues.

CMS and ONC moved quickly after the legislation passed in early 2009. By the end of that year the first set of meaningful use measures (stage 1) was out for public comment. Once these were in final regulation, a set of standards and certification criteria quickly followed, along with the development of the ONC certification program. The first set of certification criteria was designed to meet the specific goals of ARRA—stimulate innovation and expand the product market while assuring that the technology could support the individual measures of meaningful use. The result was an explosion of products, mostly new, certified to the new ONC criteria and process. As of the summer of 2012, over 1400 unique, complete EHR systems and EHR modules were listed on the Certified HIT Products List (CHPL) on ONC's web site, www.healthit.hhs.gov.

As we move through this second decade of the century, then, we can clearly see that it is one of innovation and dynamic activity on all fronts of HIT—cloud-based software, new, easy-to-use mobile hardware, less costly HIE architectures—and much promise.

Seventy years in the making, we are now about to witness a major revolution in how health and care are viewed, how they are supported by information technology, and the advances that will result as more and more health information can be shared securely and with patient permission.

Certification—What, Who, and Why

Certification is nothing more than assurance that certain characteristics of an object, person, or organization are present. It can be done at the first level, which is nothing more than the developer's personal word that the characteristics are present; at the second level, which involves an overarching organization of similar developers or persons to attest that the characteristics are present; or at the third level, which provides maximum confirmation that the characteristics are present through independent review, testing, assessment, or audit.

Applicability of Certification in the Healthcare Industry

Certification of professionals, perhaps the best-known of the certification programs relevant to healthcare, should not be confused with licensure, the latter being a legal designation with a standardized set of requirements. Certification of professionals can vary in its intensity and level of assurance, as noted above. It can be a simple signed certificate verifying attendance or participation in a particular educational program, or it can be verification that an intensive examination was administered and passed by the individual. The latter may test technical capabilities as well as written knowledge. It is therefore important to note that, without knowing the nature of the certification process involved, it is not possible to adequately judge the level of competence or expertise that an individual actually offers.

This is also true of product certification. An external, independent certifying body may grant certification status based on attestation that the product performs a certain way in a given environment by testing it according to a specified set of criteria in a laboratory setting or by testing it in the environment where it is to be used. Further, it may test each step or process independently, or it may test the integration of those steps as they work together to achieve a particular outcome. No matter what the approach, a consistent set of criteria must be used across all products tested in a specified category in a specific certification program. As in certification of professionals, for HIT product certification to truly be of value to interested parties, those parties should have clear knowledge of the criteria and the program and how they are relevant to intended use.

Certification should not to be confused with accreditation. An entity or organization may be accredited to perform certain functions (certification, for example) to specified standards. A certifying body, therefore, may be accredited by another organization that has assured that the certifying body is following all the policies and procedures recommended or required for accreditation. Some of these may be international, as in the International Organization for Standardization (ISO) guides and requirements for testing organizations, or local, as in the requirements named by a state government to conduct certification business within that state. Accreditation, then, is an assurance that the testing and/or certifying body conducts its business according to the accrediting body's external policies and procedures.

Lastly, HIT certification bodies are different and separate from the certificate authorities that provide digital certificates as part of the public-key infrastructure (PKI) assuring the secure transmittal of information between two entities.[8] The former provide assurance, as noted above. The latter provide infrastructure elements that allow transmission of information to occur securely.

HIT Certifying Bodies and Programs

As noted earlier, the first and only certifying body for HIT software until late 2010 was CCHIT, which certified EHRs systems in the ambulatory, inpatient, emergency-department, behavioral-health, and post-acute-care settings. It also developed certification programs in a number of specialties: cardiovascular medicine, dermatology, child health, clinical research, oncology, and women's health (ambulatory obstetrics.) Using a public road map, CCHIT increased the complexity of the certification process regularly so that CCHIT-certified EHRs systems would better meet the needs of those caring for patients. It tested over 300 criteria in the areas of functionality, security, and interoperability, fully certifying only those products that passed all criteria, met standards for integration of data within the system, and were already in use in a clinical setting. New products were granted provisional pre-market certification if they had not yet been implemented for use.

While this comprehensive, provider- and patient-focused approach offered buyers more assurance in their product selections and attracted both small and large developers, the federal government wished to stimulate innovation and broaden the market further to include new types of products, such as modular pieces of a complete EHR system.

Certification for Meaningful-Use Incentive Payments: The Temporary Program

In September 2010, ONC authorized two of what would ultimately be six ONC authorized testing and certification bodies (ONC-ATCBs) to certify EHR systems to the federal government's program of criteria and standards. This temporary program was developed to increase innovation and open the door to multiple new products—some of which fulfilled all of the federal government's criteria, many of which were certified as modules on the basis of fulfilling one or a limited number of criteria in addition to the criteria for privacy and security. The federal criteria were, by regulation, limited to those necessary to support the meaningful-use objectives and measures outlined by CMS and were not designed to meet the comprehensive needs of those engaged in patient care. As such, there was no requirement to test that the modules supporting individual criteria integrated with other modules or functions, security testing was less robust than in the CCHIT-certified programs, and the testing procedures were developed by the National Institute for Standards and Technology (NIST) of the U.S. Department of Commerce rather than by a public multi-stakeholder process. In spite of these limitations, the ONC certification program has been successful in meeting its goals—the nearly 2000 products listed on the Certified HIT Products List include many new products as well as upgrades of the more mature and better-known EHR systems.

The temporary nature of this first ONC certification program allowed it to get up and running quickly in order to assure that ONC-certified products could become available in time for the first meaningful-use attestation period. The lessons learned from the temporary program helped define the permanent testing and certification program that was implemented in 2012.

The Permanent ONC Testing and Certifying Bodies

The American National Standards Institute (ANSI) was named as the accrediting body for those organizations desiring to be in the permanent ONC certification program—the ONC authorized certifying bodies (ACBs)—when the temporary program sunsets. Likewise, the National Voluntary Laboratory Accreditation Program (NVLAP) was chosen to accredit those organizations desiring to perform the testing functions on which certification is based—the accredited testing laboratories (ATLs). Both certifying and testing bodies must now adhere to the ISO standards and guidelines required by ANSI and NVLAP, respectively. These accreditation processes were not available during the temporary program, but will assure a more standardized approach to both testing and certification going forward. A second difference between the temporary and the permanent program is that in the temporary approach the same ONC-authorized organization was expected to test and certify a particular EHR system or module. In the permanent program, EHR system and module developers may seek testing from one accredited organization and certification from a different accredited and authorized organization, though both processes will clearly be offered by most organizations.

 TIP ANSI and NVLAP announced five organizations each as accredited in mid-July 2012, with four organizations having dual accreditation, one with ANSI accreditation only, and one with NVLAP accreditation only.

Editions of ONC Certification Criteria

Contrary to popular belief, the various sets of ONC certification criteria that are required to be in ONC-certified health information technologies are not aligned with the various stages of meaningful use. In order to have certified EHR systems, providers must have and be using the edition of ONC certification criteria that is recognized by the secretary of Health and Human Services at the time—independent of the stage of meaningful use to which they intend to attest. Therefore, when the 2014 edition of ONC criteria become required in fiscal year 2014, every provider applying for incentive payments must either purchase new or upgrade previously certified EHR systems in order to have ONC-certified technology that will provide eligibility for any of the stages of meaningful use. Similarly, there is no alignment between the temporary and permanent certification programs and the validity of certification for the various editions of certification criteria. Sunsetting of the temporary program occurred October 4, 2012 when the new permanent program was announced and went into effect. This does not, however, invalidate the certifications conducted by the temporary ONC-ATCBS. These certifications will be valid until the new 2014 edition of certification criteria is required. Likewise, the new testing and certifying participants in the permanent program may test and certify EHR technologies to the 2011 edition of certification criteria as long as the secretary of HHS recognizes these criteria as valid for certification. Figure 31-2 depicts the relationship between editions of certified technology and meaningful-use stages.

CCHIT Certification 2010 Ambulatory EHR Certification Criteria

CCHIT

May 17, 2011

©2011 The Certification Commission for Health Information Technology

P = Previous Criterion
M = Modified
N = New for Year
O = Optional

Internal Sort Column	Criteria #	Category	Criteria	Year Introduced or Last Modified	2011 Certification	Comments	Criteria Reference	Test Script and Step Number AMB = Ambulatory Test Script SEC = Security Test Script
2011.AM.001	AM 01.01	Identify and maintain a patient record	The system shall create a single patient record for each patient.	2006	P		DC.1.1.1.	AMB 1.02
2011.AM.002	AM 01.02	Identify and maintain a patient record	The system shall associate (store and link) key identifier information (e.g., system ID, medical record number) with each patient record.	2006	P	Key identifier information must be unique to the patient record but may take any system defined internal or external form.	DC.1.1.1.	AMB 1.02
2011.AM.003	AM 01.03	Identify and maintain a patient record	The system shall provide the ability to store more than one identifier or each patient record.	2006	P	For interoperability, practices need to be able to store additional patient identifiers. Examples include an ID generated by an Enterprise Master Patient Index, a health plan or Insurance subscriber ID, regional and/or national patient identifiers if/when such become available.	DC.1.1.1.	AMB 1.03

Figure 31-2 An Example of Certification Criteria. Reprinted with permission from the Certification Commission for Health Information Technology.

Evaluation of HIT Products Beyond Certification

As complicated as it may seem, certification is not the only approach to evaluating HIT in general and EHR systems in particular. How one assesses a given technology is dependent on the goal of the assessment and how the information will be used. We have discussed some of the different goals of the various EHR certification programs developed to date. As we consider several other useful ways of evaluating HIT, it is important to recognize that they each assess a different aspect of the interaction between the technology involved and its use by clinicians. Taken together, they may be able to truly evaluate the effectiveness of HIT as its use becomes more widespread.

Goals and Approaches of Different HIT Evaluation Programs

The best approach to assessing a particular aspect of HIT depends very much on the goal of the assessment. In the same way that certification is designed to provide a level of assurance to the purchaser of the HIT product, other approaches are driven by different goals, as demonstrated by the following types of programs.

Improved Patient Safety—Monitoring for Potential Problems

In November 2011, the IOM released a report that voiced concern about the lack of evidence that EHR technology was safe for use in the clinical setting.[9] There have been, of course, anecdotes about system failures that could lead to patient harm. And there have been breaches of privacy and security that have the potential to cause harm. Given the lack of good data, however, it is difficult to determine what should be included in an assessment of the patient-safety features associated with HIT for either the inpatient or ambulatory environments. There have been reports on how HIT can help meet the safety objectives of the Joint Commission,[10] and information from the world of medical malpractice suggests how better HIT processes may improve overall patient safety,[11] but there is no data regarding how HIT might actually harm patients. This is an area that clearly needs further study, and ONC has been directed to make this a priority for 2012.

 TIP Data from malpractice claims suggest that the leading causes of these claims are poor communication, lack of documentation, and lack of follow-up after ordering referrals or procedures—all of which could be addressed by integrated functions within the EHR system and interoperability among providers and with patients.

Interoperability Testing

As federal standards for interoperability are recognized by the secretary of HHS, they will be included in the ONC standards and criteria required for certification. However, these standards must meet readiness requirements before they can be mandated in regulation. Since widespread adoption is one of those requirements, it will take some time for robust inclusion of interoperability standards for health information exchange in the ONC certification process. In the interim, progress continues in the private sector to ensure interoperability among various EHR systems, between EHR systems and patient-controlled medical devices, and between patient-controlled personal health records and EHRs. The participants in these types of health information exchanges are being tested for interoperability by a number of entities outside of the public sector, though no formal assessment program is currently recognized. This is because federally regulated standards must be mature and have a long life cycle once they are included in a rule. The industry, however, is constantly evolving these standards, attempting to harmonize where multiple standards exist, developing new ones as necessary, and testing until they are mature and widely accepted.

Usability Ratings

Usability is defined by ISO as "...the effectiveness, efficiency, and satisfaction with which the intended users can achieve their tasks in the intended context of product use."[12] From a clinician's point of view, it's what makes it easy to electronically record and retrieve reliable, well-organized information about a patient at any given moment without reliance on paper and other staff. Perhaps most important, usability is closely tied to patient safety—poor usability may result in not seeing important data, ordering the wrong medications or tests, or, worse yet, entering information into the wrong person's chart.

The science of usability has been the focus of recent work by NIST, the Agency for Healthcare Research and Quality (AHRQ), and a number of ONC grantees. There is now universal agreement that usability in the HIT environment is characterized and informed by the science of user-centric design (UCD) and both formative (done as part of the development process) and summative (comparing one system with another using standardized formats) testing. Past experience with CCHIT in objective testing and public reporting of usability ratings, current research on usability funded by ONC grants, and the practical application of new approaches to assessing usability will likely allow for more evaluation of HIT along this important axis in the near future, with new usability ratings publically available. In the interim, NIST has made available to all EHR system developers a set of principles and guidelines that can be used to increase usability in the provider setting.[12]

Performance in the Clinical Setting—Satisfaction Surveys

A number of organizations regularly survey providers with respect to their satisfaction with their HIT products. The American College of Physicians (ACP) and KLAS are the best-known sources of information related to these surveys, and both provide a trove of useful information about what appears to work well in the clinical settings and what functions could be improved. These reports on the real-life experience of HIT users offer potential EHR purchasers an important complement to the criteria-driven certification process that tests EHR systems in a laboratory setting.

Policies and Procedures—Accreditation

The most secure systems in the world will not keep information confidential if human intervention or error allows for data breaches through failure to follow accepted policies and procedures. Therefore, any discussion about HIT must include acknowledgment that it is another tool for use or abuse by individuals. Every clinical setting that employs these tools must have a sound set of policies and procedures that are understood and adopted by all that use them. Organizations such as the National Committee for Quality Assessment (NCQA) assess policies and procedures in many areas, including privacy and security, and the degree to which they are followed by provider groups interested in patient-centered medical home (PCMH) designations and accreditation as an accountable care organization (ACO).

Healthcare Reform—Internal Assessment

As providers organize themselves to successfully assume various degrees of financial risk while managing a population of patients, they will need far more HIT functionality than what is or can be available in an EHR system. Practice-management systems, financial-management systems, remote patient-centered monitoring devices, and robust data warehouses that can support advanced business analytics will also be required. These technologies will need to integrate with one other and the EHR system in ways that have heretofore been unprecedented in order to support care coordination, the selection and management of specific populations of patients, improved quality of care, state-of-the-art customer service, and business intelligence. There are many factors that will determine the success of a provider group's ability to function in this type of environment, but the "right" HIT infrastructure is foundational. Assessing this infrastructure and assuring it can meet the needs of the organization that is assuming financial accountability for care is important for both the organization itself and the payers with whom it is sharing that financial risk.

 TIP In addition to a strong HIT foundation, a successful ACO will need a governance, a solid primary case base, strong leadership with a team-oriented culture, enough financial capital to assume some risk, a significant proportion of its population in the risk environment, and enough emphasis on customer satisfaction to promote lasting patient relationships.

Certification Program Development

A good certification program in a dynamic area like HIT with its multiple stakeholders will benefit from multi-stakeholder development and program test piloting. The goal is to achieve a reasonable balance between what can be done technologically at reasonable cost and what the purchaser needs and desires. Ideally, the certification program's development process should reflect its public mission and clearly articulate how and why it may add value to both the product developer seeking certification and the purchaser of a certified product.

Scoping the Work

Scoping is mission critical, in more ways than one. The scope must be true to the mission of the certifying body or program, but also narrow enough to be practical, scalable, and marketable. For example, an outpatient obstetrics clinical record has information that is historically relevant at the time of actual delivery, but the inpatient obstetrical record requires very different functionalities and information about both mother and baby (with a record of its own at the time of birth). The inpatient record is specific to events that occurred during the entire admission, labor, delivery, and immediate post-partum period. One of the most obvious and basic differences between these two systems is the need for the inpatient system to support the ordering of IV medication doses based on vital signs, progression of labor, or level of pain. Certification criteria for an EHR system used in the ambulatory obstetrical setting should be highly specified to assure that the needed functions are achieved, but the criteria do not need to include information that would be necessary at the time of actual birth in the inpatient setting.

Criteria Development

As noted earlier, criteria in the HIT realm generally fall into several categories: functionality, security, and interoperability, with functionality further subcategorized by area, such as care coordination, patient engagement, or public-health reporting. The criteria are developed by stating the overall function and identifying each of the detailed steps necessary to achieve that function, as shown in Figure 31-3. The process is best served by convening a multi-stakeholder group of experts who can balance user need with the stage of technical development and "roadmap" criteria for future use as necessary and appropriate. Alternatively, criteria development can come under the aegis of the federal government and become part of the regulation process. Either way, the criteria should be reliable and objectively testable.

EHR Reporting Period			
FY/CY 2011	FY/CY 2012	FY/CY 2013	FY/CY 2014
MU Stage I	MU Stage I	MU Stage I	MU Stage I or MU Stage 2
All Eligible Professional (EP), Eligible Hospital (EH), and Critical Access Hospital (CAH) must have EHR technology that has been certified to all applicable 2011 edition EHR certification criteria or equivalent 2014 edition EHR certification criteria adopted by the Secretary.			All EPs, EHs, and CAHs must have EHR technology that has been certified to all 2014 edition EHR certification criteria that would support the objectives and measures, and their ability to successfully report the Clinical Quality Measure (CQM), for the MU stage that they seek to achieve.

Note: There is no such thing as being "stage-1 certified" or "stage-2 certified."

Figure 31-3 The Relationship between Certification Edition and Stage of Meaningful Use

Test Scripts or Testing Procedures

Criteria are best tested using workflows that accurately reflect how information is used in the specified setting. These can be short, criterion-specific steps in an overall workflow process (as in the ONC certification testing procedures) or a comprehensive, clinically oriented workflow that includes multiple criteria and also tests for integration of data across various functions in the system (as with CCHIT certification). The experience of clinically active users of EHR systems is invaluable in the development of these test scripts and is highly recommended.

Public Comment

Assessment programs in general benefit from some form of public input and feedback. This can be a formal governmental process or more informal processes to meet the more flexible needs of the market. Either way, the program is enriched with the added knowledge of multiple other stakeholders in the field.

Test Piloting

Before going to market or being mandated by the public sector, all HIT programs and processes should be thoroughly pilot tested. It is then, and only then, that one finds and is able to fix problems before widespread marketing or rollout. The importance of this step can best be underscored by what happened shortly after the first certifications were conducted using the ONC criteria in late 2010. Time pressures had not allowed for piloting before the first certifying bodies were authorized to commence the ONC program, using the mandated criteria and testing procedures. As the program was implemented, a number of problems were discovered, one of which was that the testing procedures included outdated medications that had been removed from the market.

These problems were rectified as they came to light, as was the confusion about the validity of the ONC certification process for the earliest EHR systems, but they are good examples of what is generally discovered and rectified during the piloting period, before developers pay for and go through a certification process. Many of the EHR systems were not programmed to include these obsolete pharmacological preparations—which were required for testing and certification only, not for actual use.

Testing of HIT Products

Once the criteria and testing scripts or procedures are accepted and published, product testing begins. Testers are selected to test each product in exactly the same way with respect to each criterion. This can be done remotely, using secure Web-based screen sharing with either a developer's or provider's laboratory. Either way, it is to the developer's benefit to be able to demonstrate an alternative path if the tester has difficulty seeing that a particular scenario, criterion, or step has been accomplished. The results of this testing process are then forwarded to the certifiers.

Final Certification of Product

International standards require that the testing and certifying arms of the entire process be distinct and separate. This is because final certification can also be dependent on a number of nontechnical factors, such as how the product is marketed or whether it is in use in the setting for which it is intended. CCHIT does not offer full certification to a product unless it is installed and being used in the clinical setting. The ONC program, on the other hand, has no such requirement.

The entire testing and certification process can require a full day of testing for a complete EHR system or only an hour or so for some of the simpler ONC modules that include only one criterion (like smoking status). The real cost of certification, however, is not in the actual testing but in assuring that the developer has included all of the coding necessary in the programming process that will allow for certification at the first attempt.

Review the Criteria

The first step for any developer is to carefully review all of the relevant criteria and testing procedures to make sure the system is programmed to meet these requirements. If not, there will need to be reprogramming or inclusion of technology that can meet the requirements. This is probably the most difficult and onerous step. Once accomplished, however, a few more steps will lead to successful certification.

Establish a Relationship with the Testing and/or Certifying Entity

The developer makes contact and establishes a relationship with an individual who will help them through the process. The developer should read and participate in all the support that is provided. Some certifying bodies offer very robust preparation manuals and communities of practice so every prospective customer comes fully prepared for a successful certification.

Practice

Prior to testing, most developers or providers seeking certification of self-built systems run through the test scenarios on their own to make sure they can do them quickly and easily when subsequently observed during the actual testing process.

 TIP Practicing is probably the most important step to take prior to scheduling the actual testing and certification.

Testing

As noted, the testers direct the developers or providers of self-built products to demonstrate how the technology meets the requirements of the criteria and testing procedures while observing how this is done. If there are questions, a tester may ask for a repeat, or the developer may choose to approach the criterion from another direction. These are all acceptable modifications. What is *not* acceptable is reprogramming of any sort to meet the criterion in question.

Certification

The vendor may market a product as certified for a specific program, but the vendor must assure that there is no confusion about the program(s) for which the product is certified. For instance, CCHIT-certified 2011 ambulatory products do *not* meet the requirement for ONC certification. ONC certification done by CCHIT may be marketed as "ONC-certified by CCHIT," or simply as "ONC-certified," but the two certification programs must be labeled differently and separately. Almost 100 comprehensive ambulatory EHR systems on the market are now certified by both ONC and CCHIT, assuring that their users are eligible for meaningful-use incentive dollars while also assuring that their functions are integrated and workflow-based to meet the needs of patient care.

Management of Updates

As a developer updates the software, renewed certification may be required. In general, vendors and developers are required to notify certifying bodies of any version changes, and the latter then determine whether recertification is warranted. Some developers consider each update a new product and certify each as a new version. Others, particularly in the case of ONC certification, bring back the updated version with the attestation that the update did not change the programming. New certification would be appropriate if new, previously untested criteria were added or if the underlying architecture is altered in any way.

The Future

In the end, we all need technologies that make it easier for clinicians to do their work, improve the interaction between clinicians and patients (either virtually or face-to-face), and allow for the secure reuse of data for purposes that benefit our society at large (surveillance, research, emergency preparedness, public health, improvements in the quality of care)—without adding burden on the delivery system.

This means that *functionality* must include the ability to integrate information from multiple sources within the technology being used at the point of care, including information coming from and going to patients. Functionality must also include the ability for information that requires reporting to be reliably and securely collated and sent to the appropriate receiver, with minimal provider intervention. It means that all information about follow-up or lack thereof comes to the attention of the clinicians. And it means that clinical decision support goes far beyond prompts and reminders, providing up-to-date information that is relevant and specific to a given patient in a nonintrusive format.

It also means that *privacy* and *security* will become more granular, allowing patients to better control which of their health data may be shared with whom. Further, as more and more health data finds its way to the cloud, new technical approaches to secure access to that data will be developed. As indicated earlier, however, security is also a human problem. Most data breaches do not occur because of technical failures. They occur because of lost computers, open or unlocked desktops, or because obsolete electronic information has not been disposed of appropriately. They can also occur because of poor patient-consent processes or different policies and procedures within the multiple settings a clinician may practice. Therefore, tight security means following a consistent set of policies and procedures designed to minimize these human-factor risks as much as it means attending to state-of-the-art technical security. One is only as good as the other.

 TIP One way to maximize security is to make sure that all personally owned systems that may be used for work-related activity are encrypted.

While we spend a good deal of time talking and working on *interoperability* and have made significant strides in the ability to send summary documents securely and easily, there is still much work to be done before we can truly reap the benefit of universal access to the data needed when it is needed and by whom it is needed. The HITSC has done a tremendous amount of work in identifying possible standards to meet this need, but many are not yet mature—not well tested and in widespread use. However, the ability of clinicians to access their patients' records from virtually anywhere on the planet is now a basic expectation when caring for patients within any sort of organized system that has electronic health information available. This is a tremendous advantage that is paving the way for more widespread demand for the use and sharing of electronic information under the appropriate privacy and security infrastructure. While true and total interoperability is still a Holy Grail of sorts, it has been recognized as a goal that we can work toward. In the interim, whatever standards are in place at any given time will continue to be part of certification processes.

Lastly, we know that other features, such as *usability, portability, attention to workflow, time efficiency,* and especially *safety,* are all important aspects of how clinicians and patients regard the HIT systems that have become part of their lives. Therefore, when we look to the future, we know that there are new technologies on the horizon—both software and hardware—that will fulfill these needs as easily (but more securely) as an iPhone full of applications meets the needs of its owner.

As our markets become even more dynamic, we will need more dynamic evaluation processes to provide the assurance that these new technologies are safe, secure, and reliable. And we will also need to assure that the trade-off between consumer protection and stimulating innovation does not sacrifice one for the other. Certification programs set in regulation every three years under these conditions will not be sustainable.

Finally, we will need to assure that we have multiple solid assessment programs for HIT in place that can be used for research purposes to better guide the development of better, more effective, more efficient, and appropriately secure ways of creating and using electronic health data. Our goal of a healthier nation is dependent on us all.

Chapter Review

Certification of healthcare IT is a simple concept with a complicated implementation when applied to the dynamic and exciting healthcare environment that we will be living in for years to come. As a basic mechanism for assuring an outside observer that a specified list of characteristics is present, early certification programs helped overcome one of the major barriers to EHR adoption among ambulatory clinicians—lack of information about what an EHR system should (and actually did) do. As the federal government moved forward with ARRA, the opportunity to stimulate the economy through support for widespread adoption of HIT that would be used in a measurable and meaningful way led to the development of federal certification programs linked to financial incentives for meeting meaningful use—and the development of hundreds of new EHR-related products. There are, however, significant limitations to these programs. Certification in the healthcare environment is a diverse, poorly understood entity in general, and certification of HIT has become even more confusing. As we educate ourselves and each other going forward, the advantages and limitations of the various methods of assessing HIT in its many forms and settings, certification included, need to be studied and better understood with respect to their effect on patients, clinicians, and the health of the public at large.

Questions

To test your comprehension of the chapter, answer the following questions and then check your answers against the list of correct answers that follows the questions.

1. What technological advancement opened the door to broad interest and use of health information technology?

   A. E-prescribing systems

   B. Personal computers

   C. Semantic interoperability

   D. Digital certificates

   E. Practice-management systems

2. Which of the following are policy levers used by the federal government?

   A. Statute and regulation

   B. Payment and reimbursement methodologies and amounts

   C. Contractual requirements

   D. Conditions of doing business with the federal government

   E. All of the above

3. Among the barriers to early adoption of EHR systems by physicians in the ambulatory sector, which one was the first to be addressed shortly after ONC was formed by presidential executive order?

 A. The cost of EHR systems

 B. The need for interoperability among various systems

 C. Privacy concerns

 D. Lack of knowledge about how to evaluate EHR systems

 E. The need for culture change in the clinical setting

4. What was the goal of the first certification program developed by CCHIT?

 A. Increase adoption by providing assurance to would-be purchasers that the technology would help support patient care processes

 B. Increase the number of products available to purchasing clinicians

 C. Standardize product development to minimize possible safety risks associated with innovation in healthcare

 D. Assure interoperability among all certified EHR systems

 E. Make EHR products more usable

5. What are the objectives of the ONC-developed certification program? Circle all that apply.

 A. Assure that the EHR systems meet safety criteria

 B. Support meaningful-use objectives and measures

 C. Stimulate new, innovative approaches to managing clinical data

 D. Support patient-care workflows and processes

 E. Stimulate the economy by expanding the EHR market

6. Which of the following is a true statement about a certified EHR system?

 A. It does what the user wants and expects.

 B. It is easy to use and makes one's work more efficient.

 C. It embeds state-of-the-art security technology.

 D. It includes a specified list of characteristics for which it has been certified.

 E. It can share data with other certified healthcare information technologies.

7. What are some of the characteristics of the ONC certification program? Circle all that apply.

 A. Testing assures that all functions within the EHR technology are integrated.

 B. Close to 2000 products have been listed as certified HIT.

 C. Testing protocols were developed by multi-stakeholder subject matter experts.

 D. Allows for some first-level certification.

 E. Applicable to all types of providers.

8. When will an eligible provider (EP) need to be using an EHR system that has been certified to ONC's 2014 edition of certification criteria?

    A. By January 1, 2014

    B. When the secretary of HHS recognizes the new criteria

    C. When the permanent certification program goes into effect

    D. By January 1, 2013 if attesting to MU stage 2 in 2014

    E. Whenever planning to attest to stage 2

9. Which of the following did the IOM report on patient safety and HIT published in November 2011 include?

    A. Recommendation that the FDA immediately start regulating EHR systems with respect to patient safety

    B. Summary of multiple studies enumerating the patient-safety hazards of EHRs

    C. Recommendation that HHS should direct ONC to develop a monitoring system to track possible patient-safety defects in EHR technology

    D. Outline of ways to assess the safety of EHRs

    E. Recommendation that patient-safety testing be added to the ONC certification program

10. Which of the following options does *not* make the inclusion of interoperability standards in the federal certification process more difficult?

    A. The HITSC, informed by its workgroups, makes recommendations to ONC about which standards are mature and ready for the regulatory process.

    B. There can be multiple standards for the same transactions.

    C. Standardized testing protocols for interoperability among all HIT products have yet to be developed.

    D. Interoperability standards are evolving in a dynamic environment; the federal regulatory process is a multi-year cycle.

    E. Many proposed interoperability standards are not yet mature—they have not been tested or widely adopted.

11. Which of the following is *not* a true statement with respect to usability and EHR systems?

    A. Usability testing will be included among the 2014 ONC certification criteria.

    B. NIST has made available a set of principles and guidelines that developers may use.

    C. There was experience with usability in the market prior to the ONC certification program.

D. ONC has funded a number of grantees to further develop usability in the clinical setting.

E. User-centric design is a science that informs good usability, particularly as it pertains to patient safety.

12. Which of the following is *not* a characteristic of accreditation programs?

A. Apply to organizations

B. Assess policies and procedures

C. May assess business integrity and evidence of leadership

D. May include an HIT assessment

E. Allow organizations to become eligible for meaningful-use incentive payments

13. In the interests of a timely rollout, which step of the certification development process was eliminated in the 2011 ONC program?

A. Scoping

B. Open public comment regarding proposed criteria

C. Testing procedure development

D. Piloting of the testing procedures

E. Soliciting of public comment on the test procedures

14. What is the most important thing a developer should do before applying for certification?

A. Review the certification criteria and testing procedures

B. Establish a relationship with someone in the testing/certification organization

C. Practice going through the test procedures

D. Prepare to reprogram if compliance with a criterion cannot be demonstrated

E. Certify before all planned updates so as not to risk successful certification

15. Which of the following are true statements?

A. Certification is a simple concept.

B. A certified EHR system meets the needs of every clinician who aspires to use it effectively and efficiently.

C. Current certification programs assure the usability and portability of patient data, integration of data within the EHR system, and that the software is safe—it will not cause patient harm.

D. Certification processes will need to become more flexible to meet the needs of a dynamic HIT environment.

E. Multiple other ways of assessing HIT are necessary to complement certification programs.

Answers

1. **B.** While ever more advances are made in both the technology and the policies associated with widespread adoption of HIT, the personal computer put the promise and the reality of the availability of electronic information in front of every individual.

2. **E.** All are methods that are used to develop and implement federal policy.

3. **D.** The Certification Commission for HIT was the first of many efforts supported by ONC to come to fruition by certifying ambulatory EHR systems in 2006 to a robust set of over 300 criteria that provided assurance to physicians that these products would meet basic needs for supporting patient care in the clinical setting.

4. **A.** The goal of CCHIT is and always has been to support clinicians interested in adopting healthcare information technologies in order to provide better care to their patients. As interoperability and usability became more standardized and testable, these aspects were included in the certification process.

5. **B, C, E.** By federal law, the ONC certification program is limited to what is necessary to support the meaningful-use incentive program. At the same time, the intent of ARRA was to stimulate the economy, which can be done through market expansion and stimulating innovation.

6. **D.** Certification brings value if one is aware of the characteristics and criteria to which the product is certified and the goal of the certification program.

7. **B, D.** The ONC program has certified over 600 unique ambulatory EHR systems, close to 100 inpatient EHR systems, and many modules and updated versions of a single EHR system. This includes first-level certification (attestation) of some of the privacy criteria. It does not certify for settings other than ambulatory and inpatient, does not test for integration of functions, and used federal expertise only in the initial development phases.

8. **A.** All EPs must be using an EHR system that has been certified to the 2014 edition of certification criteria by January 1, 2014 if they intend to apply for meaningful-use incentive payments. These criteria will be recognized by the secretary of HHS before this time, but actual use can be delayed until the 2014 date. There is no connection between the stage of meaningful use to which attestation is intended and the required edition of certified technology.

9. **C.** ONC has been directed to monitor any adverse patient safety issues that may be associated with the use of EHR systems.

10. **A.** All of the options listed make codifying interoperability standards in the certification editions more difficult except the focus and commitment with which the federal advisors hasten to bring standards to the level of maturity necessary for inclusion into the certification program.

11. **A.** Usability is not part of the 2014 ONC certification program. NIST and ONC grantees are actively pursuing how to characterize and test for usability, and user-centric design has been informing both these efforts as well as the earlier efforts of CCHIT to develop and include usability as part of its testing protocols. The latter publicly posted usability ratings for all ambulatory EHR systems certified to their criteria.

12. **E.** Only products certified by ONC-authorized testing labs and certification programs can provide eligibility for meaningful-use incentive payments.

13. **D.** NIST did not have time to pilot the testing procedures. All other steps took place, though public comment regarding the test procedures was not publicly posted, as it was for the criteria themselves.

14. **C.** Practicing for the testing processes is key to success. A developer or provider of a self-built system will *not* be able to reprogram during the testing process and should come prepared to demonstrate compliance. Further, since some upgrades may require recertification, all reasonable upgrades should be included at the time of certification.

15. **A, D, E.** Certification programs do not meet all of the needs of a using provider, nor does the current ONC program include any of the attributes listed in C, though the CCHIT certification program does.

References

1. Shortcliffe, E. & Cimino, J. (Eds.). (2006). *Biomedical informatics* (3rd ed., p. 24). Springer.

2. Weed, L. L. (1968). Medical records that guide and teach. *New England Journal of Medicine 278*, 593–600, 652–657.

3. Bowie, J. & Barnett, G.O. (1976). MUMPS: An economical and efficient time-sharing system for information management. *Computer Programs in Biomedicine 6*, 11–22.

4. Executive Order 13335. Incentives for the use of health information technology and establishing the position of the national health information technology coordinator. Accessed from www.federalregister.gov/executive-order/13335.pdf.

5. Thompson, T. & Brailer, D. (2004). The decade of health information technology: Delivering consumer-centric and information-rich health care: Framework for strategic action. Accessed from www.providersedge.com/ehdocs/ehr_articles/The_Decade_of_HIT-Delivering_Customer-centric_and_Info-rich_HC.pdf.

6. Blumenthal, D., et al. (2006). Health information technology in the United States: The information base for progress. Accessed from www.rwjf.org/files/publications/other/EHRReport0609.pdf.

7. Blumenthal, D., DesRoches, C., Donelan, K., Ferris, T., Jha, A., Raushal, R., Rao, S., Rosenbaum, S., & Shield, A. (2008). Health information technology in the United States: Where we stand, 2008. Accessed from www.rwjf.org/content/dam/supplementary-assets/2008/health-info-tech-in-the-US.pdf.

8. IOM. (November 8, 2011). Health IT for patient safety: Building safer systems for better care. Accessed from http://iom.edu/Reports/2011/Health-IT-and-Patient-Safety-Building-Safer-Systems-for-Better-Care.aspx.

9. Radecki, R. & Sittig, D. (2011). Application of electronic health records to the Joint Commission's 2011 national patient safety goals. *Journal of the American Medical Association 306*, 92–93.

10. Mangalmurti, S., Murtagh, L., & Mello, M. (2010). Medical malpractice liability in the age of electronic health records. *New England Journal of Medicine 363*, 2060–2067.

11. Redish, J. & Lowry, L. (2010). Usability in health IT: Technical strategy, research, and implementation. NISTIR 7743. Accessed from www.nist.gov/customcf/get_pdf.cfm?pub_id=907316.

12. Shumacher, R. & Lowry, L. (2010). NIST guide to the processes approach for improving the usability of electronic health records. NISTIR 7741. Accessed from www.nist.gov/manuscript-publication-search.cfm?pub_id=907313.

PART V

Healthcare IT Operations

Andre Kushniruk, Editor

Computer Hardware and Architecture for Healthcare IT

Daniel Lachance

In this chapter, you will learn how to

- Identify commonly used IT terms and technologies
- Compare and contrast electronic health record (EHR)/electronic medical record (EMR) technologies and how each is implemented
- Install and configure hardware drivers and devices
- Work with document imaging
- Classify different server types, environments, features, and limitations
- Set up a basic PC workstation within an EHR/EMR environment
- Troubleshoot and solve common PC problems

Computers have been used in the healthcare industry since the 1950s, when the primary use focused on research (which continues today). Over the next two decades, with the introduction of transistor and integrated circuit (IC) technology, prescriptions, patient billing, medical decision processes, and patient health records started to depend upon the correct hardware configurations supporting specialized software. Even today, medical professionals use specialized computer hardware and software to conduct CAT scans and MRIs, while also using handheld computing devices for bedside visits.

Terminology is key to determining which type of computer hardware component or configuration best meets a specific requirement. Current buzz phrase such as "cloud computing" are important in that they could mean offsite-hosted EMR systems and data storage, thus eliminating the need for local IT expertise and costly hardware. Some

EMR systems require a more powerful computer than others, and you may need to procure the correct equipment or identify computer systems whose hardware can be upgraded to support new software. Data requirements could dictate the retention, size, and speed of internal and external disks, or data might be stored offsite, often referred to as data being *stored in the cloud*. As you can see, a single term or phrase can have important implications.

Identify Commonly Used IT Terms and Technologies

A modern Windows computer network will consist of Windows client operating systems (such as Windows Server 2008) and domain controllers (DCs). A domain controller is a Windows server that contains the Active Directory (AD) database. The AD database contains user account information, passwords, groups, and computer accounts for computers that have joined the domain. Computers that have joined the AD domain can be centrally managed by the AD domain administrator.

Most computer networks use network cables and switches to interconnect devices; others may use wireless technologies. Wired networks use switches as a central wiring location. Figure 32-1 depicts an Ethernet network switch. Ethernet switches commonly have 24 RJ-45 ports, allowing for up to 24 devices to be plugged in. Often there are one or two additional high-speed ports used to interconnect switches, thus allowing more than 24 devices to exist on a local area network (LAN). Routers, both wired and wireless, are plugged into switches just like any other computer, thus allowing connectivity to other networks such as the Internet. Modern wireless routers often have a few RJ-45 ports, which means they also function as a mini switch.

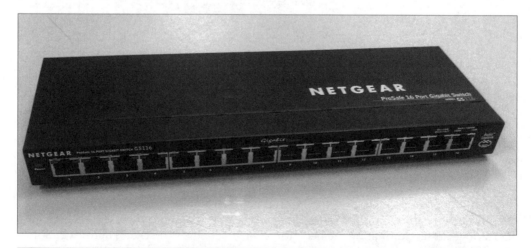

Figure 32-1   A 16-port Netgear Ethernet switch

Compare and Contrast EHR/EMR Technologies and How Each Is Implemented

Cloud computing refers to using computing resources, such as an EMR system or data storage, that are hosted offsite. Companies offering cloud computing software services are called *application service providers* (ASPs). This eliminates local server hardware and IT staff dedicated to server management onsite to support this infrastructure. Often, all that is needed on your client stations is a web browser and a connection to the Internet via your Internet service provider (ISP). Depending on the volume of data and how quickly it must be accessible, a fiber Internet connection may be required. On the provider side, the hosted software solution might be a virtualized server. As opposed to installing an operating system on a dedicated physical machine, there could be many virtualized operating systems (virtual machines) running concurrently on a single physical host computer.

Inversely, client-server EMR systems imply client workstations connected to an EMR server onsite, meaning it is the local IT staff's responsibility. The upside is faster network speeds than a cloud EMR solution and local organizational control over your EMR data. Some EMR systems (as well as any software) may expose application programming interfaces (APIs), which allow a developer to create custom or additional functionality.

Another variation of connecting to an EMR system might be using a dumb terminal that connects to a mainframe. A dumb terminal is essentially a screen and keyboard that runs a program that runs on the central mainframe computer. Although still in use today, on modern computers, a terminal server plays the same role as a mainframe computer: the server runs applications locally using its computing resources, and users connect to that application from their computers via remote access, or terminal client, software. Figure 32-2 shows the Windows Remote Desktop Connection screen. These clients are often referred to as *thin clients*, since they need little processing power and storage to run applications hosted on a terminal server.

Install and Configure Hardware Drivers and Devices

Hardware devices, whether internal to a computer or external (a peripheral), require a software driver installed in the operating system. Most times the operating system will detect new hardware and install the appropriate driver, but not always. Drivers are provided on CD by the manufacturer, or you can download them from the manufacturer's web site. Care must be taken to ensure the correct driver is installed for the model of hardware present. A 64-bit installation of Windows Server 2008 requires a 64-bit printer driver; the 32-bit printer driver for Windows Server 2008 will not work. Microsoft publishes a list of hardware that will work with its operating systems; this list is called the Hardware Compatibility List (HCL).

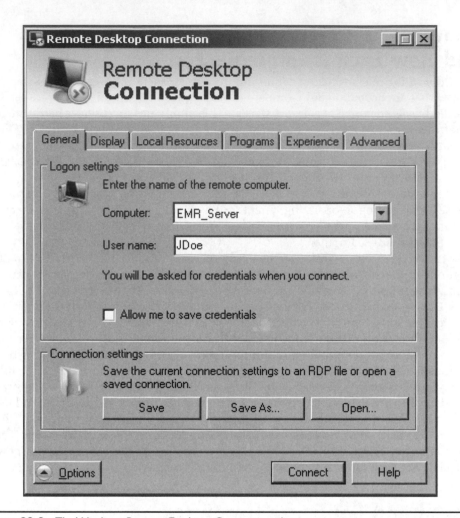

Figure 32-2 The Windows Remote Desktop Connection client

Central Processing Unit

The central processing unit (CPU) is often referred to as the "brains" of a device. Servers, desktops, laptops, tablets, smartphones, and many more types of devices all have a CPU. Internal CPU speed is often measured in either gigahertz (GHz, or billions of operations per second) or millions of instructions per second (MIPS); a faster CPU means more power drawn as well as more heat generated. Today's CPU chips are multicore, meaning a single physical CPU chip may actually house, for example, four internal separate CPUs (referred to as *quad core*).

The CPU is also referred to as a *microprocessor*; however, the term "microprocessor" can also be applied to task-specific circuitry, such as the graphics processing unit (GPU), which may be on an expansion video card.

Motherboards and Bus Slots

The main circuit board found in a computer is the motherboard. Specific motherboards can accept specific CPUs, and care must be taken to ensure they both match and run at the fastest possible speeds together. Motherboards also contain one or more expansion card slots (bus slots).

Modern systems might have a single Peripheral Component Interconnect (PCI) slot and several Peripheral Component Interconnect Express (PCIe) slots. PCI cards have a maximum throughput of 500 megabytes (MB) per second, often expressed as MBps. PCIe slots come in many forms such as X1, X8, and X16. X1 has a data throughput of 500MBps bidirectionally or 250MBps unidirectionally. X16 has a maximum bidirectional throughput of 8 gigabytes per second (GBps), which is derived from 500MBps multiplied by 16.

Remember that any computer component that has a faster speed draws more power, which increases heat. Adequate power supplies inside the computer must be considered, especially when upgrading older computers to newer internal components with a higher power draw. For example, a newly upgraded computer may have components that, in total, require 600 watts of power. If the 450-watt power supply is not upgraded, the machine will not turn on! In a given room, plugging in several computers and medical equipment might require different AC wall outlets to be on separate electrical circuits; otherwise, the power draw may be too great, resulting in nothing powering on.

Random Access Memory

Motherboards and some specialized expansion cards have random access memory (RAM) slots. RAM is electronic memory where the operating system (OS), application software, and any documents you are working on exist. More RAM means you can run modern operating systems and application software, run multiple programs concurrently, and have more documents open concurrently. The specifications for a given EMR system might require locally installed software on a computer with a minimum of 4GB RAM. For example, you can find out how much RAM a Windows Server 2008 computer has by clicking the Start menu, right-clicking Computer, and choosing Properties; then look for Installed Memory (RAM), as shown in Figure 32-3. Bear in mind some EMR systems may not require locally installed software. Instead, the only requirement might be a modern web browser such as Firefox or Internet Explorer. In this case, the EMR system is hosted elsewhere (the cloud) and as such may have lesser hardware requirements.

 TIP   Note that 32-bit computers cannot address more than 4GB of RAM.

Data stored in RAM requires electricity. Permanent data storage requires a storage medium such as a hard disk. Modern computers may also use solid-state drive (SSD) technology, meaning there are no moving parts like there are in hard disks. No moving parts means less wear and tear, noise, power draw, and heat, and often it means faster data access times, which comes at a price premium.

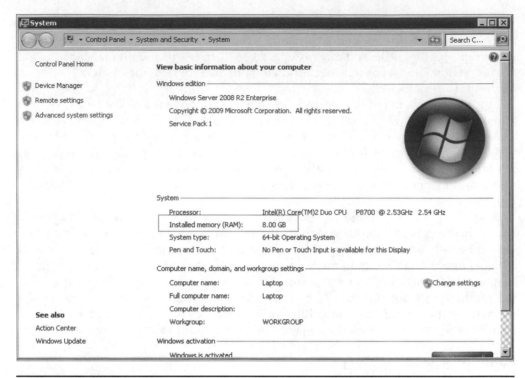

Figure 32-3   Viewing the amount of installed RAM on a Windows system

Data Storage

Hard disk storage can be internal or external and is not dependent upon electricity for data retention like RAM is. Modern computers typically use Serial Advanced Technology Attachment (SATA) hard drives.

High-end workstations and servers might use SATA or Small Computer Systems Interface (SCSI) hard disks. Older systems typically used Integrated Drive Electronics (IDE) hard disks. Table 32-1 summarizes the three disk technologies.

Additional storage can be achieved by locally plugged in external hard disk storage, including flash drives (often called *thumb drives*). Handheld medical devices, much like smartphones, digital cameras, portable media players, and tablets, often have a small amount of internal data storage capacity that can be transferred externally at a later time. Some equipment may allow the use of removable storage media such as secure digital (SD) cards.

CDs, DVDs, and Blu-Ray optical discs can store data or software installation files. Writing to, or *burning*, optical media requires a writable drive, for example, a DVD writer. Operating system installations are often made available on a bootable DVD. Table 32-2 lists the maximum capacity of each.

Standard	Throughput	Description
IDE	Up to 133MBps	Used by older desktops and laptops, with either a 40- or 80-wire data cable and Molex power connector. Motherboards in the past often had both a primary and secondary IDE pin connector. Each allowed up to two IDE devices where one device was designated as the master and the other as the slave.
SATA	Up to 750MBps (SATA 3.0), 3Gbps (eSATA)	Common in today's computers. Uses a seven-wire data cable and a SATA power connector. The number of SATA connectors depends on the motherboard. Some computers have an eSATA port for external SATA drive connectivity.
SCSI	Up to 640MBps	Many SCSI standards have been developed over the decades; Ultra640 is one of the newest. A SCSI card or Host Bus Adapter (HBA) is required and may be built into the motherboard's chipset. Newer SCSI standards allow up to 16 SCSI devices on a single SCSI bus. Both ends of the SCSI bus must be terminated, and each SCSI device requires a unique SCSI ID.

Table 32-1 Hard Disk Standards

Media Type	Maximum Capacity
CD	Up to 800MB
DVD	Up to 17GB (double-sided dual layer), but most commonly 4.7GB
Blu-Ray	Up to 50GB (dual layer)

Table 32-2 Optical Disc Standards

Yet another data storage medium is backup tapes, which require a tape drive for reading and writing to the tapes. There are many tape standards, for example, Digital Linear Tape (DLT), which can store up to 800GB of data on a single tape. Backing up data is critical because hard disks will fail at some point. Most backup software checks the archive bit (a file attribute) to determine whether a file has changed and must be archived. Performing a full system backup clears the archive bit (the files have just been backed up and do not need to be archived). When a file is changed, the operating system turns on the archive bit, which means the file needs to be archived (backed up). Table 32-3 lists backup types.

Onsite backup of data can be an effective component of a multiple-level backup system that also involves offsite or online backup. In addition to tape, CD/DVD, hard drive, or other media can be used for onsite backup. Offsite backup can be handled via secure courier service, which is the process of transporting backup data on physical media offsite to a secure location.

 CompTIA EXAM TIP Incremental backups clear the archive bit.

Backup Type	Description
Daily (full)	Backs up all files in the specified location and clears the archive bit. Takes the longest to back up but is the quickest to restore.
Differential	Backs up only files that have changed since the *previous full backup* (files with the archive bit turned on) and does not clear the archive bit.
Incremental	Backs up only files that have changed since the *previous incremental or full backup* (files with the archive bit turned on) and clears the archive bit. Takes the least amount of time to back up but the longest to restore.

Table 32-3   Common Backup Types

Peripherals

Devices plugged into computers to achieve additional functionality are called *peripherals* and, sometimes, *input/output* (I/O) devices. A keyboard is considered an input device, while a printer is considered an output device. External hard disks, printers, and electrocardiography (EKG) machines, for example, are peripherals. Most modern peripherals plug into a Universal Serial Bus (USB) port, shown in Figure 32-4.

Up to 127 USB devices can be plugged into a USB port using USB hubs. Smaller USB devices such as flash drives draw their power from the USB port, where other USB devices such as large-storage-capacity hard disks or EKG devices have their own external power supply. There are many types of USB-connected devices, including the following:

- Storage devices
- Keyboards and mice
- Printers and document scanners
- Barcode scanners
- Signature pads
- EKG devices

Table 32-4 lists the three USB standards. Take note that the throughput is expressed in bits per second (bps) versus bytes per second (Bps).

Other equipment may physically connect to a computer in other ways. Some equipment may connect via a serial port (often referred to as an RS-232 port) or a PS/2 port. Modern computer keyboards and mice connect via USB ports, but older computers use PS/2 ports for keyboards and mice. A barcode scanner used by a pharmacist to scan a prescription label might connect to a computer via a PS/2 or USB port, or it might connect wirelessly. A modern computer may have many USB ports but not have a serial port, while specific medical equipment may require a serial port connection. A USB-to-serial adapter may be used in this situation. Adapters are available for all types of connections.

Rivaling USB, some systems have an IEEE 1394 (often referred to as FireWire) port. Devices such as video cameras and hard disks can connect to FireWire ports. Up to 63 devices can be daisy-chained together on a single FireWire bus for transfer speeds of either 400MBps or 800MBps (FireWire 400 and FireWire 800, respectively).

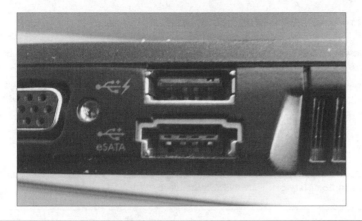

Figure 32-4 A USB (top) and eSATA (bottom) port on a laptop

Standard	Maximum Throughput
USB 1.0	12Mbps
USB 2.0	480Mbps
USB 3.0	5Gbps

Table 32-4 USB Standards

 CompTIA EXAM TIP There can be 127 devices on a USB bus and 63 on a FireWire bus.

Tracking/Auditing Software

Healthcare IT technicians are frequent users of IT asset tracking and auditing software. This class of software has evolved as devices serviced by the IT department have grown exponentially in recent years. The software can now scan workstations and other devices such as printers, routers, and switches across the healthcare enterprise connected over the LAN or VPN. The scan provides details about hardware and software installed in all workstations.

Network Transfer of Data

Most computing devices including modern medical equipment will have not only physical connectors to transmit their data but also network connectivity, both wired and wireless. For example, a laptop computer or an EKG device could transmit data across a network in any of the ways shown in Table 32-5.

Network Standard	Maximum Throughput	Description
RJ-45 port allowing a network cable to be plugged in	Up to 10Gbps	Wired networking; offers the best speed and security.
Wi-Fi 802.11b/g/n	Up to 200Mbps	Wireless; 802.11b speed is 12Mbps, 802.11g speed is 54Mbps, 802.11g speed is up to 200Mbps. Maximum range is typically in the 100-foot range.
Bluetooth	Up to 2Mbps	Wireless; maximum range is typically in the 30-foot range.

Table 32-5   Common Network Transmission Standards

 TIP   Wi-Fi and Bluetooth are wireless technologies and therefore are susceptible to environmental conditions (such as electrical storms and heavy snowfall) and other interference.

Exercise 32-1: Match the Definition to the Terms

Definition	Term
Centrally stores data and facilitates backup	Incremental
Allows 63 devices to be daisy-chained	USB
A modern Wi-Fi networking standard	Bluetooth
Centrally stores multiple records	File server
Can be used to wirelessly synchronize data between devices	Database server
Allows up to 127 devices to be daisy-chained	FireWire
Type of backup that does not clear the archive bit	PS/2
Type of keyboard connector	Differential
Type of backup that clears the archive bit	802.11n

Document Imaging

Documents used in the medical industry such as birth records, results of examinations, clinical research, and so on, can be converted to digital format for ease of transmission and searching. Inversely, having a hard copy of a prescription or patient medical information is still important in some cases. Modern printers are often called *all-in-one* devices, because they might be a printer, photo copier, scanner, and fax machine all at the same time. Some medical equipment will have these capabilities built into the medical device. Medical images can also be scanned at various quality levels. This is often referred to as *EMR scanning*. The following devices are commonly used to achieve document imaging:

- Flatbed scanner
- Handheld scanner

- Photocopier

- Smartphone app

A scanned document or image can be saved in a variety of file formats. Optical character recognition (OCR) is a method of converting a picture of text into editable and searchable text. Table 32-6 describes common file formats.

The quality of a scanned document or image depends on a variety of attributes such as dots per inch (DPI). For display on a computer monitor, 72 DPI may be suitable, but for print, 600 DPI may be required. Color depth determines how many shades of colors are viewable; 48-bit color depth is superior to 24-bit color depth. Resolution, as it relates to document imaging, determines the number of pixels per inch (PPI) of a scanned document. Scanning at 24,000 PPI generates a much larger file than scanning at 5,400 PPI. Various scanned file formats have different rates of compression to reduce storage space. Scanning devices may have their own limited internal memory, or they might allow external storage and may even transmit scanned data across a network to a storage location. The need for a physical file room is virtually nonexistent when using document imaging to digitize patient information to an EMR system.

Assuming PDF will be the saved file format of a scanned document, bookmarks, hyperlinks, custom tags, and annotations can be added throughout the file and can be indexed, thus making the content searchable for quick retrieval in the future. Additional data about the file (referred to as *metadata*), such as who scanned the document or when it was scanned, can also be stored within the file and is also searchable. PDF files have their own security model that controls what can be done with the document content. Figure 32-5 shows the document security settings for a PDF file.

File Type	Description
Tagged Image File Format (TIFF)	Uses data tags that can be indexed and are searchable. Can store text and images within a single file, even multipage documents; useful for various patient documents. Multiple edits do not reduce image quality. Requires a plug-in for web browser viewing.
Portable Document Format (PDF)	Can store text and images within a single file, even multipage documents; useful for various patient documents. Uses a security model to control the content within the PDF file. Uses data tags that can be indexed and are searchable, as well as bookmarks and hyperlinks. PDFs are typically smaller in size than TIFF files depending on how many fonts are embedded in the PDF file. A plug-in is required for web browser viewing. PDF is accepted as a standard for long-term archiving.
Joint Photographic Experts Group (JPEG)	Natively viewable in a web browser; best used to store photographs because of its unlimited color palette.
Graphics Interchange Format (GIF)	Natively viewable in a web browser; best used to store computer-generated images. Has a limited color palette compared to JPEG. Best used to efficiently store images with large areas of the same color.

Table 32-6 Common Scanning File Formats

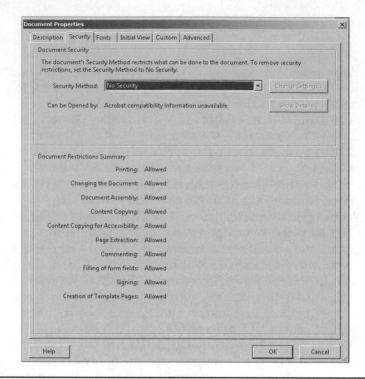

Figure 32-5 Document security settings for a PDF file

Classify Different Server Types, Environments, Features, and Limitations

Servers are powerful computers fulfilling one or more specific roles. Networking operating systems (NOSs) such as Red Hat Linux or Windows Server 2008 can be installed on regular desktop computers or laptops; however, proper server-class hardware tends to give the best results. This is because server-class hardware has more RAM, storage capacity, and faster CPUs than a desktop or laptop computer. Depending on how the server will be used, more RAM than normal might be required. For example, a locally hosted EMR application server serving hundreds of users needs more RAM (and processing power and, most likely, more disk space!) than a locally hosted file server serving a few dozen users. Servers often duplicate power supplies and disk systems to make the server highly available. In the event of a power outage, it is imperative the server shut down gracefully to prevent potential file corruption or damage to hardware components. An uninterruptable power supply (UPS) solves this problem; it has a bank of batteries and several electrical outlets to allow critical devices to be plugged in. It is also common for servers to have multiple network interface cards (NICs) as well as USB, FireWire, and external SATA (eSATA) ports.

Modern network appliances may have a NOS preinstalled and preconfigured to serve a specific function. Many organizations run NOSs as virtual machines using virtualization software such as VMware, Microsoft Hyper-V, or Citrix XEN. Figure 32-6 shows Microsoft Hyper-V. This allows more than one virtual server to run on a single physical computer at the same time.

The configuration of the NOS and the software installed really determines the server role.

- **File server**   Shares folders and files to network users. The NOS controls access to this resource. Management and backup of these files is performed centrally on the server.

- **Print server**   Shares printers to network users. Print jobs are first spooled to the print server and then despooled to the physical print device. The NOS controls access to the printers.

- **Database server**   Allows network users to access one or more databases that contain tables, which contain records. The NOS may authenticate users, but the database software has its own security model.

- **Application server**   Hosts a specific application, such as an EMR system, for multiple user network access. In a client-server EMR environment, this server would be the responsibility of local IT staff. ASPs, or cloud computing providers, host application servers for their clients, so the servers are their responsibility.

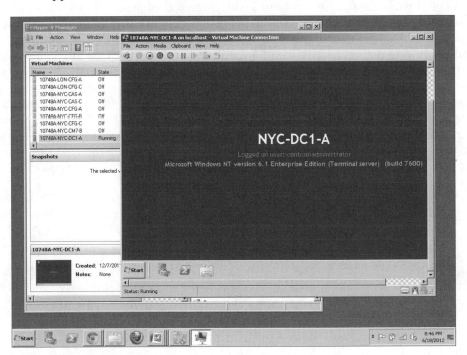

Figure 32-6   Microsoft Hyper-V Manager with a running virtual machine, NYC-DC1-A

Server software requires the correct NOS, version, and updates. For example, an EMR system designed to run on Windows Server 2003 may not run on Windows Server 2008 and most likely will not run on Red Hat Linux Enterprise Server. Server software will sometimes require other prerequisite software to be installed and configured in a specific manner. These issues are irrelevant if your EMR system is hosted by an ASP; it is their responsibility.

Server disk storage may physically exist inside the server, the server might access disk storage on a storage area network (SAN), or both! A SAN hosts high-speed, high-capacity disks that are centrally managed on a storage network that various servers can access. Users access the server, for example, to update a patient electronic record in an EHR system, and the server writes that data to disks stored on the SAN. Storing an echocardiogram in an EHR, for example, takes more space than storing medical documents, since an echocardiogram would be stored as video content. The NOS, and often the server-based application software, can restrict how much space is consumed by users, how large stored data can be, and how long data is retained before it must be archived.

Set Up a Basic PC Workstation Within an EHR/EMR Environment

A workstation requires either room temperature or slightly cooler to operate properly. Thin client workstations are computers with limited configuration flexibility and processing power; they are useful when the EHR/EMR client software will be run on the server side. Often the thin client OS is installed into computer chips (firmware) rather than being installed on a hard disk. Care must taken to ensure fans and vents are not obstructed; otherwise, the system will overheat, and modern systems will simply shut down. Once all hardware components are plugged in (including the power supply and network cable!), if the machine does not have a preinstalled OS, you can manually install the OS or use a mechanism such as disk imaging to apply an OS image captured from a reference system.

The way in which the EMR system is accessed will determine the type of hardware and software you need. A workstation accesses an EMR system in three ways.

- Application software installed on the workstation communicates with the EMR system over specific network channels (ports); these ports must be allowed to travel through firewalls.

- A web browser, and possibly web browser plug-ins such as a PDF viewer. Web browsers use standard port numbers (80 and 443) that most firewalls allow.

- A remote access client such as Windows Remote Desktop (formerly called Terminal Services). The user launches and interacts with the EMR system locally, but all processing occurs on the EMR application server. Windows Remote Desktop Protocol (RDP) uses port 3389.

Troubleshoot and Solve Common PC Problems

Sometimes software and hardware fail. Files become corrupt, cables become disconnected, and software updates need to be applied—quite a variety of problematic sources. Troubleshooting methodology dictates the following:

1. *Identify the problem.* If providing telephone support, be careful; make sure you and your client use proper terms (try to avoid too much computer jargon, though!). Ask for specific error codes and error messages. Can you duplicate the problem? What is the scope: a single station, a single printer, or everybody on the network?

2. *Determine probable cause, and test possible solutions.* First, reboot the computer. This solves many inexplicable computer problems. Then test the easy stuff! Might the power cable be disconnected? Does the printer toner or printer ink ribbon need to be changed? Is the keyboard layout changed to a different language? Does the station have a valid IP address? Does the logged-in user have the proper permissions? The list is endless. If you determine the issue should be escalated to a different technician, then do that.

3. *Ensure the problem is solved.* Sometimes fixing one thing breaks something else. Thoroughly test your fix and have the user test the fix; until you both agree the problem is solved, it is not.

4. *Document your solution.* Most organizations have a knowledge base used by technicians and help desk staff to document the problem and solution. This knowledge base can be searched in the future when the same problem occurs.

Hardware and Software Problems

Some hardware has a life expectancy, especially hard disks. It is only a matter of when they will fail, so data backups, discussed earlier in this chapter, are of paramount importance. Multiple hard disks can be arranged in a redundant array of independent disks (RAID) array to increase performance or fault tolerance. For example, RAID 1 (disk mirroring) duplicates all hard disk writes so that if something happens to one hard disk, the other has an up-to-date copy of the files.

Peripherals such as mice, keyboards, scanners, printers, and so on, may have problems with their power supplies or data connection cables. For USB devices, make sure the cable is plugged in snugly. Remember that the OS may detect the hardware you've plugged in, but it may not have a driver so that you can use the hardware. Visit the vendor web site for the most up-to-date driver for your hardware.

Software vendors occasionally release patches for their software. A patch corrects a problem of some kind; compare this with an update. Updates may also correct problems, but they can also add functionality. A hotfix addresses a very specific problematic issue, and sometimes the hotfix is not made downloadable to the public; you might receive an e-mail from the vendor with a link to the hotfix in response to your request. Over time, patches, updates, and hotfixes can be built into a service pack (SP). For example, as of this writing, Windows Server 2008 has SP2. The Windows OS has built-in update capabilities, as shown in Figure 32-7. If your settings are grayed out, it means your machine is configured via Group Policy settings on an Active Directory domain controller.

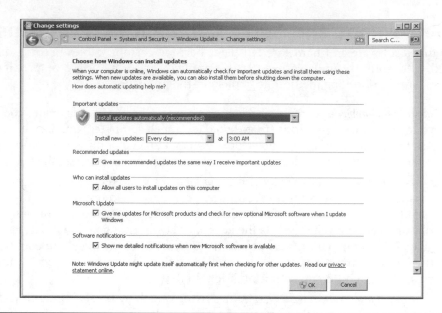

Figure 32-7 Windows update options

In addition to the basic hardware and software problems that can arise, in the healthcare IT environment we must also be keenly aware that such problems occur in the context of complex healthcare activities that are being carried out, often in life-critical settings and situations. For example, a range of problems can occur in e-prescribing (i.e., the use of electronic tools to prescribe medications). For instance, controlled substances can and are commonly prescribed by physicians for legitimate reasons, both in the inpatient and outpatient settings that use e-prescribing. The US Department of Justice defines controlled substances as:

> Drugs and other substances that are considered controlled substances under the Controlled Substances Act (CSA) are divided into five schedules. Substances are placed in their respective schedules based on whether they have a currently accepted medical use in treatment in the United States, their relative abuse potential, and likelihood of causing dependence when abused.
>
> —Source: http://www.deadiversion.usdoj.gov/schedules/ index.html#define, accessed 11/14/12)

There are five schedules. Examples of the drugs in the first two schedules include heroin in Schedule I and meperidine (Demerol), a synthetic narcotic, in Schedule II. The e-prescribing system treats a controlled substance like any other drug or medication, thus there are no particular interface issues unique to ordering a controlled substance through e-prescribing per se. There is, however, a more mundane but no less important issue than an interface issue associated with e-prescribing, which is printing prescriptions. Many states require controlled substance prescriptions to be written on paper and do not allow electronic signature. Furthermore, controlled substance prescriptions are commonly required to be written on special paper, often with holograms on the paper. Thus it is a common challenge for HIT technicians to limit controlled substance prescription printing from many computers in a busy office practice or hospital unit to a limited number of printers with locked-down cassettes in which the controlled substance grade paper resides.

Some other common problems that may arise include the entry or retrieval of improperly formatted patient demographics, improperly formatted data, inadvertent deactivation of medications, and a range of errors resulting from failure of hardware or software communication links and processing components (such as fax machines, local networks, and the Internet) during complex healthcare work processes. It is important to identify such errors immediately and isolate the source of the problems. Complicating matters, the interactions between the system's hardware and software, and the complexity of healthcare activities, may lead to errors that might not be easily detectable until such systems are installed and "live" health data is being transmitted and processed. In addition, standard information technologies are typically interfaced with a range of complex medical devices and monitors, which requires isolating the failure to the original source (for example, the main computer systems or the interfacing technologies, devices, or wireless networks). Such problems need to be identified, escalated as expediently as possible, and reported to the management of healthcare organizations, as well as to vendors of healthcare IT where appropriate.

There is often a complex interaction between healthcare IT (e.g., EMRs and EHRs) and medical devices (e.g., infusion pumps, bar code scanners, and patient monitors). If it is suspected that a medical device is malfunctioning, a number of practical steps can be taken, including checking whether the power is on, checking the network connection, checking that all input/output (I/O) devices are functioning correctly (the most common issues being the device driver not being enabled or being out of date), checking whether the device is interfacing correctly with other systems and software (such as EMRs), and if necessary, checking all configuration settings. With healthcare software such as EMR software, a number of clinical problems can occur and may be reported by clinicians, such as storage or retrieval of incorrect patient data, data from the wrong patient appearing in a record, incomplete data, and delays in updating data in patient records and systems. It is important to locate and isolate affected modules or fields, determine the type of file or data affected, and escalate the problem to the proper support level (e.g., hospital IT management, or a vendor, in the case of serious problems that can rectified locally). In addition, hospitals require the development of fail-safe downtime procedures to ensure continued functioning of the healthcare institution in the case of major healthcare IT system failure or electrical blackouts. Due to the increase in wireless transmissions of patient data in healthcare settings, it is important to ensure patient and health data is being transmitted properly and without error. This may involve having end users complete system performance surveys, checking access point placements, and rolling out advanced healthcare network monitoring software (which is increasingly being adopted in hospitals and healthcare settings).

Server load and utilization may need to be checked to ensure proper and efficient access to information across a healthcare setting. This involves a variety of computer systems and technologies, especially if clinicians report lengthy access and response times from problem reports or from survey results. Load and utilization can also be analyzed using network-monitoring software to analyze throughput, rate of transmission, and errors in transmission of data over time. This data provides useful reporting to management which can alert the organization to potentially serious issues in data transmission.

Many of the issues with hardware, devices, operating systems, application software, and basic network problems are the responsibility of a desktop support technician. In a healthcare organization, a desktop support technician sets up, maintains, and troubleshoots end user devices in healthcare clinical and business environments. This person must have good communication skills, a professional demeanor, and the ability to liaise effectively between people in Information Services (IS) and a diverse group of end users. Typical responsibilities for the desktop support role include new equipment setup, imaging and deployment, application troubleshooting, trouble ticket management, documentation of technical procedures, and research regarding new products for improved clinical and business processes. Typical operating systems, hardware, and network applications that the healthcare desktop support technician or analyst should have expertise in includes: Windows XP, Windows 7/8, Mac OS, laptops, desktop computers, iPads, Citrix Client, Cisco VPN Client, Remote Desktop, and Wireless Network Client.

Chapter Review

This chapter introduced common computing hardware components that the HIT professional must understand to support computing devices in a healthcare environment. Gone are the days when only a few elite people had the skills and knowledge to work with medical equipment and software. Web-based EMR systems hosted locally or by an ASP (private versus public cloud) have become the norm, along with using handheld wireless devices to access these systems. The smallest rural medical practice up to the largest hospitals and research facilities are now demanding a standard of competence from their IT support staff; this is the purpose of the HIT certification.

Questions

To test your comprehension of the chapter, answer the following questions and then check your answers against the list of correct answers at the end of the chapter.

1. Which piece of hardware allows multiple network devices to be plugged in?

   A. Router

   B. NIC

   C. Switch

   D. Domain controller

2. EMR systems can be hosted by which third-party entity?

   A. ISP

   B. NIC

   C. SAN

   D. ASP

3. A user clicks an icon on their desktop and then types https://intranet.acme.us/emr to launch an EMR application. This user is using a thin client workstation. Which term best describes the type of EMR client station?

   A. Web browser client

   B. Terminal Services client

   C. Remote Desktop client

   D. ASP client

4. To which of the following does the IEEE 1394 standard apply?

   A. USB

   B. 802.11g

   C. RAID

   D. FireWire

5. Which of the following provides the fastest data transfer rate?

   A. USB 3.0

   B. FireWire 800

   C. IDE

   D. SATA 3.0

6. Which of the following provides the fastest data transfer rate?

   A. Bluetooth

   B. 802.11g

   C. Gigabit Ethernet

   D. 802.11n

7. A medical modeling program uses very intense video imagery. Which type of interface would provide the best video throughput?

   A. PCIe

   B. PCI

   C. USB 2.0

   D. FireWire 800

8. You are asked to convert a patient paper chart to an EMR. What type of hardware should you use?

   A. Printer

   B. NIC

   C. Scanner

   D. USB keyboard

9. Your organization hosts a local EMR application server. The server uses RAID 1 and is a domain controller. You have been asked to propose a data backup strategy that allows the quickest nightly backup using a minimum of storage. Which backup type should you suggest?

   A. Daily

   B. Differential

   C. Incremental

   D. Full

10. Which type of backup clears the archive bit? (Choose all that apply.)

    A. Daily

    B. Differential

    C. Incremental

    D. Full

11. You are an IT technician for a small rural medical clinic. The attending physician asks for the fastest type of external hard disk storage available for her state-of-the-art laptop. What should you recommend?

    A. eSATA

    B. IDE

    C. USB 2.0

    D. FireWire 400

12. You are scanning patient records and would like to include images and searchable annotations. The saved file must have its own control over who can print its content. Which file format should you use?

    A. GIF

    B. JPEG

    C. TIFF

    D. PDF

13. Your manager has asked you to create a tutorial for new employees to learn the EMR system. You have decided to use computer screen–capture still images and descriptive text to be published on the intranet web site. What file format would be best suited for computer-screen still images?

    A. GIF

    B. JPEG

    C. TIFF

    D. PDF

14. Which file formats are *not* natively viewable in most web browsers? (Choose all that apply.)

    A. GIF

    B. JPEG

    C. TIFF

    D. PDF

15. After troubleshooting a software application problem, you discover that the vendor has a link on its web site to download a script file that solves the problem. When you click the link, instead of downloading the script file, you are asked to provide your e-mail address so that you can be sent the script file. What term best describes this script file?

    A. Service pack

    B. Hotfix

    C. Update

    D. Patch

Answers

1. **C.** Network devices plug into a switch so that they can communicate. Routers interconnect different networks; network devices do not plug directly into a router. NICs allow devices to communicate on a network. Domain controllers are Windows servers that can service domain user logon requests; they hold a copy of the Active Directory database that replicates to other domain controllers.

2. **D.** Application service providers (ASPs) provide application services to their clients. The hardware and software installation, configuration, and maintenance are the responsibility of the ASP, not the client; the client pays a fee to use the service, such as an EMR system. A NIC allows connectivity to a network. SANs are specialized high-speed storage networks used by servers. ASPs provide hosted software solutions for their clients.

3. **A.** HTTPS is a web browser protocol. Even though some applications other than web browsers can use HTTPS, a web browser client is the best answer. Terminal Services and Remote Desktop clients do not normally use HTTPS; they normally use Remote Desktop Protocol (RDP). ASP client is a possible answer, but web browser client is the best answer.

4. **D.** The IEEE 1394 standard is also known as FireWire. USB, 802.11g, and RAID are not referred to as the IEEE 1394 standard.

5. **D.** SATA 3.0 is rated at 750MBps (6Gbps), USB 3.0 at 625MBps (5Gbps), FireWire 800 at 100MBps (800Mbps), and IDE at 133MBps.

6. **C.** Gigabit Ethernet is a wired network standard with speeds up to 1Gbps. The Bluetooth transfer rate is up to 2Mbps, 802.11g wireless is up to 54Mbps, and 802.11n is up to 200Mbps.

7. **A.** PCI Express (PCIe) uses lanes for data throughput. A X1 (single lane) has bidirectional throughput of 500MBps. PCIe X16 would have bidirectional throughput of 8GBps. This is much better throughput than PCI (500MBps), USB 2.0 (480Mbps), or FireWire 800 (800Mbps).

8. **C.** Scanners can digitize physical paper documents such as patient charts. Printers do the opposite; they take digital data and print onto a physical medium such as paper. NICs allow connectivity to a network. A USB keyboard plugs into a USB computer port (older keyboards have a different plug that plugs into a computer PS/2 keyboard port).

9. **C.** Incremental backups back up only those files that have changed since the last backup, whether it was a full (daily) or incremental. Full (daily) backup will back up all files whether or not they have changed. Differential backups archive file changes only since the last full backup.

10. **A, C, D.** Only differential backups do not clear the archive bit. The archive bit is a file attribute that determines whether a file must be backed up. Changes to a file turn on the archive bit, which means the file must be backed up, but performing a differential backup does not turn on the archive bit.

11. **A.** eSATA (3Gbps), USB 2.0 (480Mbps), and FireWire 400 (400Mbps) are external disk interfaces; IDE is only internal.

12. **D.** PDF files can include text, images, and annotations and can have their own security model, such as who can print the document. GIF files are best used with computer screenshots or images consisting of few colors. JPEGs and TIFFs do not have their own security model.

13. **A.** GIF files are best used with computer screenshots or images consisting of few colors. JPEGs and TIFFs are best used for high-resolution images with many colors. PDFs can contain images as well as searchable text and have their own security model.

14. **C, D.** GIF and JPEG files can be viewed using any web browser. TIFF and PDF files require a web browser plug-in to be viewable within the web browser.

15. **B.** Hotfixes are solutions to very specific problems and are not normally publicly downloadable like service packs might be. Many vendors will send you an e-mail message with details on how to obtain the hotfix.

CHAPTER 33

Programming and Programming Languages for Healthcare IT

Alex Mu-Hsing Kuo, Andre Kushniruk

In this chapter, you will learn how to
- Explain the importance of programming for healthcare information technology
- Describe operating systems and their functions
- Identify the differences between interpreted and compiled programming languages
- Use object-oriented programming languages
- Apply web markup and scripting languages
- Understand simple HTML and XML statements

In the world of computers, a *program* is a sequence of instructions or machine codes telling the computer how to perform specific tasks. Machine code is the computer's primitive language and consists of sequences of binary 1s and 0s that the computer processor (e.g., made by Intel or AMD) understands. To simplify the process of programming, a wide variety of higher-level programming languages have been developed. A programming language can be defined as a set of notations designed for writing programs to communicate instructions to a computer. Many programming languages are in existence today, such as BASIC, Perl, Fortran, COBOL, C, and Java. An understanding of healthcare information technology requires knowledge about programming and programming languages that can be used for implementing healthcare information systems (HISs). As this chapter will illustrate, there are a range of different programming languages that have been used to create software in healthcare. They generally fall into one of two categories: interpreted languages (e.g., Basic and Perl) or compiled languages (e.g., Fortran and COBOL). With a compiled language, a compiler is a computer program (or set of programs) that transforms the language source codes into machine-specific instructions (a binary form known as *object code*) before being saved as an executable file. With interpreted languages, the code is saved in the same format that it was created in. Next, an interpreter immediately translates the high-level instruction into an intermediate form, which the interpreter then executes. The interpreter analyzes and executes each line of source code in succession, without looking at the entire program (see Figure 33-1). Basically, interpreting code is slower than running the compiled code because the interpreter must analyze each statement in the program each time it is executed and then perform the desired action. Nevertheless, the compiled code simply performs the entire program, which is more efficient and has higher performance.

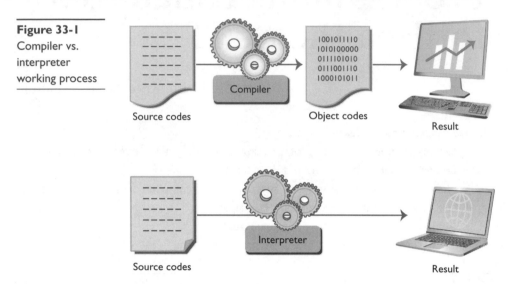

Figure 33-1
Compiler vs. interpreter working process

Languages and Virtual Machines

Modern computer systems consist of a number of layers, starting with the underlying hardware layer (the hardware that the computer software runs on), moving up to layers dealing with operating systems, and finally moving up to layers dealing with running application software (e.g., applications written for business or healthcare). The evolution of computer systems can be characterized by the invention of many languages, which were developed over time to specifically make programming and human interactions with computers easier. Initially computer systems were programmed in machine language (1s and 0s, as mentioned earlier in this section). Programming at the machine level was tedious and difficult, and as a result, assembly languages appeared early in the evolution of computer systems. Assembly languages use symbolic instructions, such as "Load a register with a value from memory location A," which in a specific assembly language might look like LOAD R0 A. The limitations of assembly languages are that they require knowledge of a computer's specific architecture, such as the central processing unit (CPU) registers or memory locations, and will run only on specific types of computers (IBM mainframe, Mac, PC, etc.). To make interacting with computers simpler, operating systems began to evolve that would take care of low-level functions of running computer software so that programmers could focus on the task they want to carry out, rather than worrying about how to interact with underlying hardware and lower levels of hardware and software.

Operating Systems

Operating systems have evolved to make writing programs and running computer systems easier by handling lower-level computer functions instead of operating at the machine or assembly language level. Essentially, an operating system creates a virtual layer or machine, where functions or operations are simulated with software rather than actually existing in the hardware. The functions of an operating system are as follows:

- **Process management** A process is an individual program or operation, such as a word processing application being run on a PC. Each process needs resources to run to completion (e.g., CPU time, memory, files, and input/output devices), and the operating system manages this.

- **Memory management** For a program to be executed, it has to be mapped to memory addresses and loaded into computer memory; this is also handled by the operating system.

- **Storage management** The operating system provides a uniform and logical view of the storage of information in files and maps files onto physical media.

- **Protection and security** The operating system controls access to processes and access by users to computer resources.

- **Distributed system management and processing** Network operating systems allow for the sharing of files and resources across an entire network.

There are many types of operating systems, with Microsoft Windows being one operating system that has been used extensively for HISs. Hospitals and health organizations have widely adopted Microsoft operating systems, initially running Microsoft DOS and now Microsoft Windows. The Mac OS has also become widely used in HIT. In addition, open source operating systems are common; these operating systems have been made available in source-code format rather than compiled binary code. Linux and Unix are examples of this type of operating system. The C language was created in conjunction with the development of the Unix operating system, and it allowed for an efficient and modular approach to the development of that operating system. The C language itself also became a widely used type of programming language, as will be described in the next section.

High-level languages have been designed to become somewhat independent of the underlying hardware and operating system as well as to make programming easier. For example, high-level languages like Fortran and C were developed so that instructions written in those languages would run on a variety of different machines, with only a few minor changes, as long as the machine is running a compiler (e.g., a C compiler for a particular machine) or interpreter that is able to convert the general high-level programming language instructions down to the appropriate low-level machine instructions on a particular machine (e.g., a PC or a Mac).

In healthcare, the issue of the interoperability of systems is critical. If operating systems and applications are not interoperable, electronic data cannot be exchanged. Although the cross-platform exchange of data between systems such as Windows and Mac has improved, it's important to carefully consider the ability of different hardware and software to seamlessly exchange health data.

The C Language

C is a general-purpose compiled language initially developed by Dennis Ritchie between 1969 and 1973 at Bell Labs. It was designed to provide language constructs that map efficiently to machine instructions, and to require minimal runtime support.[1]

To edit a C program, the very first thing is to find a text editor to edit the C source codes. Several text editors are available for editing a C program, such as Adobe Dreamweaver, Microsoft WordPad, Notepad, and TextPad. Among them, TextPad (www .textpad.com) is a powerful, general-purpose editor for Microsoft Windows that can edit plain-text files. It is very easy to use, with all the features that a power C programmer requires. The second tool you will need is a C compiler that you can use to compile the program. Examples are GNU C compiler (gcc), MINGW compiler, and Code: Blocks for Windows. Now, we will use a very simple example to explain how to edit and run a C program. We use TextPad to edit the program. At the very beginning of the C program is the syntax *#include <stdio.h>*. It links the standard input/output (I/O) library to the program so that the program can interact with the screen, keyboard, and file system of the computer. In C, libraries are files of already-compiled code, which you can merge with your program at compilation time. Each library comes with a number of *associated header files* (.h), which make the functions easier to use.

The second line of the program is *main()*. Every C program must contain a function called *main()*. It is the start point of the program. The *main()* function declares the start of the function, while the two curly brackets (lines 3 and 6) after *main()* show the start and finish of the function. Curly brackets in C are used to group statements into a function or in the body of a loop. Such a grouping is known as a *compound statement* or a *block*.

The most common type of instruction in C is a *statement*, which is the smallest independent unit in the language. You write statements in order to convey to the compiler that you want to perform a task. Statements in C are terminated by a semicolon. C-language syntax is case sensitive. Most C programs are in lowercase letters. For example, the fourth line in this program, *printf("Hello World!\n");*, will print the words "Hello World!" on the screen. The text to be printed is enclosed in double quotes. The \n at the end of the text tells the program to print a newline as part of the output. Line 5, *printf("This is my first C program.");*, is used to write out the text "This is my first C program." on the screen.

After finishing the source code editing, we save it as MyProgram.c (with .c as the file extension). Now, we are able to use a C compiler (e.g., gcc) to compile the program. For example, the compilation command on Unix is *cc -o MyProgram MyProgram.c*. At this point, if there are errors in the program, the compiler will show the error information on the screen. We should then correct these errors in the program and recompile the program. If there are no more errors in it, the compiler will return no error messages and will create an object file called *MyProgram* (in Unix, the default object filename is *a.out*). Then, we can execute the object file to see the output, as shown in Figure 33-2.

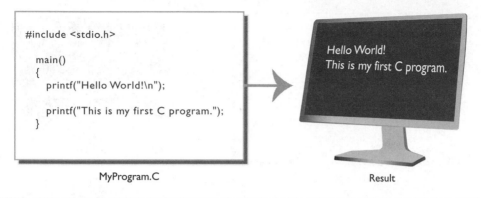

```
#include <stdio.h>

  main()
  {
    printf("Hello World!\n");

    printf("This is my first C program.");
  }
```

MyProgram.C

Hello World!
This is my first C program.

Result

Figure 33-2 A simple C program printing two lines of text

The C++ Language

Since the C programming language was developed, new approaches to programming have appeared. One of the most significant advances has been the concept of object-oriented programming. C++ is an object-oriented programming language developed as an extension to the C language by Bjarne Stroustrup at Bell Labs in 1983. It is now one of the most popular programming languages and is implemented on a wide variety of hardware and operating system platforms. Object-oriented programming is focused around the concept of *objects*, which represent things around you. An object can be a person, place, or thing. For example, an object can be used to represent a patient. The Patient object can have a number of attributes (e.g., Name, Address, Patient Number). In addition, using the concept of classes, objects can be classified or organized into hierarchies. For example, a Patient may be classified as either an In-Patient (if the patient is the hospital) or an Out-Patient (if the patient is outside the hospital). In-Patient and Out-Patient are said to be *subclasses* of the parent class Patient. C++ added these object-oriented features to its syntax with the ability to define classes, such as a Patient class, which for the Patient class would look something like this:

```
Class Patient
{
      // Here would go the statements defining the class in detail
      // could specify attributes like Name, Address, Patient Number
      // could also specify the operations that could be done on Patient
objects
}
```

The C++ syntax and program development processes are very similar to those of the C language. You can use any text editor to edit a C++ program file. If you are on a Unix machine, you would save the file with the filename *xxx.C* (make sure it ends with .C, not .c—it is case sensitive!), while if you are on a Windows operation system, you would save the file with file extension *.cpp*. For example, you use TextPad to edit a C++ program called *MyProgram.C* (Figure 33-3).

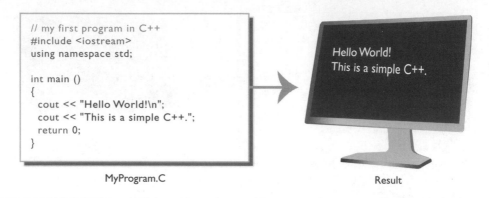

```
// my first program in C++
#include <iostream>
using namespace std;

int main ()
{
  cout << "Hello World!\n";
  cout << "This is a simple C++.";
  return 0;
}
```

MyProgram.C

Hello World!
This is a simple C++.

Result

Figure 33-3   A simple C++ program printing out two lines of text

In the program, the first line, *// my first program in C++*, beginning with two slashes (//) is a comment line. It does not affect the behavior of the program. You can use comments to include short explanations or definitions within the program to help the reader understand the programming logic.

The second line beginning with a hash (#), *#include <iostream>*, is a directive for the preprocessor. It is not a regular code line with expressions but indications for the compiler's preprocessor. In this case, the directive *#include <iostream>* tells the preprocessor to include the *iostream* standard file. This specific file includes the declarations of the basic standard I/O library in C++, and it is included because its functionality is going to be used later in the program.

The third line, *using namespace std;*, includes all parts of the namespace in C++. A namespace is created to set apart a portion of code with the goal to reduce, or otherwise eliminate, confusion. This is done by giving a common name to that portion of code so that when referring to it, only entities that are part of that section would be referred to. The namespace *std* includes all standard C++ libraries. The *iostream* library we mentioned earlier is part of the *std* namespace. Therefore, when we use the *std* namespace, we don't need to include the extended name of the *iostream* file.

The fourth line, *int main ()*, is the point at which the C++ program starts its execution, independently of its location within the source code. It does not matter whether there are other functions with other names defined before or after it. The *main()* function is always the first one to be executed in any C++ program. For that same reason, it is essential that all C++ programs have a *main()* function. Similar to C, the two curly brackets (lines 5 and 9) after *main()* show the start and finish of the function.

The sixth and seventh lines, *cout << "Hello World!\n";* and *cout << "This is a simple C++.";*, will write out the words "Hello World!" and "This is a simple C++." on the screen, respectively. The *cout* is the name of the standard output stream in C++. It is declared in the *iostream* standard file within the *std* namespace.

The eighth line, *return 0;*, is a return statement that causes the *main()* function to finish. A return code of *0* for the *main()* function is generally interpreted to mean the program worked as expected without any errors during its execution. This is the most usual way to end a C++ console program.

Next, we will use a compiler (e.g., gcc for a Unix machine) to compile the program. At the Unix prompt, we type the following command:

```
g++ MyProgram.C -o MyProgram
```

Then, a file called *MyProgram* is located in the same directory containing *MyProgram.C*. To run the program, we simply type *MyProgram* at the Unix prompt. Two lines of words will display on the screen, as shown in Figure 33-3.

There are several advantages to using C++, as follows:[2]

- C++ is a third-generation language that allows programmers to express their ideas at a high level as compared to low-level assembly languages.

- C++ also allows a programmer to get down into the low-level workings and fine-tune as necessary. For example, it allows the programmer strict control over memory management.

- C++ is a language with international standards. After years of development, the C++ programming language standard was ratified in 1998 as ISO/IEC 14882:1998. The standard was amended by the 2003 technical corrigendum, ISO/IEC 14882:2003. The current standard extending C++ with new features was ratified and published by ISO in September 2011 as ISO/IEC 14882:2011. Code written in C++ that conforms to the international standards can be easily integrated with preexisting codes and allows programmers to reuse common functions. This will dramatically reduce program development time.

- Since C++ is an object-oriented language, this makes programming easier and allows easy reuse of code or parts of code through inheritance.

- As mentioned at the beginning of this section, C++ is a very widely used programming language. Many tools and study resources are available for C++ program development.

The Java Language

Java is an object-oriented programming language originally created by Sun Microsystems. The language syntax is very similar to C or C++, but Java has a simpler object model and fewer low-level facilities.[3] To design a Java program, all source code is first edited in plain-text files with *.java* as the file extension. The programmer can use any text editor (e.g., Adobe Dreamweaver, Microsoft WordPad, Notepad, or TextPad) to edit the codes. Those source files are then compiled into *.class* files by a Java compiler. The *.class* file contains *bytecodes*, which are the machine language of the Java Virtual Machine (Java VM or JVM). Then, the just-in-time code generator converts the bytecode into the native machine code, which is at the same programming level. Because the Java VM is available on many different operating systems, the same *.class* files are capable of running on different operating systems, such as Microsoft Windows, Mac OS, or Linux (see Figure 33-4).[4] In other words, the same Java application is able to run on multiple platforms through the Java Virtual Machine.

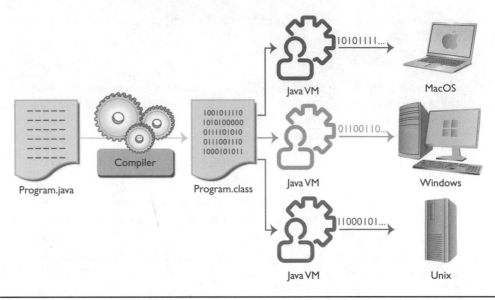

Figure 33-4 An overview of the Java programming process

To run a Java program, you need two tools: the Java Development Kit (JDK) SE and a text editor. In the example of Figure 33-5, we use TextPad to edit the source codes (*HelloWorld.java*). The Java programming language *compiler* (*Javac*) can translate (press Ctrl+1) the source codes into bytecodes (*HelloWorld.class*) that the Java Virtual Machine can understand. Then, the Java application *launcher tool* uses the Java Virtual Machine to run (press Ctrl+2) the program. It will then display the greeting "Hello Java World!"

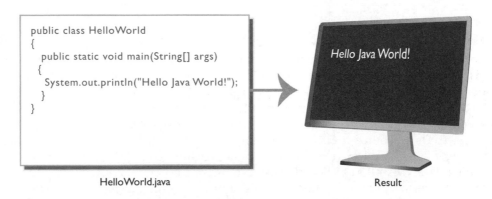

Figure 33-5 A simple Java program printing "Hello Java World!"

In conclusion, using Java as a system developing tool has the following benefits:[5]

- **Object oriented**   Java program can be easily extended because it is an object-oriented programming language. In Java, everything is an object.

- **Platform independent**   When a Java program is compiled into platform-independent bytecode, rather than compiled into platform-specific code such as C or C++, the bytecode can be distributed over the Web and interpreted by the JVM on whichever platform it is being run.

- **Architecture neutral**   The Java compiler generates an architecture-neutral object file format, which makes the compiled code executable on any processors that have the Java runtime system.

- **Portable**   The architecture-neutral and implementation-independent characteristics of Java make it very portable.

- **High performance**   With the use of just-in-time compilers, Java enables high performance.

- **Multithreaded**   With Java's multithreaded feature, it is possible to write programs that can do many tasks simultaneously. This design feature allows developers to construct interactive applications that run very smoothly.

- **Distributed and dynamic**   Java is designed for a distributed environment on the Internet and is considered to be more dynamic than C or C++. Also, Java programs can carry an extensive amount of runtime information that can be used to verify and resolve accesses to objects at runtime.

- **Easy to learn**   Java is designed to be easy to learn. If you understand the basic concept of object-oriented programming (OOP), then you can easily master Java.

HyperText Markup Language (HTML)

HTML is a markup language for describing web pages, not a programming language like Java or C++. Markup tags (also called *elements*) are the major components in an HTML document (usually called a *page*). They are keywords (tag names) surrounded by angle brackets, as in <html>. HTML tags normally appear in pairs like <html>...</html>. *Tags* and *elements* are often used to describe the same thing. Additionally, the tag names are not case sensitive.

An HTML page can be considered a document tree that could contain four main parts, as follows:[5]

- **Doctype (optional)**   The first tag to appear in the source code of a web page is the *doctype* declaration. The <!doctype> is not an HTML tag. It is an optional part that provides the web browser with information (a declaration) about what kind of document it is and what HTML version is used in the page so that the browser can display the document correctly.

- **HTML** Immediately after the <!doctype> comes the <html> element. It is the root element of the document tree, and everything that follows is a descendant of that root element.

- **Head (optional)** The <head> tag is used for text and tags that do not show up directly on the page. It is a container for all the head elements. Elements inside <head> can include scripts, instruct the browser where to find style sheets, provide meta information, and more.

- **Body** The <body> tag is used for text and tags that are shown directly on the page. This is where the page shows the contents. Everything that you can see in the browser window is contained inside this element, including paragraphs, lists, links, images, tables, and more.

An HTML element is everything from the start tag to the end tag. There are rules for editing HTML elements.[5]

- HTML elements normally come in pairs like <h1> and </h1>.

- An element starts with a start, or opening, tag (e.g., <h1>) and ends with an end, or closing, tag (e.g., </h1>). The end tag is written like the start tag, with a forward slash before the tag name.

- The element content is everything between the start and end tags (e.g., <h1>*Introduction to HTML*</h1>).

- Some HTML elements have empty content. An empty element is closed in the start tag, as in
 (="
</br>").

- Most HTML elements can have attributes. Attributes provide additional information about HTML elements. Similar to elements, there are several rules for editing attributes.[5]

  - Attributes are always specified in the start tag.

  - Attributes come in name and value pairs, as in name="value".

To understand the HTML document structure and how different elements or attributes work, it's useful to consider a simple web page with typical content features, as shown in Figure 33-6. In this example, the author uses the HTML5 doctype for the document. The <title> tag shown in the browser toolbar defines the page title as "Alex's Home Page." It is required in all HTML/XHTML documents.

The text between <body> and </body> is the visible page content. Here, the text "Introduction to HTML" between <h1> and </h1> is displayed as a heading. The text "Edited by Alex Kuo" between <p> and </p> is displayed as a paragraph, and the tag <font> specifies the font size (4), font face (verdana), and color (red) of the text. Size, face, and color are attribute names of this tag, while 4, verdana, and red are values for each attribute, respectively.

The <a> tag creates a link to another document by using the href attribute. In this example, the hyperlink text is "Visit W3Schools," and the URL for the link is http://www.w3schools.com/.

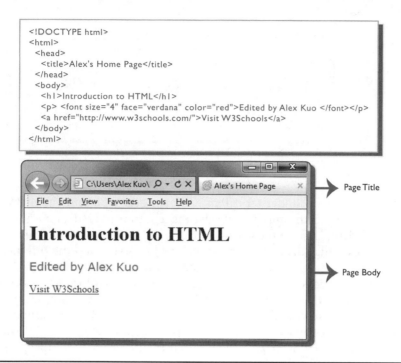

```
<!DOCTYPE html>
<html>
 <head>
  <title>Alex's Home Page</title>
 </head>
 <body>
  <h1>Introduction to HTML</h1>
  <p> <font size="4" face="verdana" color="red">Edited by Alex Kuo </font></p>
  <a href="http://www.w3schools.com/">Visit W3Schools</a>
 </body>
</html>
```

Figure 33-6 A simple HTML document and the corresponding web page

In real application, you would use a text editor to edit an HTML document and save it as *xxx.html* (*.html* is the file extension of an HTML document). Then, you would use a web browser (e.g., Microsoft Internet Explorer, Google Chrome, or Firefox) to read the HTML document and display it as a web page. The browser does not display the HTML tags but uses the tags to interpret the content of the page.

Web-based HTML content can be enhanced with multimedia on a variety of software platforms. For example, Adobe Flash is an animation program/platform that can be used to enhance web pages with video, animation, and interactivity. It can be used to stream audio and video, and flash animations have been used for broadcasts, games, and advertising. Flash content can be displayed on computer systems using Adobe Flash Player, which is a freely available plug-in for web browsers.

Extensible Markup Language (XML)

XML is a markup language much like HTML. However, it is different from HTML, which was designed to display data with a focus on how data looks. XML was created to structure, store, and transport data. So, an XML is nothing more than a plain-text document. Any software that can handle plain text can also handle XML.[6]

The tags used in HTML are predefined. However, XML tags are designed to be self-descriptive and not predefined. Document authors must define their own tags. For example, the tags in Figure 33-7 are not predefined in any XML standard. These tags are defined by the author.

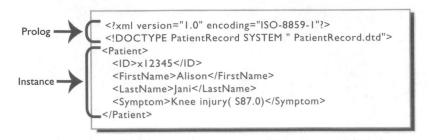

Figure 33-7 A simple XML with author-defined, self-descriptive tags

It is also important to understand that XML is not a replacement for HTML. The main objective of XML is to simplify data sharing and transport (data interoperability). In the real world, one of the most time-consuming challenges for computer system developers is to exchange data between incompatible systems over the Internet because computer systems and databases contain data in incompatible formats. XML data is stored in plain-text format. This provides a software- and hardware-independent way of storing data. Also, exchanging data as XML greatly reduces this complexity, since the data can be read by different, incompatible applications as well as by humans.

An XML document consists of two parts: the prolog (also called the *XML declaration*) and instances (also called *XML elements*). The first line in an XML document always is the prolog that defines the version (in this example, 1.0) and the encoding used (ISO-8859-1 = Latin-1/West European character set). The elements in an XML document form a document tree (Figure 33-8). The tree starts at the root (<bookstore>) and branches (<book>) to the lowest level of the tree. All elements can have subelements (child elements, such as <title>, <author>, etc.).

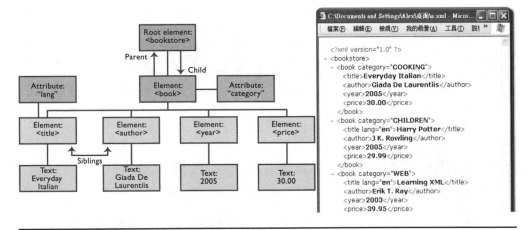

Figure 33-8 An XML tree structure

There are two types of XML documents: well-formed and valid XML. A *well-formed* XML document has XML syntax as follows:

- The document must have a root element (e.g., <bookstore>).

- All elements in the document must have a start tag and a closing tag (e.g., <book> ... </book>).

- Tags are case sensitive (e.g., <BOOKSTORE> ≠ <bookstore>).

- Elements must be properly nested (<bookstore> <book> ...</bookstore></book> is not a correct XML structure).

- XML attribute values must be quoted (e.g., <book category="COOKING">).

A *valid* XML document is a well-formed XML document that also conforms to the rules of a document type definition (DTD) or schema. Therefore, a valid XML must be a well-formed document. However, it may not be true that a well-formed XML is a valid document (Figure 33-9).

Figure 33-9
Two types of
XML document

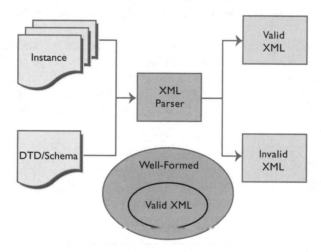

There are several benefits to using XML.[5,6]

- XML is a W3C Recommendation standard, endorsed by software industry market leaders.

- XML tags are designed to be self-descriptive and not predefined. New tags can be created as they are needed.

- Tags, attributes, and elements provide context information that can be used to interpret the meaning of content. For example, <price>30.00</price> represents a book's price as $30, thus opening up new possibilities for highly efficient search engines, intelligent data mining, agents, and so on. This is a major advantage over HTML or plain text where context information is difficult or impossible to evaluate.

- XML supports multiple data formats and can easily map existing data structures such as relational databases to XML. This is very beneficial to data interoperability.

- Information coded in XML is easy to read and understand and can be processed easily by computers.

Active Server Pages (ASP)

Active Server Pages (ASP) is a powerful tool for making dynamic and interactive web pages. It is a server-side script language developed by Microsoft that runs inside the Microsoft Windows Internet Information Services (IIS) server. When you use a browser to read an HTML document, the browser at the client computer interprets the tags and displays it as a web page on the browser. However, when an Internet Explorer browser reads an ASP file, IIS passes the request to the ASP engine at the server. The ASP engine reads the ASP file line by line and executes the scripts in the file. Scripts may access any data or databases and return the results to the browser as plain HTML (see Figure 33-10).

An ASP file can contain text, HTML, XML, and scripts, and it has the file extension *.asp*. The ASP commends are surrounded by the symbols <% and %>. Similar to C, C++, Java, HTML, and XML editing, you use a text editor to edit an ASP file and save it as *xxx.asp*. For example, in Figure 33-11, the *<% response.write ...%>* command in the *ASPtest.asp* file is used to output the text "Hello ASP. I like you." to the browser.

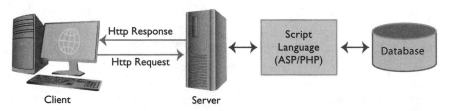

Figure 33-10   An ASP working process

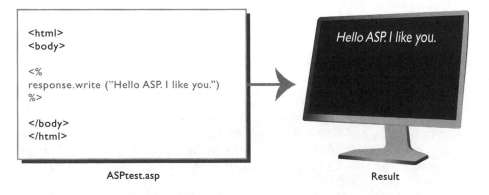

Figure 33-11   A simple ASP file and the corresponding result in a browser

Figure 33-12 shows a more complex ASP file that accesses a Microsoft Access database and converts the data stored in a Student table to an XML document.

There are several benefits to using ASP, as follows:[5]

- ASP can be used to dynamically edit, change, or add any content on a web page.

- ASP customizes a web page to make it more useful for individual users.

- ASP responds to user queries or data submitted from HTML forms.

- Programmers can easily use ASP to access any data or databases and return the results to a browser.

- ASP provides good application security (since ASP code cannot be viewed from the browser).

- ASP can minimize network traffic because the scripts are run on the server side.

- Compared with CGI and Perl, ASP is easier to learn.

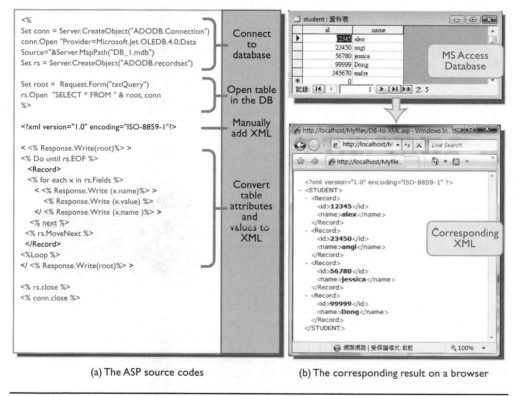

(a) The ASP source codes   (b) The corresponding result on a browser

Figure 33-12   A more complex ASP to convert database data to an XML document

Hypertext Preprocessor (PHP)

Hypertext Preprocessor (PHP) is also a server-side scripting language where scripts are executed on the server and returned to the browser as plain HTML, like ASP. PHP runs efficiently on different platforms (Windows, Linux, Unix, etc.) and is compatible with almost all servers used today (Apache, IIS, etc.). It supports many databases, such as MySQL, Informix, Oracle, Sybase, Solid, PostgreSQL, Generic ODBC, and more.[7]

A PHP document has a file extension of *.php* and can contain text, HTML tags, and scripts. A script always starts with *<?php"* and ends with *"?>*. The script can be placed anywhere in the PHP document. Each code line in it must end with a semicolon, which is a separator and is used to distinguish one set of instructions from another. For example, in Figure 33-13, the *<?php echo "Hello PHP. I love you."; ?>* command will output the text "Hello PHP. I love you." to the browser.

In Figure 33-14 (a), the PHP script accesses a Microsoft Access database and converts the data stored in a Student table to an XML document (Figure 33-14 (b)), the same database and result shown in Figure 33-12 (b)).

There are several benefits to using PHP, as follows:[5]

- PHP is open source software that can be downloaded and used freely.
- PHP runs efficiently on different platforms and supports many databases (e.g., MySQL, Informix, Oracle, Sybase, Solid, PostgreSQL, and Generic ODBC).
- PHP is compatible with almost all servers used today (e.g., Apache, IIS, etc.).
- PHP is easy to learn and runs efficiently on the server side.

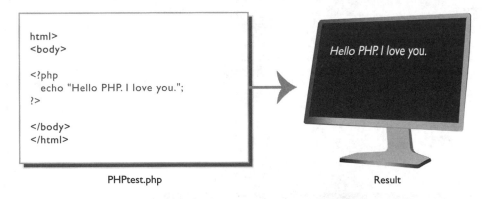

```
html>
<body>

<?php
   echo "Hello PHP. I love you.";
?>

</body>
</html>
```

PHPtest.php

Hello PHP. I love you.

Result

Figure 33-13 A simple PHP file and the corresponding result in a browser

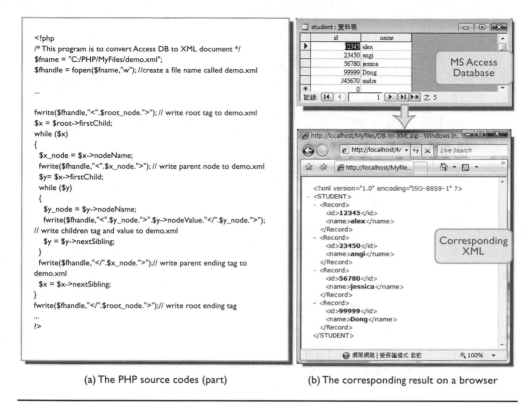

```php
<?php
/* This program is to convert Access DB to XML document */
$fname = "C:/PHP/MyFiles/demo.xml";
$fhandle = fopen($fname,"w"); //create a file name called demo.xml

...

fwrite($fhandle,"<".$root_node.">"); // write root tag to demo.xml
$x = $root->firstChild;
while ($x)
{
  $x_node = $x->nodeName;
  fwrite($fhandle,"<".$x_node.">"); // write parent node to demo.xml
  $y= $x->firstChild;
  while ($y)
  {
    $y_node = $y->nodeName;
    fwrite($fhandle,"<".$y_node.">".$y->nodeValue."</".$y_node.">");
// write children tag and value to demo.xml
    $y = $y->nextSibling;
  }
  fwrite($fhandle,"</".$x_node.">");// write parent ending tag to
demo.xml
  $x = $x->nextSibling;
}
fwrite($fhandle,"</".$root_node.">");// write root ending tag
...
?>
```

(a) The PHP source codes (part)   (b) The corresponding result on a browser

Figure 33-14 A more complex PHP script to convert database data to an XML document

Chapter Review

This chapter provided you with an overview of a number of languages that are often used in the development of software in the healthcare industry. For details on any one of the languages, the reader is referred to the many books and manuals available. The chapter began with a discussion of compiled versus interpreted programming languages and also discussed the importance of operating systems. A number of high-level programming languages were described, including C, C++, and Java. Although not a programming language, the Hypertext Markup Language (HTML) is integral to understanding how web applications work and was also discussed, along with XML for structuring, storing, and transferring data. Finally, the chapter discussed Active Server Pages (ASP), a powerful tool for making dynamic and interactive web pages, and PHP, a popular scripting language. All of the languages described in this chapter are used in creating many different types of HIT applications, and their use and application in healthcare will continue to grow.

Questions

1. A compiler is a _____.

   A. set of machine codes

   B. programming language

   C. program that transforms language source codes into machine-specific instructions

   D. sequences of binary 1s and 0s

2. You can use _____ to edit a C program.

   A. Microsoft Word

   B. TextPad

   C. Microsoft PowerPoint

   D. Microsoft Excel

3. C++ is _____.

   A. an object-oriented programming language

   B. a first-generation language

   C. a markup language

   D. by Sun Microsystems

4. In Java, _____.

   A. the syntax is not similar to C++

   B. *bytecodes* are the machine language of the Java Virtual Machine

   C. the same program cannot run on different machines

   D. you use Microsoft Word to edit the source program

5. HTML is a _____.

   A. markup language

   B. general-purpose programming language

   C. machine language

   D. network protocol

6. Which of the following statements is correct?

   A. XML was designed to display data with a focus on how the data appears.

   B. The tags used in XML are predefined looks.

   C. XML tags are designed to be self-descriptive and not predefined.

   D. A well-formed XML is also a valid XML document.

7. Active Server Pages (ASP) is a _____.

    A. markup language to display data on a web page

    B. machine language

    C. text editor

    D. server-side script language for making dynamic and interactive web pages

8. What is the purpose of Hypertext Preprocessor (PHP)?

    A. It was designed to protect data security.

    B. It defines an XML structure.

    C. It cannot run efficiently on different computer platforms.

    D. It is a server-side scripting language where the scripts are executed on the server and returned to the browser as plain HTML.

Answers

1. **C.** A compiler is a program that transforms language source codes into machine-specific instructions. The code is then saved as an executable computer-readable file.

2. **B.** You can use TextPad to edit a C program. Adobe Dreamweaver, Microsoft WordPad, and Notepad are other editors that can be used to edit C programs.

3. **A.** C++ is an object-oriented programming language that is currently one of the most popular programming languages and is implemented on a wide variety of hardware and operating system platforms.

4. **B.** In Java, *bytecodes* are the machine language of the Java Virtual Machine.

5. **A.** HTML is a markup language for describing web pages. HTML is not a programming language like Java or C++.

6. **C.** XML tags are designed to be self-descriptive and not predefined. Document authors must define their own tags.

7. **D.** Active Server Pages (ASP) is a server-side script language for making dynamic and interactive web pages.

8. **D.** Hypertext Preprocessor (PHP) is a server-side scripting language where the scripts are executed on the server and returned to the browser as plain HTML.

References

1. King, K. N. (2008). *C programming: A modern approach, second edition*. Norton.

2. Overland, B. (2011). *C++ without fear: A beginner's guide that makes you feel smart, second edition*. Prentice Hall.

3. The Java Tutorials. Accessed from http://docs.oracle.com/javase/tutorial.

4. Java Tutorial. Accessed from www.tutorialspoint.com/java/java_overview.htm.

5. W3School.com. Accessed from www.w3schools.com.

6. Fawcett, J., Ayers, D., & Quin, R. E. (2012). *Beginning XML, fifth edition*. Wrox.

7. Gilmore, W. J. (2012). *Beginning PHP and MySQL: From novice to professional, fourth edition*. Apress.

CHAPTER 34

Databases, Data Warehousing, and Data Mining for Healthcare

Alex Mu-Hsing Kuo

In this chapter, you will learn how to
- Explain what a database is and why it is important in healthcare information technology
- Explain what data warehousing and data mining are
- Develop and manage a web-based database application, a data warehouse system, or a data mining project
- Identify and explain issues for developing database applications, data warehouse systems, or data mining projects in healthcare

Healthcare Databases

Healthcare is the most data-intensive industry in the world.[1,2] Patient information stored in health information systems (HISs) can be used by healthcare professionals for patient care, for treatment advice, and for surveillance of a patient's health status; it can be used by healthcare researchers in assessing clinical treatment, procedures, and effectiveness of medications; and it can be used by administrative personnel in cost accounting and by managers for planning. The challenge for a traditional HIS is how to make data useful for clinicians and empower them with the tools to make informed decisions and deliver more responsive patient services.

A healthcare database is a collection of related patient health data organized to facilitate its efficient storage, querying, and modification to meet the healthcare professional's needs.[3] Nowadays, many healthcare environments have applied database technologies to improve work efficiency and reduce healthcare costs. The following are some important database application areas in healthcare:[3,4]

- **Solo practice** General practitioners (GPs) find that most of their needs for HISs are focused on patient data management, schedule keeping, and billing. The data management functions of modern databases allow GPs to easily maintain and retrieve patient health information and reduce paperwork as well as documentation errors.

- **Group practice** The operation of a group practice where several healthcare professionals cooperate in providing care creates many problems regarding access to medical records. Data for the record is generated at multiple sites, but the entire record should be complete and legible whenever and wherever it is retrieved. Databases that store large volumes of data over long periods of time from patients (and from other clinical sources) provide support to healthcare teams for accessing and analyzing patient data during the process of providing patient care.

- **Clinical research** Databases are usually involved in the study of medications, devices, diagnostic products, or treatment regimens (including information about the safety and effectiveness of drugs intended for human use). This data may be used to inform decision making for the prevention, treatment, and diagnosis of disease. When studies become moderate to large in terms of their populations and observation period, a database approach becomes essential.

- **Service reimbursement** Perhaps the largest databases in use that are related to healthcare are those associated with reimbursement for health services. Requirements for inquiry and audit are generating the need for more complete medical encounter information. This leads the healthcare providers who handle reimbursement accounting to consider database technologies.

- **Health surveillance** This refers to the collection and analysis of health data about clinical syndromes that have a significant impact on public health. Data from databases can be used to detect or anticipate disease outbreaks. Then, governments can drive decisions about health policy and health education. Surveillance databases serve an important role as collections of disease reports as well as patient behavior.

- **Healthcare education** Databases are also used for healthcare education. Such databases contain medical student and laboratory data so that students can receive appropriate assignments, be matched to the patient population, and have their progress tracked.

- **Electronic health records (EHRs)** Databases are at the core of EHRs, which are designed to allow users (e.g., physicians, nurses, and other health professionals) to store and retrieve patient data electronically. Data available to users in the EHR is stored in and retrieved from databases.

Database Basics

Before database systems were developed, data was stored in traditional electronic files. Traditional file-processing systems have several drawbacks such as program-data dependency, duplication of data, limited data sharing, lengthy development times, and excessive program maintenance.[1] Database technologies have evolved since the 1960s to ease increasing difficulties in maintaining complex traditional information systems with a large amount of diverse data and with many concurrent end users. Over the past few decades, there has been an increase in the number of database applications in business, industry, healthcare, education, government, and the military.

A database model (database schema) is the structure or format of a database, described in a formal language supported by the database management system (DBMS). Several different database models have been used in DBMSs: the hierarchical model, the network model, the relational model, and the object-oriented model have been proposed since the concept of a DBMS was first created.[1] Among them, the relational database model is the most commonly adopted model today and is widely used in the healthcare industry. Thus the remainder of this chapter will focus on the relational database model.

The relational database model is a collection of *relations* that refer to the various tables in the database. The *table* is the basic data structure of the relational model. A table includes three components:

- **Name**   Used to uniquely identify a table
- **Column (also called attribute/field)**   A set of data values with particular data types (e.g., CHAR, NUMBER, DATE, etc.)
- **Row (also called instance/tuple/record)**   A set of related data, in which every row has the same structure

In a table, the *primary key* (PK) is a column (or combination of columns) that is used to uniquely identify a record in a table (e.g., an employee number in an employee database). The *foreign key* (FK) identifies a column in one table that refers to a column (usually a PK) in another table. For example, in Figure 34-1, the table name is called EMPLOYEES with many columns and rows (this is a database table for a hospital employee database). Each column would record, respectively, the employee's ID (EMPLOYEE_ID), first name (FIRST_NAME), last name (LAST_NAME), and whatever else is important to the employee. For example, in Figure 34-1, reading across the rows from the top down, you can see that the first employee has the EMPLOYEE_ID of 100, has the FIRST_NAME Steven, and has the LAST_NAME King. The second row describes the information for EMPLOYEE_ID 101. The columns represent the fields (or attributes) of each employee record. A healthcare database consists of data stored in many such tables (that are linked together through foreign keys).

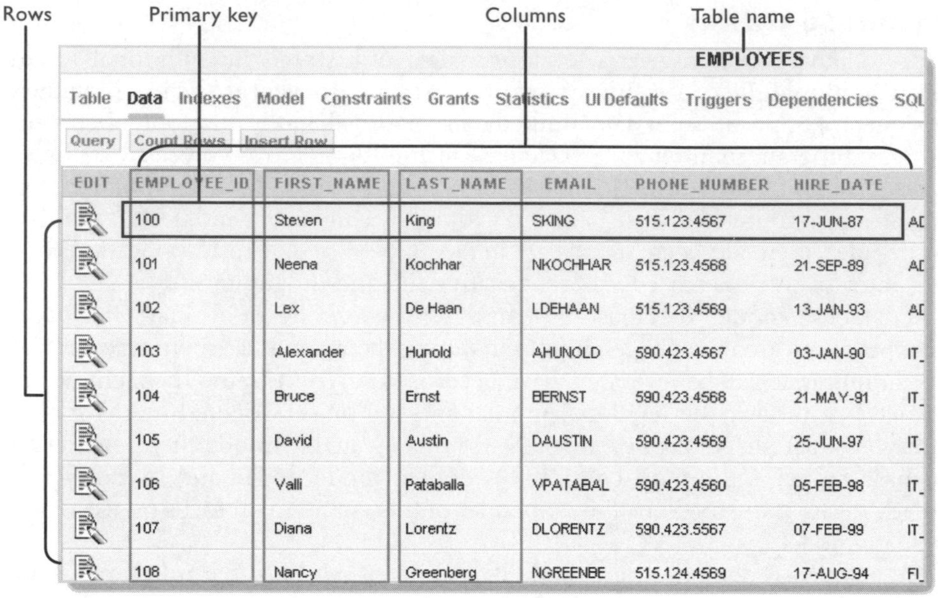

Rows   Primary key   Columns   Table name

EMPLOYEES

Table **Data** Indexes Model Constraints Grants Statistics UI Defaults Triggers Dependencies SQL

Query Count Rows Insert Row

EDIT	EMPLOYEE_ID	FIRST_NAME	LAST_NAME	EMAIL	PHONE_NUMBER	HIRE_DATE	
	100	Steven	King	SKING	515.123.4567	17-JUN-87	AD
	101	Neena	Kochhar	NKOCHHAR	515.123.4568	21-SEP-89	AD
	102	Lex	De Haan	LDEHAAN	515.123.4569	13-JAN-93	AD
	103	Alexander	Hunold	AHUNOLD	590.423.4567	03-JAN-90	IT_
	104	Bruce	Ernst	BERNST	590.423.4568	21-MAY-91	IT_
	105	David	Austin	DAUSTIN	590.423.4569	25-JUN-97	IT_
	106	Valli	Pataballa	VPATABAL	590.423.4560	05-FEB-98	IT_
	107	Diana	Lorentz	DLORENTZ	590.423.5567	07-FEB-99	IT_
	108	Nancy	Greenberg	NGREENBE	515.124.4569	17-AUG-94	FI_

Figure 34-1 A relational database table structure

A database management system is a set of software programs that control the organization, storage, management, and retrieval of data in a database. Structured Query Language (SQL) is a nonprocedural programming language that enables a user to manage a (relational) database. Using SQL statements, the user can query tables to display data, create objects, modify objects, and perform administrative tasks. SQL statements are divided into three categories:

- **Data Definition Language (DDL) statements** These statements create, alter, and drop database objects.

- **Data Manipulation Language (DML) statements** These statements query, insert, update, and delete data in tables.

- **Data Control Language (DCL) statements** These statements commit or roll back the processing of transactions.

For example, the following DML statement retrieves all employee_id, first_name, last_name, job_id, and salary data from the EMPLOYEES table in Figure 34-1:

```
SELECT employee_id, first_name, last_name, job_id, salary
FROM Employees;
```

Database Application Development Process

A healthcare database application design process usually includes four stages (Figure 34-2):

- **Stage 1** Analyze the business scenario and extract business rules.
- **Stage 2** Design an entity relationship diagram (ERD) based on the business rules extracted from stage 1.
- **Stage 3** Select a database model (e.g., Oracle DB) and create a physical database (tables, views, functions, etc).
- **Stage 4** Choose a development tool (e.g., Oracle APEX) to implement the application.

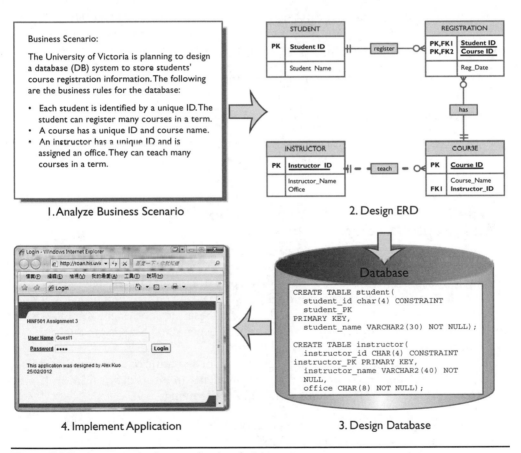

Figure 34-2 A generic database application design process

Analyzing the Business Scenario and Extracting Business Rules

Business rules describe the operations, definitions, and constraints that are intended to embody the business structure or to control or influence the behavior of an organization. Many database system developers believe that clear business rules are very important in database modeling because they govern how data is stored and processed. To model a database, the system analyst needs to do the following:[1]

- Identify and understand those rules that govern patient's health data.

- Represent those rules so that they can be unambiguously understood by system developers.

- Ensure the rules are consistent (a rule must not contradict other rules).

For example, the Island Medical Program at the University of Victoria (UVic) is planning to design a database (DB) system to store each medical student's course registration information. The following are some business rules for the database:

- Each medical student is identified by a unique ID. The student can register a maximum of five courses in a term.

- A course has a unique ID and course name and can be taught by only one instructor.

An instructor has a unique ID and is assigned an office. They can teach a maximum of two courses in a term.

Modeling Database: Entity Relationship Diagram Design and Normalization

The next step is to model the database. Data modeling is the process of creating a data model by applying formal data model descriptions using data modeling techniques. Several techniques have been developed in the past decades for the design of data models, such as the entity relationship model (ERM), IDEF-1X, object-relational mapping, object role model, and relational model. For database model design, the ERM is the most commonly used tool for communications between database system analysts, programmers, and end users during the analysis phase.

The ERM produces a type of conceptual schema or semantic data model that is used to organize a relational database and its requirements in a top-down fashion (for an example, see Figure 34-3). It contains three major elements:

- **Entities**   A person, place, or object about which the data is collected (the boxes in Figure 34-3 labeled STUDENT, INSTRUCTOR, etc.).

- **Attributes**   Type of information that is captured related to the entity (the fields inside each box in Figure 34-3).

- **Relationships**   The associations and connections between the entities. Depending on the cardinality and modality, a number of relationship symbols are introduced (the lines connecting the boxes in Figure 34-3).

When people design an ERM, they usually use an entity relationship diagram to serve as a blueprint for database programmers to follow the business rules to build a physical database. This is very similar in building construction. An architect designs a building blueprint, and workers follow the information contained in it to erect the structure. For example, based on the business rules extracted in the previous section, I used Microsoft Office Visio 2007 to construct the ERD shown in Figure 34-3.

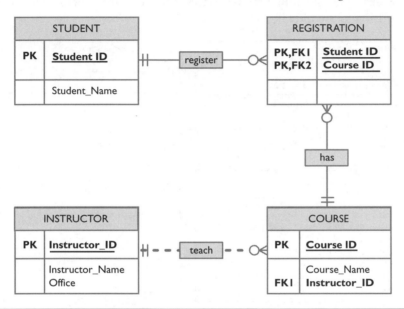

Figure 34-3   The ERD for UVic course registration system

Creating a Physical Database Using Structured Query Language

After creating the ERD, programmers are able to create a physical database based on the blueprint. Physical database design requires several decisions that will affect the integrity performance of the database system. The information needed for this process includes the following:

- **Table/column name**   Usually uses a singular noun or noun phrase, and the name should be specific to the organization (e.g., a university DB uses STUDENT for the table name and uses student_id for the column name in the table to store the student's ID number)

- **Data format**   Defines the data type (e.g., NUMBER, CHAR, DATE, etc.) for each column to minimize storage space and maximize data integrity
- **Constraints**   Specify the number of instances (e.g., an instructor can teach a maximum of five courses) or value range (e.g., a course score is between 0 and 100) for one column
- **Default value**   Is the value a column will assume (e.g., default value for score is 0) if a user does not provide data

Then, database programmers use SQL to create a physical database with several tables. For example, the four CREATE statements shown in Figure 34-4 create four tables according to the ERD in Figure 34-3.

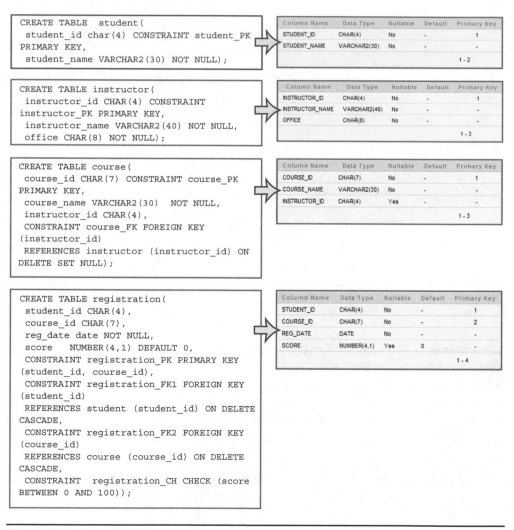

Figure 34-4   Four CREATE statements

Implementing a Healthcare Database Application

The last stage for the database application development is to choose a tool to implement the application. For example, in developing a web-based healthcare database application, there are several available tools for this purpose, such as Hypertext Preprocessor (PHP), Active Server Pages (ASP)/ASP.NET, Process and Experiment Automation Realtime Language (PEARL), Oracle Application Express (APEX), Java, and C++. Among them, Oracle Application Express is a free, rapid web application development tool for an Oracle database (Oracle is one of the most widely used DBMSs in healthcare today). Using only a web browser and limited programming experience, a database application designer can develop and deploy professional applications that are both fast and secure. For example, using APEX, a page is the basic building block of an application. When you build an application in Application Builder, you create pages that contain user interface elements, such as tabs, lists, buttons, items, and regions. Then, you add controls to a page on the page definition. For example, based on the tables created in stage 3, I developed a simple web-based database application for health informatics course registration using APEX, as shown in Figure 34-5. In this application, users can use any Internet browser (e.g., Internet Explorer, Firefox, Chrome) to log into the application (http://roan.his.uvic.ca:8080/apex/f?p=140; username=guest, password=guest). The home page will show all the students' registration information. The user also can click the tabs at the top of the page to view or edit student profiles, instructor backgrounds, and course descriptions.

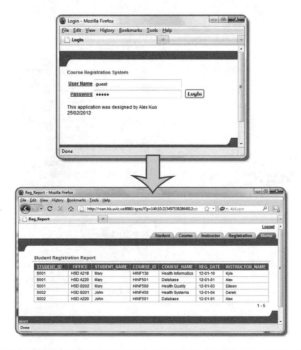

Figure 34-5   A simple APEX application for online course registration

Use Case 34-1: A Simple Web-Based Healthcare Database Application

MINISHELL is a student group project that was undertaken for the course Database Design in HIT (H501) at the School of Health Information at the University of Victoria.[1] It is an electronic health record system utilizing APEX in an Oracle database system. The goal was to create a usable system that would meet user needs from an EHR perspective of both an inpatient and ambulatory population. The required functionalities included giving the system the ability to support workflow in an emergency department, operating room, hospital clinic, or ward setting. Recognizing the diverse population of users and uses that this represents, the developers had to ensure that comprehensive patient records (including all aspects of a patient's past and current medical history) were available.

The group developing MINISHELL followed the four-stage design process described earlier to implement the application. Microsoft Visio 2003 was used to draw the ERD that included 15 tables (Figure 34-6). Patients and their allergies can be tracked easily through allergy, patient_allergy, and patient tables. Each patient can be visited zero to many times by the practitioner. In each visit, zero to many drugs might be prescribed, and zero to many tests might be ordered. The tables Allergy, Diagnosis, Unit, Facility, Test_Result, Source_tbl, Treatment, Provider, Drug, and Family_doctor play the role of parent tables, and the five tables patient, Patient_Allergy, Visit, Prescription, and Order are child tables, which connect to parent tables through foreign keys.

When a healthcare practitioner logs into the system (http://roan.his.uvic .ca:8080/apex/f?p=100; username=HG3, password=nurse1), the practitioner will see the home page shown below. From this page the practitioner can admit patients, and view their admission history, treatment history, and prescription lists by clicking the links on the left side of the screen. The healthcare practitioner can also enter allergies, prescriptions, and treatment orders for the patient.

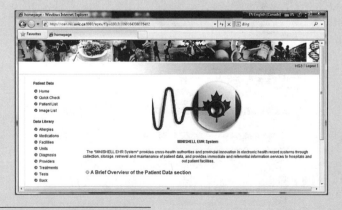

---

1. A data analyst (Elham Sedghi), three registered nurses (Michelle Henness, Nicole Michaud Hamilton, Shabana Kapadia), a social worker (Lida Kam), and a QA analyst (Maryam Katani) designed and implemented this database application under the supervision of Dr. Alex Kuo.

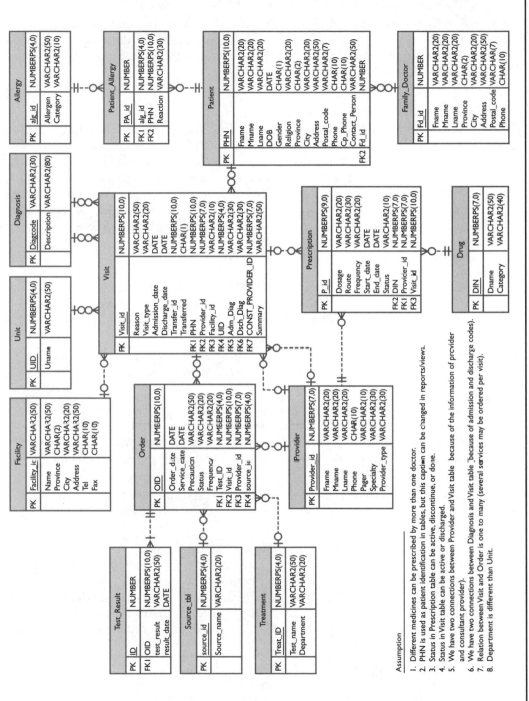

Figure 34-6 The ERD of the MINISHELL EHR

Assumption

1. Different medicines can be prescribed by more than one doctor.
2. PHN is used as patient identification in tables, but this caption can be changed in reports/views.
3. Status in Prescription table can be active, discontinue, or done.
4. Status in Visit table can be active or discharged.
5. We have two connections between Provider and Visit table because of the information of provider and consultant provider).
6. We have two connections between Diagnosis and Visit table because of admission and discharge codes).
7. Relation between Visit and Order is one to many (several services may be ordered per visit).
8. Department is different than Unit.

Database Administration and Security

When developing databases, database administration is an important topic that needs to be taken into account in order to ensure that critical health data is managed efficiently and effectively. Another key concept when developing databases for storing and using sensitive health data is security.

Database Administration

Database administration refers to a set of functions for logical and physical database design and for dealing with management issues, such as ensuring database performance, data security and privacy, data backup and recovery, and database availability.[1] A database administrator (DBA) must have a sound understanding of current hardware and software (e.g., operation systems [OSs] and networking) architectures, security/privacy policies, and data processing procedures to ensure enough disk space is always available, backups are performed regularly, indexes are maintained and optimized, and database statistics are up-to-date.

The main database administration tasks are as follows:[4]

- **Managing database memory**   One of the most important aspects of managing a database is to make sure that there is always enough disk space. As the data size grows, the DBA needs to evaluate whether to allocate more memory to the database.

- **Managing users**   The task includes creating/dropping user accounts, locking and unlocking user accounts, resetting account passwords, granting administrative privileges, and assigning quotas.

- **Monitoring the database for performance issues**   When problems occur within a system, it is important to perform an accurate and timely diagnosis before making any changes to the system. If there is a problem, the DBA may look at the symptoms, analyze statistics, and immediately start changing the system to fix those symptoms.

- **Backing up databases**   As with any database, backups need to be scheduled, executed, and monitored. Details of the process will be discussed in the next section.

- **Executing data security/privacy policies**   Security policies define the rules that will be followed to maintain security in a database system. A security plan details how those rules will be implemented. A security policy is generally included within a security plan. To maintain database security, a DBA follows the organization security plan to grant privileges to enable the user to connect to the database, to run queries and make updates, and to create schema objects.

Database Security

Database security refers to protecting the data against accidental or intentional loss, destruction, misuse, or disclosure to unwanted parties. Some common data security issues include the following:

- **Theft and fraud**   This occurs when any person uses another person's means of access to view, alter, or destroy data. In some cases, the thief can access a computer room to steal database hardware.

- **Data breaches**   A data breach is the intentional or unintentional release of confidential data (e.g., patient's health records) to unauthorized third parties.

- **Loss of data integrity**   Data integrity is imposed within a database at its design stage through the use of standard rules and procedures and is maintained through the use of error checking and validation routines. When data integrity is compromised, data will be invalid or corrupted.

- **Loss of availability**   Loss of availability means that data, applications, or networks are unavailable to users and may lead to severe operational difficulties of an organization.

Database security management must establish administrative policies and procedures, create physical protection plans, institute backup and recovery strategies, and apply hardware or software technologies to protect data. Security countermeasures can be categorized into technical and nontechnical methods,[1,5] as described in the following lists.

Technical data security methods include the following:

- **Integrity controls**   Data is kept consistent and correct by means of controls that a database administrator puts on the database. This may involve limiting values a column may hold, constraining the actions that can be performed on the data, or triggering the execution of certain procedures to track access to data (e.g., recording which user has done what and accesses which data). The tracking or auditing of who accesses patient data (and for what purposes) is especially important given the sensitivity of personal health data.

- **Authentication**   This refers to a way of identifying a user (a person or a software program) by having the user provide a valid ID and password before the access is granted. The process of authentication is based on each user having a unique set of criteria for gaining access.

- **Authorization**   This refers to verifying that the user has authority to access a database object (e.g., table, procedure, or function) before allowing the user to access it. In other words, this determines which actions an authenticated principal is authorized to perform on the database. The tasks required to control authorization are also referred to as *access management*.

For example, a user called Alex wants to log in to the www.CyberHealth.com server to use the EHR that can be accessed from that site. In this example, authentication is the mechanism whereby the system running at www.CyberHealth.com should securely identify the user Alex. The authentication must provide answers to the following questions:

- Who is the user Alex?
- Is the user Alex really who he represents himself to be?

To answer these questions, the server depends on some unique bits of information known only to Alex. It may be as simple as a password or public key authentication or as complicated as a Kerberos-based system. If the authenticating system can verify that the shared secret was presented correctly, then the user Alex is considered authenticated. What's next? The server running at www.CyberHealth.com must determine what level of access Alex should have. For example, is Alex authorized to view a specific patient's data? Is Alex authorized to modify the patient's data? Is Alex authorized to delete the patient's data? In this example, the server uses a combination of authentication and authorization to secure the system. The system ensures that the user claiming to be Alex is really Alex and thus prevents unauthorized users from gaining access to secured resources running on the EHR at the www.CyberHealth.com server.

- **User-defined procedures** User-defined procedures or interfaces allow system designers to define their own security procedures in addition to the authorization rules.

- **Data encryption** This refers to mathematical calculations and algorithmic schemes that transform plain text into cybertext, in other words, converting text into a form that is not readable to unauthorized parties. Using encryption, a key specifies the particular transformation of plain text into cybertext, or vice versa, during decryption. The following are two common encryption methods for data protection:

- **Secret-key encryption, also known as symmetric-key cryptography** This refers to a class of algorithms for cryptography that use trivially related, often identical, cryptographic keys for both decryption and encryption. Examples of popular and well-respected symmetric algorithms include AES, Blowfish, CAST5, RC4, TDES, and IDEA.

- **Public-key encryption, also known as asymmetric-key cryptography** In public-key cryptography, a user has a pair of cryptographic keys: a public key and a private key. The private key is kept secret, while the public key may be widely distributed. Incoming messages would have been encrypted with the recipient's public key and can be decrypted only with the recipient's corresponding private key. Examples of popular and well-respected public-key algorithms include RSA, ElGamal, Knapsack, ECC, and Diffie-Hellman.

- **Firewall** This refers to an integrated collection of security measures designed to prevent unauthorized electronic access to a networked computer system. It is also a device or set of devices configured to permit, deny, encrypt, decrypt, or proxy all computer traffic between different security domains based upon a set of rules and other criteria.

- **Intrusion detection system (IDS)** This refers to software and/or hardware designed to detect unwanted attempts at accessing, manipulating, and/or disabling of computer systems, mainly through a network, such as the Internet.

- **Data masking** This refers to the process of obscuring (masking) specific data within a database table or column to ensure that data security is maintained and sensitive customer information is not leaked outside of the authorized environment. Common methods of data masking include encryption, masking (e.g., numbers for letters), substitution (e.g., all males names = Alex), nulling (e.g., ####), or shuffling (e.g., zipcode12345 = 51432).

Nontechnical data security methods include the following:

- **Personnel controls** This refers to exerting control over who can interact with a resource. The resource can be database data, an application, or hardware. Activities such as monitoring to ensure that personnel are following established security practices can be carried out. Standard job controls, such as separating duties so no one employee has responsibility for an entire system or keeping system developers from having access to production systems, should also be enforced (particularly in healthcare, where the data stored can be considered to be sensitive).

- **Physical access controls** These limit access to particular computer rooms in buildings and are usually part of controlling physical access. Sensitive equipment (hardware and peripherals) must be placed in secure areas (e.g., locked to a desk or cabinet). Also, an alarm system can avoid a brute-force break-in.

- **Maintenance controls** The healthcare organization should review external maintenance agreements for all hardware (e.g., server, networks) and software (e.g., source codes) that the database system is using to ensure system performance and data quality.

- **Data privacy controls** Breaches of confidential data (e.g., patient health data) could result in loss of user trust in the organization and could lead to legal action being taken against the healthcare organization. Information privacy legislations play a critical role in protecting user data privacy. For example, the U.S. Health Information Portability and Accountability Act (HIPAA) is a federal law enacted to ensure that the freedom of patients to choose healthcare insurers and providers will not come at the expense of the privacy of their medical records.[6]

Database backup and recovery are mechanisms for restoring databases quickly and accurately after loss or damage. A DBMS should provide four basic facilities for the backup and recovery of a database:[1]

- Backup facilities that provide periodic backup copies of the database (backup data should be kept offsite at safe locations)

- Journalizing facilities that maintain an audit trail of transactions and database changes

- A checkpoint facility by which the DBMS periodically suspends all processing and synchronizes its files and journals to establish a recovery point

- A recovery manager that allows the DBMS to restore its original condition if needed

Data Warehouses for Healthcare

The need to analyze large amounts of health data is becoming increasingly important to managers, healthcare organizations, and healthcare researchers. In response to this, new ways of organizing health data have been developed to help health professionals and managers query health data. As a consequence, in recent years the concept of a data warehouse (DW) has emerged in healthcare.

What Is a Data Warehouse (DW)?

Healthcare is information dependent and cannot be provided efficiently without data regarding the patient's past and current conditions. Patient health records provide the who, what, when, where, and how of patient care, and they are the resources needed for further decision support and knowledge discovery. Unfortunately, in the real world, clinical data comes from many different sources, e.g., patient visits, test results, laboratory reports, diagnoses, therapy, medication, and procedures. This data is usually stored in distributed and heterogeneous databases. For example, a patient's registration data is stored in a Microsoft Access database, a laboratory report in a Sybase database, diagnosis information in an IBM Informix database, and medication information in an Oracle database. Healthcare professionals need to integrate the data from several transaction information systems (databases) to provide quality treatment and patient care. However, heterogeneous data and distributed data repositories make clinical decisions difficult (Figure 34-7). A data warehouse (DW) integrates (extracts, transforms, and loads [ETL]) data from several transaction information systems into a staging area. It is believed that a DW can provide healthcare professionals with clinical intelligence that enables them to better understand problems, discover opportunities, and measure performance.[7]

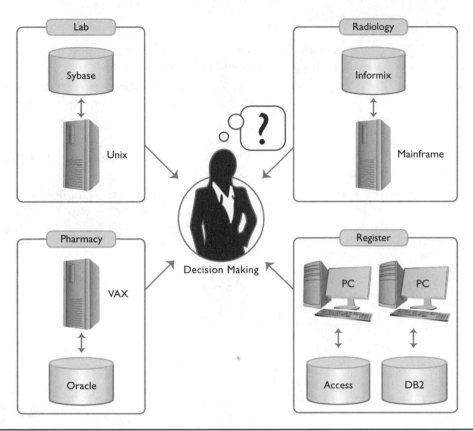

Figure 34-7 Heterogeneous data and distributed data repositories make clinical decision making difficult.

Bill Inmon defined the data warehouse as "a subject oriented, integrated, nonvolatile and time-variant collection of data in support of management's decisions."[8] In other words, a data warehouse is a repository of an organization's electronically stored data designed to facilitate reporting and analysis. This classic definition of a data warehouse focuses on data storage. However, the means to retrieve and analyze data; to extract, transform, and load data; and to manage the dictionary data are also considered essential components of a data warehousing system.

The Differences Between a DW and OLTP

Online Transaction Processing (OLTP) refers to a set of programs that help users manage transaction-oriented applications in industries, such as banking, airlines, supermarkets, and manufacturing. These transaction-oriented applications include data entry and retrieval transactions. Data warehouses are different from OLTP based on the following five aspects.[9]

Design Objectives

- OLTP is a software system that facilitates and manages transaction-oriented applications, typically for data entry and retrieval transaction processing.

- A DW is a decision-making-oriented repository. It is mainly used for decision analysis, with strong interoperability between different computer systems.

Data Types

- OLTP contains department detail, short-period data, snapshot, and/or ongoing status of business.

- A DW consists of an enterprise-level, integrated, time-variant, and nonvolatile collection of data. Data often originates from a variety of sources. It may include five types of data (Figure 34-8): current operational data, legacy data, lightly digested data, heavily digested data, and metadata.

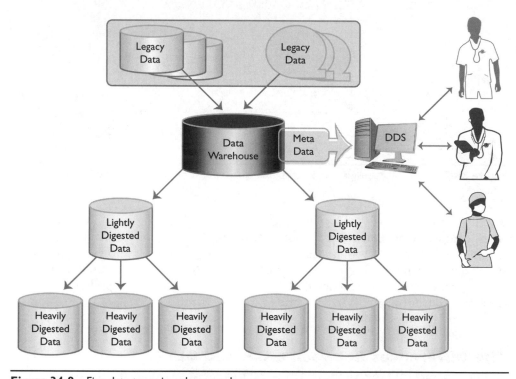

Figure 34-8   Five data types in a data warehouse

Functionalities

- OLTP provides online query, modify, insert, and delete functions. Efficiency and steadiness are major goals for OLTP.

- DW is subject-oriented and supports a variety of decision analysis functions as well as strategic operational functions.

Data Structures

- OLTP usually contains many relational tables and is highly normalized.

- A DW uses a star schema to store data. The star schema consists of a few "fact tables" (possibly only one, justifying the name) referencing any number of "dimension tables." The fact table holds the main data while the smaller dimension tables describe each value of a dimension and can be joined to fact tables as needed (Figure 34-9).

Analytical Capabilities

- OLTP helps users control and run fundamental business tasks. It possesses limited analytical capabilities.

- A DW enables users to analyze different dimensions of multidimensional data. For example, it provides time series and trend analysis views.

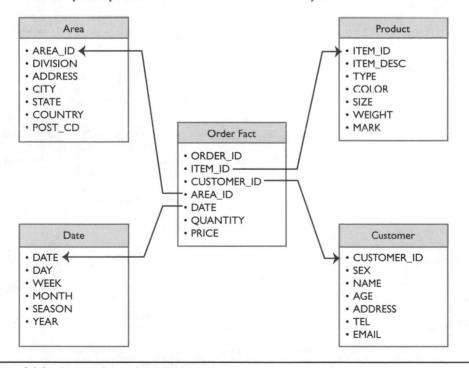

Figure 34-9 A star schema data structure

Data Warehouse Models

Data warehousing supports a variety of decision analysis functions as well as strategic operational functions. Data often originates from a variety of sources (different types of databases), formats, and types, and it is generally consolidated, transformed, and loaded into one or more instances of a database management system to facilitate a broad range of analytical applications. A data warehouse may consist of a single large enterprise-wide database to which users and administrators connect directly, or it may incorporate several smaller systems, called *data marts*, each of which addresses a specific subject area within the overall warehouse. Online Analytical Processing (OLAP) is the core component of data warehousing and analytics. It gives users the ability to interrogate data by intuitively navigating from summary to detail data.

In real applications, you can use four aspects to categorize a data warehouse model:

1. Categorized by functionalities (enterprise DW vs. department DW)

   - An enterprise DW (also called EDW, Figure 34-10) supports a variety of decision-analysis functions as well as strategic operational functions.

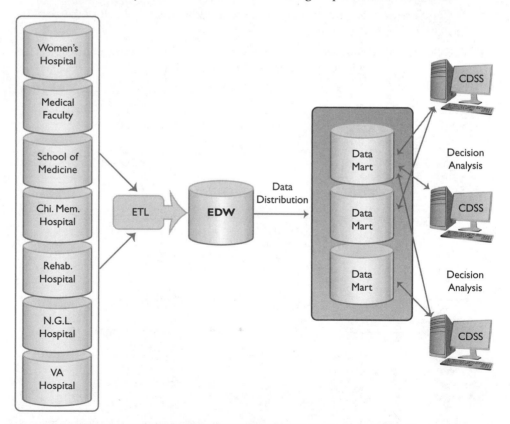

Figure 34-10 Enterprise DW vs. department DW (data mart) model. (CDSS refers to Clinical Decision Support System.)

- A department DW (also called a data mart, a subset of EDW) is usually oriented to a specific purpose or major data subject that may be distributed to support businesses and contains analytical data designed to focus on specific business functions for a specific community within an organization.

2. Categorized by storage location (centralized DW vs. distributed DW)

- A centralized DW consists of a single large enterprisewide database. Data often originates from a variety of sources and is loaded into one or more instances of a database management system to facilitate a broad range of analytical applications. The main benefit of this model is that data is more consistent and easy to maintain. However, the major concern of this model is that it has high development and maintenance costs (based on the data level and security level).

- A distributed DW (Figure 34-11) usually consists of several department DWs (data marts). This model is suitable for companies doing distributed business operations.

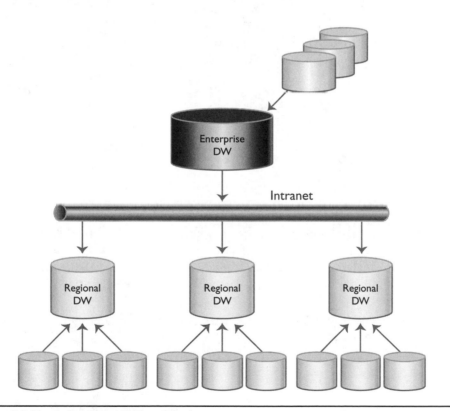

Figure 34-11 A distributed DW model

3. Categorized by topology (physical DW vs. virtual DW)

- A physical DW stores all aggregate data in a physical storage location. The DW consists of five types of data: current operational data, legacy data, lightly digested data, heavily digested data, and metadata.

- A virtual DW does not store data in a physical storage location. This model is a virtual (conceptual) DW that uses an intranet/Internet to connect all distributed databases (Figure 34-12).

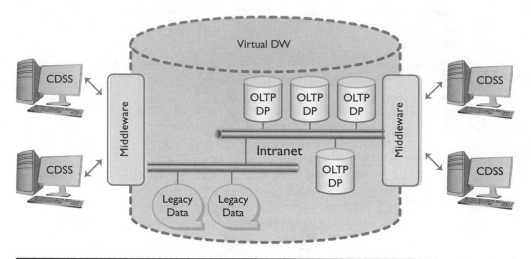

Figure 34-12 A virtual DW model

4. Categorized by data status (dynamic DW vs. static DW)

- A dynamic DW consists of a snapshot DW and a longitudinal DW (Figure 34-13). It can be applied to an organization that needs both short-term tactical analysis and long-term strategic analysis. This model requires high development and maintenance costs. Therefore, it is seldom used in real applications.

- A static DW is an EDW or a data mart that consists of a nonvolatile (static) collection of data.

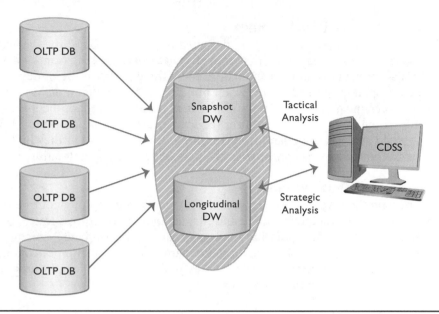

Figure 34-13 A dynamic DW model

A Healthcare Data Warehouse Life Cycle

The classical system development life cycle (SDLC) is not suitable for data warehouse development.[8] The data warehousing industry is in agreement that the data warehouse life-cycle model should consist of the following five major phases.[10,11,12]

Phase 1: Requirement Analysis

All IT systems of any kind need to be built to suit user needs. A system must be usable. If the system is not used, there is no point in building it. To become a real organizational asset leveraged throughout healthcare systems, user requirements must be carefully analyzed and defined before implementing a data warehouse. The system analyst talks to the user to understand the details of the processes, the business, the data, and the issues; arrange site visits to get firsthand experience; discuss the meaning of the data, the user interface, and so on; and document them. The system analyst also lists the nonfunctional requirements such as performance and security.

Phase 2: System Design

Key activities in this phase are to determine the data warehouse model; design the extraction, transformation, and loading system; and draw the front-end applications. Tasks typically include cataloging the source system, defining key performance indicators and other critical business metrics, mapping decision-making processes underlying information needs, and designing the logical and physical schema.

Phase 3: Prototype Development

This phase builds the three parts that are designed in previous phase: the data stores, the ETL system (including data quality system and metadata), and the front-end application. With some caution and consideration, these three parts can be built in parallel. The most important consideration when building in parallel is to define accurate interfaces between the parts. The primary objective of prototype development is to constrain and in some cases reframe end-user requirements by showing opinion leaders and heavyweight analysts in the end-user communities precisely what they had asked for in the requirement analysis phase or in the previous prototyping iteration.

Phase 4: System Deployment

Deployment typically involves two separate deployments: the deployment of a prototype into a production-test environment and the deployment of a stress-tested, performance-tested production configuration into an actual production environment. Once a user-approved DW is ready, the development team puts all the components in the production boxes (the ETL system, the data stores, and the front-end applications) and deploys the system for actual production use.

Phase 5: System Operation

This phase involves the day-to-day maintenance of the data warehouse. The operations team continues to administer the data warehouse and to support the users. There are basically three types of support: helping new and existing users using the system, administering new users and their access rights, and solving errors or problems that happen when using the data warehouse. Users will also have enhancement requests: to add more data to the data warehouse (or change existing data), to add a feature to the front-end applications, or to create new reports or new data structures. In such cases, the development team may include these requests in the next release.

Data Mining for Healthcare

As the amount of stored health data increases exponentially, it's increasingly recognized that such data can be analyzed or "mined" to uncover new and important patterns. In this section, I explore the role of data mining in identifying and revealing important patterns or trends in health data.

What Is Data Mining?

Data mining (DM) is different from OLAP that focuses on the interactive analysis of data and typically provides extensive capabilities for visualizing the data and generating summary statistics.[13] Data mining is "an integral part of knowledge discovery in database (KDD), which is the overall process of converting raw data into useful information."[14] In other words, it is the process of automatically discovering useful information in large data repositories (e.g., data warehouses). The data mining process consists of four major transformation phases,[15] as shown in Figure 34-14.

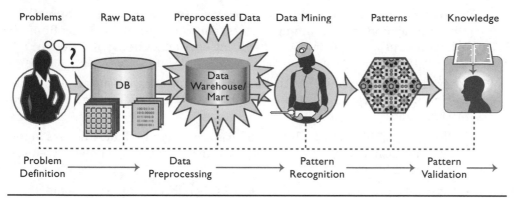

Figure 34-14 A generic process of data mining

1. **Problem definition phase** A healthcare data mining project starts with an understanding of the healthcare problems. Data mining experts, business experts (healthcare setting managers), and domain experts (healthcare professionals) work closely together to define the project objectives and the requirements from a healthcare quality improvement perspective. The project objective is then translated into a data mining problem definition. In the problem definition phase, data mining data and tools are not yet required.

2. **Data preprocessing phase** The original or "raw" data provided for data mining often needs certain levels of preprocessing before it can be input to a data mining algorithm. The purpose of preprocessing is to transform the raw data into an appropriate format for subsequent analysis. The tasks involved in data preprocessing include fusing data from multiple sources (files, spreadsheets, or database tables), cleaning data, integrating data, and transforming data.

Real-world data tends to be incomplete (lacking attribute values or certain attributes of interest or containing only aggregate data), noisy (containing errors or outlier values that deviate from the expected), and inconsistent (e.g., containing discrepancies in the department codes used to categorize items). Data cleaning routines attempt to fill in missing values (e.g., fill in most probable value), smooth out noise (e.g., apply binning, regression, clustering algorithms to remove noisy data), and correct inconsistencies in the data (e.g., correct a patient's age that might be listed as −25 or 154).

Data integration involves merging data from multiple sources inside/outside heterogeneous databases, data cubes, or flat files into a coherent data store (e.g., data warehouse) for further data mining processing. This task usually encounters many interoperability issues. Kuo et al.[16] described several interoperability issues and approaches to deal with the issues.

For example, data from multiple data resources may need to be transformed into forms appropriate for mining, such as transforming patient gender from male/female data to M/F or 1/0, normalizing data values from $-100\sim100$ to $-1.0\sim1.0$, or categorizing age ranges from $0\sim130$ to youth/middle-age/senior.

3. **Pattern recognition phase**   This phase involves choosing the proper data mining algorithm to discover the patterns. Basically, these algorithms can be divided into four types:

   • **Clustering**   This refers to the task of discovering groups and structures in the data that are in some way or another similar, without using known structures in the data.

   • **Classification**   This refers to the task of generalizing a known structure to apply to new data. In other words, it predicts one or more discrete variables, based on the other attributes in the data set.

   • **Regression**   This refers to predicting one or more continuous variables, such as profit or loss, based on other attributes in the data set. It attempts to find a function that models the data with the least error.

   • **Association**   This refers to finding correlations between different attributes in a data set. The most common application of this kind of algorithm is for creating association rules, which can be used in a market basket analysis. For example, the Apriori association algorithm can produce association rules that indicate what combinations of medications and patient characteristics lead to adverse drug reactions (ADRs).[17]

Choosing the best algorithm to use for a specific analytical task can be a challenge. While you can use different algorithms to perform the same business task, another algorithm may produce a different result, and some algorithms can give more than one type of result.

4. **Pattern validation phase**   Pattern (rule) validation is the process of assessing how well the mining models perform against real data. It is important that the mining team validates the discovered patterns before deploying them into a production environment. There are several approaches for validating the patterns.[18] The following are some examples:

   • **Using statistical validity to determine whether there are problems in the data or in the model**   A number of statistical methods can be used to evaluate the data mining model quality or pattern accuracy, such as cross-validation and receiver operating characteristic (ROC) curves.

   • **Separating the data into training and testing sets to test the accuracy of patterns**   It is common for the data mining algorithms to find patterns in the training set that are not present in the general data set. To deal with the so-called over-fitting issue, the validation uses a test data set that the data mining algorithm was not trained on. The learned patterns are applied to the data set, and the resulting output is compared to the desired output.

- **Asking domain experts to review the results of the data mining to determine whether the discovered patterns have meaning in the targeted business scenario** In a health data mining project, physicians and healthcare domain experts will be involved in the validation process to interpret the accuracy of the patterns.

Applications of Data Mining in Healthcare

In recent years, data mining has received considerable attention as a tool that can be applied to healthcare research and management. To perform descriptive and predictive analysis, data mining employs various analysis methods, which include clustering, classification, regression, and association analysis (as discussed in the previous section), to discover interesting patterns in the given data set that serve as the basis for estimating future trends. For example, Kuo et al. proposed an association analysis algorithm for the detection of adverse drug reactions in healthcare data.[17] The Apriori algorithm was used to perform association analysis on the characteristics of patients, the drugs they were taking, their primary diagnosis, co-morbid conditions, and the ADRs or adverse events (AE) they experienced. This analysis produced association rules that indicate what combinations of medications and patient characteristics lead to ADRs. Cheng et al. proposed the use of classification algorithms to help in the early detection of heart disease, a major public health concern all over the world.[19] Balasubramanian and Umarani identified the risk factors associated with high levels of fluoride content in water, using data mining algorithms to find meaningful hidden patterns to support meaningful decision making about this real-world health hazard.[20] The Concaro et al. study[21] focused on the care delivery flow of diabetes mellitus and applied a data mining algorithm for the extraction of temporal association rules on sequences of events. The method exploited the integration of different healthcare information sources and was used to evaluate the pertinence of care delivery flow for specific pathologies in order to refine inappropriate practices that lead to unsatisfactory outcomes.

In research of data mining applied to cancer detection and treatment, Luk et al.[22] used Artificial Neural Network (ANN) and Classification And Regression Tree (CART) algorithms to distinguish tumor from nontumor liver tissues. Eventually, they revealed that these classification algorithms were suitable for applying the building of a tissue classification model based on the hidden pattern in the proteomic data set. In addition, ANN and CART algorithms generated good predictive abilities for differentiating between tumor and nontumor tissues for liver cancer. Cao et al. proposed the use of data mining as a tool to aid in monitoring trends in clinical trials of cancer vaccines. By using data mining and visualization, medical experts could find patterns and anomalies better than just looking at a set of tabulated data.[23] Many other real data mining applications in healthcare have been described.[24] Kalish has also described many real-world examples of how data mining has helped to reduce healthcare cost.[25]

Despite the benefits of applying data mining to the healthcare quality improvement, Shillabeer and Roddick[26] have indicated several inherent conflicts between traditional applications of data mining and applications in medicine. Perhaps the most challenging issues for the application of this technology to healthcare are data security and privacy. Therefore, an organization must formulate clear policies regarding the privacy and security of patient health records before embarking on data mining, and it must enforce those policies with its partner-stakeholders and agencies.

Chapter Review

Healthcare is the most data-intensive industry in the world today. Health information systems can be used by healthcare professionals to improve healthcare services and reduce costs. The challenge for HISs is how to make data useful for clinicians and empower them with the tools to make informed decisions and deliver more responsive patient services.

In this chapter, I first discussed the requirements for databases in healthcare and the basics of relational databases, database models, database administration, and security. I then described the steps involved in developing healthcare databases and illustrated this with an example of developing a web-based healthcare database application. I then discussed two important and emerging database applications: health data warehousing and data mining.

A data warehouse (DW) integrates data from several transaction information systems into a staging area. It is believed that DWs can provide healthcare professionals with clinical intelligence that will enable them to better understand clinical problems, discover opportunities, and measure the performance of healthcare systems.

Data mining (DM) is the process of automatically discovering useful information from large data repositories (e.g., data warehouses). In recent years, data mining has received considerable attention as a tool that can be applied in healthcare research and management.

A case study was also used to help you learn about the concepts of databases, data warehouses, and data mining in healthcare.

Questions

To test your comprehension of the chapter, answer the following questions and then check your answers against the list of correct answers at the end of the chapter.

1. What is a database model?
   A. A file processing system
   B. The structure of a database
   C. A set of mathematic algorithms
   D. A database management system (DBMS)

2. Finish the following sentence. In the relational database model, _____.
   A. a table name is used to uniquely identify a column
   B. the primary key is used to identify a column in one table that refers to a column in another table

    C. tables are the basic unit of data storage

    D. Data Control Language (DCL) statements can commit or roll back the processing of transactions

3. What is a database management system (DBMS)?

    A. A set of software programs to control the organization, storage, management, and retrieval of data in a database

    B. A nonprocedural programming language

    C. A data security mechanism

    D. A set of Data Definition Language (DDL) statements

4. What is the most commonly used tool for data modeling database?

    A. Entity relationship model

    B. IDEF-1X

    C. Object role model

    D. Spiral developing model

5. Which of the following statements is correct?

    A. Authorization is a way of identifying a user before the access is granted.

    B. Integrity controls keep the data consistent and correct by means of controls that a database administrator puts on the database.

    C. Data breaches mean that data, applications, or networks are unavailable to database users.

    D. Data security is not important in the database system design.

6. Finish the following sentence. Secret-key encryption _____.

    A. is also known as asymmetric-key cryptography

    B. uses a public key and a private key for both decryption and encryption

    C. is software designed to detect unwanted attempts of accessing database recourses

    D. is also called symmetric-key cryptography

7. Finish the following sentence. A distributed data warehouse _____.

    A. stores all aggregated data in a single physical storage location

    B. is also called Online Analytical Processing (OLAP)

    C. usually consists of several department data marts

    D. consists of snapshot and longitudinal databases

8. What is *not* the reason for creating a data mart?

   A. Lower cost

   B. More business functions

   C. Improving end-user response time

   D. Creating collective view by a group of users

9. Finish the following sentence. Data mining (DM) _____.

   A. is also called Online Analytical Processing

   B. focuses on the interactive analysis of data

   C. is a network protocol

   D. is the overall process of converting raw data into useful knowledge

10. Finish the following sentence. In a data mining project, pattern validation _____.

   A. is the process of assessing how well the mining models perform against real data

   B. is not important

   C. is the data extraction, transformation, and loading process

   D. is a method to clean data in the database

Answers

1. **B.** A database model is the structure of a database.

2. **C.** In the relational database model, tables are the basic unit of data storage.

3. **A.** A database management system (DBMS) is a set of software programs to control the organization, storage, management, and retrieval of data in a database.

4. **A.** The most commonly used tool for data modeling database is an entity relationship model (ERM).

5. **B.** Integrity controls keep the data consistent and correct by means of controls that a database administrator puts on the database.

6. **D.** Secret-key encryption is also called symmetric-key cryptography.

7. **C.** A distributed data warehouse usually consists of several department data marts.

8. **B.** Creating a data mart is not for providing more business functions.

9. **D.** Data mining is the overall process of converting raw data into useful knowledge.

10. **A.** In a data mining project, pattern validation is the process of assessing how well the mining models perform against real data.

References

1. Hoffer, J. A., Prescott, M. B., & McFadden, F. R. (2005). *Modern database management, seventh edition.* Pearson.

2. Hey, T. & Tansley, S. (Eds.) (2010). *The fourth paradigm: Data-intensive scientific discovery.* Microsoft Research.

3. Collen, M. F. (2011). *Computer medical databases: The first six decades (1950–2010).* Springer-Verlag London Ltd.

4. Oracle Database Express Edition 2 day DBA. Accessed from http://docs.oracle.com/cd/E17781_01/server.112/e18804/toc.htm.

5. Wiederhold, G. (1981). Database technology in healthcare. *Journal of Medical System, 5,* 175–196.

6. The Health Insurance Portability and Accountability Act of 1996 (HIPAA) privacy and security rules. (1996). Accessed from www.hhs.gov/ocr/privacy.

7. Akhtar, M.U., Dunn, K., & Smith, J.W. (2005). Commercial clinical data warehouses: From wave of the past to the state of the art. *Journal of Healthcare Information Management, 12,* 20–26.

8. Inmon, W. H. (2005). *Building the data warehouse, fourth edition.* John Wiley & Sons.

9. Data warehouse models, class note: HINF 310: Electronic records and decision support systems. School of Health Information Science. (2012).

10. Understanding the data warehouse lifecycle model. (2003). Accessed from http://hosteddocs.ittoolbox.com/MD041005.pdf.

11. Kimball, R., Ross, M., Thornthwaite, W., Mundy, J., & Becker, B. (2008). *The data warehouse lifecycle toolkit, second edition.* John Wiley & Sons.

12. Rainardi, V. (2011). *Building a data warehouse with examples in SQL Server.* Apress.

13. What is OLAP? An analysis of what the often misused OLAP term is supposed to mean. Accessed from www.bi-verdict.com/fileadmin/dl_temp/98d5e8f68f1177bdde5871afc66f8c9e/fasmi.htm?user_id=.

14. Tan, P. N., Steinbach, M., & Kumar, V. (2005). *Introduction to data mining.* Addison-Wesley.

15. Fayyad, U., Piatetsky-Shapiro, G., & Smyth, R. (1996). The KDD process for extracting useful knowledge from volumes of data. *Communications of the ACM, 39,* 27–34.

16. Kuo, M. H., Kushniruk, A. W., & Borycki, E. M. (2011). A comparison of national health data interoperability approaches in Taiwan, Denmark and Canada. *Electronic Healthcare, 10,* 14–25.

17. Kuo, M. H., Kushniruk, A. W., Borycki, E. M., & Greig, D. (2009). Application of the Apriori algorithm for adverse drug reaction detection. *Studies in Health Technology and Informatics, 148*, 95–101.

18. Richesson, R. L. (2012). *Clinical research informatics.* Springer.

19. Cheng, T. H., Wei, C. P., & Tseng, V. S. (2006). Feature selection for medical data mining: comparisons of expert judgment and automatic approaches. *Proceedings of the 19th IEEE Symposium on Computer-Based Medical Systems,* IEEE Computer Society, Washington, DC.

20. Balasubramanian, T. & Umarani, R. (2012). Clustering as a data mining technique in health hazards of high levels of fluoride in potable water. *International Journal of Advanced Computer Sciences and Applications, 392*, 166–171.

21. Concaro, S., Sacchi, L., Cerra, C., & Bellazzi R. (2009). Mining administrative and clinical diabetes data with temporal association rules. *Studies in Health Technology and Informatics, 150*, 574–578.

22. Luk, J. M., Lam, B. Y., et al. (2007). Artificial neural networks and decision tree model analysis of liver cancer proteomes. *Biochemical and Biophysical Research Communications, 361*, 68–73.

23. Cao, X., Maloney, K. B., & Brusic, V. (2008). Data mining of cancer vaccine trials: A bird's-eye view. *Immunome Research, 4*.

24. Canlas Jr., R. D. (2009). *Data mining in healthcare: Current applications and issues.* Carnegie Mellon University.

25. Kalish, B. M. (2012). Digging for dollars: Data mining is an evolving tactic that can help reduce health care costs. *Employee Benefit Adviser, 10*, 36.

26. Shillabeer, A. & Roddick, J. (2007). Establishing a lineage for medical knowledge discovery. *ACM International Conference Proceeding Series, 70*, 29–37.

Networks and Networking in Healthcare

Roman Mateyko

In this chapter, you will learn how to
- Explain how telecommunications networks are evolving with the advent of the Internet
- Describe key data networking concepts
- Describe the functions a data network performs using the OSI model of communications
- Describe how data flows in a wired or wireless network
- Describe HL7 and its use in transmitting healthcare data

This chapter is a brief tour through the topic of data networks and their use in healthcare. The topic of data networks is broad, deep, and constantly evolving. Many books have been written about data networks, so the best that a single chapter on the topic can do is give you an appreciation of key concepts, components, and approaches associated with data networks.

Telecommunications and Healthcare

The topic of data networks falls under the more general area of data communications. Data communications has roots in both telecommunications and computer science. Telecommunications is a broad topic area with relevance to healthcare. Doctors, nurses, and patients have been using telephones and telephone networks to talk to each other since the beginning of telephone service. Ambulances have used radio networks to communicate to hospitals to inform them of the state of patients in their care. Television networks have been used to inform citizens about the status of epidemics. The Internet and wireless networks of tomorrow have the potential to radically change the way healthcare is delivered.

From Voice to Data Networks and the Global Internet

For most of the past century, telecommunications was characterized by the emergence of special-purpose networks. First came the telegraph, which used a series of dots and dashes to communicate. Then came the voice network, which for most of the twentieth century was the truly global network. It consisted of end devices—telephones—that were attached by wire to a central office switch. Telephone systems were owned and operated by telephone companies. The voice network was engineered to transport voice conversations. Then came radio networks, which eliminated the need to run wire, made it possible to broadcast information to the masses, and made it possible to communicate with an ambulance rushing a patient to a hospital. Radio networks were then followed by television broadcast networks, which added the dimension of moving images to sound transmission. These networks had television sets as end devices connected to a cable head end. In the last third of the twentieth century, data networks emerged. Some were public, and some were private. They were controlled by enterprises, academic institutions, governments, and common carriers, and these networks transported data. Finally, cellular networks appeared. They made it possible for subscribers to place a voice call to anybody, anywhere and anytime, and then to check their e-mail on handheld devices such as the iPhone. Each of these networks had a specific function, but they presented a challenge to the providers of those networks in that they were independent networks, created especially for the traffic they carried and costly to manage on an individual basis.

The holy grail of the telecommunications industry has been the integration of these different networks into one. This has been attempted a number of times in the context of new technologies such as the Integrated Services Digital Network (ISDN) in the 1980s and then the Broadband Integrated Services Digital Network (BISDN) in the early 1990s; neither succeeded in totality. But then the Internet emerged to become the global network. Technological advances in the last 20 years have made it possible to carry data, voice, and video traffic over the Internet and over networks based on Internet technologies. It looks like the Internet will be the single network that carries it all.

Today different networks exist in the typical hospital setting: voice networks, pager networks, Wi-Fi networks, hardwired LANs, ambulance radio networks, Bluetooth body monitoring networks, the Internet, and cellular networks. Each network has to be considered individually when it comes to planning, implementing, and operating, and these networks have to interoperate, which is sometimes a technical challenge. Healthcare will benefit greatly when the businesses needs that these separate networks fulfill can be accomplished using the Internet.

A single chapter cannot do the topic of data networks justice. However, since convergence will one day mean that Internet-type networks will carry all types of traffic (data, voice, and image) and interconnect all types of devices, then the focus of this chapter on Internet type networks will give you the fundamentals you need to understand communications in the healthcare setting.

Data Communications Concepts

This section deals with the fundamental communications concepts that are key to understanding why healthcare networks are built the way they are and how they work.

Connectivity: The Geometrical Nature of Networks

Data networks make it possible for people or machines to communicate with each other, and these networks do it in the most efficient way possible. This efficiency is achieved by using technology and by making intelligent trade-offs.

Figure 35-1 shows how the number of connections increases as the number of end-points of a network grows. The relationship is geometric ($\sim n^2/2$). What this tells you is that it takes a lot of connections to make sure that many people or things can talk to each other in a network. And if you think about it, the maximum number of simultaneous conversations that you can have is n/2. (If you have an odd number of end points, then it is $(n-1)/2$, which means in the case of an even number of connections that $n^2/2-n$ connections are dormant.) If you were to use copper wires to connect these endpoints, you would be wasting a lot of copper, and that was what happened in the early days of telephony until innovations such as the switch board and telephone switch were invented.

Figure 35-2 shows what happens when humans apply technology. The many connections are replaced with N connections into a box or piece of technology that magically ensures each end node can talk to any other end node. At one point in time, in voice networks, the stuff in the box was a set of relays and gears that connected one telephone to another, and the box was called a *mechanical central office switch*. Today the stuff is a special-purpose computer built of silicon chips running a software program called a *router*, or *switch*, that routes messages from one end node to another or to a

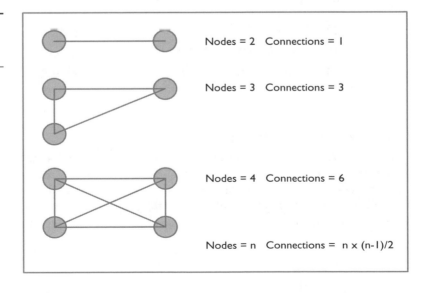

Figure 35-1
The connectivity problem

Nodes = 2   Connections = 1

Nodes = 3   Connections = 3

Nodes = 4   Connections = 6

Nodes = n   Connections = n x (n-1)/2

Figure 35-2
Technology
applied to the
connectivity
problem

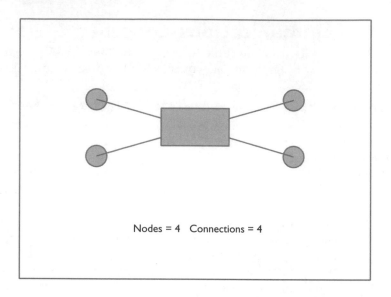

Nodes = 4   Connections = 4

network of these devices, also called the Internet, that routes messages globally. The efficiency that the technology in the box provides is traded off against the possibility that if too many messages are being sent through this box or combinations of boxes, some of them will be dropped; thus, the system has limited capacity, and that limited capacity is usually statistical in nature.

Exercise 35-1: Plotting Connectivity

Plot the equation n*(n–1)/2 in a spreadsheet to see how the number of connections increases and compare the two approaches.

1. In column A of the spreadsheet, put the numbers 1-25.

2. In column B, put the equation n*(n–1)/2.

3. In column C, put the equation N/2. Chart these to see the relationship. You can either ignore the odd numbers or use the equation (n–1)/2.

Communication Models

Data networks originated as the need for computers to exchange information arose. In the case of the early Internet, universities needed to interconnect their computers to share research data. In the case of private data networks built by corporations and healthcare organizations in the latter part of the past century, these organizations needed a way to interconnect computers and users to computers supplied to them by computer manufacturers such as International Business Machine (IBM) and Digital Equipment Corporation (DEC). These computer manufacturers developed their own data network technologies and sold them alongside their computers. The problem occurred when information had to be shared across two or more data networks that were based on different computer manufacturers' technology. For example, two hospitals, each having data networks based on different computer manufacturers' technology, needing to exchange patient data would either have to somehow custom interconnect their networks or have to perform the exchange manually.

The computer community recognized this as a problem and developed two models of computer communications to solve it. These models defined a set of standards that described the functions of modern data communication systems; these models were the Open System Interconnect (OSI) seven-layer model (also called the *OSI stack*) and the Internet five-layer model. The OSI model was a product of the International Standards Organization (ISO) standardization process. The OSI model, though widely accepted, was never fully implemented because of the popular emergence of the Internet. The OSI model is used today in a theoretical way and is part of jargon used by network professionals. Figure 35-3 shows the two models side by side. The Internet model is implemented by the global Internet and by networks based on Internet technologies.[1]

In both models, data in digital form (binary 1s and 0s) sent from an application residing in a transmitting device is passed down from the topmost layer—the application layer, which is the layer that interacts with a human—and is then encapsulated with control information from the layer below it until it reaches the physical layer where the binary 1s and 0s are turned into a physical representation—a pulse of light or electricity. Other than the physical layer, the functions of the other six layers are implemented in software. This process is then performed in reverse in a receiving device until it gets to the human at the application layer at the other end. In the model, the layer below performs a service to the layer above it. Each layer in the transmitter is said to have a virtual connection with each layer in the receiver, other than the physical layer, which has a physical connection. What follows is a brief description of each layer.

Figure 35-3

Comparison of OSI and Internet communications models

OSI Layer	Internet Layer
Application	Application
Presentation	
Session	
Transport	Transport
Network	Network
Data Link	Data Link
Physical	Physical

Physical Layer

Layer 1, or the physical layer, is responsible for converting the logical 1s and 0s coming from layer 2 into some type of physical signal such as a burst of electrons (voltages) or photons (light pulses).

Data Link Layer

Layer 2, or the data link layer, is responsible for controlling when a device should transmit (also known as *media access*), delimiting the message boundaries of the continuous string of 1s and 0s coming from layer 1 into packets, and ensuring that the transmission is error free by detecting and sometimes correcting errors.

Network Layer

Layer 3, or the network layer, is responsible for routing messages along the best route possible by building routing tables and assigning network addresses to devices attached to the network.

Transport Layer

Layer 4, or the transport layer, is responsible for error checking; flow control; sequencing packets; establishing, maintaining, and terminating conversations; and packetizing larger messages into smaller messages.

Session Layer

Layer 5, or the session layer, is responsible for initiating, managing, and terminating a communication session; initiating any adjunct services such as logging onto devices, file transfer, or security; and recovering from transport layer interruptions.

Presentation Layer

Layer 6, or the presentation layer, is responsible for displaying, formatting, and editing inputs and outputs (from the application layer). This layer makes it possible to display the same data on different terminal types. This layer may also be responsible for encryption.

Application Layer

Layer 7, or the application layer, is the interface between the human using the network and the network. A suite of applications exist at this layer such as HTTP (also called the Web), e-mail, the Domain Name System (DNS), and File Transfer Protocol (FTP).

Communications Protocols

Communications protocols define messages, message formats, and the rules for exchanging those messages between computers and communication devices. Imagine two computers communicating with each other, and associated with each computer is the seven-layer OSI model. As mentioned, each layer in one computer communicates virtually with each layer in the other computer according to a communications protocol.

Figure 35-4 shows the message format of a generic protocol data unit (PDU). A PDU is associated with a communications protocol. The information in the PDU is represented by 1s and 0s. Other than the physical layer, each layer in the OSI model has a PDU associated with it.

NOTE Network professionals commonly call the data link PDU a *frame* and the network PDU a *packet*.

Each portion of the PDU is called a *field* and has a specific role. The two delimiters at each end of the PDU tell the system where the PDU starts and stops. Delimiters are analogous to capital letters and periods in a sentence. The destination address tells the system where the PDU is going, and the source address tells the system where the PDU has come from. The control information field carries in it codes that tell the system what to do. For example, one of those codes could signify that a transmitter wants to start a conversation with a receiver in a similar way that the alert tone on a cellular phone alerts a caller to an incoming call. The payload carries the message that is being transmitted. In the OSI model, the payload is usually the PDU from the layer above it. Examples of the types of messages that could be transmitted in the payload at the application layer in a healthcare setting include information about a patient's medication, a transmission of a medical image, or real-time data coming from a patient-monitoring device such as a heart rate monitor. The payload could also contain HL7 information as described in the previous section of this chapter. Finally, the error check field is a type of quality control on the frame. The transmitter performs an algorithm that mathematically relates the information in the transmitted PDU to the error check field. The receiver performs that algorithm on the received PDU and then checks to see whether the value it calculated is the same as that sent in the error check field. If it is not, the same PDU is said to be in error, and some type of error correction is invoked such as retransmitting the PDU.

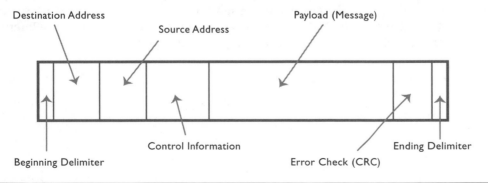

Figure 35-4 Generic PDU

Data and Signals

In computer systems, information and data are represented as 1s and 0s; this is a logical representation. This is also true of all the layers of the OSI model except for the physical layer. At the physical layer, the logical 1s and 0s become something that is real or physical, such as a burst of electrons or photons. The presence or absence of these bursts can signify a 1 or a 0. A chart of the amplitude or power of these bursts over time is referred to as a *signal*.

Figure 35-5 shows two signal types. The first is a sine wave, and the second is a pulse signal; 1s and 0s can be encoded in sine waves by varying amplitude, frequency, and phase. In pulse signals, a 1 can be represented by the presence or absence of a pulse.

Information is transmitted through a network when these signals representing 1s and 0s travel through wires, fibers, and by radio propagation; each is considered a different transmission media. Each type of media has its own physical characteristics that affect those signals. Two such key characteristics are susceptibility to noise and maximum capacity, also called *bandwidth*.

Susceptibility to noise relates to how easily external signals not associated with the transmitted signal can get induced into the media and thus distort the transmitted signal. This distortion leads to errors. In the case of the pulse signal, there may be a spike of noise that causes an empty spot where there is no signal to look like a pulse. The receiver then interprets that noise burst as a 1 that is not what the receiver sent and is therefore an error. Maximum capacity relates to how much information transmission media can carry. For example fiber optic media can carry much more information than can copper media and a coaxial cable can carry more information than a 26-gauge telephone cable.

Digitization

Digitization is the process of representing something like an image or sound using discrete samples and then being able to reconstruct it with a certain level of fidelity. Sampling of music and then storing those samples as binary digits on a plastic disc is how music is distributed using CDs. A similar thing is done with medical imaging associated with picture archival and communication systems. Binary digits or 1s and 0s are the same things that data networks transport. Given that images and voice signals can be sampled, those samples can be carried by data networks. This is how the Internet will become the single network carrying data, voice, and video traffic.

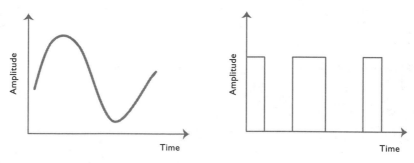

Figure 35-5 Examples of signals

Throughput

A measure of how much data can be moved through a network successfully is called *throughput*. Throughput is measured in bits per second. Usually people will use the term *bandwidth* and state it in terms of bits per second. In data networks, throughput can be affected by many things; one of those is the capacity of the transmission medium that places an upper limit on throughput. Another is the latency through the network. Latency is often the result of how digital signals are transmitted and processed by hardware and software in devices that make up the network. For example, as a packet encounters a router in its path across the network, it is read into the receive buffer of a router, analyzed, and put out onto the transmit buffer of that router. Every time this happens, a small delay is added to the packet's journey. For a given amount of information transmitted, the longer it takes to transmit that information because of all these delays, the lower the throughput.

Addressing in Data Networks

If one device, the transmitter, wants to send information to another device, the receiver, it must know where to send that information. That means the receiver must have some type of identifier that distinguishes it from other, possibly similar receivers on the network. That identifier is usually called an *address*. In TCP/IP networks there are four types of addresses to consider.

MAC Addresses

Media Access Control (MAC) addresses exist at the data link layer. They are usually depicted as six groups of two hexadecimal numbers and are 48 bits long; see Figure 35-6. They exist in hardware, are assigned by device manufacturers, and are therefore fixed. They are also referred to as *Ethernet addresses* since they are what appear in the source and destination address field of Ethernet PDUs.

IP Addresses

IP addresses exist at the network layer. They are depicted as four groups of up to three decimal numbers separated by dots and are 32 bits long; see Figure 35-6. They exist in the software configuration of a network device and are either assigned manually by an administrator or assigned through a process called Dynamic Host Configuration Protocol (DHCP). These addresses are also broken down into the network part and host part, the delineation depending on the class of address.

Currently IP version 4 addresses exist in the global Internet. IP version 6 addresses are now being introduced and should supplant IP version 4 addresses in time. IP version 6 addresses contain 128 bits and therefore have a much greater address space than their IP version 4 counterparts. The world's adoption of IP version 6 addresses will become critical because the IP version 4 address space is just about exhausted.

IP addresses are sometimes associated with subnet masks; see Figure 35-6. Subnet masks are a pattern of 1s and 0s that subdivide a range of IP addresses for routing and administrative purposes.

Figure 35-6
Sample network
addresses

Address Type	Example
Datalink (Ethernet)	07-13-54-ac-76-cc
Network Layer (IP Address)	143.56.98.101
Subnet Mask	255.255.255.192
Port Address	80 (Web Browsers)
Hostname (Web)	www.somename.com

IP addresses are assigned to organizations by the Internet Corporation for Assigned Names and Numbers (ICANN).

IP addresses can be either dynamically assigned (i.e., each time a client logs in, a different IP address gets assigned), or they can be static (i.e., a client has a fixed or constant IP address assigned by a network administrator). Servers using DHCP grant IP addresses to clients dynamically and for a limited time interval. DHCP is used to obtain configuration information, including an IP address. Two advantages of dynamic IP addressing are that there are fewer risks for security (because a new IP address is generated for each login), and that network configuration is automatic so it does not require an administrator. However, static IP addressing can be a more reliable way to ensure secure access to files stored on an organization's network computers.

Transport Control Protocol (Layer 4) Port Addresses

Port addresses exist in layer 4 of the TCP/IP communications model. These port addresses are 16 bits long, and each port address is uniquely associated with an application. Port addresses 0 through 1023 are considered well-known ports, and the remaining port addresses are available for dynamic assignment. For example, web browsers use port address 80, and mail applications use port address 25. When an application is transmitting a message, it identifies to the TCP software which source port address it is sending from and which destination port address it is sending to. The TCP software then puts these in the source and destination fields of the layer 4 PDU it builds.[1]

Hostname

Hostname addresses exist at the application layer. They are usually depicted as a group of letters separated by dots. The letters usually form meaningful words such as www .google.com; see Figure 35-6. Hostnames reside in software in the host and also in Domain Name System servers. DNSs are databases that relate IP addresses to hostnames for the purpose of address resolution. DNSs form a domain name system; somewhat like the white pages, they relate human-friendly names to computer-understandable names, which are the addresses. ICANN manages the Internet domain system and authorizes private companies to assign domain names.

Address Resolution

Address resolution occurs at various levels when a sender is transmitting a message to a receiver. For example, when a user clicks a link in a web browser (the sender), a browser request message is sent to a web server (the receiver). That request is eventually placed into a packet at layer 3; however, that packet needs a destination IP address. That IP address is supplied by resolving that hostname through the Domain Name System to an associated IP address. That IP address is then placed in the destination field of the IP packet and sent into the network. At the other end, as that packet emerges on the LAN to which the web server (the receiver) is attached, the packet is placed in a data link frame, which needs a MAC destination address in order for it to arrive successfully. This MAC address is resolved to the IP address through the Address Resolution Protocol (ARP).

To determine what MAC address is associated with the destination IP address, the device sends a broadcast message to the LAN with the destination IP address in its payload. All the devices on the LAN receive that message, but only the device whose IP address matches replies. This reply has the MAC address of the replying device embedded in it. This MAC address is then used as the destination address for the data link frame, which transports the web request to the server.

End devices have caches that store these address resolutions temporarily. For example, a workstation will have a DNS cache and an ARP cache.

The World Wide Web as an Example of a Network Application

The World Wide Web (WWW) is one of the most popular network applications in use today and is increasingly used for transmitting healthcare data. It is an example of a client-server architecture where the client is a web browser such as Firefox and the server is a web server running a program such as Apache. The presentation and descriptive markup language that is used to generate web pages is HyperText Markup Language (HTML). The protocol used by the client to request a web page and by the server to respond to that request is HyperText Transfer Protocol (HTTP). The addressing mechanism that is used to locate a web page is called a *universal resource locator* (URL).

HTTP is a textual protocol that defines the rules and format for message exchange. For example, HTTP defines a request command that is used to request information from a server. The PDU for this command has a request line, a request header, and a request body. HTTP is an application protocol using the underlying services of TCP. When a link is clicked in a browser, it opens a TCP session with the host identified in the URL and sends that request via port 80 of the TCP PDU. The URL identifies the protocol (HTTP, FTP, or HTTPS) in use, the network location (host and port), and the path name to the data object on the server. The server then responds with an HTTP response. The PDU for a response is composed of a response status field, a response header, and the response body that contains the web page the client requested.[2]

PANs, LANs, MANs, and WANs

Data networks can be categorized according to physical extent, anywhere from centimeters to kilometers. The range of a given data network often dictates the type of underlying technology used and the design of the communications protocol that is needed. The way TCP/IP networks are designed is that the network and transport layers or TCP/IP are abstracted from the lower layers. Thus, TCP/IP rides on top of the two lowest layers and provides an end-to-end service for devices attached to the network.

PANs

Personal area networks (PANs) span the human body and the area near the human body. The communications technologies used here are typically Wi-Fi and Bluetooth, which are wireless technologies. The technology used includes network interface cards (NICs) which provide wireless interfaces for devices such as laptops, heart rate monitors, and tablets. The management of these networks usually falls to a healthcare unit in the organization where staff members evaluate, select, purchase, deploy, and provide operational support for these devices.

LANs

Local area networks (LANs) span rooms or buildings. Here wireless transmission and wired transmission are used. The communications technologies employed are typically Wi-Fi and Ethernet, also known as IEEE 802.3. The equipment includes NICs, hubs, switches, wireless access points, and file and print servers. Here again, the deployment model is usually local with the organization's staff evaluating, selecting, purchasing, deploying, and providing operational support for these devices.

MANs

Metropolitan area networks (MANs) are on the order of city blocks and urban areas. Again, wireless and wired technologies are used. Examples for physical transport include 26-gauge copper telephone wire, cable plant, short-haul fiber optic, point-to-point microwave, and cellular networks. The communications technologies include Ethernet, ADSL, LTE, and WiMAX. Small ISPs, local carriers, and regional carriers tend to provide services at this level. Organizational staff manages contracts and service levels with suppliers of these services and interconnect their managed network infrastructure (PANs and LANs) to these networks.

WANs

Wide area networks (WANS) are on the order of large cities, province and states, and countries. Wireless and wired technologies are used as transport. Examples of transport technologies include point-to-point long-haul microwave, long-haul fiber systems, and satellites. Communications technologies include wide area Ethernet over fiber, wave length division multiplexing (WDM), legacy carrier technologies such as Asynchronous Transfer Mode (ATM), Optical Carrier (OC), and Time Division Multiplexing (TDM). Regional and national carriers operate at this level. Organizational staff manages contracts and service levels with suppliers of this service and interconnect their managed network infrastructure to these networks.

The foregoing categories of networks can create a context for the reader to think about how healthcare information is communicated in the healthcare system. For example, monitoring devices on a patient can be continuously sending data via a PAN that connects to a device in the LAN. As the patient moves through a hospital, those monitoring devices connect and reconnect to various LANs that exist in that hospital. The application that analyzes that data may be running on a server located across the city from the hospital, and thus the data is gathered and then sent via a MAN to that server to be processed. The analysis of that real-time patient data may trigger a need for the patient to undergo a diagnosis by a specialist who is located in another city. That specialist and the patient would use a WAN to set up and use a video-conferencing system to perform that diagnosis.

How a Network Works

This section will describe how a typical TCP/IP network works. It will discuss application and network architectures and describe the components used to implement those architectures and the protocols used. It will also describe two examples of data transfer: one device communicating with another device on the same LAN and one device communicating with another device on another LAN across a WAN.[1]

Application Architectures

Two fundamental application architectures exist on a network: peer to peer and client server. In a peer-to-peer architecture, all devices on a network are equal and can perform the same function; there is no master. A peer-to-peer model works well when there are a limited number of users and has the advantage of being simple but the disadvantage of not being scalable. Also, the traffic pattern on peer-to-peer networks is random because any device may be talking to any other device. An example of a peer-to-peer application is instant messaging (IM). The first example later in this section (see Figure 35-7) will follow the data flow between two workstations (W1 and W2) exchanging an IM message on LAN1.

In client-server architecture, there are many clients and one server. That server performs a set of centralized functions for those clients. An example of client server architecture is the Web. A web server has multiple web browsers or clients sending requests to it for web pages. It acts like a file server in that it is a central store of web pages. The client and server do not need to be on the same LAN; they just need to be connected to the network, as shown in Figure 35-7. A client-server model has the advantage of being able to scale and provide greater control but the disadvantage of unnecessary overhead for small scale. The second example later in this section will follow the data flow from a web browser to a web server. Here workstation W1, which is the client and is running a web browser, sends HTTP requests to server S2, the server, through LAN1 and across the WAN and then through to LAN2 (also shown in Figure 35-7).

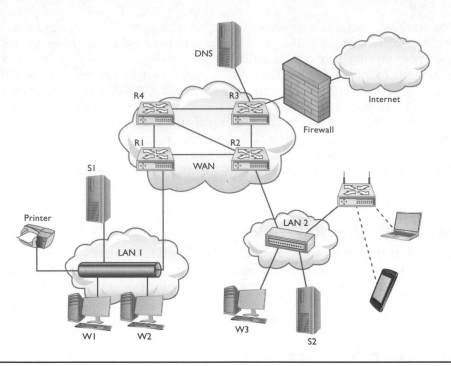

Figure 35-7 How a network works

Network Architectures and Implementations

Network architectures vary according to the needs of the network. Networks used for healthcare purposes are different from networks used for business purposes. The architecture associated with Figure 35-7 is a simplified version of a WAN architecture, which is one that you may find in a healthcare setting.

Wide Area Network

The network in Figure 35-7 shows an implementation of a typical network architecture. There is a WAN that interconnects two LANs (LAN1 and LAN2) and then interconnects both to the Internet. A MAN or backbone network could serve the same function as the WAN in the diagram except that it would have different geographic scope and use different technology. The WAN in Figure 35-7 consists of routers interconnected with communication circuits. Routers move messages (PDUs) according to a set of instructions that each has, called a *routing table*. Routing tables are dynamically built using routing protocols. These routing protocols are software programs that optimize the path that messages take by analyzing changes occurring in the network such as addition or deletion of networks or circuits, the utilization of circuits, and latency across circuits. Common routing protocols include Routing Internet Protocol (RIP) and Open Shortest Path First (OSPF). Routers are said to implement layers 1 to 3 of the OSI stack.

There are two more connections pictured in Figure 35-7, one to the Internet and one to a domain name server. Most modern networks connect to the Internet, and they usually do this using a special routing protocol called Border Gateway Protocol, whose job it is to make the rest of the Internet aware of the existence of the network by advertising its IP addresses. A firewall is also positioned between the Internet and the network. The firewall protects the network by filtering out unwanted traffic. The job of the domain name server is to resolve hostnames to IP addresses for this network.

 NOTE Domain name servers are part of a globally interconnected hierarchical network that stores and distributes all hostname and IP address pairs.

Local Area Network

The purpose of a LAN is to interconnect a set of devices that are within physical proximity. A LAN makes it possible for users to share resources such as print, file, and fax servers. Attached to the WAN in Figure 35-7 are two LANs depicting two different architectures. LAN1 shows a bus architecture, and LAN2 shows a star architecture. These are physical architectures. The bus architecture of LAN1 is rarely used today. This architecture was implemented using a single coax cable that attached to each device. LAN2, the physical star, is the way most LAN topologies are implemented today where wires spread out from a central switch to all devices. Also attached to router R2, via the central switch, is a wireless access point, which shows how a wireless network could overlay a wired network.

From a network perspective, LANs are seen as broadcast domains where broadcasts of layer 2 PDUs or frames are generated by one device wanting to communicate with another device on the LAN. Although LAN1 and LAN2 differ at the physical layer, they function similarly at the data link layer. Broadcasts are characteristic of most LAN protocols and in particular of the widely adopted Ethernet protocol (802.3), which uses Carrier Sense Multiple Access with Collision Detection (CSMA/CD). In Ethernet, there are a set of devices connected to a common infrastructure such as a shared coaxial cable or the backplane of a hub or switch. If one device wants to transmit to another device, it enters the MAC address of that device in a frame and then transmits that frame bit by bit onto the communications medium. All devices receive that broadcast frame, but only the device to which it is addressed recognizes it and then "reads" it in; other devices on the LAN ignore the broadcast. Because the transmitter is transmitting the frame, it also listens for any corrupted transmissions. If it detects one, it stops its own transmission and assumes another transmitter tried to transmit at the same time, which caused the collision. If there are no collisions, the receiver takes the frame and passes it up the OSI stack until it gets to the application layer where the message is delivered to the application. If there is a collision, each device that was trying to transmit simultaneously waits a different amount of time, the duration of which is determined randomly, and then the devices retry their transmissions.

Attachments to the LAN include end devices such as workstations, printers, servers, hubs, switches, and routers. To participate in the LAN, each device needs a network interface card and, in the case of a wired LAN, a cable attaching it to a hub or switch. End devices such as workstations and servers implement the complete OSI stack. They also run application-layer software, which in the example is instant messaging client software. Alternatively, a user at W1 may be sending messages to a web server such as the server S2 in LAN2. Both these are done at the application layer. Those messages, however, are sent down the stack to each layer and to the physical layer where pulses of electricity or light emanate from the interface across the network, and then the inverse process occurs at W2 or at the server. In contrast, devices such as routers are said to communicate at the bottom three layers of the OSI stack. For example, W3 and the server will be communicating to the switch at layer 2 and below.

LANs provide the same function in a healthcare setting except in addition to workstations, servers, and printers, there could be health-specific devices, such as patient monitors, infusion pumps, and ventilators, attached to the LAN. Note that healthcare LANs have unique requirements such as needing to be robust and secure. They must be robust because missing patient data, especially real-time monitoring data, can affect patient safety. They must be secure because of the privacy requirements associated with patient data.[3]

Device Configuration

Before an end device can start communicating, it must be configured. This configuration can happen either manually or automatically. The manual method involves having a network administer configure the device or provide information for the user to do so. The automatic method involves using the Dynamic Host Configuration Protocol (DHCP). In either case, the following minimal information is configured on an end device: its IP address, a subnet mask, the IP address of its DNS server, and the IP address of the LAN gateway. Routers R1 and R2 are also called *gateway routers* because they are the gateway out of the LAN onto the bigger network. The address of the DNS server is needed to decode the hostname into an IP address. The subnet mask is used by the device to discern whether the destination address of a PDU it is sending resides on the local LAN. If not, then the PDU is forwarded to the gateway. The combination of IP address and subnet makes it possible for the device to determine whether it should be sending information to the gateway on the LAN for which it has the IP address.

 NOTE The end device already knows its MAC address because it is assigned by the equipment manufacturer and exists in hardware.

An End-to-End Network

The application layers of two devices that are communicating across a network are abstracted from that network. The complexity of the underlying network is hidden from them. The sending application and device usually determine the location of the destination application and device based on resolving a hostname to an IP address. Knowing that IP address and the port to which the application wants to connect (destination port address), the sending device software sets up a circuit that connects it virtually to the destination device. Then the reverse occurs, and a bidirectional communication channel is established between the two applications at both ends of the network. Neither device knows there may be LANs, WANs switches, and routers in the path. Furthermore, TCP ensures a reliable transmission by having the transmitter resend PDUs that the receiver detects are in error. This mode of communication is also known as *connection-oriented communications*.

> **NOTE** You should understand that this is a highly simplified explanation of the mechanism of transmission and error recovery; much detail has been omitted.

Ping is a useful network administration utility that can be used to check whether a host can be reached on an Internet Protocol (IP) network. It can also be used to assess how long it takes for messages to be sent from an originating host computer to a computer receiving the messages. Another useful TCP/IP utility is Tracert, also known as "Traceroute". Tracert is a Microsoft Windows command-line tool that can be used to find the route of packets of information moving through a network to reach a host. By tracing the path of messages, tracert can be used to test and troubleshoot problems in networking.

Use Case 35-1: A Device Communicating with Another Device on the Same LAN

In this example, device W1 will be sending an instant message to device W2 (see Figure 35-7). Let's assume that W1 has already resolved W2's IP address through a previous DNS request. (Note that W1 would have used the DNS's IP address that is stored in its configuration to reach the DNS to resolve W2's IP address.) Upon creation of the message by the user, the IM software tells the TCP layer which destination port address to use. The destination port field, source port field, and other fields of the TCP PDU including the payload where the IM message resides are filled in. The TCP PDU is then moved to the network layer where it is encapsulated with layer 3 information such as W2's IP address as the destination address and W1's IP address as the source address. Layer 3 checks the destination address against the gateway address and the subnet mask and determines that the IP address is on LAN1. This layer 3 PDU is then handed down to layer 2 and encapsulated with layer 2 information. The software searches for W2's IP address in its ARP cache; if it finds it, it places W2's MAC address in the destination field. If not, it does an ARP as described in the previous section and places W2's MAC address in the destination field. Finally, it places its own MAC address in the source field.

The data link then broadcasts the layer 2 PDU to all devices attached to the LAN and, assuming there is no collision, W2's layer 2 software recognizes its MAC address and stores W1's PDU in its input buffer. The other devices on the LAN disregard this PDU since the destination MAC address does not match their MAC address. W2's data link then discards the layer 2 information and sends the layer 3 PDU up to the network layer. Similarly W2's layer 3 software passes the layer 4 PDU up to layer 4. Layer 4 checks to see whether there were any errors and, if not, inspects the destination port address and passes the payload to the IM software, which passes it onto the user at the application layer.

Use Case 35-2: A Device Communicating with Another Device on Another LAN Across a WAN

In this example, W1 will be sending an HTTP request to the web server S2 on LAN2 (see Figure 35-7). The user on W1 enters a URL with S2's domain name in it. Let's assume W1 has made a similar HTTP request previously and holds S2's hostname and IP address in its DNS cache. The HTTP request is formed and sent to W1's layer 4 with the destination port of 80. The layer 4 PDU is formed and placed in the layer 3 PDU's payload along with the S2's IP address as the destination address. Layer 3 then uses the subnet mask to compare the PDU's destination address with the gateway IP address stored in its configuration. It determines that the PDU's destination address is not on the local LAN. Knowing this, the software places the PDU in a layer 2 frame, which has the gateway's (R1) MAC address set as the destination address. (If W1 didn't have the gateway MAC address in its cache, it would issue an ARP to determine it.) W1's datalink then transmits the layer 2 PDU, which finds its way to the gateway router R1.

The software in router R1 removes the layer 3 PDU from the layer 2 PDU payload and discards the rest of the layer 2 PDU. Whereas layer 2 is responsible for ensuring that one device can communicate to another device on a LAN, layer 3 is responsible for determining the best path a given PDU will take to traverse the network. Referring to the diagram, a PDU starting out on R1 can take any number of paths to get to LAN2: R1-R4-R3-R2, R1-R2, or R1-R4-R2. Unlike what happens at layer 2, routers do not broadcast PDUs at layer 3; they route PDUs, and they do this based on information they have stored in routing tables. Thus, router R1 processes the layer 3 PDU by inspecting its destination IP address and matches it with a routing table entry and determines which of the many paths it should take.

When that determination is made, it puts the layer 3 PDU back in a layer 2 PDU payload and sends it on one of the two ports associated with the three paths leaving router R1. Let's assume that path R1-R2 is the path chosen. The PDU then moves along the path from R1 to R2, which could be a WAN circuit such as a fiber-optic channel. It arrives at R2, and R2 repeats the process of discarding the layer 2 information and looks at the destination address of the PDU. According to its routing table, the destination address is on the router port associated with LAN2.

Router R2 then creates a layer 2 PDU with a destination MAC address equal to that of S2's MAC address based on an ARP table lookup using the IP address in the PDU. The layer 3 PDU is placed into the payload of the layer 2 PDU. The layer 2 PDU is then broadcast on LAN2 and received by S2 since it is addressed to S2. S2 then moves the PDU up to the application layer where the web server responds.

 NOTE The network-layer packet or layer 3 PDU that is created at the source is never modified as it moves across the network. In contrast, layer 2 PDUs are created and destroyed.

CompTIA EXAM TIP   A service-level agreement (SLA) is a contract between an Information Technology (IT) service provider and a customer (for example, a hospital) that specifies what services the IT provider will furnish and almost always contains specific measures of the services to be provided. SLAs are commonly used for network service providers or ISPs, and contain such measures as percentage of time services will be available and how many simultaneous users can be served. Information Services (IS) departments in healthcare and other industries have adapted the SLA idea for internal, department-to-department agreements. An internal SLA specifies what the IS department's responsibilities are, primarily around implementing, maintaining, and communicating the status of the IT services. In an internal SLA, the receiving department is also responsible for notifying the IS department (in a manner that is timely, complete, and accurate) of service failures or issues, and then assisting the IS department in the resolution of these failures or issues.

Exercise 35-2: Checking Configuration Information

Query your device for configuration information and relate it to the previous section.

1. If you are running a Windows operating system, you should enter the command-line window and then enter the command **IPCONFIG /ALL**.

2. Then look at the information displayed and pick out the configuration information for your workstation.

3. What is its IP address, subnet mask, gateway address, MAC address, and DNS address? Some clients have other interface information; what is it?

CompTIA EXAM TIP   Many small medical office practices still connect to the Internet via an Internet modem. Some Internet modems connect via an Ethernet network cable, but most now connect via Universal Serial Bus (USB). The Internet modem cable plugs into a router via the WAN or Internet jack. After connecting the cable, the HIT technician should turn the modem off and back on to allow the router to recognize it.

Wireless Networks

The term *wireless networks* can be used in many contexts. For example, you could consider a satellite network a wireless network. However, this chapter is about data networks in healthcare and the wireless networks that are dramatically changing how healthcare is done and that give patients, nurses, and doctors the ability to move around in the work setting. These are Bluetooth, Wi-Fi, and cellular networks. Since the practitioner will likely manage Wi-Fi networks, the focus of this chapter will be primarily on Wi-Fi networks.

The first thing to consider about wireless networks such as Wi-Fi is that they use the electromagnetic spectrum (radio waves) as a medium of transmission, and this medium places limitations on the bandwidth available for transmission. In a given space and at a given frequency band, only one signal can be transmitted; two would interfere with each other. Whereas running these signals in separate cables that are properly shielded will not lead to these signals interfering with each other, radio spectrum is shared, limited, and subject to interference.

The second thing to consider about wireless networks is that they are wireless; they have no cable, there are no connectors, and there are no ports to attach to. That means a user doesn't have to plug into anything or call anybody to provision a port on a network for them; they can connect to the network just by turning their wireless interface card on. This makes it possible for clinicians, doctors, and nurses to move from patient to patient, or from room to room, maintaining a connection with the network. A network can be created in a building almost instantaneously without needing to run cables. But this also means anybody else can connect to the wireless network as well, and if the wireless network extends to the parking lot of the hospital, they don't even have to gain access to the building. Anybody with an air interface can listen to the radio transmission and read what is being transmitted in plain text. This is especially critical in the healthcare setting where the data that is being transported includes primarily patient data, care data, diagnosis, and treatment data. This data has to be kept private. For this reason, wireless networks have to be secured using various techniques such as encrypted transmission.[3]

The third thing to consider about wireless networks is that in the healthcare setting their utility is very evident. They make it possible for doctors to be more productive. For example, when visiting multiple patients on their rounds, they have access to clinical information systems; they don't have to head back and forth to some tethered terminal to get their records. And when they leave the hospital and realize they forgot to do something like order pharmaceuticals for a patient, they can pull over in their cars, turn on their smartphones, and place that order remotely.[3]

Wireless Applications and Issues in a Healthcare Setting

Wireless networks enable a number of healthcare applications including biomedical devices, voice communications, real-time location-based services, guest access, and clinical access. Each of these applications provides benefits to the healthcare systems; however, some create new considerations.

Patients who need to use monitoring devices are no longer tethered by cables; instead, these devices communicate wirelessly and thus enable those patients to be mobile. Patients can have a heart monitor put on in the hospital and then go home, all while having their hearts continuously monitored. The foregoing is a benefit for the patient; however, a new concern is introduced. Unlike the cable where the possibility of having an interruption in the transmission of data is unlikely, a patient leaving a hospital and going home will traverse any number of networks: an 802.11 network in the hospital, a cellular network in the car, and then a Wi-Fi network attached to the Internet at home. As handoffs to each of the different networks occur, the biomedical system has to deal with possible data interruptions and synchronization problems.[3]

Wireless technologies increase health practitioner productivity by enhancing voice communications. They make it possible to immediately contact a doctor through the use of cellular phones or voice-enabled smartphones. They determine the availability of staff through presence technology. They facilitate collaboration through conferencing technologies. However, wireless technologies, which are in the unlicensed band, are susceptible to interference and need to coexist seamlessly with legacy systems such as high-quality voice and nurse call systems.

Wireless technologies enable real-time location services for hospitals. By using 802.11-configured devices or RFID tags, hospitals can locate things such as lost heart rate monitors or staff members who are urgently needed and not responding to their cellular phones.[3]

Guest access (the provision of Internet connectivity to patients or to a patient's associates) makes it possible to connect at a time when it is especially critical to have access to the Internet. Guest access also brings with it a number of considerations: authentication, resource control, logging, and control of access infrastructure.

WLAN Topology

Figure 35-8 shows the typical topology of a WLAN. It is similar to a typical LAN topology except the transmission medium is radio spectrum. It consists of an access point, a radio spectrum, and the wireless NICs that are terminated in end devices. The AP functions as a repeater and a distribution point connecting the end devices via radio spectrum to the wired network. As a repeater, it repeats frames sent by end devices to their destination. Most of the time, the traffic pattern has a star shape moving from the end device through the AP onto the wired network to some destination. Distribution is done via antennas that are attached to the AP. The two basic types of Wi-Fi antenna are omnidirectional and directional. An omnidirectional antenna has a donutlike radiation pattern. A directional antenna's radiation pattern is focused in one direction. With the right combination of antennas on multiple APs, a consistent coverage pattern can be arranged.[1]

802.11 Standards

The 802.11 set of standards define how wireless LANs are to be implemented, their modulation techniques, and their protocols. These standards work in the 2.5GHz band and in the 5GHz band (which is also called the instrument, scientific, and medical

Figure 35-8
WLAN network

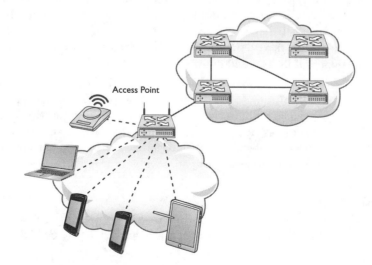

(ISM) band and is an unlicensed band in most countries). Within each band are channels that make it possible to isolate the transmission of multiple APs in the same space. The 2.4GHz band is shared with devices such as microwave ovens, cordless telephones, and Bluetooth, and therefore 802.11b and 802.11g devices that operate in the 2.4GHz band suffer from interference. These standards use direct-sequence spread spectrum (DSSS) and orthogonal frequency-division multiplexing (OFDM) modulation techniques. The media access control mechanism is Carrier Sense Multiple Access with Collision Avoidance (CSMA/CA). Here, rather than sending out a message and sensing if a collision occurred, the transmitter waits for a signal from the AP that it is clear to send a signal before it sends the message.[4]

802.11a

This standard covers wireless WLANs in the 5GHz range. There are eight channels in this frequency range, and each channel runs at 54Mbps. NICs can be located a maximum of 300 feet from the AP. This is a legacy standard and is being supplanted by newer standards.

802.11b

This standard covers WLANs in the 2.4GHz range. There are three channels in this range, with each channel running at 11Mbps. The maximum range is 450 feet. This standard is also being supplanted by newer standards.

802.11g

This standard covers WLANs in the 2.4GHz range. There are three channels in this range, with each channel running at 54Mbps. The maximum range is 300 feet. It is backward compatible with the A and B versions. WLANs based on this standard are commonplace today.

802.11n

This standard covers WLANs in the 2.4GHz range and the 5GHz range. The speed the WLAN can achieve is up to 600Mbps with a range of 450 feet. This standard achieves such high speeds partly because it uses a novel approach to antenna design that takes advantage of multipath propagation. The antennas used in this standard are called *multiple-input multiple-output antennas* (MIMO).

 CompTIA EXAM TIP Wireless site surveys are one approach to use when planning and designing a wireless network. Required wireless coverage ranges, data rates, network capacity, and other factors are taken into account during a site visit. Testing for RF interference, analysis of building floor plans, and other techniques lead to optimum placement of wireless access points.

Security

Unlike wired networks where network access is physical (you need to plug a cable into a port and that port is in a room that has a door that may be locked), wireless networks can be accessed by anyone who is within range of the wireless signal. Therefore, wireless networks need to be secured, especially if they happen to be carrying sensitive patient data. There are different ways of securing wireless networks, and some are more or less secure than others.

Not broadcasting the service set identifier (SSID) is a less secure way of securing a wireless network. To get on the network, the user needs to know the SSID. When the user enters it, upon getting prompted by the system, the user sends it to the AP. What makes it less secure is that the SSID is stored in plain text, which means anybody sniffing the WLAN can get the SSID. Another less secure way of securing the LAN is MAC filtering. When MAC filtering is used, only a specified set of MAC addresses are given access to the network. The reason it is less secure is that a hacker sniffing frames on a wireless network can read a MAC address and then use that MAC address to gain entry into the network.

Wireless Equivalent Privacy (WEP) was the original security mechanism associated with 802.11. It required the user to manually enter a key, which would be used to encrypt transmitted data. Manual key entry limits scale and exposes WLANs to security breaches (keys being stored on sticky notes). Thus, WEP was replaced by Wi-Fi Protected Access (WPA) and then WPA2 (also known as 802.11i). 802.11i uses the Advanced Encryption Standard (AES) and is considered a more secure way of securing wireless LANs.[4,7]

Other security measures that can be considered for healthcare networks include the following:[3,7]

- Antenna and signal gain design that limits the WLAN footprint to the true usage perimeter.

- Policies preventing attachment of wireless devices to the enterprise network.

- Avoiding meaningful names for the WLAN SSID since this provides readily accessible information to hackers.

- Implementing intrusion detection methods on the WLAN. For example, the issuance of multiple incorrect SSID frames could trigger an event.

- Recognizing that the WLAN will always be a less secure network and then treating it as such by isolating it from the core network and placing appropriate safeguards, such as firewalls, between it and the core network.

Bluetooth

Also known as 802.15, Bluetooth covers data exchange over very short distances in the ISM band (2.4GHz to 2.48GHz). It supports fixed and mobile devices and is used in PANs. Bluetooth uses a modulation scheme called *frequency-hopping spread spectrum* (FHSS). Depending on which version of Bluetooth is being used, the data rate varies from 1Mbps to 3Mbps. The protocol used is a master-slave protocol where a master can control up to seven slaves. Examples of devices that use Bluetooth are laptops, wireless phones, iPhones, and GPS. Bluetooth can be used to transmit short-range health sensor data.[1]

WAP, WML, and HTML5

Wireless Application Protocol (WAP) is a standard that describes how browsers and servers communicate with each other over a wireless mobile network and defines an environment for application development. This standard includes a layered architecture similar to the OSI stack where the bottom layer, Wireless Datagram Protocol (WDP), is an adaptation layer to different wireless network technologies. The four layers above the WDP layer are then consistent for all communication devices and provide for interoperability. Figure 35-9 shows these layers. The Wireless Session Protocol is analogous to a stripped-down version of HTTP. The Wireless Application Environment (WAE) originally included the Wireless Markup Language (WML), again analogous to HTML and based on XML.[5]

HTML5, the newest version of the Web's markup language, has as some of its design objectives to support the development of cross-platform mobile applications and to run in low power and small form factor devices such as iPhones and iPads and to support multimedia applications found on these devices.

Figure 35-9 WAP protocol suite[5]		
WAE	Wireless Application Environment
WSP	Wireless Session Protocol
WTP	Wireless Transport Protocol
WTLS	Wireless Transport Layer Security
WDP	Wireless Datagram Protocol
Wireless Data Network Infrastructure	

Cellular

Cellular networks provide users with the ultimate ability to be untethered anywhere, and it is possible that one day they will become the ultimate access method for telecommunications.

LTE

Long-term evolution (LTE) is the newest cellular network standard and has gained global acceptance. The designers of LTE had the following objectives in mind: take advantage of emergent digital signal processing techniques and modulation techniques, and use an IP transport fabric. The upload peak rate of LTE is approximately 75Mbps, and the download peak rate is 300Mbps. The multiplexing techniques used are frequency division duplexing and time division duplexing. Voice can be carried on the LTE networks using Voice over IP technologies, but there are also hybrid methods available to carry voice. LTE has a low data transfer latency of 5 milliseconds. LTE can support cell sizes that range from 10 meters up to 100 kilometers. There is backward compatibility with previous cellular systems.[6]

Transmission of Healthcare Data (HL7)

In this final section of the chapter, I will describe HL7, which is both a standards organization and a standard. The "L7" in HL7 refers to layer or level 7 of the OSI stack and relates to the healthcare applications that reside at the application layer.

According to www.hl7.org, "Founded in 1987, Health Level Seven International (HL7) is a not-for-profit, ANSI-accredited standards developing organization dedicated to providing a comprehensive framework and related standards for the exchange, integration, sharing, and retrieval of electronic health information that supports clinical practice and the management, delivery and evaluation of health services. HL7's 2,300+ members include approximately 500 corporate members who represent more than 90% of the information systems vendors serving healthcare."[10]

HL7 is a framework for exchanging data in healthcare and was a response to the costs associated with writing interfaces for the growing number of healthcare applications. Since the nature of healthcare applications is that they are unique, each interface is therefore different. That means for a given application a developer needs to write an interface for every other application that the application will interface with. With HL7, a developer just needs to follow the standard for message exchange and knows that the application will interface with any other application that follows the HL7 standard.

There are two versions of the HL7 standard in existence today: HL7 v2 and HL7 v3. HL7 version 3 is an improvement over HL7 v2 since the people who defined it had the advantage of seeing what worked and didn't work for HL7 v2. They also had the advantage of incorporating innovations in computing methodologies, best practices, and technological innovation such as XML in the intervening time between the HL7 v2 release and the start of HL7 v3's development. Having said that, the majority of HL7 implementations today are according to HL7 v2, and there are two reasons for this. The first is that HL7 v2 was around for ten years, and it captured the initial investments in application development at that time. Second, one of the objectives of HL7 V2 was to have high adoption rates, and to do that, the designers purposely left about 20 percent of the standard flexible. Furthermore, HL7 v2 was focused on clinical interfaces and applications, whereas HL7 v3 is focused on medical informatics.[9]

Many of the functions and business processes in healthcare lend themselves to automation. This includes exchanging data between various suborganizations and systems within hospitals, between various political entities such as governments, and for use in health informatics. HL7 tries to standardize what are essentially unique healthcare models for hospitals, clinics, and labs. The value of HL7 comes from the network effect; the more people who use it, the greater its value becomes; and the greater its value becomes, the more people who use it. As the number of applications that use HL7 increases, the motivation for those applications that have not yet adopted it, to adopt it, increases.[9]

HL7 v2

Development on HL7 v2 began in 1987. Its design reflects the healthcare information concerns of the time, which were admissions, discharges, transfers, orders, and reports, and the design of HL7v2 reflects this. HL7 v2 is also a flexible standard, meaning it can be added to over time, and this is why a key design principle of HL7 v2 is its backward compatibility.

The key HL7 v2 design concepts are message syntax, segment structure, fields, delimiters, data types, and vocabulary. In HL7 v2, messages are triggered by events. There are different message types, and each message is composed of segments. Each segment has a three-character identifier that comes first, followed by fields, which contain components and subcomponents. Delimiters separate these components and subcomponents. An example of a message type is the ORM message. ORM stands for an order message. Examples of delimiters include the field separator (|) and the component separator (^). Each segment has a definition table.[8]

The patient identifier (PID) segment is a very common segment across message types. It has a number of components, such as PID-5 (patient name) and PID-7 (date/time of birth). For example, a patient name would be represented as |john^doe|. Another example of a segment is the AL1 (allergy) segment, which contains information about patient allergy information, including codes for allergy type and severity. The BLG segment contains information about billing, such as the charge type, when to charge, and the reason for the charge. The IN1 (insurance) segment contains information about insurance policy coverage, for example, insurance plan and company ID. The MSH (message header) segment is contained in every HL7 message, and contains the source of the message, its purpose, and its destination. The OBR (observation request) segment contains information about exams, diagnostic studies, and observations and assessments specific to a result or order. As a final example, the SCH (schedule activity information) segment contains information about scheduled appointments. The Z segment is a special segment that enables developers to create their own segments, thereby allowing flexibility for "local" extensions to HL7 v2.

Segments contain fields. An example of a field within a segment is the Healthcare Provider Type Code field, which contains information to identify what type of provider cared for a patient. This field can be contained in an HL7 message within various segments, for example, the BLG segment. HL7 recommends using the Health Care Provider Taxonomy values—derived from another standard, ANSI ASC X12—in this field. For example, 207PS0010X is the code for Sports Medicine; an emergency physician with special knowledge in sports medicine.

Data types are another HL7 v2 design concept. Data types define the values, formats, and vocabulary that fields, components, and subcomponents can have. Data types are also categorized as simple and complex. Simple data types contain a single value, whereas complex data types may contain more than one, and each of those can be a different data type. An example of a simple data type is DT or date. Its format is YYYY[MM[DD]]. An example of a complex data type is SAD or street address, which includes the house number and street.[8]

HL7 v3

Development on HL7 v3 started in 1992 with an aim to improve upon HL7 v2. The development team had at its disposal the accumulated knowledge learned from the many existing implementations of HL7 v2 and was able to apply new IT best practices. It addressed the need for the following: a consistent application data model, the need for formal methodologies to model data elements and messages, well-defined application and user roles, a consistent data model, and precision in the standard.[9]

A key goal of the HL7 v3 development work was to create a more rigorous standard than HL7 v2, that would lend itself to vendor conformance testing. HL7 v2 made vendor conformance testing difficult because there were a lot of HL7 v2 variants. These variants resulted from the flexible design of HL7 v2, which made it possible to have optional data elements and segments. This left it up to implementors to ensure conformance.

HL7 v3 combines object orientation and a Reference Information Model (RIM) to create HL7 v3 messages. This results in a standard that is extensible, is current, can be conformance tested, is abstracted from technology, and covers healthcare exhaustively. At the top of the RIM backbone, there are three main classes:[8]

- Act, which refers to something that has happened or will happen
- Role, which is a position, job, or competency
- Entity, which is something that is living or nonliving

The meaning of each class is determined by structural attributes. These three are linked using the association classes ActRelationship, Paticipation, and Rolelink. As in HL7 v2, there are data types defined such as name and addresses. Figure 35-10 shows an example of patient identifier coding in HL7 v2 and HL7 v3. The purpose of this example is to convey the structural difference in how the information is coded; it is not necessarily an accurate depiction. Note that HL7 v3 has adopted the XML style.

Note that despite advances in the development of HL7 and the need for the implementation of such standards, the volume of network transmissions in healthcare is increasing rapidly, with large amounts of healthcare data now being transmitted wirelessly. This increasing volume creates the potential for problems. For HL7 messages, problems may include incomplete data transmission, data being transmitted in wrong segments, deactivated threads or nodes, missing or incomplete patient data in key segments, data out of order and potentially misread, scrambled or timed-out messages (for example, due to fax or network failure), all potentially leading to medical error. In healthcare, network administrators must be keenly aware of the potential for such issues.

```
HL7 v2
PID|||000-00-1111||Doe^John^H^^^^ 121 Smith Dr.^^Someroad
Somestate^xx^00012||(999)555-5555|(666)666-6666||||AC00000000|| CR
HL7 v3
    <patient>
        <patient>
            <id root="1.23.456.7.899876.5432" extension="12345"/>
            <patient_Person>
                <id root="1.23.456.7.899876.5432" extension="12345"
assigningAuthorityName="xx" validTime="2012-06-21"/>
                <nm xsi:type="dt:PN" use="L">
                    <family/>
                    <given>John</given>
                    <given>Doe</given>
                </nm>
            </patient_Person>
        </patient>
    </patient>
```

Figure 35-10   Comparison of HL7 v2 and v3 coding

CompTIA EXAM TIP Remote Authentication Dial In User Service (RADIUS) is a remote network access protocol. It acts as a gatekeeper by verifying identities via pre-determined usernames and passwords. A RADIUS server can enforce user policies and restrictions.

EMR/EHR Outbound Communication

Electronic medical records (EMR) systems—otherwise known as electronic health records (EHR) systems—frequently need to interoperate with one of many other systems within a healthcare organization, and also with systems outside of the organization. In the vast majority of cases in the United States, this is accomplished by system-to-system software interfaces that comply with HL7 standards. Let's see how this works with a Bolling example. Some EMRs have a billing module that interacts directly with other modules, such as the ADT. If a healthcare entity uses that billing module within its EHR, no interface from the EHR to the billing module is required. Quite a few billing systems, independent of a healthcare entity's EHR, predate the current EHR and the billing departments have often prevailed over the IT department to maintain the independent billing system. Some of these billing systems are subsystems or modules of Practice Management systems. In some cases, a particular EHR does not have a billing module. When an independent billing system is preferred or required, an interface between the EHR and billing system is required. HL7 handles EHR-to-billing-system outbound communication with the BLG segment. In many cases the technical management of these interfaces is managed by a third system known as an interface engine.

Chapter Review

Internet and wireless technologies are changing how telecommunications services work and are provided in healthcare. The Internet holds the promise of converging voice, video, and data traffic onto a single network. Wireless technologies promise to extend connectivity to people anywhere and at any time. These changes are also motivating healthcare innovations as telecommunications is applied to problems in clinical settings, making it possible for clinical staff to work differently and sometimes do things they couldn't do before.

This chapter focused on TCP/IP networks since they will likely be the transport network of the future. Concepts necessary to the understanding of how TCP/IP networks work were introduced: connectivity, communications models, communication protocols, throughput, addressing, applications, and PANs, LANs, MANs, and WANs. To understand how networks work, it is useful to know how data flows. The chapter covered two examples of data transfer: transfer between two workstations on the same LAN and data transfer between a workstation and server on a different LAN. Wireless networks offer the benefits of mobility to clinicians, which makes the provision of services to patients more efficient and effective. The predominant wireless WLAN technologies and standards were covered.

Questions

To test your comprehension of the chapter, answer the following questions and then check your answers against the list of correct answers at the end of the chapter.

1. How many connections would be needed to fully connect six people?

    A. 6

    B. 15

    C. 12

    D. 18

2. ARP is associated with what process?

    A. The process of resolving domain names to hostnames

    B. The process of resolving domain names to IP addresses

    C. The process of resolving IP addresses to MAC addresses

    D. The process of resolving IP addresses to layer 4 port addresses

3. Throughput is _____.

    A. determined by dividing the amount of information transferred by the time it takes to transfer the information

    B. determined by dividing the bandwidth by the time it takes to transfer the information

    C. is always constant; it is the delay in the network that changes

    D. None of the above.

4. A PDU has what basic structure?

    A. A beginning and ending delimiter with a payload between these two delimiters

    B. A beginning and ending delimiter, source and destination address fields, a control field, a payload field, and an error check field

    C. Source and destination address fields and a payload

    D. A control field and a payload

5. Which layer of the OSI model is responsible for determining the best route through a network?

    A. Network layer

    B. Physical layer

    C. Session layer

    D. None of the above

6. With a client-server architecture, _____.

    A. there are one or more clients that request the services of one server

    B. each device is a client and a server

    C. there are one or more servers that request the services of clients

    D. it is better to work at a small scale since there is little overhead

7. For a device to communicate on a TCP/IP network, it needs what information?

    A. Firewall address, MAC address, DNS server, IP address, subnet mask, and gateway address

    B. IP address, DNS name, IP address, subnet mask, and gateway address

    C. IP address, MAC address, DNS server, IP address, subnet mask, and gateway address

    D. IP address, MAC address, subnet mask, and gateway address

8. While a network-layer PDU traverses the network, _____.

    A. its destination MAC address never changes

    B. the source IP address is matched to the last gateway it passes

    C. its destination IP address is changed to that of the first router it encounters

    D. its source and destination addresses do not change

9. IT staff employed by a healthcare organization would play which role associated with a WAN?

    A. Plan and build the WAN

    B. Provide operations support for the WAN

    C. Design components of the WAN such as the fiber-optic transmission system

    D. Manage contracts and service levels with suppliers of WAN services

10. What is different about wireless networks versus wired networks?

    A. A wireless network is constrained to a 1-meter radius versus a wired network that can span rooms or city blocks.

    B. The OSI stack is different for a wireless network versus a wired network.

    C. Wired networks use radio waves to communicate.

    D. Wireless networks use radio waves to communicate.

11. What is the key benefit that wireless networks provide to healthcare?

    A. They make it possible for patients to surf the Internet in their beds.

    B. They are more secure than wired networks.

    C. They give caregivers mobility and thus make them more productive.

    D. They make it easier for network managers to do their jobs.

12. What two key concerns do healthcare organizations have with respect to wireless networks that most other organizations do not?

    A. Using omnidirectional antennas and directional antennas

    B. Choosing radio that use direct-sequence spread spectrum and orthogonal frequency-division multiplexing

C. Protecting the confidentiality of patient data and ensuring there is no data loss because of network interruptions in order to keep patients safe

D. Using both SSID hiding and MAC filters for improved security

13. What is the most secure method used to protect wireless networks?

A. SSID

B. WPA2

C. Big Mac filtering

D. WEP

14. HL7 is mainly a _____.

A. messaging standard

B. an XML variant

C. a programming language

D. None of the above

15. HL7 v2 _____.

A. is no longer used

B. has the majority of implementations because vendors discounted prices greatly

C. is exhaustive and rigorous because it has an RIM

D. has the majority of implementations because adoption was a design goal and the developers purposely made it flexible in order to get that adoption

Answers

1. **B.** n*(n−1)/2 = 6*(6−1)/2 = 15.

2. **C.** The ARP cache, which is developed as ARP requests are made, is a table of records where IP addresses are associated with MAC addresses.

3. **A.** Throughput is information bits transferred divided by the time to transfer them.

4. **B.** There are seven basic fields: a beginning and ending delimiter, source and destination address fields, a control field, a payload field, and an error check field.

5. **A.** The network layer is responsible for routing and therefore figuring out the best path through the network.

6. **A.** Client-server by definition is many-to-one since the resources are centralized in the server.

7. **C.** The minimal set is IP address, MAC address, DNS server, IP address, subnet mask, and gateway address.

8. **D.** While a network-layer PDU traverses the network, its source and destination addresses do not change, which is how the end-to-end capability of TCP/IP is guaranteed.

9. **D.** Healthcare staff would manage contracts and service levels; having any role in the deployment or operation of a WAN is far beyond the interest of healthcare organizations whose purpose is to provide healthcare services.

10. **D.** Wired networks use wires, and wireless networks depend on radio waves.

11. **C.** The key differentiator is that wireless networks make it possible for users to use devices without cables.

12. **C.** Protecting the confidentiality of patient data and ensuring there is no data loss because of network interruptions in order to keep patients safe is of paramount importance to healthcare organizations.

13. **B.** WPA2 is currently the most secure standard.

14. **A.** HL7 defines how healthcare information is transmitted, so it is a messaging standard.

15. **D.** HL7 v2 has the majority of implementations because it was the first and only standard until HL7 v3 was written and also because it was flexible, which made it easily adoptable.

References

1. Fitzgerald, J. & Dennis, A. (2009). *Business data communications and networking, tenth edition*. Wiley.

2. Schulzrinne, H. (1996). World Wide Web: Whence, wither, what next? *IEEE Network Magazine, 10.*

3. Cisco Medical-Grade Network (MGN) 2.0 – Wireless Architectures (2010). Cisco Systems. Accessed October 9, 2012, from http://www.cisco.com/en/US/docs/solutions/Verticals/Healthcare/MGN_wireless_adg.html

4. Hiertz, G., et al. (2010). The IEEE 802.11 universe. *IEEE Communications Magazine, 48.*

5. Danielyan, E. (2003). WAP: Broken promises or wrong expectations? *The Internet Protocol Journal, 6.*

6. Parkvall, S., et al. (2011). Evolution of LTE toward IMT-Advanced. *IEEE Communications Magazine, 49.*

7. Bragg, R., et al. (2004). *Network security: The complete reference*. McGraw-Hill/Osborne.

8. Benson, T. (2010). *Principles of health interoperability HL7 and SNOMED: The book*. Springer.

9. The HL7 evolution comparing HL7 versions 2 and 3. Accessed on July 1, 2012, from www.corepointhealth.com.

10. Health level seven international. Accessed on July 1, 2012, from www.hl7.org/about/index.cfm?ref=nav.

Systems Analysis and Design in Healthcare

Andre Kushniruk, Elizabeth Borycki

In this chapter, you will learn how to

- Describe the importance of good systems analysis and design for healthcare information technology
- Implement systems design and analysis principles and methods
- Utilize the systems development life cycle (SDLC)
- Apply traditional approaches to systems analysis and design
- Employ object-oriented approaches to systems analysis and design
- Describe trends in systems analysis and design in healthcare

Increased information demands are leading to the development of more advanced healthcare information systems (HISs) and healthcare information technology. This chapter introduces the main concepts and techniques of modern systems design and analysis as applied to HISs. At the core of successful system development in healthcare is good systems analysis and design. This involves the selection and use of appropriate methods of analysis for assessing the information needs of a healthcare organization. System design involves specifying in detail how the components of systems will work together to provide useful functionality. As you will see, this needs to be based on an in-depth understanding of healthcare problems and the needs of healthcare professionals.

This chapter aims to describe the role and importance of systems analysis and design in rapidly changing healthcare environments. Approaches to systems analysis and design will be described, including traditional structured approaches to systems development and modeling of system requirements and design. Additionally, newer approaches such as object-oriented (OO) systems analysis and design will be described. Different design and implementation strategies and methodologies will be described, with an emphasis on understanding their advantages and disadvantages as they relate to healthcare. The reasons for the success and failures of HISs will be discussed, along with consideration of designs that might have helped to avoid failures. Approaches to system design will also be discussed in the context of a variety of healthcare information systems, ranging from electronic health record (EHR) systems to decision support systems. It has become increasingly clear that engineering information systems in healthcare is complex and requires the careful and informed application of appropriate methods and approaches to developing information systems. In this chapter, we will discuss the need for improving the development of information systems, and we will provide you with the background for understanding the complexity of HIT. We will also introduce a range of methods that can be used for improved systems analysis and design.

Systems Analysis and Design in HIT

A system can be defined as a collection of interrelated components (subsystems) that work together as a whole to achieve an outcome.[1] There are many types of systems, ranging from biological systems to political systems. A health information system is a collection of interrelated components or subsystems that input and process data to produce an output that is needed for healthcare tasks. For example, EHRs have been designed to support physicians' use of information in dealing with patients.[2] An EHR might consist of the following subsystems: patient scheduling, medications, documentation, laboratory information, and diagnostic imaging. As shown in Figure 36-1, these subsystems could be broken down further into subsystems (e.g., the medication subsystem can be broken down into a computerized physician order entry [CPOE] subsystem and a medication administration [MAR] subsystem). In addition, computer systems contain both manual and automated processes, which is an essential consideration, where some parts of the system involve manual activities (such as the entry of patient data by a clinician into a system using a keyboard) and some parts are automated or internal to the system (such as the automated application of decision rules for the detection of adverse drug interactions).

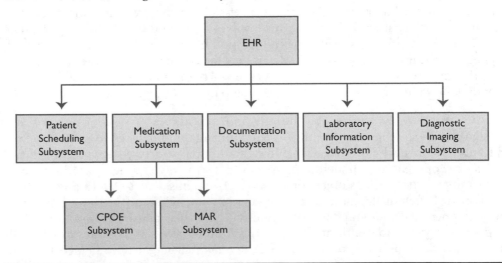

Figure 36-1 Subsystems of an electronic health record system

The System Development Life Cycle (SDLC)

A systems development project is a planned undertaking that produces an HIS. The development of any new information system involves analysis, design activities, and implementation activities. *Systems analysis* refers to the process of understanding and specifying in detail what the HIS should do. The results of a systems analysis form the foundation or basis for a specific system design. *System design* refers to the process of specifying in detail how the components of the HIS should work together to achieve desired functionality. A *systems analyst* is an IT professional who uses analysis and design techniques to solve healthcare problems using HIT.

A central concept in HIS development around which activities, methods, and approaches are considered is the systems development life cycle (SDLC). The SDLC is a term used to describe the process and stages in the development of new HISs. The SDLC provides guidance to HIS developers by providing structure, methods, and a checklist of activities needed to successfully develop an HIS. As shown in Figure 36-2, the typical phases in the SDLC are the following:[1]

1. Planning phase
2. Analysis phase
3. Design phase
4. Implementation phase
5. Support phase

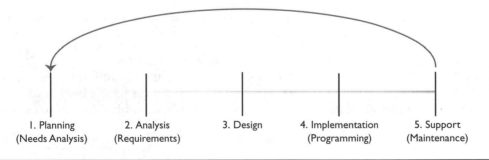

Figure 36-2   The systems development life cycle

The Planning Phase

The first phase—the Planning phase—involves coming up with the initial idea for an HIS development project. This includes identifying a healthcare problem that needs to be addressed and defining what aspects of the problem can be improved using healthcare information technology. During this phase, a feasibility study may be undertaken where the objectives and scope of the project are presented, the current problems with the existing situation are considered, and a recommended HIS solution is proposed. This phase may involve input from a manager and systems analysts working together to come up with a proposal for an organization to develop an HIS. At this point, if the project appears to be worth pursing (i.e., the projected benefits outweigh the costs), the project will then move into the Analysis phase.

The Analysis Phase

In the Analysis phase, a detailed assessment of the current situation is undertaken to determine where and how an HIS can be applied to solve healthcare problems. This may involve systems analysts going into a particular hospital setting (such as an emergency department or clinic) and collecting information about information gaps and problems that might be improved through the use of HIT. During this phase, the systems analysts involved in the project begin to gather information about the requirements for the new HIS that will be developed. This includes determining *technical requirements* for the HIS. Some examples of technical requirements include the following:[1]

- The HIS must run in a Windows 7 environment.
- The response time of the system to user queries must be less than one second.
- The data in the system must be backed up at the end of each day.

The *functional requirements* of the HIS describe the specific functions the HIS should support, with some examples of functional requirements for an HIS including the following:[1]

- The system will allow physicians to enter medication orders.
- The system will allow nurses to view medication orders.
- The system will provide automated alerts when entering a medication that the patient is allergic to.

Nonfunctional requirements make up the third major category of requirements for HIS; they include requirements for the system that are neither technical nor functional but are essential, such as the requirement that the system have a high level of usability and that the system functions can be learned easily by users with minimal prior computer experience.[3]

 CompTIA EXAM TIP Systems analysis refers to describing what a system should be able to do and involves specifying system requirements (i.e., technical, functional, and nonfunctional requirements).

Requirements gathering is a major activity that occurs during the Analysis phase. This may involve a team of analysts whose aim is to understand the current work situation and determine the requirements for the new HIS. This includes describing each of the following (see Figure 36-3):

- The physical environments in which the newly developed system will be deployed

- The different types of interfaces to other computer systems (e.g., laboratory or other data may need to be obtained directly from other systems)

- User and human factors considerations that will need to be addressed

- The actual functionality of the system

- The level of quality assurance (i.e., how error free must the system be)

- The security considerations

- Technical considerations

Systems analysts use a range of methods to obtain the requirements of an HIS, including the following:

- Distributing questionnaires to stakeholders and end users (e.g., to physicians, nurses, and allied professionals who will be users of the system being developed) to assess issues with current systems and requirements for new ones

- Reviewing organizational documentation, existing reports, forms, and procedure descriptions

- Conducting interviews with end users (e.g., physicians, nurses, allied health professionals)

- Observing current work practices (e.g., watching health professionals in an emergency setting to determine requirements for a new emergency room information system)

From the software engineering literature, as well as from the growing literature describing HIS implementations worldwide, there are two key points that need to be considered. One key consideration is that weak analysis of system requirements (i.e., performing an incomplete requirements analysis before proceeding with system design) will lead to "shortchanged user requirements," which have been highly associated with failed projects, because incomplete requirements form an insufficient base for design of effective systems.[4] The complexity of the environments where an HIS is deployed,

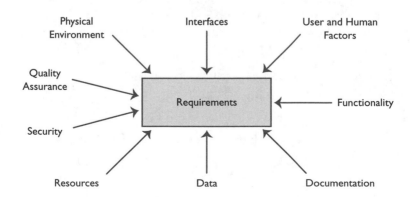

Figure 36-3
Summary of types
of requirements
in an HIS

the many and varied uses, and users of systems (ranging from clinics to hospitals to users of systems including physicians, nurses, and allied health professionals) all make gathering "sufficient" information about requirements difficult and challenging. The literature is full of examples of system development that has led to HISs that have not met user needs, that have not worked, or that had to be "turned off." The other key consideration for an HIS is that research in software engineering has indicated that perhaps the single greatest factor in the failure of complex systems is a lack of end user input and involvement.[4] To avoid system failure and to ensure effective system design, consultation with end users should begin in the systems analysis phase and continue throughout the whole SDLC through completion of the system's development and testing. This will be described in the following sections.

Use Case 36-1: Conducting Interviews to Determine Problems with a Hospital System

In this case study, we will examine the interview protocol that was created for gathering requirements about a new HIS that was to be implemented in order to replace an existing system, which had been reported to have a number of problems. In this example, a set of questions was created that were to be asked of physicians in the clinic where the new system would be implemented. The questions focused on understanding what the problems with the existing system were. The following is the set of questions that was developed for this purpose:

- How often do you use the current system?
- For what purposes?
- Have you had any problems using the system?
- Can you give me some examples of problems you have encountered?
- Are there new features you would like to see in an improved system?

These questions were used to drive interviews with 20 physicians who were the end users of the current system. The interviews were recorded and transcribed for analysis in order to identify all problems with the current system that needed fixing. The following is the transcript from one of the first physicians interviewed (with responses in bold):

Systems analyst: How often do you use the current system?

Doctor: About two or three times a day.

Systems analyst: For what purposes?

Doctor: To check the values of the patient for abnormal levels.

Systems analyst: Have you had any problems using the system?

Doctor: Well, I am finding that the data presented is not correctly updated and also that I have problems accessing the system from home.

Systems analyst: Can you give me an example of the data not being current?

Doctor: Yes, some of the records do not contain reports that were generated at other hospitals, and the data from this hospital sometimes is mixed up with data from other patients.

Systems analyst: Really, can you show me an example?

Doctor: Yes I'll show you this one I just printed out.

Systems analyst: Anything else?

Doctor: Yes, X-ray reports do not show on the system for at least several days.

Systems analyst: Are there new features you would like to see in an improved system?

Doctor: I would like to see guidelines about how to interpret abnormal lab values presented to me on the screen when an abnormal value appears.

Based on an analysis of all 20 interviews, it was clear a number of problems or themes kept reappearing from the interviews, such as the problem of information not being updated correctly and data being incorrectly displayed, as well as long delays in getting patient data. Based on these findings (and results from other forms of requirements gathering, including giving out questionnaires to both physicians and nurses), the requirements were specified for a new system that would replace the old one and that would address these issues. Specifically, the new system would be required to provide more timely updates of patient information, always present correct patient data, have a reduced period of time for providing physicians with reports, and have online guidelines for users to help them in interpreting abnormal lab values.

In general, the activities involved in conducting requirements analysis include the creation of a report, or a requirements specification, with a number of major sections, including the following:[5]

- **Analysis method** A list of end users consulted and a description of the methods used to obtain requirements (e.g., observation, interviews, or questionnaires).

- **Statement of user requirements** The objectives of the system, as well as all the technical, functional, and nonfunctional requirements that are listed. The potential impact of the system on end users and the need for training are discussed.

- **Statement of system constraints** The constraints of the system when it will be implemented in the real setting of use.

- **Documentation** Summaries of interviews and questionnaire results, as well as a set of diagrams describing the system requirements.

The requirements specification includes a number of key diagrams in the Documentation section. These diagrams form the basis or foundation upon which the sound design of the system will be based. The diagrams included in the report will depend on what type of approach is being used to collect and specify system requirements, as will be described.

There are many approaches and tools that are used to aid in collecting and specifying system requirements. One such approach is known as the *traditional*, or structured, approach to systems analysis and design. This approach includes a number of different diagramming techniques and tools. One such diagram that has traditionally been used in structured systems analysis is known as the *data flow diagram* (DFD); see Figure 36-4 for a simple HIS example of a DFD, along with a key indicating the

Data Flow Diagram Symbols:

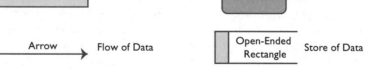

Data Flow Diagram:

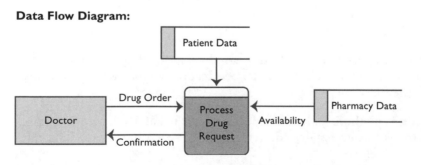

Figure 36-4 Data flow diagram symbols and simple example

meaning of the symbols used in the diagram. In the diagram, computer processes are depicted as rounded rectangles, while data stores or entities that are used by the processes are depicted using open-ended rectangles. The arrows show the flow of data from external agents into and out of processes, and the type of data is labeled on the arrows. In this example, Drug Order data flows into the Process Drug Request process from the Doctor, and data labeled Confirmation flows back to the Doctor after the drug request is processed. This type of diagram can be used to show how information flows and is processed in a healthcare organization to describe the current, or "as is," situation. It can also be used to describe how information will flow in the proposed HIS that will replace the current situation.[1]

Other types of diagrams and tools associated with traditional structured analysis include entity relationship diagrams (ERDs) that describe the relationship among the "things" of interest for designing a system such as patient data, pharmacy data, and so on, that are depicted as boxes in the ERD and labeled as shown in Figure 36-5. In this figure, there are three entities: Patient, Doctor, and Patient Record. Within each box representing an entity are its attributes. For example, within the entity Patient, the attributes are Name, Address, and Patient Number. Each Patient is associated with (can have) only one Patient Record (in this hospital system), and likewise each Patient Record can be associated with only one Patient. The two small vertical lines on the horizontal line between Patient and Patient Record indicate this relationship. Likewise, there is the line connecting Patient and Doctor, showing there is relationship between these two entities, with crow's-feet markings (the small circles with three small lines coming from them) to indicate that Patients can have zero or more (could be many) Doctors and alternatively that Doctors can have or be associated with zero or more Patients. These diagrams are very important in that they form a blueprint for creating and designing the databases that underlie HISs, with entities in such diagrams being implemented as relational database tables.[1]

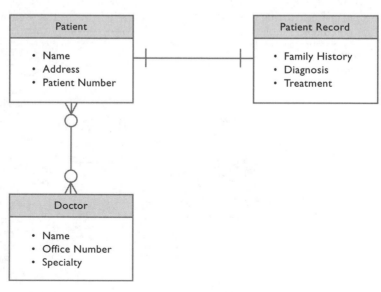

Figure 36-5 Example of an entity relationship diagram

CompTIA EXAM TIP Entity relationship and data flow diagrams are examples of diagrams associated with structured systems analysis.

In contrast to traditional structured systems analysis and design, more recent approaches have appeared including object-oriented (OO) systems analysis and design, which defines a newer set of associated diagramming techniques and tools to support work in the analysis phase.[6] OO systems analysis and design involves using a set of diagrams that are defined in the Unified Modeling Language (UML). UML diagrams have become a standard way of representing user requirements for many HISs and are commonly used to represent key aspects of current and proposed HISs in terms of system requirements. One such UML diagram that is commonly used to describe HIS requirements is known as the *use case diagram*.[6]

Figure 36-6 illustrates a use case diagram for a computerized physician order entry system. In the diagram, a figure represents an *actor* (i.e., a type of user of the system to be developed), in this case a physician. The main outer circle represents the automation boundary, which separates the computer system to be developed from manual parts of the system and end users outside of the automation boundary. In Figure 36-6, the three smaller circles inside the larger circle represent three use cases, which are the individual activities that the system can carry out. The arrows from the physician to the three use cases indicate that the actor is involved in each of the use cases (i.e., the physician user initiates each of the use cases). In the diagram there are three use cases shown: Order New Medication, Review Medication, and Stop Medication. Note that this type of diagram indicates who the users of the system will be (i.e., the actors) and also indicates what they can use the system to do. Since this diagram is constructed in the Analysis phase, it describes what the system will do, not how it will be done. (The description of how the system will carry out the functions illustrated in the use case diagram will be described during the Design phase, which follows the Analysis phase.) This type

Figure 36-6
Use case diagram
for CPOE system

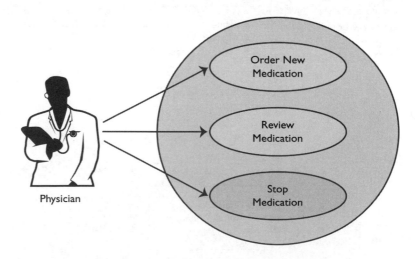

Use Case 36-2: Representing Requirements for an HIS in UML

Based on requirements gathered during the Analysis phase, a patient record and scheduling system are being designed for use in a doctor's office by receptionists, nurses, and doctors. The receptionist will use the system to enter new patient information when first-time patients visit the doctor and to schedule all appointments. The nurses will use the system to keep track of the results of each visit and to enter information about patient care. The nurses will also be able to print patient reports or the history of a patient's visits. The doctors will primarily use the system to view the patient's history and enter patient diagnostic and treatment information, as well as print patient information. Figure 36-7 shows the use case diagram for describing the requirements for the system based on this description. The three actors (i.e., receptionist, nurse, and doctor) are represented as figures, while the use cases (i.e., the activities the system will need to carry out based on the earlier description) are represented as the smaller circles within the larger circle representing the entire system.

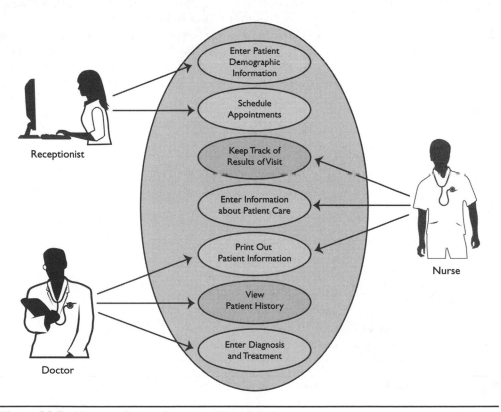

Figure 36-7 Use case diagram for patient record system

of diagram is increasingly used in order to give a clear view of system requirements. Each use in the diagram can be expanded to include a detailed text description of how the actors and the use case interact (i.e., scenarios describing in detail the interactions between the user and the system in carrying out a use case like Order New Medication).

Another diagram initially developed during the Analysis phase when using the OO approach to systems analysis and design is called the *class diagram*.[6] The class diagram is used to represent the "objects" in the work environment that need to be modeled and included in the HIS being developed. Objects have some surface-level similarities to the entities in the ERD described earlier, from a traditional structured systems analysis and design standpoint. However, the class diagram is different from the ERD in a number of important ways. For example, in developing clinical decision support (CDSS), in Figure 36-8, you can see that there are several types, or classes, of objects that need to be understood and modeled. In the figure there are three classes of objects depicted in rectangles: Clinical Decision Support, Drug Alert, and Drug Reminder. Each class of objects has its own attributes. For example, the attributes of Clinical Decision Support are Invocation Style, Message Text, and Message Format, thus indicating that all types of clinical decision support have a particular way of being invoked, have some text to be displayed to users, and have some particular format for messages to users. The classes Drug Alert and Drug Reminder are subclasses of Clinical Decision Support, which is shown by the arrow with a triangle leading up to Clinical Decision Support. This means they *inherit* all of the attributes of Clinical Decision Support. Thus, Drug Alert and Drug Reminder are types of Clinical Decision Support and have all the features of their superclass Clinical Decision Support. In addition, Drug Alert and Drug Reminder have their own attributes specific to them. For example, every Drug Alert has an Urgency Level and an associated Drug Alert Rule.

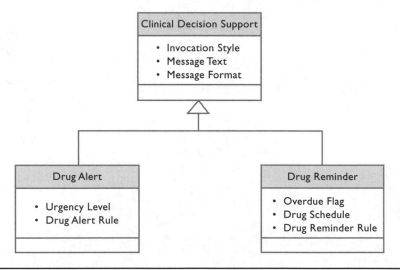

Figure 36-8 Class diagram for clinical decision support components

The Design Phase

The results of the Analysis phase provide a foundation for the Design phase of an HIS. Obtaining the "right" information from the Analysis phase is critical to the success of HIS design. Based on the requirements gathered during the analysis, the design of the system is specified during the Design phase. The design can be considered the blueprint that specifies how the system will work. This is in contrast to the Analysis phase, which focuses on what the system will be able to do; in the Design phase, you move on to the consideration of *how* the system will do it. System design also involves the intensive use of diagramming and modeling techniques, as will be described. A wide range of design approaches and methodologies can be used to drive the design of complex systems such as an HIS. These range from traditional structured approaches to object-oriented approaches.[1] There are a number of considerations to keep in mind when moving from the Analysis phase to the Design phase, including the following:

- Has there been sufficient requirements gathering on which the design can be based?

- Will there continue to be sufficient end-user feedback during the design of the system?

- Is the appropriate design methodology being used for designing the system?

The design of an HIS includes the specification of the following:

- Designing the application architecture (i.e., describing how each system activity and function specified from the Analysis phase is carried out)

- Designing and integrating the network needed (i.e., specifying how the various parts of the system will communicate)

- Designing the user interface (i.e., specifying how users will interact with the system)

- Designing system interfaces (i.e., specifying how the system will work with other systems)

- Designing the underlying database (i.e., specifying how the system will store data)

As will be discussed, it is often recommended that an HIS design be carried out using an iterative approach that includes developing prototypes (partially working, limited versions of the system design) that can be quickly shown to end users to gain input and feedback into design (well before the design is finalized).[7] The result of the Design phase is essentially the "blueprint" for the HIS; this includes a range of models and diagrams that specify the needed components of the system and provides detail on how they will work and interact. One of the most commonly used diagrams used for traditional structured HIS design is known as a *structure chart*, as depicted in Figure 36-9. The structure chart shows the modules of a system and their relationships. A module, which is represented by a box in the figure, is an identifiable component of a system that performs a desired function. This diagram shows a top-down hierarchical depiction of modules of a system. For example, the top module called Create New Medication Order has three immediate submodules below it: Record Medication Information, Process Medication Order, and Produce Confirmation. In turn, the module Record Medication Information can be broken down into the four modules below it: Enter Med Name, Enter Med Dose, Enter Med Route, and Enter Med Frequency. The lines in the chart show the calling structure from high-level modules down to ones at the bottom of the chart. For example, in Figure 36-9 you can see that from left to right, the top, or *boss*, module Create New Medication Order will first invoke or call Record Medication Information (e.g., in order to obtain input from the user about the medication to be recorded); then the boss module will call Process Medication Order (in order to actually process the medication order, check for drug interactions, send the information about it to a medication database, etc.), which is finally followed by the boss module calling the module Produce Confirmation (which displays to the end user a confirmation that the order has been made). It should be noted that some of these modules will themselves likely need to be broken down further. For example, Process Medication Order could be broken down to multiple submodules during the design process. This is known as *stepwise refinement*.

Using the object-oriented approach to systems design, an important type of diagram is called the *sequence diagram*.[6] With each use case developed during the Analysis phase, a corresponding sequence diagram is created to show how the use case actually works. For example, Figure 36-10 shows a corresponding sequence diagram for the use case Order New Medication (listed as one of the use cases from Figure 36-6). An important part of sequence diagrams is the concept of sending "messages" to objects that are needed to carry out functions required in a certain sequence over a period of time. The

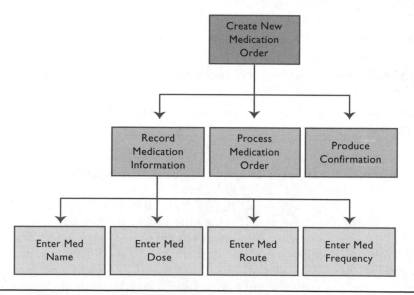

Figure 36-9 Structure chart for the activity Create New Medication Order

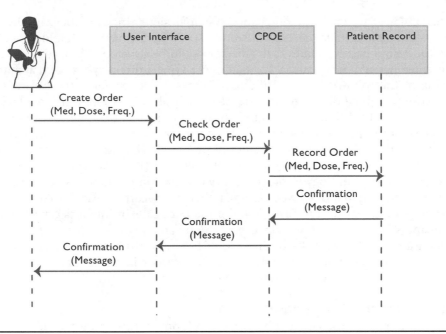

Figure 36-10 Sequence diagram for entering medications into a CPOE

sequence diagram shows how the user initiates the interaction with the CPOE by first sending the message Create Order to the User Interface object, as shown in the top-left horizontal arrow from the actor to the User Interface object. The Create Order message includes in it the parameters for the following: the name of the medication to be ordered (i.e., Med), the dose, and the frequency (Freq). Next, the User Interface object sends the message Check Order to the CPOE object. That object in turn sends a Record Order message to the Patient Record object. Next, notice the arrows going in the other direction from the Patient Record object back to the CPOE object, back to the User Interface object, and finally back to the user, providing the user with a confirmation of the order. This simple example shows that the sequence diagram can elaborate on and provide design details for how a single use case works by showing how different system components interact with each other by sending messages to each other in sequence over time to carry out an activity such as CPOE.

You should consider many principles of good design when developing HISs. For example, the concept of designing components of systems so that they are modular is one of the most important concepts. By good modularity we mean that the components or modules of a system have high *cohesion*, which means that each module focuses on one task and does that task well, as opposed to carrying out many functions. If a module is associated with more than one main task, it should be broken up or decomposed into submodules. Additionally, good modularity is associated with *loose coupling*, where the system modules do not interact closely with each other but are somewhat self-contained and do not inadvertently cause side effects with other modules.[1] There are a range of other good system design principles; for example, design patterns have emerged as sets of templates to speed up OO system development.[8] One group of design patterns states that systems should be developed in layers that can be easily interchanged or modified. For example, a typical three-layer system architecture consists of the following layers:[1] the user interface, or *view layer*; the business logic layer (containing the programming logic to run applications); and the data layer (the underlying database that the system reads and writes data to). The user interface, or view layer, is the part of the system that the user interacts with. If it is designed in a modular and self-contained way, with only a few well-defined connections and easily locatable interfaces to the layer immediately below it (the business logic layer), then as user interface technology improves, a new user interface can be added to the system easily by replacing that one layer. However, this will become difficult to do, or next to impossible to do easily, if the system's user interface calls or interacts extensively with the business logic layer below it. Likewise, if there are only a few clear and easily identifiable interfaces between the business logic layer and the underlying database layer, a new, more modern type of underlying database can be installed that will not require extensive reprogramming of the layers above it.

The Implementation Phase

Upon completion of the Design phase, the development project moves into the Implementation phase, where the design is translated into a working system by building running program code. This is the phase where the software of the HIS is constructed (or programmed), integrated with the required hardware, tested, and made ready for use in healthcare settings. The approach taken for implementation will depend on the system analysis and design methodology chosen and the type of programming languages and programming tools available. For example, if the traditional structured approach was used with the system analysis and design, then diagrams such as the structure charts would be developed to show how modules work together. In transitioning from design to implementation, the modules contained in the structure chart, as shown in Figure 36-9, are described in detail in terms of the programming code needed to carry out the function of each module. For example, the corresponding pseudo-code (English-like specification of programming steps) for the top-level boss module Create New Medication Order in Figure 36-9 would serve to "call" the three modules directly below it (Record Medication Information, Process Medication Order, and Produce Confirmation). To do this, the pseudocode corresponding to this top-level module might look like the following:

Do until no more orders

Call module Record_Medication_Information;

Call module Process Medication_Order;

Call module Produce_Confirmation;

This programlike code will be translated into the actual programming language used to implement the HIS such as with the C programming language or Java. Likewise, all the modules specified during the Design phase and represented in diagrams such as structure charts will be elaborated during the Implementation phase with programming code, as shown in Figure 36-11. This will eventually lead to a set of fully functional modules or a fully functioning HIS.

Top-down development refers to starting the development process (programming) with the module at the top of the structure chart. In contrast, *bottom-up development* refers to starting with the modules at the bottom of the structure chart, elaborating those modules with programming code first.[1] With the object-oriented OO methods, we approach this a slightly different way typically, by *scheduling* (i.e., elaborating with code) use cases. The first use cases to be scheduled are those that are judged by the developers to be most critical, risky, or important in the development of the HIS, such as a use case that other components of the HIS may rely on or that must work in order for all the other functions of the system to work.[8] We then proceed with developing use cases judged to be less critical, once the main or most critical ones have been shown to work, at least as partially working prototypes.

These resulting program codes that correspond to different modules (or use cases) in the system's design can be tested individually through unit testing, where code corresponding to a module is tested on its own or tested altogether with integration testing. Testing software systems and HISs in particular is an important area, and we refer you to complete books on this topic.[9] Here, we will briefly define two main approaches to testing of HIS software: black-box testing and white-box testing. *Black-box testing*, also known as *testing with blinders on*, refers to testing a system by giving the system specific inputs and then testing to determine whether the right outputs result.[10]

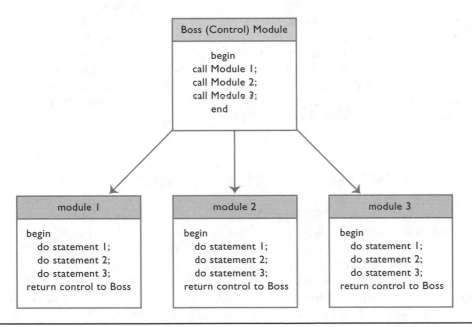

Figure 36-11   Example of a structure chart, with pseudocode programming statements

For example, you may black-box test a clinical decision system that produces drug alerts in response to the entry of drugs that a patient might have an allergy to. You can do this by creating a list of drugs to be inputted into the system that should trigger the system to output drug alerts. The output of the system, in this case alerts, would then be compared to expected outputs to determine whether the system is working properly for all test cases (i.e., the system produces alerts when expected and does not produce alerts when not expected to). Black-box testing does not require that the testing team have knowledge of the underlying computer processes or software and is often used to test commercial vendor-based systems in hospitals when they are initially installed to check their correctness and safety. In contrast, *white-box testing*, also known as glass-box testing, requires knowledge of underlying program code and internal aspects of a system. With this type of testing, specific parts of the software's underlying logic are "stepped through" (examined by a team of programmers and analysts) to determine whether the computer logic is working as expected.[10] It is important to note that as important as white- and black-box testing are, HISs are typically deployed in healthcare contexts that are much more varied and complex than other types of computer applications and also require extensive user acceptance testing, usability testing, and testing in the real setting of use.[11] These methods focus on user interactions to determine whether the HIS is usable, safe, and enjoyable (or not) to use in real and complex healthcare settings.

The Support and Maintenance Phase

Once the HIS has been put into place in a healthcare setting, the ongoing process of support and maintenance of the system begins. The system may be in place for a long period of time; however, over time, there are always changes that need to be made to improve it, make it more efficient, or make it more likely to be adopted. Furthermore, HISs are inevitably replaced over time as their hardware or software becomes obsolete. Therefore, over time new systems analysis has to be conducted to determine requirements for system modification or termination. Thus, system development is seen as being cyclical, where the progress from planning to support/maintenance then eventually begins again when existing systems need to be updated or replaced. This is depicted in Figure 36-2 by the arrow going back from the Support/Maintenance phase to the Planning phase.

Trends and Issues in HIS Analysis and Design

Approaches to the development of complex systems such as HISs have evolved considerably over the past few decades. The traditional model for developing systems is often called the *classic waterfall life cycle*. This approach to the SDLC involves the stages described earlier (Planning, Analysis, Design, Implementation, and Support) following one another in such a way that one follows the other in strict sequential order (see Figure 36-12). Once Analysis is complete, the requirements are finalized, and the project moves to the Design phase. Once the Design phase is complete, the project moves to the Implementation phase, and once that phase is complete, the project moves to the Support phase. The approach is like a waterfall, since as the development process

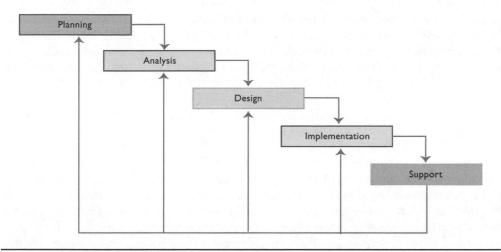

Figure 36-12 The classical "waterfall" life cycle

moves down to the next phase, it is difficult to go back to the previous phase. Therefore, the project "flows" downward. At each phase, the results, or the requirements specification produced from the Analysis phase, are typically "signed off" as complete by both the developer and the client before moving to the next phase. After the system is in place, the up arrows in the figure indicate that parts of the process may need to be modified or updated. This is typically costly and difficult to do once the system has been implemented. This type of model has been used successfully for many types of IT applications, particularly for traditional software applications such as standard business systems such as payroll applications.[1] For more complex types of applications such as complex EHRs, decision support systems, patient applications, or public health informatics systems, this approach has the drawback of expecting that most if not all user requirements can be gathered once and for all during the Analysis phase. Likewise, once the design of the system is set in the Design phase, it may be difficult and costly to try to go back to the Analysis phase as the project moves on and the Analysis phase has already been signed off as completed. In applications that are complex and that may require some piloting or experimentation, this approach may not be the best. Likewise, applications such as advanced EHRs, clinical decision support systems, and many emerging types of health applications typically require continual user evaluation and input, particularly if they are highly interactive systems.[7]

An alternative to the classic waterfall approach is known as *rapid prototyping*. This approach, which has become increasingly popular as systems become more complex, involves cycles of design, construction, and refinement of prototypes (which are incomplete but partially working versions of the system) and evaluation with end users (see Figure 36-13). In this approach, it is not assumed that initial requirements will be completely obtained at the very beginning of the development process but rather that enough requirements need to be gathered in order to start developing a working and testable prototype that is then evaluated to determine whether more requirements and design are needed (i.e., the arrow going from the Evaluation box back to the

Requirements Gathering box in Figure 36-13). This cycling may continue until no more iterations are needed, such as when an evaluation indicates that final engineering of the system can be carried out or until time or money runs out. Variations of this may involve setting a fixed length of time for each iteration (an approach known as *time boxing*), in which testable and continual progress can be demonstrated in developing software components.[12]

We refer you to other books to obtain details about the many possible variations of the previous models for carrying out the SDLC.[4] Because HIS development is complex, a thorough understanding of the options in selecting approaches to developing such systems is becoming ever more critical. Some of these variations include combining the advantages of rapid prototyping with the classic waterfall approach. For example, for applications where there is uncertainty about whether technical requirements can be met, as in some complex HIS initiatives, a first phase of rapid prototyping might be appropriate in order to assess whether the system is technically feasible and to gain information that can be used in planning out a more fixed development process. In this case, after obtaining information about technical and user requirements from building prototypes, the classic waterfall approach can be initiated in order to develop and complete the HIS. The advantages here include a better ability to estimate the time and difficulty of the different stages of the waterfall approach as well as the reduction of the risk of system development failure. Prototyping may determine that a planned HIS may not be as achievable as initially conceived before going in to an expensive and difficult-to-modify waterfall development phase. Many of these ideas are now incorporated in OO systems analysis and design, with approaches such as Agile programming where there is considerable flexibility in the ordering and sequencing involved in developing

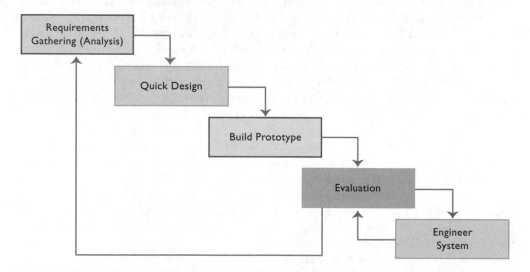

Figure 36-13 Rapid prototyping

a system; the Unified Process, which employs time boxing as described earlier; and Extreme Programming, which involves carrying out fast and iterative cycles of system development. For more information about these approaches, we recommend you look at McConnell and other sources.[4]

As a final consideration, it should be noted that in HIT, many organizations, particularly hospitals or health authorities, may be involved in a combination of "building" system components and "buying" and subsequently integrating system components. This distinction is often referred to as the *buy versus build* distinction, where the management of healthcare organizations must decide which parts of an HIS will be developed and programmed from scratch and which will be purchased either as completed software systems or as software components to be integrated with existing healthcare IT. This has a number of implications, including deciding whether a healthcare organization has the capability to develop a system or whether it is better to purchase a completed solution from an HIT vendor. A related decision is with regard to what extent a healthcare organization's HISs should be purchased from the same vendor versus buying systems from a variety of different vendors (also known as the *best-of-breed* approach). Regardless of whether you are involved in development of HIT and HIS from scratch such as developing healthcare IT applications from planning through to design and implementation or whether you working in an organization considering buying a completed off-the-shelf HIT or HIS, an understanding of the principles of health information systems analysis and design is essential for successfully deploying information technology that has a good chance of supporting and improving healthcare.

Chapter Review

The development of HISs is complex, and systems that are used in healthcare settings must be carefully designed to meet the intended needs safely and efficiently. The core of development of an effective HIS is good systems analysis and design. This involves understanding the information needs of healthcare professionals, including the technical, functional, and nonfunctional requirements for a new HIS. In addition, the concept of the systems development life cycle is central to systems analysis and design, because it provides a framework from which to consider the development of systems, from the initial Planning phase all the way through to the Analysis and Design phases and then finally to the implementation and deployment of the system in a healthcare facility. In this chapter, we described a variety of diagramming and modeling tools that are routinely used to support HIS analysis and design. The traditional, structured approach includes data flow diagrams, entity relationship diagrams, and structure charts. The alternative approach, known as OO systems analysis and design, employs use case, class, and sequence diagrams. It is important for anyone engaged in systems analysis and design in HIT to be familiar with these approaches, tools, and methodologies. In addition, it is becoming increasingly important for those designing HISs to have an understanding of the trends in the analysis, design, and testing of HISs.

Questions

To test your comprehension of the chapter, answer the following questions and then check your answers against the list of correct answers at the end of the chapter.

1. Systems analysis involves which of the following?

    A. Designing the components of a system

    B. Testing a system for correctness

    C. Obtaining system requirements

    D. Constructing a system

2. Which is an example of an object-oriented diagram that depicts overall system requirements?

    A. Sequence diagram

    B. Use case diagram

    C. Data flow diagram

    D. Entity relationship diagram

3. What does the SDLC do?

    A. Provides guidance in system development

    B. Provides a checklist of activities

    C. Provides a set of stages for system development

    D. All of the above

4. What does the classic waterfall life cycle do?

    A. Assumes that most requirements can be obtained early on in the SDLC

    B. Allows for flexibility in carrying out systems analysis and design activities

    C. Allows for easily redoing phases

    D. Is well suited for the development of complex interactive HIT application

5. Black-box testing refers to what?

    A. Testing the internal logic of a health information system

    B. Testing system components in isolation

    C. Testing system components in an integrated manner

    D. Testing systems without considering underlying program logic

6. The requirement that a system be easy to use would be an example of what?

    A. Technical requirement

    B. Nonfunctional requirement

    C. Functional requirement

    D. Incomplete requirement

7. What is rapid prototyping?

   A. It involves iterative cycles of development and testing.

   B. It is often associated with object-oriented development approaches.

   C. It is useful in designing complex or highly interactive systems.

   D. All of the above.

   E. None of the above.

8. What are objects?

   A. They are entities.

   B. They are usually very difficult to represent.

   C. They can be organized into classes.

   D. They are static.

9. Lack of user input into design has been shown to be the biggest factor leading to failed information systems.

   A. True

   B. False

10. Healthcare information testing requires much more extensive testing than conventional business applications.

    A. True

    B. False

Answers

1. **C.** Systems analysis involves obtaining system requirements to determine how existing problems might be improved through the use of HIT and other means.

2. **B.** An example of an object-oriented diagram that depicts overall system requirements is a use case diagram.

3. **D.** The systems development life cycle (SDLC) involves the following phases: Planning, Analysis, Design, Implementation, and Support. It involves activities and phenomena such as guidance in system development, a checklist of activities, and a set of stages for system development.

4. **A.** The classic waterfall life cycle assumes that most requirements can be obtained early on in the SDLC and that those requirements remain fundamentally static and stable during the entire SDLC.

5. **D.** Black-box testing refers to testing systems without considering underlying program logic.

6. **B.** The requirement that a system be easy to use is an example of a nonfunctional requirement. Another nonfunctional example is that the system functions can be learned easily by users with minimal prior computer experience.

7. **D.** Rapid prototyping involves iterative cycles of development and testing, is often associated with object-oriented development approaches, and is useful in designing complex or highly interactive systems.

8. **C.** Objects can be organized into classes so they can be included in the HIS being developed.

9. **A.** Lack of user input into design has been shown to be the biggest factor leading to failed information systems.

10. **A.** Healthcare information testing requires much more extensive testing than conventional business applications because of the high complexity of healthcare operations/clinical care and the risk of adverse patient outcomes that HIT may contribute to if not tested very thoroughly.

References

1. Satzinger, J. W., Jackson, R. B., & Burd, S. D. (2002). *Systems analysis and design in a changing world.* Course Technology – Thomson Learning.

2. Shortliffe, E., & Cimino J. (2006). *Biomedical informatics: Computer applications in health care and biomedicine.* Springer.

3. Cysneiros, L., & Leite, J. (2004). Nonfunctional requirements: From elicitation to conceptual models. *IEEE Transactions on Software Engineering, 30,* 328–350.

4. McConnell, S. (1996). *Rapid development: Taming wild software schedules.* Microsoft Press.

5. Martin, M. P. (1991). *Analysis and design of business information systems.* MacMillan.

6. Satzinger, J. W., & Orvik, T. U. (2001). *The object-oriented approach: Concepts, system development, and modeling with UML.* Course Technology – Thomson Learning.

7. Kushniruk, A. W. (2002). Evaluation in the design of health information systems: Applications of approaches emerging from systems engineering. *Computers in Biology and Medicine, 32,* 141–149.

8. Larman, C. (2002). *Applying UML and patterns: An introduction to object-oriented analysis and design and the unified process.* Prentice-Hall.

9. Patton, R. (2001). *Software testing.* Sams Publishing.

10. Kaner, C., Falk, J., & Nguyen, H. (1999). *Testing computer software.* John Wiley and Sons.

11. Kushniruk, A., Borycki, E., Kuo, M. H., & Kuwata, S. (2010). Integrating technology-centric and user-centric testing methods: Ensuring healthcare system usability and safety. *Studies in Health Technology and Informatics, 157*, 181–186.

12. Ambler, S. W. (2002). *Agile modeling: Effective practices for eXtreme programming and the unified process.* John Wiley and Sons.

CHAPTER 37

Healthcare Information Technology Project Management

Brian Gugerty

In this chapter, you will learn how to

- List several project team member and project stakeholder roles and communication strategies
- Describe how a project manager works with a project team and stakeholders to develop SMART project objectives
- Construct a work breakdown structure for a healthcare IT project
- Effectively estimate project activity durations and schedule project resources
- Manage project resources and stakeholders to maintain project scope, time, quality, and budget parameters
- Monitor and control the project in the executing phase
- Describe principles and practices to effectively close out a healthcare IT project

Today's healthcare enterprises are increasingly complex, and healthcare information technology is essential to making their operations more effective and efficient. Project management is one tool that can be used to maximize the effectiveness of information technology within healthcare enterprises. In this chapter, I will define a project and project management techniques in broad, cross-industry terms, as well as begin to convey how project management works within HIT initiatives.

A *project* is a temporary venture undertaken to create a unique product, service, or result. A project has a defined beginning and end with specific objectives to be achieved at the completion of the project. The end of a project is reached when the project's objectives have been achieved, when it is determined that its objectives will not or cannot be met, or when the need for the project no longer exists.[1] Projects have a clearly specified objective or scope of work to be performed, a predefined budget, and usually a temporary organization whose work concludes when the project ends. While the project is temporary, the product, service, or result created is usually meant to be long lasting or permanent. Some examples of projects include building a house, installing a new process, developing software, implementing an electronic health record, and revamping a healthcare organization's intranet. Any type of ongoing or continuous work such as manufacturing or planning the monthly schedule of nurses on a hospital unit is not a project because these tasks follow their respective organization's existing procedures and are ongoing.

A *program* is a group of projects that relate to each other and are managed together so that they can achieve benefits and goals that may not be achieved by managing them separately. A program may include additional work outside of the projects in the program that is necessary for achieving the program goals but is not part of the projects within the program. While a project may be part of a program, it can, and often does, operate independently of a program. On the other hand, a program always has projects.

Project management is the application of knowledge, skills, tools, and techniques to project activities in order to meet the project requirements.[1] In other words, project management is the facilitation of the planning, scheduling, and controlling of all activities that must be done to meet a project's objectives.

Use Case 37-1: Establishing the Background Story–Tree Healthcare System

You are a project manager employed by Tree Healthcare System, a not-for-profit integrated healthcare delivery network with ten hospitals. The CIO and senior VP of patient-care services at Tree have just assigned you to what they term the eMAR Implementation Project. You are to implement the electronic medication administration record (eMAR) module of the Acme electronic health record system (*including* the use of barcoding for both positive patient ID and medication identification) at Oak Medical Center, a 650-bed University Teaching Hospital at Tree. This will be the first implementation of this module at Tree Healthcare System and will be used as the "pilot" and "proof of concept" for the other hospitals, including standardization of medication administration processes and the corresponding workflow changes.

Tree has selected Acme as its electronic health record (EHR) provider. Most of Tree's hospitals already have five to six of Acme's EHR modules implemented. Future plans call for each facility to have all 12 of Acme's modules implemented within three years.

Oak Medical Center has already implemented several other clinically related, non-Acme systems; the most relevant to this eMAR implementation project is the Beta Drug Dispensing System, which it currently uses for all PRN and controlled substance medication dispensing and charging. Routine medications are currently dispensed from the pharmacy using a traditional cart fill process. Medications are currently charged when dispensed and credited if returned.

I will revisit the Tree Healthcare System use case at various points throughout this chapter.[2]

The Project Management Institute, PMBOK, and PMP

The Project Management Institute (PMI) is a not-for-profit membership association for the project management profession. PMI works to advance the project management profession by developing globally recognized standards, certifications, research programs, and professional development opportunities. PMI's standards for projects, programs, and portfolio management are the most widely recognized standards in project management across industries including healthcare.

PMI has published *A Guide to the Project Management Body of Knowledge (PMBOK Guide)*, which is a recognized standard for the project management profession and provides guidelines for managing individual projects. I will use the *PMBOK Guide Fourth Edition* to direct this chapter's discussion of project management for healthcare IT professionals.

PMI offers a certification called Project Management Professional (PMP). The PMP is considered the most important, industry-recognized certification for project managers. The PMP demonstrates that the holder of the certificate has the experience, education, and competency to lead and direct projects. PMI believes that project managers with this certification benefit from increased marketability to employers and higher salaries. As an additional resource to PMI members, PMI has created "communities of practice," which are online communities for professionals in a wide variety of industries to meet online and in other forums with other professionals in the same industry to discuss ideas and grow their community's understanding of project management. There is a healthcare community of practice that focuses on bringing an international focus to implementing project management knowledge in the healthcare industry.

Other Project Management Resources

An organization that provides training in project management is the Lewis Institute. I will use examples provided by the Lewis Institute to help you better understand project management. While the *PMBOK Guide* is a recognized standard for the project management profession, the Lewis Institute does a very good job of explaining project management concepts clearly and simply. Another reliable source of information on healthcare IT project management topics is the Healthcare Information Management Systems Society (HIMSS). You can search on project management at himss.org and find many resources on Healthcare Information Technology Project Management.

Major Project Management Constraints/Objectives

Four major variables can act as constraints, as well as objectives, in project management. These variables are

- **P** *Performance* requirements, both technical and functional
- **C** Labor and other *costs* to do the project activities
- **T** *Time* required to complete the project activities
- **S** *Scope* or magnitude of the job to be done

These variables directly affect the successful management and completion of a project. This is particularly true in the healthcare industry where quality is of the utmost importance. In this discussion of P, C, T, and S, you can think of performance as the equivalent to quality in HIT projects. Because a high degree of quality or performance is required in healthcare services, the costs associated with the HIT projects may be high as well. In other industries where quality or performance is less important than the cost of the product or service, a project may be able to be completed with lower costs. The project management triangles shown in Figure 37-1 illustrate the relationship between performance (quality), cost, time, and scope of a project.

The performance (P) or quality lines in the two triangles in Figure 37-1 are the same length. One of the most powerful aspects of the P, C, T, S "formula" is that it reminds the project manager that if the scope of a project increases, the amount of time and budget required to complete the project will also increase. Figure 37-1 can be described as follows: holding steady for the *performance* or quality of completing the project activities and objectives, an increase in *scope* will lead to an increase in both *time* until project completion and the *cost* of the project. So, when an enthusiastic stakeholder or project team member says, "We can add computerized physician order entry to the electronic medication project and make an even bigger impact," the project manager can use the P, C, T, S formula to interject the hard realities of this change into the discussion in order to keep the project on track. The project manager needs to constantly monitor "scope creep" to ensure that the costs, time, and performance remain at acceptable levels. Throughout the course of the project, the project manager will need to make a variety of decisions in order to help maintain the scope of the project. The project management triangle is a very helpful tool in doing so.

 HIT PRO EXAM TIP If the scope of a project increases, the amount of time and budget required to complete the project will also increase. A project manager needs to make sure these increases remain at acceptable levels, or he will be faced with scope creep, which may jeopardize the project's success.

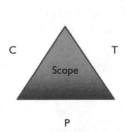 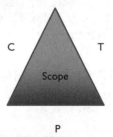

Figure 37-1 Project management triangle illustrating the P, C, T, S relationship

Healthcare Project Critical Success Factors

Within healthcare project management are many interrelated elements, or success factors, that must be kept in balance in order to achieve project success.

The foundation of successful project management is the people who manage or work on the projects themselves. Their levels of communication, leadership, negotiation, team building, decision making, and motivation combine to direct the trajectory of a project. Adding to this foundation is the culture of an organization and its values, beliefs, attitudes, behaviors, traditions, and structure. The methods employed by the organization to work both on a routine, or continuous, basis and on a project basis influence the success of a project. And, planning and information management are critical to the success of a project. The approach to a project needs to be well-defined, appropriate processes must be determined, and the work schedule needs to be developed properly.

Another critical factor to a HIT project's success is control over the project by the project manager. All projects need to be controlled and directed properly in order to track the progress of the project, compare it to the original plan, take necessary corrective action, and monitor the performance of all parts of the project to ensure the project is completed in accordance with the project goals and strategies outlined in the project initiating phase.

HIT projects need to be held to very high-quality standards, maybe not quite as high and exacting as the nuclear power industry, but oftentimes the quality does need to be close or equal to that level of exacting quality. Skimping on a barcode-assisted medication administration implementation may have fatal consequences, whereas skimping on the quality of certain parts of a house you are building will not. For example, opting for the lower-end shower for the guest bathroom instead of the most expensive one will hardly be noticed. Administering the wrong medication to a patient could cause a patient to become ill or even be fatal. Thus, finding a way to maintain high quality throughout the life cycle of a HIT project is a critical success factor.

Peter Drucker, one of the best-known and widely influential management theory and practice writers and consultants, characterized the modern medical center as "the most complex business and social arrangement in the history of mankind."[3] There are many different organizational divisions and many, many roles in a modern healthcare enterprise. HIT projects often involve many different clinical disciplines such as doctors, nurses, respiratory therapists, and others; operational departments such as laboratory, pharmacy, radiology, and others; and both internal IT technicians and professionals and external IT consultants and vendors. Moreover, there are a huge number of regulations in the healthcare industry, and there are a wide variety of payment mechanisms that are highly complex. More and more, large-scale HIT projects impact most of these divisions and roles in a healthcare center and deal with many regulations and billing challenges. For a HIT project, effectively dealing with healthcare organizational and operational complexity and the many people involved in healthcare organizations is a critical factor for success.

Project Team Roles and Stakeholders

The people, or organizations, who are actively interested in and involved with a project and who may affect or be affected by the results of the project are considered the project's stakeholders. A stakeholder may use their position of power to steer the project, its deliverables, and the project team members in a certain direction. The project team itself needs to identify the stakeholders and understand their expectations of the project in order to manage their influence as well as expectations so that they can ensure a successful outcome of the project.[4]

Effective Communication in Projects

Effective communication in all projects is essential to their overall success. Project managers spend most of their time communicating with the team members and stakeholders in order to ensure the project is planned and executed in accordance with the project's objectives and strategies. The project manager is responsible for making sure relevant information is available to team members and stakeholders, managing stakeholder expectations, and reporting on the performance of the project.[1]

A project manager is responsible for a wide range of forms of communications in a project, including the following:

- Internal (within the project) and external (customer, other projects, the media, the public)
- Formal (reports, memos, briefings) and informal (e-mails, ad hoc discussions)
- Vertical (up and down the organization) and horizontal (with peers)
- Official (newsletters, annual reports) and unofficial (off-the-record communications)
- Written and oral
- Verbal and nonverbal (voice inflections, body language)

The communication skills that a project manager, team member, or stakeholder possess can directly affect the effectiveness of the communications within a project as well as the success of a project. The following communication skills are important to have and will lead to more effective communications:

- Listening actively and effectively
- Asking questions to ensure better understanding of situations
- Fact finding to find or confirm information
- Setting and managing expectations
- Persuading a person or organization to perform an action
- Negotiating to achieve mutually acceptable agreements between parties
- Resolving conflict
- Summarizing, recapping, and identifying next steps[1]

It is important to hone or develop these skills so that you can be an effective communicator and project manager.

Process Groups

Project management is achieved through the application of standardized processes to project activities in order to meet the project's requirements. PMI has identified 42 project management processes and has incorporated these into five categories, or *process groups*, by which all projects should be managed. These five process groups are as follows:

- Initiating
- Planning
- Executing
- Monitoring and Controlling
- Closing

These project management processes apply across all industries. There is wide-ranging belief and acceptance that using these project management processes will improve the chances of a project's success.

The Project Life Cycle

Projects vary in both their size and complexity. But, regardless of the size or complexity of a project, all projects follow very similar life-cycle structures.

- Starting the project (initiating phase)
- Organizing and preparing (planning phase)
- Carrying out the project work (executing phase)
- Closing the project (closing phase)

Project phases are an element of a project's life cycle. PMI describes processes that align with the project life-cycle phases. Monitoring and controlling processes occur at every phase of a project. Figure 37-2 describes the relationship between the phases and processes.

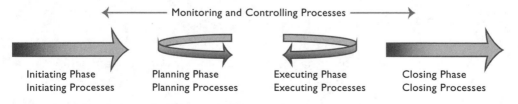

Figure 37-2 Project phases and processes

Project Initiation

While some may *not* consider the project initiating phase as important as some of the other phases of a project, such as project execution, this cannot be further from the truth. The time spent at the beginning of the project in the initiating phase is incredibly important to the success of a project. The more careful project initiation and planning that is done, the better a project's chances of success are. Projects usually don't fail at the end because of the work done on the project in the executing phase, but they often fail because not enough effective time and effort was spent in the beginning to properly initiate a project. The initiating phase often begins with a fuzzy charge from a superior to a project manager, such as "Implement an EHR." Then, with thoughtful planning, a project charter and problem and mission statements are created, and finally SMART project objectives are set and prioritized. When a project manager has clear, well-defined project objectives, she can exit the initiating phase and is well on her way to successful project completion.

Project Charter and Scope

Before any work on a new project can begin, it's advisable to create, and have approved, a project charter. The *project charter* is a high-level document that outlines the objectives and requirements of the project and serves as the official authorization for the project. PMI's initiating process group consists of the processes that need to be performed in order to define a new project or even to start a new phase in an existing project. The initiating process group defines the scope of the project, identifies the project's stakeholders and project manager, secures the financial resources necessary to begin the project, and obtains the required authorization to begin the project or phase. The project manager and the project management team help write the project charter, which is then approved and officially authorized by the project initiator or sponsor.[1]

Project Charter

In Chapter 9, which discussed project management from the executive perspective, you learned about project charters. This chapter will help deepen your understanding of project charters by discussing them as they relate to the role of the project manager.

The organization initiating a project assigns a project manager to the project. The project manager is integral to the success of the project because it is their responsibility to see that the project achieves the objectives outlined in the project charter. The project manager must focus on the following:

- Achieving specified project objectives
- Controlling the assigned project resources to meet project objectives
- Managing the four project management variables (as well as risk): performance, cost, time, and scope (PCTS)

The project manager must constantly monitor all of these areas in order to ensure that the project is progressing in accordance with the project charter, is reaching milestones, and finally achieves the goals outlined in the project charter. As discussed, efficiently balancing the competing demands of the project's overall scope, schedule, budget, quality requirements, available resources, and risk will lead to successful project completion. It is the project manager's responsibility to manage all of these factors to reach the successful completion of the project.

Project Scope Statement

Following the development and authorization of a project charter comes a more detailed description of the project and its goals through a *project scope statement*. The project scope statement is essential to the project's progress and builds upon the major factors such as required deliverables, known or assumed risks and constraints, and other variables that are identified in the project charter. Additionally, the project scope statement takes into account any other risks, constraints, or variables that may not have been known at the time the project charter was written. When the project scope statement is being developed, more information regarding the specific details of the project is available, so the scope can be defined more clearly and with greater accuracy.[1] The *PMBOK Guide* defines the project scope statement in the following way:

> The project scope statement describes, in detail, the project's deliverables and the work required to create those deliverables. The project scope statement also provides a common understanding of the project scope among project stakeholders. It may contain explicit scope exclusions that can assist in managing stakeholder expectations. It enables the project team to perform more detailed planning, guides the project team's work during execution, and provides the baseline for evaluating whether requests for changes or additional work are contained within or outside the project's boundaries.[1]

The *PMBOK Guide* outlines the following sources of information that the project management team uses to help develop the project scope statement:

- Project charter
- Requirements documentation (describes how individual requirements meet the business and clinical needs for the project)
- Organizational process assets (examples include policies, procedures, and templates for a project scope statement and files and lessons learned from previous project)
- Expert judgment (examples include other units within the organization, consultants, stakeholders, industry groups, and subject-matter experts)
- Product analysis
- Alternatives identification[1]

When a project scope statement includes a sufficient level of detail and information to define the project, the project management team has a better chance of being able to successfully manage the project.

Project Problem/Vision/Mission Statements

Because proper project initiation is critical to the success of all projects, I will also walk through the principles the Lewis Institute uses to teach project initiation. Depending on the project and the project manager's and project team's preferences, the steps outlined here can substitute for the PMI scope statement process. The creation of these "statements" is best led by the project manager but with the full participation of project team members and, when appropriate, stakeholders. The project initiating phase includes the following components:

- **Project problem statement** A problem statement defines the problem at hand and the reason for initiating a project and helps to develop a suitable solution for the problem. It's a good starting point to then go on to construct a project's vision and mission.

- **Project vision** The project vision provides a clear picture of what the final result will look like. The project vision communicates a shared understanding of the project's goals or endpoints to the project's team members and stakeholders. The project vision will answer the following questions: "What will the final result of this project look like?" and "How will the project deliverables affect our customers?"

- **Project mission statement** The project mission statement describes the overarching goal or objective that the project manager and project team is hoping to achieve and reminds the team of the ultimate purpose of the project. The mission statement should satisfy the needs of the project team, customers, and stakeholders. Additionally, the mission statement can help motivate or even inspire the team to work together to reach successful completion of the project. Important questions that you should ask as you develop the mission statement are "What are we going to do?" and "Whom are we doing it for?" and sometimes "How will we do it?"

Use Case 37-2: Sample Problem/Vision/Mission Statement

Figure 37-3 shows Tree Healthcare System's eMAR implementation project problem/vision/mission statement all bundled up on one diagram.

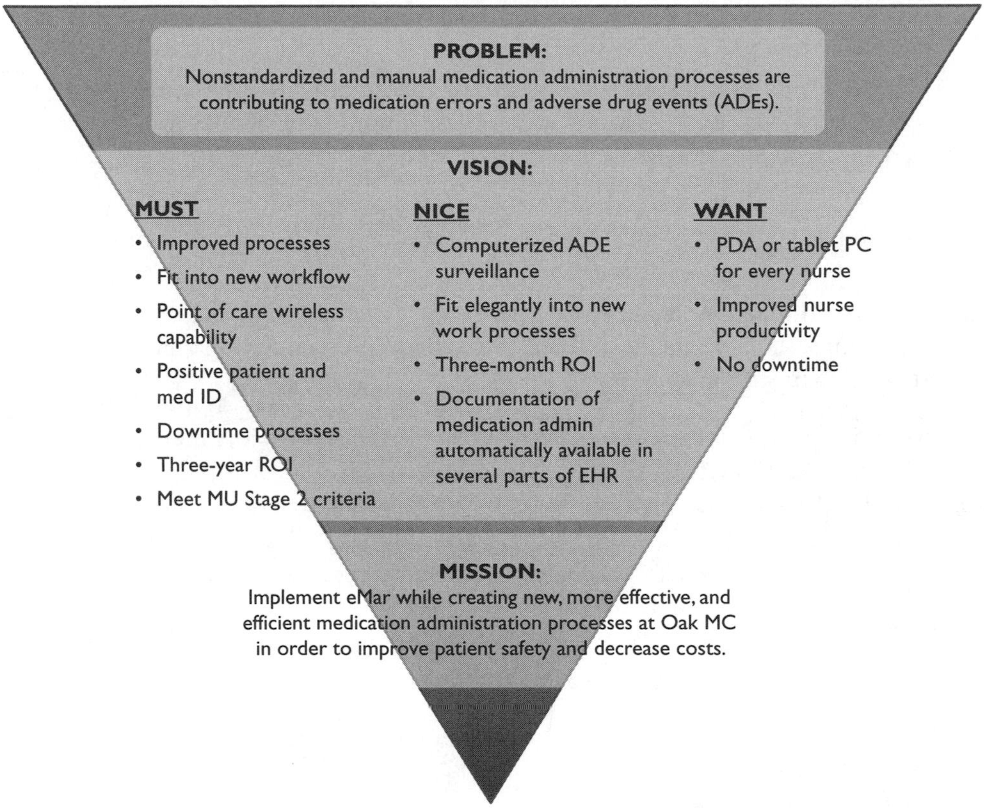

PROBLEM:
Nonstandardized and manual medication administration processes are contributing to medication errors and adverse drug events (ADEs).

VISION:

MUST	NICE	WANT
• Improved processes	• Computerized ADE surveillance	• PDA or tablet PC for every nurse
• Fit into new workflow	• Fit elegantly into new work processes	• Improved nurse productivity
• Point of care wireless capability	• Three-month ROI	• No downtime
• Positive patient and med ID	• Documentation of medication admin automatically available in several parts of EHR	
• Downtime processes		
• Three-year ROI		
• Meet MU Stage 2 criteria		

MISSION:
Implement eMar while creating new, more effective, and efficient medication administration processes at Oak MC in order to improve patient safety and decrease costs.

Figure 37-3   Use case project problem/vision/mission statement

SMART Project Objectives

The project scope statement or problem/vision/mission statement exercises done by the project team ready the team to craft project objectives that will guide the project and be used to determine project success. Within a project, the project management team will undertake project activities in order to reach the desired objectives or end of the project or phase. During the project initiating phase, you should ask the following questions of the stated project objectives: "What is our desired outcome?" and "How will we know when we achieve it?" By answering these questions, you will be able to ensure that the planned project activities will lead you to the desired end state of the project. It is important to note that the objectives should not state how they are achieved. The methods that will be used to achieve the project objectives will be developed in the next phase of the project life cycle, planning. The common acronym SMART is a helpful tool you should utilize when developing project objectives. Project managers utilize SMART goals as a way to ensure that project phases and results are successful.

- **S**   Specific. Project objectives need to be specific and unambiguously explain what the project's objectives and plans are.

- **M**   Measurable. An objective needs to be measurable in order to make sure the team is making progress towards successful completion of the project.

- **A**   Attainable. An objective needs to be able to be achieved with a reasonable amount of effort.

- **R**   Relevant. The objective needs to be important to the organization or make a positive impact on a particular situation.

- **T**   Time-limited. A deadline for project and/or phase completion needs to be set in order to help the team focus their efforts on completing their tasks in a timely manner.

Developing SMART project objectives helps ensure that project managers can successfully plan, schedule, and control all of the activities that must be done to meet a project's objectives.

HIT PRO EXAM TIP   Project objectives need to be specific, measurable, attainable, relevant, and time-limited (SMART) in order for the project to be well planned, scheduled, and controlled.

Use Case 37-3: Sample Objectives

Here are Tree Healthcare System's eMAR implementation project objectives:

- New medication administration processes clearly defined and well understood by all relevant clinical professionals

- Streamlined medication administration workflows that complement other clinical workflows

- Highly informative information about medication administration available in multiple parts of the EHR

- Adequate access of wireless devices for peak demand times

- Positive patient and medication ID approaching 100 percent

- Valid three-year ROI confirmed at go-live and after one year

- Decreased adverse drug events

- Tested downtime procedures in place

Planning a Healthcare IT Project

With the project charter approved, the problem/vision/mission statement written, and SMART project objectives set, a project manager and her team are well on their way to planning a successful healthcare IT project. The next step in successful project management that I will discuss is critical to the project and must be completed before work on the project begins. A project implementation plan must be developed before the team can begin project execution. While the project initiators or sponsors may be eager to begin the actual work of the project, it is in the best interest of the project and its stakeholders to carefully plan the work that is to be done. If you take the time up front to properly plan, you will save time and avoid costly errors in the long run. A rule of thumb is that one hour spent on planning saves three hours on execution. Equally important as developing the execution plan, the project manager needs to make sure that there is a shared understanding of what is going to be done by the entire project team. Project planning will answer the following questions:

- What must be done?
- How should it be done?
- Who will do it?
- By when must it be done?
- How long will it take?
- How much will it cost?
- How good does it have to be?[5]

If the project manager can ensure that he has developed a strong plan for the work to be done in the project as well as a shared understanding of the plan, then he has demonstrated control over the project and will be able to continuously assess the project's progress and take action to correct any deviations. Without a plan, there is no control.

The Work Breakdown Structure (WBS)

One of the most important tools in project planning is the work breakdown structure (WBS). The purpose of the WBS is to organize and define the total scope of the project.

WBS Defined

Taking the project's objectives and required deliverables into account, the WBS is a diagram that outlines the actual work that needs to be accomplished by the project team. The WBS establishes the interactions between all of the various components of the project and its deliverables.[1] The process of creating the WBS breaks the project's work and deliverables down into smaller, more manageable components, which helps the project manager maintain control of the project and helps provide clear direction to the team as to what work needs to be done. A WBS creates a visual representation of the project in its entirety and is a very valuable communication tool for the project manager, project team members, and project stakeholders.[6]

WBS Principles

Before you can successfully create a WBS, you must understand the difference between a project deliverable and a project activity. A project deliverable is the output or product that is created by the project's activities. A project activity is what you need to do in order to produce the deliverable or product. A WBS is a collection of all important project activities.

 HIT PRO EXAM TIP   An *objective* is a desired end state, and a *task* (project activity) is the action that leads to the desired end state.

To create a WBS for a project, the project manager will need to take the project scope statement, the project requirements from the organization initiating or sponsoring the project, and the organizational processes assets, such as policies, procedures, WBS templates, and files and lessons learned from previous projects, and break them down into smaller, more manageable components or levels until the work and deliverables are defined at the work package level. It is usually advisable to recruit the project team members and sometimes certain stakeholders into the process of creating the WBS, but ultimately, the project manager (PM) is responsible for creating a comprehensive and effective WBS. Figure 37-4 shows the levels of the WBS.

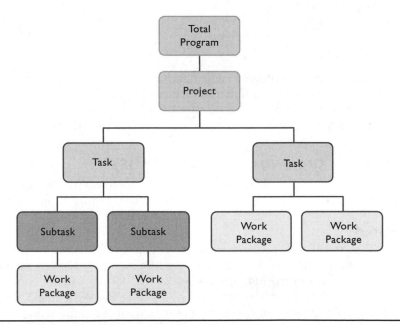

Figure 37-4   Project management work breakdown structure

Below the Project level, all of the components are called *project activities*. Colloquially many people call project activities *tasks*. But, since Task is a level in a WBS, it's better to call all of the components of work to be done in a project *project activities*.

How many levels should you break the work down to? That depends. WBSs in the construction industry and engineering projects commonly involve many levels, up to 20 in some cases. More than four levels (Project, Task, Subtask, and Work Package) are often unnecessarily complex for HIT projects. The rule of thumb is to break down the project only as far as you need to easily manage it. For example, if you have a great network engineer with whom you have worked with on other projects, you might simply have a task that says "Manage network" with no subtasks below it. On the other hand, if you have a new network engineer on the project, you might need to have "Assess, plan new components, and test network" as a subtask, and you may even break down those subtasks further into work package activities so that together you and the new network engineer can effectively manage all the important activities related to the network infrastructure for the project.

Use Case 37-4: Sample WBS

Figure 37-5 represents a partial WBS for the Tree Healthcare System eMAR implementation project. Other tasks include Design, Test, Train, Deploy, and Maintain.

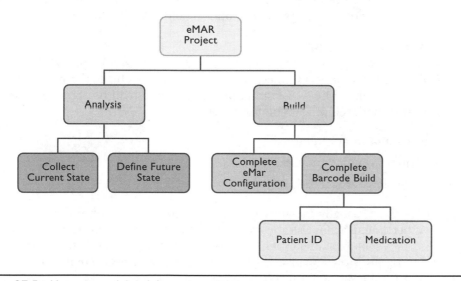

Figure 37-5   Use case work breakdown structure example

The work package level is the lowest level in the WBS. Very simply, the work package groups project activities that fit together logically and that can then be assigned to one person or team to execute. Once the work package level has been reached, a project manager can dependably estimate the cost of the project, develop an accurate schedule for the work to be completed, and, finally, better manage and control the work.[1] For the WBS to be an effective tool for the project manager, it must answer the questions outlined earlier as well as ensure a shared understanding among the project team of the objectives.

 HIT PRO EXAM TIP The project manager can reasonably estimate the cost of the project, develop an accurate schedule for the work to be completed, and effectively manage and control the project activities *after* a WBS has been created all the way down to the work package level.

Another important principle in constructing WBSs is that a WBS tells you nothing about sequencing. Sequencing of project tasks or activities comes in the next step, scheduling of project resources.

Estimating Time, Cost, and Resources

Once the project manager has created the WBS all the way down to the work package level, she can begin estimating the time, costs, and resources necessary to successfully achieve the project's objectives. After these estimates have been created, the project manager can develop a realistic schedule, budget, and plan for the project.

Key Points About Estimating

Taking the time to properly plan a project's activities increases the probability that the team will achieve the project's objectives. If the project has been planned well to this point, then most likely time, cost, and resource estimates will be accurate. Here are a few key points for developing accurate estimates:

- Understand what is required.
- Prioritize activities and tasks.
- Decide who needs to be involved.

In HIT projects, usually the greatest resource expenditure is on the time of project team members (clinical analysts, business analysts, network engineers, clinical application specialists, subject-matter experts, hardware/device technicians, and others). Thus, the main thing the project manager will be estimating is project activity duration. This will account for the vast majority of resources and cost in most HIT projects.

Essentially, what you are estimating is the probable project activity duration. The bell curve applies here. In a project with 100 activities, some of your estimates will be over, and some of your estimates will be under the actual time required to complete those tasks. If you, your project team, and the stakeholders have done your very best to estimate the duration of each of the project activities, the over/under will average out, and your overall estimate will be reasonably accurate. A word about padding: *padding*, or increasing a project activity's estimated duration time, is common. But, padding at the work package or subtask levels or overall project level inevitably leads to more cost because of the well-known "student effect"—the project activities fully consume the allotted time. Therefore, padding should be avoided.

How do you estimate project activity durations? One way is to look at historical records of similar project activities done in similar projects in the past. How long did the project activity actually take? Another way is to ask the person who will be responsible for doing the project activity. They usually have the best idea of how long it will take, and if they don't know right away, a series of questions by the project manager or dialogue with other team members will help you develop a reasonable estimate. If you have used the methods described earlier for estimating, then chances are you will have a relatively accurate estimate of the work and will complete the project successfully.

Developing the Project Schedule

With the work necessary to achieve the project's objectives defined, the WBS created, and the project activities and costs estimated, the project manager is now ready to develop the project schedule. The project manager will need to take into account the project activities, estimated time to complete the activities, required resources, and project delivery date to develop the project schedule. This is an important step in the process and one that may have several revisions throughout the life of the project. The project schedule outlines the target start and finish dates for all project activities and milestones. A milestone is an identifiable or noteworthy event that marks significant progress on the project.[7] Time and resource estimates will need to be reviewed, and often revised, to create an approved project schedule that will serve as a baseline to track project progress.

Purpose of Scheduling

If the project manager is able to continuously maintain a realistic schedule as project work develops and changes, he will be able to keep the project moving forward and will be able to inform team members and stakeholders of the project's status. Without having an accurate project schedule and without monitoring the progress of the project's activities and revising the schedule, as needed, it will be hard for a project manager to have good control of the project and will make completing the project on time and on budget almost impossible. If the project manager sees the project deviating from the schedule, he can take appropriate measures to get the project back on track or make any necessary updates to the project's budget and scope.

Introduction to Scheduling Techniques

In project management there are many different techniques that can be used to help develop and maintain an accurate project schedule. I will discuss several of them here. One area that is outside the scope of this chapter is a detailed discussion of project management software. Microsoft Project and many other good project scheduling and management software application products are readily available. In the vast majority of projects you will be part of or manage in HIT, a software application tool will be used to develop and maintain the project schedule. They have many helpful features that greatly simplify creating a schedule. What I will provide here are principles, practices, and advice that will ideally make your use of these essential products more powerful and effective.

Several analytical techniques underpin the algorithms of project management scheduling software that produces Gantt chart–like project schedules. By far the most common scheduling analytical technique is the critical path method. To use a PM software scheduling application that employs the critical path method in a project with interdependent activities in order to develop a chartlike depiction of the project schedule, a project manager needs to know the following:

- All project activities that are required to complete the project (from WBS)
- The time each activity will take to complete
- The relationship between all activities

The project manager will then be able to calculate the critical path, which is the longest path (in time) from project start to project finish. The critical path indicates the minimum time necessary to complete the entire project.[8] The longest path in the diagram is the critical path, and any activity on this path is considered a critical activity and must be executed on time to keep the overall project end date on time. Oftentimes in a project there will be activities that are not on the critical path; these are referred to as *slack* or *float* activities. Slack or float activities have the flexibility to be delayed without delaying the total project beyond its target completion date.[9] When the float of an activity or path is negative, meaning there is no flexibility, it is called *supercritical*. As a general rule, two critical paths in one project should be avoided. And, any activities that have any risk associated with them should have float.[9]

Scheduling Resources in Projects

All projects rely on a variety of resources to actually do the work outlined in the project documents. Resources include but are not limited to people, materials, equipment, and money. Without adequate resources, a project will have difficulty reaching the target completion date or may not achieve its objectives. At this point in the project, the project manager must identify the resources required for successful project completion and then plan, or schedule, the resources so that the team can work effectively.

Resource allocation is the process of assigning the necessary resources that have previously been identified to each project activity in the plan. Some activities may require more than one resource, and depending on the nature of the activity, the amount of resources required may vary at different points throughout project execution. The project plan may need to be revised to account for resource availability.

Scheduling resources before any work begins on a project allows the project manager to see where resources may be overloaded and make adjustments to the project plan.

Resource Leveling

The process of revising a plan's schedule (start and finish dates) in order to account for resource availability is called *resource leveling* and is used to optimize the distribution of work among resources.[1] Resource leveling is important to successful project management because while the assumption has been made earlier in the plan that there are unlimited resources available to a project, this is hardly ever the case. Most likely, at some point in a project the demand for a resource, or resources, will outweigh the availability of the resource(s). Resource leveling helps the project manager handle this problem and keep the project on track. Figure 37-6 illustrates two types of resource leveling techniques: *time-critical leveling* and *resource-critical leveling* and the differences between them.[9]

Figure 37-6
Time-critical vs. resource-critical resource leveling

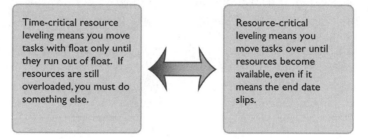

Time-critical resource leveling means you move tasks with float only until they run out of float. If resources are still overloaded, you must do something else.

Resource-critical leveling means you move tasks over until resources become available, even if it means the end date slips.

Resource-leveling techniques are applied to project schedules that have already been analyzed by the critical path method and can often lead to changes in the critical path as well as potentially other parts of the project.[1]

Factoring in Resource Availability

To create a schedule, the project manager will need to begin by inputting the actual time it will take to complete each project activity. Then, resource availability must be factored into the schedule to determine the duration (in calendar time) it will take to complete the project work. The project manager needs to make sure they know the actual availability of their team members when developing a schedule; without this, she cannot create a meaningful schedule.[9] When factoring in resource availability, it is important to understand that people's productivity can be affected by the following three factors:

- P   Personal. People must take breaks.
- F   Fatigue. They get tired.
- D   Delays. They are waiting for something.

It has been found that in a standard eight-hour day, you will get only about 80 percent, or 6.4 hours, of productive work from a person. This loss in productivity comes from P, F, and D.[9] Additionally, breaking tasks down into smaller segments can add time to the project schedule because there is setup time associated with starting each new segment of a task. If the project manager can prioritize tasks and have team members working on fewer project activities at one time, setup time will be decreased, which will help the overall project schedule. One suggestion for this is to give each team member a "priority-one" activity and a backup activity. When there is a break in the work on the "priority-one" activity, team members can move to their backup activity.

Use Case 37-5: Sample Schedule

The Tree Healthcare System eMAR implementation project's project team successfully initiated the project and developed a comprehensive view of the project activities in the form of a WBS. They then went on to create a schedule using the principles and best practices of project management. Figure 37-7 shows a high-level schedule for Tree's eMAR project. It shows the project activities only at the task level. In a project like this, there would be more than 100 activities at the subtask and work package levels. Such a detailed schedule is beyond the scope of the introductory nature of this chapter.

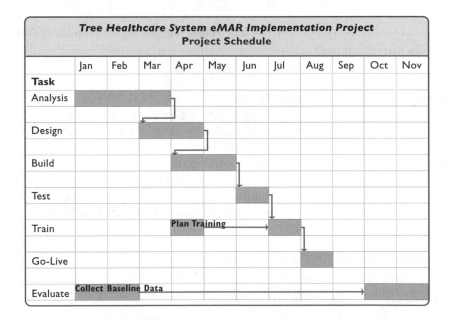

Figure 37-7 Tree Healthcare System eMAR Implementation Project schedule

Executing, Monitoring, and Controlling HIT Projects

The project charter and problem/mission/vision statements have been written, the objectives have been outlined, the WBS has been created, and the time, cost, and resources have been estimated; in addition, a schedule has been developed, and resources have been allocated. So, execution of the project's deliverables is ready to begin. All of the careful, thoughtful planning that has been done up front will help ensure that execution goes smoothly, according to plan, and that the project objectives are achieved. The executing phase of a project includes completing the work outlined in the project plan in order to meet the project requirements, coordinating resources, and performing the activities in the plan.[1] Additionally, during the executing phase the project manager will need to constantly monitor the progress of the project and make any necessary changes to the plan in order to keep the project moving in the direction of achieving its objectives.

Execution Principles, Issues, and Opportunities

The executing phase of the project is the time when the work that has been planned for the project actually gets completed, a large portion of the project's budget is spent, and the plan may be updated or a new plan baseline is established as a result of the work being done. These changes may be made because activity durations varied from the expectations in the plan or there were changes in resource availability or productivity or from other unanticipated risks that may have arisen once execution began. If the changes are of a large enough scale, change requests will need to be initiated and subsequently approved so that the project management plan or documents can be revised and new baselines established if necessary.[1] During the course of the executing phase, the project manager is responsible for managing the team to perform the work necessary to achieve the project's objectives. Some of the project manager's responsibilities include the following:

- Acquiring the project team, tracking their performance, and helping improve their skill sets

- Performing quality assurance audits

- Distributing important information to the team and stakeholders

- Managing stakeholder expectations[1]

 CompTIA EXAM TIP During project execution, the project manager is responsible for seeing that the work that needs to be done to achieve the project objectives is completed according to the plan and, if not, for initiating project change requests.

Monitoring Progress in Projects

Throughout the course of the executing phase, the project manager is also responsible for monitoring the progress of the project. Monitoring the project includes tracking, reviewing, and controlling the progress and performance of the project as well as identifying and mitigating any risks that may have developed during the progress of the project; strong risk management is important to the success of the project for the following reasons:

- Improves project performance
- Ensures quality does not take a backseat to cost and schedule
- Reveals developing problems early
- Determines what needs to be done to mitigate identifiable risks
- Identifies areas where other projects should be managed differently
- Keeps clients informed of status
- Reaffirms organization's commitment to the project

Project Control and Evaluation

Project control is achieved by comparing where one is with where one is supposed to be and then taking corrective action to resolve any discrepancies that exist. The project manager controls the direction of the project and helps ensure its success by regularly, and consistently, monitoring the project's performance and measures that against the project's plan and objectives. If the project manager sees the project progressing in a different way than outlined in the plan or she sees any stalling, she needs to initiate any necessary changes to the plan.[1] Just like in all of the other phases of project management, there are systematic review techniques that the project manager should use.

Kinds of Evaluation Reviews

I suggest three kinds of evaluation reviews that the project manager can use during the course of the project to systematically ensure that the project is progressing according to plan and will achieve its objectives. Table 37-1 lists them.

Review Type	Purpose
Status	PCTS okay? Critical path?
Design	Does it work? If not, can we make it work?
Process (also called Lessons Learned)	Done well? What could be done better?

Table 37-1   Types of Project Management Evaluation Reviews

- **Project status review**   The project status review should occur weekly on shorter projects and monthly on longer projects. This review looks at the current status of the project. Specifically, it reviews the P, C, T, S of the project using something called an *earned-value analysis* that I will discuss in the next section. The future status of the project is also considered in this review, including deviations to the schedule, or C, P, S. The status of critical tasks must be updated at this time. Any risk factors contributing to problems in the project need to be identified and solutions need to be developed, if possible. And finally, risk management principles should be applied, if necessary.

- **Project design review**   The project design review examines a product, service, or software design to see whether it meets the project requirements. The questions that need to be asked are "Does it work?" and "Can we make it work?"

- **Project process review**   The project process review happens at major project milestones or at completion of the project; it evaluates whether the project was done well and what needs to be improved, and it develops a list of "lessons learned" from the project that can be applied to future projects.

Earned-Value Analysis

Oftentimes a project management team will use a *schedule* report to review the progress of a project. Unfortunately, this will not provide the team with a true picture of the project's status because it does not take into account the effort or work that has been put into the project, which may be greater than anticipated but slowing down the overall progress. To properly assess the status of the project and account for any deviations from the plan, the project manager should conduct an *earned-value analysis*. The earned-value system is an integrated cost-schedule tracking system that looks at the project's P, C, T, S to help the project manager, team, and stakeholders understand the true status of the project. An earned-value analysis integrates the following factors in order to accurately assess the project's performance and progress:

- **Cost variance**   Any difference between the estimated cost of an activity and the actual cost of an activity

- **Schedule variance**   Any difference between the scheduled completion of an activity and the actual completion of that activity

To determine the cost and schedule variances, the project manager will need to use the following equations:

$$Schedule\ variance = BCWP - BCWS$$

$$Cost\ variance = BCWP - ACWP$$

where:

- **Budgeted Cost of Work Scheduled (BCWS)** The budgeted cost of work scheduled to be done in a given time period

- **Budgeted Cost of Work Performed (BCWP)** The budgeted cost of work actually performed in a given time period (aka earned value)

- **Actual Cost of Work Performed (ACWP)** The amount of money actually spent for completing the work in a given time period

Using the earned-value analysis will help provide a clear and realistic understanding of the project's progress as well as an understanding of why it may not be progressing according to the plan. With the click of a button, Microsoft Project and other project-scheduling software products produce earned-value analysis data once the schedule is updated with percent activity completion across all project activities.

Use Case 37-6: Sample Project Status Meeting

The project status meeting one month into the executing phase of the Tree Healthcare System eMAR implementation project had the following findings:

- Most project activities, including all critical path activities, begun to date were on schedule.

- The Plan Training Curriculum activity did not start when it had been planned to start because of an illness of the education director.
  - This activity had significant float, so it was rescheduled to start one week after the status meeting with no untoward effect on the project.

- The earned-value analysis indicated that the project was spending somewhat more than the plan had called for to maintain the on-schedule performance.
  - To be somewhat overspent this early into the executing phase presented an opportunity for the PM and project team to study why several team members were working overtime to keep the project on schedule and to propose a solution. If this pattern had been allowed to continue, the project may have come in on time, but it would have been very significantly over budget.

- Potential risks identified for the project during the initiating phase were reviewed. It was determined that none of those risks had manifested at that point and that no new risks were identified.

HIT PRO EXAM TIP An earned-value analysis looks at the project's P, C, T, S to help the project manager, team, and stakeholders understand the true status of the project, and it integrates cost and schedule variances in order to accurately assess a project's performance and progress.

Changing the Plan

If after conducting project evaluation reviews and an earned-value analysis the project manager finds that there has been a significant change (+/– 5%) in P, C, T, S, then the project manager may need to initiate an official change in the project's process. The project manager will need to fill out an official project change form or document to request the change in the project by outlining where the change has occurred and why and how the project will be amended if the change is approved.

Closing the Project

You have now seen how a healthcare IT project progresses from the initiating phase to the planning phase and then on to the executing phase, with its emphasis on monitoring and controlling processes. All that is left is to confirm that all aspects of the project's activities are finished so that the project can be officially complete. At the time of project closing, the following activities may take place:

- The project is accepted by the project initiator or sponsor.
- A post-project review is conducted.
- Lessons learned are documented.
- Any necessary updates are applied to the organizational process.
- Project notes are filed for use in future projects.
- Any other close-out procedures required by the project sponsor or organization are performed.

Additionally, the entire project management team should look at how the team has worked together to achieve the project's objectives. Specifically, the following team processes should be evaluated:

- Leadership
- Decision making
- Problem solving
- Communications
- Meetings

- Planning
- Giving feedback to team members and others
- Conflict management

Once a project is complete, it is important for the project team to take some time to conduct a post-mortem analysis to evaluate what went well throughout the course of the project as well as what did not go well during the project. Through this analysis, the team will develop a list of lessons learned regarding the project specifically, as well as about project management in general, and will look to carry these lessons learned over into future projects.

Use Case 37-7: Closing Out the Sample Project

The Tree Healthcare System eMAR implementation project post-mortem analysis was remarkable for the following:

- **P** Performance/quality
  - There was acceptable user satisfaction with the eMAR as delivered as measured by a valid and reliable survey.
  - Adverse drug event rates decreased slightly but not statistically significantly, which was considered acceptable.
  - The project team members and stakeholders were very satisfied with the processes and outcomes of the project.
- **C** Cost
  - There was a 5 percent budget overrun that was considered acceptable by management, especially since the PM, aided by earned-value data, alerted management more than two months before project completion that this overrun and its magnitude would be likely.
- **T** Time
  - The project started and ended on time.
- **S** Scope
  - The project manager successfully avoided several attempts at increasing scope.

The project documents, including the initiating phase reports, WBS, schedules, status reports, and project post-mortem analysis, were archived for reference for future projects.

Chapter Review

In this chapter, I took the rather extensive subject of project management and broke it down into an easy-to-understand explanation in order to provide you with the knowledge necessary to understand how essential project management is to healthcare IT. Given the constraints of this book, I did not go into as much detail or explanation of some of the specific techniques described in the chapter, such as the WBS, critical path method, earned-value analysis, and others. I highly recommend the Project Management Institute's *A Guide to the Project Management Body of Knowledge*, the Lewis Institute, and the Healthcare Information Management Systems Society (HIMSS) as sources for additional information on the subject.

In this chapter, I covered the four phases of a project (initiating, planning, executing, and closing) and broke out the major activities in each phase as they apply to healthcare information technology so that you are better equipped to work in project management in the healthcare industry. At the start of the project, or the initiating phase, you will develop a project charter and outline the project's scope and mission. Then you will need to develop SMART objectives and finally prioritize the project's objectives. After you do this, you will move into the planning phase where you will develop the WBS and estimate the time, cost, and resources needed for the project. Once you've created the WBS and have strong project activity duration estimates, you can develop the project's schedule and schedule/allocate resources for the project utilizing the critical path method and resource leveling techniques I described. Then you are ready to move to the executing phase and begin monitoring and controlling processes in earnest. In this phase, the project "work" gets done, and you will be responsible for monitoring the progress of the project and maintaining control over the project. I described several types of evaluation reviews, including an earned-value analysis that will help you monitor and control the project's trajectory. I also described how to make changes to the plan, if and when necessary. Once the work of the project is complete (and ideally the objectives have been met), you can move on to closing the project. In this phase of project management, you will conduct a post-mortem analysis of the project to see what went well and what did not, and you can develop a list of lessons learned that can be applied to other projects in the future.

You learned that a project is a temporary activity that is undertaken by a team in order to create a unique product, service, or result in a defined time period, and project management is the organization or facilitation of all of the planning, scheduling, and monitoring or controlling of all the activities or tasks that must be done to meet the project's goals or objectives. Utilizing the project management process and techniques described in this chapter will significantly increase your chances of managing projects successfully and will help you to be a more valuable asset to an organization. The project management process can be applied to projects in all industries, not just healthcare. You can take the skills you have learned here and apply them in many different situations and ideally be successful at whatever it is you've set out to accomplish.

Questions

To test your comprehension of the chapter, answer the following questions and then check your answers against the list of correct answers at the end of the chapter.

1. Project management techniques are useful tools for healthcare IT project managers to have because it helps them do what?

    A. Teach their project team how to cut corners so they can get their work done more quickly

    B. Manage computer projects better

    C. Facilitate the planning, scheduling, and controlling of projects

    D. Execute healthcare IT projects without having to create a plan

2. What are some examples of good communication strategies for project team members and stakeholders?

    A. Fact finding for better information, close-mindedness, and not listening to a variety of people

    B. Asking questions, listening actively, resolving conflict, and managing expectations

    C. Strong argument skills and persuading others to achieve project goals

    D. Listening actively, turning away from someone who is talking, answering questions, and reading

3. Scope creep is good for healthcare IT projects because it helps the scope of the project increase slowly.

    A. True

    B. False

4. What is the purpose of a work breakdown structure?

    A. To create a diagram of all the people on the project team and what work they will do

    B. To break the project down so that the scope of the project is decreased and the project can be executed more quickly

    C. To create a visual representation of the project so everyone can understand the purpose of the project

    D. To break the project's work and deliverables down into smaller, more manageable components, which helps the project manager maintain control of the project and helps provide clear direction to the team as to what work needs to be done

5. What two processes occur during all phases of a project's life cycle?

    A. Monitoring and controlling

    B. Watching and listening

C. Executing and closing

D. Planning and finishing

6. During the executing phase, what are the project manager's responsibilities?

   A. Acquire the project team, tracking their performance and helping to improve their skill sets

   B. Perform quality assurance audits

   C. A and B

   D. None of the above

7. For a project manager to accurately estimate the time, cost, and resources necessary to achieve a project's objectives, what will the project manager need to do?

   A. Understand what is required and decide who needs to be involved

   B. Prioritize project activities

   C. All of the above

   D. None of the above

8. The process of moving project activities out until resources are available, even if it means the project end date slips, is called what?

   A. Time-critical leveling

   B. Scheduling adjusting

   C. Resource-critical leveling

   D. Project leveling

9. For a project manager to determine the critical path, what does a project manager need to know?

   A. All project activities that are required to complete the project (from the WBS)

   B. The time each activity will take to complete

   C. The relationship between all activities

   D. All of the above

   E. None of the above

10. An earned-value analysis looks at the project's performance, cost, time and scope status to help the project team understand the status of the project and integrates both cost and schedule variances to assess a project's progress and performance.

    A. True

    B. False

Answers

1. **C.** Project management knowledge and techniques are useful tools for healthcare IT project managers to have because it helps them with facilitating the planning, scheduling, and controlling of projects.

2. **B.** Some examples of good communication strategies for project team members and stakeholders are asking questions, listening actively, resolving conflicts, and managing expectations.

3. **B.** False. Scope creep is to be avoided in all types of projects.

4. **D.** The purpose of a work breakdown structure is to break the project's work and deliverables down into smaller, more manageable components, which helps the project manager maintain control of the project and helps provide clear direction to the team as to what work needs to be done.

5. **A.** The monitoring and controlling process groups occur during all phases of a project's life cycle.

6. **C.** Some of the project manager's duties are acquiring the project team, tracking their performance, and helping improve their skill sets, as well as performing quality assurance audits.

7. **C.** For a project manager to accurately estimate the time, cost, and resources necessary to achieve a project's objectives, the project manager will need to understand what is required, decide who needs to be involved, and prioritize activities and tasks.

8. **C.** The process of moving tasks out until resources are available, even if it means the project end date slips, is called *resource-critical leveling*.

9. **C.** For a project manager to determine the critical path, a project manager needs to know all project activities that are required to complete the project (from WBS), the time each activity will take to complete, and the relationship between all activities.

10. **A.** An earned-value analysis looks at the project's P, C, T, S to help the project team understand the status of the project and integrates both cost and schedule variances to assess a project's progress and performance.

References

1. *A guide to the project management body of knowledge (PMBOK guide), fourth edition.* (2008). Project Management Institute.

2. Murphy, J. and Gugerty, B. (2007). Healthcare IT project management workshop. The Summer Institute in Nursing Informatics, Baltimore, Maryland.

3. Drucker, P. (1986). *Management tasks, responsibilities, practices.* Truman Talley Books.

4. Project Management Docs. (2012). *What is a stakeholder?* Accessed on June 2012 from http://www.projectmanagementdocs.com/articles/what-is-a-stakeholder.html.

5. Lewis, J. (2010). *Project planning, scheduling, and control.* McGraw-Hill.

6. Work breakdown structure: Purpose, process and pitfalls. Accessed from http://www.projectsmart.co.uk/work-breakdown-structure-purpose-process-pitfalls.html.

7. Mantel, S. J., Meredith, J. R., Shafer, S. M., & Sutton, M. M. (2001). *Core concepts of project management.* John Wiley & Sons.

8. Levy, F. K., Thompson, G. L., & Wiest, J. D. (1963). The ABC's of the critical path method. *Harvard Business Review, 41,* 413–423

9. Lewis, J. (2003). *The project manager's pocket survival guide.* McGraw-Hill.

PART VI

Appendices

CompTIA Healthcare IT Technician Exam Objective Map

The following table maps each official CompTIA Healthcare IT Technician exam domain to the corresponding chapters in which the information pertinent to the domain is covered.

Chapter Number	Chapter Title
Domain 1.0	**Regulatory Requirements**
11	Health Information Technology and Healthcare Policy
12	Navigating Health Data Standards and Interoperability
13	Regulatory Aspects of Healthcare IT: Legal Best Practices and Requirements
14	The Electronic Health Record as Evidence
29	Architectural Safeguards
30	Healthcare Cybersecurity Technology
Domain 2.0	**Organizational Behavior**
1	Overview of Health Care in the United States
5	An Overview of Processes Associated with Healthcare Delivery Within Provider Organizations: Focus on the Ambulatory Setting
6	An Overview of Processes Associated with Healthcare Payment Within Ambulatory Provider Organizations
10	Communication Skills in Healthcare IT, Building Strong Teams for Successful Healthcare IT
14	The Electronic Health Record as Evidence
18	HIT Connectivity and Interoperability Opportunities and Challenges
26	Physical Safeguards, Facility Security, Secure Systems and Networks, and Securing Electronic Media
27	Healthcare Information Security: Operational Safeguards

HIT Pro Exams Objective Maps

The following tables map each official HIT Pro exam domain to the corresponding chapters in which the information pertinent to the domain is covered.

Practice Workflow & Information Management Redesign Specialist Exam

Chapter Number	Chapter Title
Domain I	*Fundamentals of Health Workflow Process Analysis and Redesign*
20	Organizational Success Factors in Healthcare Informatics Implementation
21	Fundamentals of Health Workflow Process Analysis and Redesign
22	Reporting Requirements and Regulatory and External Factors Affecting Healthcare IT
Domain II	*Usability and Human Factors*
16	Human Factors in Healthcare IT
19	Fundamentals of Clinical Decision Support
32	Computer Hardware and Architecture for Healthcare IT
Domain III	*Health Management Information Systems*
4	The Role of Information Technology in Healthcare
8	The Role of Healthcare IT in Improving Population Health
11	Health Information Technology and Healthcare Policy
22	Reporting Requirements and Regulatory and External Factors Affecting Healthcare IT
29	Architectural Safeguards

Clinician/Practitioner Consultant Exam

Chapter Number	Chapter Title
Domain II	*Quality Improvement*
7	Using Healthcare IT to Measure and Improve Outcomes
17	Build- and Implementation-Related HCIT Success Factors
20	Organizational Success Factors in Healthcare Informatics Implementation
21	Fundamentals of Health Workflow Process Analysis and Redesign
22	Reporting Requirements and Regulatory and External Factors Affecting Healthcare IT
Domain III	*Working with HIT Systems*
15	Core HCIT Functionality
16	Human Factors in Healthcare IT
18	HCIT Connectivity and Interoperability Opportunities and Challenges
24	Building Trust
Domain IV	*Health Information Management Systems*
15	Core HCIT Functionality
17	Build- and Implementation-Related HCIT Success Factors
18	HCIT Connectivity and Interoperability Opportunities and Challenges
34	Databases, Data Warehousing, and Data Mining for Healthcare
Domain V	*Planning, Management, and Leadership for Health IT*
9	Strategic Leadership and Management of Health Information Technology in Provider Organizations
Domain VI	*History of Health*
4	The Role of Health Information Technology

Implementation Manager Exam

Chapter Number	Chapter Title
Domain I	*Project Management*
37	Healthcare Information Technology Project Management
Domain II	*Fundamentals of Health Workflow Process Analysis and Redesign*
20	Organizational Success Factors in Healthcare Informatics Implementation
21	Fundamentals of Health Workflow Process Analysis and Redesign
22	Reporting Requirements and Regulatory and External Factors Affecting Healthcare IT

Implementation Support Specialist Exam

Chapter Number	Chapter Title
Domain III	*Vendor-Specific Systems*
15	Core HCIT Functionality
16	Human Factors in Healthcare IT
17	Build- and Implementation-Related HCIT Success Factors
19	Fundamentals of Clinical Decision Support
20	Organizational Success Factors in Healthcare Informatics Implementation
22	Reporting Requirements and Regulatory and External Factors Affecting Healthcare IT
34	Databases, Data Warehousing, and Data Mining for Healthcare
Domain IV	*Working with Health IT Systems*
15	Core HCIT Functionality
16	Human Factors in Healthcare IT
18	HCIT Connectivity and Interoperability Opportunities and Challenges
24	Building Trust
Domain V	*Installation and Maintenance of Health IT Systems*
15	Core HCIT Functionality
36	Systems Analysis and Design in Healthcare
Domain VI	*Information and Computer Science*
25	Risk Assessment and Management
26	Physical Safeguards, Facility Security, Secure Systems and Networks, and Securing Electronic Media
27	Healthcare Information Security: Operational Safeguards
30	Healthcare Cybersecurity Technology
32	Computer Hardware and Architecture for Healthcare IT
33	Programming and Programming Languages for Healthcare IT
34	Databases, Data Warehousing, and Data Mining for Healthcare
35	Networks and Networking in Healthcare
36	Systems Analysis and Design in Healthcare
Domain VII	*Terminology in Health Care and Public Health Settings*
12	Navigating Health Data Standards and Interoperability
18	HCIT Connectivity and Interoperability Opportunities and Challenges

Technical/Software Support Staff Exam

Trainer Exam

About the CD-ROM

The CD-ROM included with this book comes with MasterExam software, select artwork from Chapter 25, and a link to download the Adobe Digital Editions ebook version of this book.

System Requirements

The MasterExam software requires Windows 2000 or newer and Internet Explorer 6.0 or newer and 20MB of hard disk space for full installation. The artwork from Chapter 25 requires Adobe Acrobat Reader. The Adobe Digital Editions ebook requires the Adobe Digital Editions software.

Installing and Running MasterExam

If your computer CD-ROM drive is configured to autorun, the CD-ROM will automatically start up upon inserting the disc. From the opening screen, you can install MasterExam by clicking the MasterExam link. This will begin the installation process and create a program group named LearnKey. To run MasterExam, use Start | All Programs | LearnKey | MasterExam. If the autorun feature does not launch your CD-ROM, browse to the CD-ROM and click the *LaunchTraining.exe* icon.

Exploring MasterExam

Once you have loaded the MasterExam software, you will find one practice exam for the CompTIA Healthcare IT Technician exam. Six HIT Pro practice exams, one for each exam, are available for download via the Bonus MasterExam link. To download any of the HIT Pro practice exams, you will need to complete a free online registration. To do so, simply click the Bonus MasterExam link on the CD-ROM's main launch page and follow the directions provided.

For each MasterExam practice exam, the number of questions, the type of questions, and the time allowed are intended to be an accurate representation of the actual exam environment. You have the option to take an open-book exam, including hints and answers; a closed-book exam; or the timed MasterExam simulation.

When you launch a MasterExam practice exam, a digital clock display will appear in the bottom-right corner of your screen. The clock will continue to count down to zero unless you choose to end the exam before the time expires.

Removing MasterExam

MasterExam is installed to your hard drive. For best results when removing Master-Exam, use the Start | All Programs | LearnKey | Uninstall option.

Artwork

Enlarged versions of Table 25-1 and Figure 25-1 are included on the CD-ROM so that you can view them in more detail. Table 25-1 is printable so that you can use the risk register.

Free Adobe Digital Editions Ebook

The contents of this book are available as a free ebook download in the form of a secured Adobe Digital Editions file. You should read this entire section and review the Adobe Digital Editions system requirements as well as the Adobe Digital Editions online FAQ on www.adobe.com before you begin.

The CD-ROM contains a link to download the Adobe Digital Editions software and a link to the McGraw-Hill ebook download web page.

Installing Adobe Digital Editions

You must have the Adobe Digital Editions software installed to open, view, and navigate the free ebook. You can download the latest version of Adobe Digital Editions for free from the Adobe web site, www.adobe.com, or you can use the version included on the CD-ROM.

You must download and install Adobe Digital Editions before attempting to download the free ebook file. Please review the Adobe Digital Editions FAQ on the Adobe web site before installing Adobe Digital Editions to check your computer and device compatibility and the system requirements (minimum system requirements are listed in a moment).

Ebook Readers for Apple iOS

Ebook reader software is available online that will allow you to view the free ebook on an Apple device. The Bluefire Reader for Apple iOS application is one of the more popular examples and supports Adobe Digital Editions ebook DRM. You can visit www .bluefirereader.com to learn more about Bluefire Reader and to download the application. Customer support for Adobe Digital Editions should be directed to Adobe Systems, Inc. Customer support for Bluefire should be addressed to Bluefire Productions, LLC. McGraw-Hill does not warrant that the use of any ebook reader software will ensure the free ebook will operate on your device.

Adobe Digital Editions System Requirements

The minimum system requirements for Adobe Digital Editions are listed here. Be sure to check the Adobe web site for the most up-to-date system requirements.

- **Windows** Microsoft Windows XP with Service Pack 2 (Service Pack 3 recommended), Windows Vista (32-bit or 64-bit), or Windows 7 (32-bit or 64-bit); Intel Pentium 500MHz processor; 128MB of RAM; 800x600 monitor resolution.

- **Mac** PowerPC: Mac OS X v10.4.10 or v10.5; PowerPC G4 or G5 500MHz processor; 128MB of RAM. Intel: Mac OS X v10.4.10, v10.5, or v10.6; 500MHz processor; 128MB of RAM.

- **Supported browsers and Adobe Flash versions for Windows** Microsoft Internet Explorer 8, Mozilla Firefox 3, Google Chrome for Windows; Adobe Flash Player 9 or 10. For Mac: Apple Safari 4, Mozilla Firefox 3; Adobe Flash Player 9 or 10.

Free Adobe Digital Editions Ebook Download Procedure

To complete the download, follow these steps:

1. First, download and install the Adobe Digital Editions software on your computer.

2. Next, follow the link to the ebook download web page, http://books.mcgraw-hill .com/ebookdownloads/9780071802796. You are required to provide your name, a valid e-mail address, and your unique access code in order to download the ebook.

3. You can find your unique access code on the label that is adhered to the inside flap of the CD-ROM envelope. The CD-ROM envelope is inside the paper sleeve bound into the back of this book.

4. Upon submitting this information on the ebook download web page, an e-mail message will be sent to the e-mail address you provided. Follow the instructions included in the e-mail message to download your free ebook.

 WARNING The unique access code entitles you to download one copy of the free ebook. The unique access code can be used only once. Unless you set up additional computers in Adobe Digital Editions with an Adobe ID before you download the free ebook, the ebook will be usable only on the computer on which it was downloaded. If you don't want to set up an Adobe ID, be sure to download the ebook to the computer or device you intend to read it on.

Help

A help file is provided through the help button on the CD-ROM's main page in the lower-left corner. An individual help feature is also available through MasterExam.

Technical Support

Technical support information is provided here by feature.

Free Ebook Download Support

For questions regarding the operation of Adobe Digital Editions and the free ebook download, e-mail techsolutions@mhedu.com or visit http://mhp.softwareassist.com.

LearnKey Technical Support

For technical problems with the MasterExam software (installation, operation, removal), please visit www.learnkey.com, e-mail techsupport@learnkey.com, or call toll free at 1-800-482-8244.

McGraw-Hill Content Support

For questions regarding book content, please e-mail customer.service@mcgraw-hill .com. For customers outside the United States, e-mail international_cs@mcgraw-hill.com.

INDEX

Numbers

10 X 10 Program, AMIA, 218
2.4GHz band, 802.11 standards, 854
2.5GHz band, 802.11 standards, 854
3DES (Triple DES), 715, 717
45 CFR Part 1603, 275–276
45 CFR Part 164, Subpart C. *See*
Security Rule, HIPAA
45 CFR Part 164, Subpart E3. *See*
Privacy Rule, HIPAA
5GHz band, 802.11 standards, 854
802.11 wireless standards, 252,
853–854

A

A (Addressable) implementation
specification, 285
ACA. *See* PPACA (Patient Protection
and Affordable Care Act) of 2010
acceptance of risk, 598
access control
accountability and, 666–668
balanced, 667–668
basic, 674–676
database security, 813–814
database security with
physical, 815
at highest level of
confidentiality, 672
key fobs for, 615–617
medical ethics and court order
sources of, 671
medical record regulations
and, 671
multilevel data confidentiality
and, 670–671
operational safeguards for
EHRs. *See* operational
safeguards, EHRs
operational safeguards for
HIEs. *See* operational
safeguards, HIEs
overview of, 668–669
patient privacy, 282–283,
672–674
physical safeguards. *See*
physical safeguards
privacy consent and, 673–674
purpose of use, 672

roles and permissions as,
668–669
security technology safeguards,
286, 580
truth tables for, 669–670
XACML for, 685
access points, WLANs, 853
accountability
innovative adoption and, 455
maintaining with access
control, 666–667
maintaining with audit
control, 667
as professional value, 44
accountable-care organizations.
See ACOs (accountable-care
organizations)
accreditation, certification vs., 738
Accredited Standards Committee
(ASX) X12, 251
Accredited Standards Committee
X12, 332
ACM (Association from Computing
Machinery), 714
ACOs (accountable-care
organizations)
integrated care delivery model,
336
Medicare Shared Savings
Program, 35–36
operational safeguards for,
647–648
payment reform coupled to,
35, 526
performance measurement
regulations, 138
Pioneer program, 36
population health initiatives
of, 154
reimbursement incentive
models, 464
Active Server Pages (ASP) language,
794–795, 809
active surveillance reporting, public
health, 155
activities, project deliverables vs.
project, 904–906
acute care, 11–14

ACWP (Actual Cost of Work
Performed), earned-value
analysis, 914
AD (Active Directory), 760
ADDIE model, training program,
544
Addressable (A) implementation
specification, 285
addressing, in data networks,
842–843
ADEs (adverse drug events),
avoiding, 437–438
administration, database, 812
administrative agencies
HIPAA and HITECH rules, 275
types of, 299–301
administrative processes, EMRs
(electronic medical records), 358
administrative simplification
provisions, HIPAA, 275–276
administrators of healthcare
organizations, 11
admissibility, EHR discovery vs., 309
Adobe Digital Edition, 936–937
Adobe Flash, 791
ADT (admission, discharge, transfer)
system, 359
adult care nurse practitioners
(ANPs), 10
adult learning, educational
training, 547
Advanced Encryption Standard
(AES) algorithm, 717, 855
Advanced Primary Care Practice
Demonstration, Medicare, 35
adverse events
FDA monitoring reports
of, 696
healthcare litigation triggers,
324
healthcare quality and, 5
from medical device software,
641–642
AES (Advanced Encryption
Standard) algorithm, 717, 855
Agency for Healthcare Research and
Quality (AHRQ), 136, 230
aggregated data, HIT for population
health, 159